Nutrition

Maintaining and improving health

Nutrition

Maintaining and improving health

Fourth edition

Geoffrey P Webb BSc MSc PhD
Nutrition writer, and consultant at the School of Health,
Sport and Bioscience, University of East London, London, UK

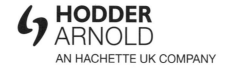

HODDER
ARNOLD
AN HACHETTE UK COMPANY

First published in Great Britain in 1994 by Butterworth Heinemann
Second edition 2002 and third edition 2008 by Hodder Arnold

This fourth edition published in 2012 by

Hodder Arnold, an imprint of Hodder Education, a division of Hachette UK
338 Euston Road, London NW1 3BH

www.hodderarnold.com

Hachette UK's policy is to use papers that are natural, renewable and
recyclable products and made from wood grown in sustainable forests. The
logging and manufacturing processes are expected to conform to the
environmental regulations of the country of origin.

Whilst the advice and information in this book are believed to be true and
accurate at the date of going to press, neither the author nor the publisher can
accept any legal responsibility or liability for any errors or omissions that may
be made. In particular (but without limiting the generality of the preceding
disclaimer) every effort has been made to check drug dosages; however it is
still possible that errors have been missed. Furthermore, dosage schedules are
constantly being revised and new side-effects recognized. For these reasons
the reader is strongly urged to consult the drug companies' printed
instructions before administering any of the drugs recommended in this book.

British Library Cataloguing in Publication Data
A catalogue record for this book is available from the British Library

Library of Congress Cataloging-in-Publication Data
A catalog record for this book is available from the Library of Congress

ISBN-13 978-1-4441-4246-4

1 2 3 4 5 6 7 8 9 10

Commissioning Editor:	Naomi Wilkinson
Project Editor:	Mischa Barrett
Production Controller:	Francesca Wardell
Cover Design:	Lynda King
Cover image © Corbis	

Typeset in Berling Roman 9.5 pts by Datapage (India) Pvt. Ltd.
Printed and bound in Spain by Graphycems

What do you think about this book? Or any other Hodder Arnold title?
Please visit our website: www.hodderarnold.com

For my daughter Kate Webb on the understanding
that she dedicates her first book to me.

Accessing the resources on the companion website

Resources supporting this book are available online. These include:

- An outline of a course based on this text with cross references to the book
- PowerPoint slides that give the framework of this course of lectures
- Answer plans for sample short-note and essay-type exam questions
- References with links to free copies of many of the sources cited
- A comprehensive glossary of terms.

To access these materials go to www at www.hodderplus.co.uk/nutrition-webb and click on 'additional resources' in the right hand menu.

The first time you visit the website, you will need to register with your serial number.
Serial number prs6285fgt (There is a link for this below the log in box.)

Once you have registered you will not need the serial number but can log in using your email address and the password you set up during registration.

CONTENTS

Preface   xi
Acknowledgements   xiv

PART 1 – CONCEPTS AND PRINCIPLES

1. **Changing priorities for nutrition education**   **3**

   Identification of the essential nutrients   3
   Adequacy: the traditional priority in nutrition   5
   The current priority: diet as a means to health promotion or disease prevention   7
   Is intervention to induce dietary change justified?   16
   Effecting dietary change   23
   Concluding remarks   29

2. **Food selection**   **30**

   Introduction and aims of the chapter   30
   The biological model of food   31
   Dietary and cultural prejudice   32
   Food classification systems   33
   Non-nutritional uses of food   38
   The hierarchy of human needs   39
   A model of food selection: the 'hierarchy of availabilities' model   41
   Physical availability   42
   Economic availability   43
   Cultural availability   56
   'Gatekeeper' limitations on availability   62

3. **Methods of nutritional assessment and surveillance**   **64**

   Introduction and aims of the chapter   64
   Strategies for nutritional assessment   64
   Measurement of food intake   65
   Tables of food composition   72
   Dietary standards and nutrient requirements   75
   Clinical signs for the assessment of nutritional status   85
   Anthropometric assessment in adults   86
   Anthropometric assessment in children   92
   Estimating fatness in animals   94
   Biochemical assessment of nutritional status   95
   Measurement of energy expenditure and metabolic rate   98

4. **Methods to establish links between diet and chronic disease**   **102**

   Introduction and aims of the chapter   102
   Strategic approaches: observational versus experimental   102
   Features and problems of epidemiological methods   104
   Cross-cultural comparisons   107

Time trends 110
Migration studies 112
Cohort studies 112
Case–control studies 115
Cross-sectional studies 117
'Experiments' of nature 118
Animal experiments 118
Human experimental studies 121
In-vitro studies 132
Scientific honesty 133

5. Dietary guidelines and recommendations **134**

The range of 'expert reports' and their consistency 134
Variations in the presentation of guidelines and recommendations 136
'Food' recommendations 137
Energy and body weight 139
Recommendations for fats, carbohydrates, protein and salt 140
Alcohol 143
How current UK diets compare with 'ideal' intakes 146
Other nutrients 147
Willingness to change 147
Some barriers to dietary change 149
Aids to food selection 150
Concluding remarks 154

6. Cellular energetics **156**

Introduction and aims of the chapter 156
Overview of metabolism 156
Metabolism of glucose and the monosaccharides 158
Metabolism of fatty acids and glycerol 160
Metabolism of amino acids 161
The pentose phosphate pathway 161
Overview of macronutrient handling in the gut 162

PART 2 – ENERGY, ENERGY BALANCE AND OBESITY

7. Introduction to energy aspects of nutrition **167**

Sources of energy 167
Units of energy 167
How energy requirements are estimated 168
Variation in average energy requirements: general trends 170
Energy content of foods 171
Sources of dietary energy by nutrient 172
Energy density 174
Nutrient density 176
Sources of dietary energy by food groups 177
Starvation 178
Eating disorders 182
Cancer cachexia 185

8.   Energy balance and its regulation   **187**

    The concept of energy balance   187
    Physiological regulation of energy balance   188
    The 'set point' theory   189
    Is energy expenditure regulated?   189
    External influences on food intake   192
    Control of energy intake   192
    The leptin story   198

9.   Obesity   **202**

    Defining obesity   202
    Prevalence of obesity   203
    Consequences of obesity   211
    The metabolic syndrome or 'syndrome X'   219
    Causes of obesity   219
    Prevention and treatment of obesity in populations   229
    Obesity treatment in individuals   232
    'Aggressive' treatments for obesity   237

PART 3 – THE NUTRIENTS

10. Carbohydrates   **245**

    Introduction   245
    Nature and classification of carbohydrates   246
    Dietary sources of carbohydrates   247
    Sugars   248
    Artificial sweeteners   250
    Diet and dental health   252
    Starches   255
    Non-starch polysaccharide   257
    Resistant starch   260
    The glycaemic index   261
    Dietary factors in the aetiology of bowel cancer   262
    Dietary factors in heart disease   266

11. Protein and amino acids   **268**

    Introduction   268
    Chemistry and digestion   268
    Intakes, dietary standards and food sources   270
    Nitrogen balance   271
    Protein quality   274
    The significance of protein in human nutrition   278
    Concluding remarks   284

12. Fats   **285**

    Nature of dietary fat   285
    Types of fatty acid   287
    Sources of fat in the human diet   291
    Roles of fat in the diet   294

Blood lipoproteins   300
Digestion, absorption and transport of dietary lipids   301
Transport of endogenously produced lipids   303
The diet–heart hypothesis   304
Fish oils   317
Other natural oils used as supplements   322

13. The micronutrients   **324**

Scope of this chapter   324
Overview of dietary supplements   325
Food fortification   329
Assessment of the micronutrient adequacy of British adults   330
Anti-oxidants and the oxidant theory of disease   335
Do high anti-oxidant intakes prevent heart disease, cancer and other chronic diseases?   341
Use of substances other than essential nutrients as dietary supplements   346

14. The vitamins   **357**

General concepts and principles   357
Vitamin A (retinol)   361
Vitamin D (cholecalciferol)   365
Vitamin E (α-tocopherol)   371
Vitamin K (phylloquinone)   372
Thiamin (vitamin B_1)   374
Riboflavin (vitamin B_2)   376
Niacin (vitamin B_3)   377
Vitamin B_6 (pyridoxine)   380
Vitamin B_{12} (cobalamins)   381
Folate or folic acid (vitamin B_9)   383
Biotin   389
Pantothenic acid   389
Vitamin C (ascorbic acid)   390

15. The minerals   **393**

Introduction   393
Chromium   394
Copper   395
Fluoride   396
Magnesium   396
Manganese   397
Molybdenum   398
Phosphorus   398
Potassium   398
Selenium   399
Zinc   400
Iodine and iodine-deficiency diseases   402
Iron and iron-deficiency anaemia   405
Calcium storage and uptake   410
Calcium and bone health   414
Sodium and disease   421
Review of evidence for a salt–hypertension link   427

PART 4 – VARIATION IN NUTRITIONAL REQUIREMENTS AND PRIORITIES

16. Nutrition and the human lifecycle	**435**
Introduction	435
Nutritional aspects of pregnancy	437
Lactation	448
Infancy	449
Childhood and adolescence	462
The elderly	469
17. Nutrition as treatment	**484**
Diet as a complete therapy	484
Diet as a specific component of therapy	488
Malnutrition in hospital patients	496
18. Some other groups and situations	**507**
Vegetarianism	507
Racial minorities	513
Nutrition and physical activity	519

PART 5 – THE SAFETY AND QUALITY OF FOOD

19. The safety and quality of food	**533**
Aims of the chapter	533
Consumer protection	533
Food poisoning and the microbiological safety of food	540
Bovine spongiform encephalopathy	554
Food processing	560
The chemical safety of food	564
Functional foods	573
Index	584

The *Glossary* and *References* are available online at **www.hodderplus.co.uk/nutrition-webb**

PREFACE

It was 20 years ago, while a visiting professor at the University of North Florida in early 1992, that I took the first tentative steps towards producing the first edition of this book. My aim was to produce a comprehensive text covering all aspects of nutrition for students at various academic levels but who had no previous academic experience of studying nutrition. I aimed to make the book accessible to students from different academic backgrounds who might have limited background knowledge of biochemistry and/or the physical and mathematical sciences. My main focus was on the role of diet and nutrition in promoting health in people living in affluent countries – hence the title, *Nutrition: A health promotion approach*. Despite this title, the book contained only a brief discussion of health promotion theory and health promotion as a discipline in its own right. So, in order to make the general health-promoting aims of the book clear – but without implying a substantial component of health promotion theory – a new title has been chosen: *Nutrition: Maintaining and improving health*.

I have not ignored the nutritional issues and problems of the developing world, but the bulk of discussion is aimed at students living and intending to work in the affluent countries of Europe, North America and Australasia. I have tried to avoid writing yet another science-based but prescriptive guide to healthy eating; rather I have sought to identify the current consensus on major issues and topics in nutrition and to critically discuss and evaluate the evidence that underpins these views – and where appropriate to discuss alternative opinions. I have included a substantial section dealing with the methods used to study nutrition, not just to help prepare students who might want to carry out these procedures, but also to empower all students to be able to read, understand and critically evaluate the scientific literature.

How has the book changed over 20 years? Each new edition has been larger than its predecessor, and this fourth edition must be close to double the length of the first. The sections dealing with energy aspects of nutrition and the micronutrients are now much more extensive, and there are short sections dealing with a variety of topics not covered in the first edition, including dietary supplements, functional foods, superfoods, meta-analysis, and the scale and implications of world population growth. There are bullet-point summaries of 'key points' at the ends of each major section in the book, and feedback from my own students suggests that these are a popular 'student-friendly' addition to the text. Some of the changes in the book have been driven by changes in nutrition itself, but many more have been driven by changes and development of the author. These developments have been accelerated by researching and writing scholarly articles and other books on topics such as weight control, nutrition of the elderly, and dietary supplements and functional foods.

What has happened in nutrition over the last 20 years? There has been a marked tendency to medicalize eating – a blurring of the boundaries between nutrition and pharmacy. Food and food components are increasingly being consumed in the often vain hope that they will prevent or treat diseases or slow the ageing process. A third of British adults take dietary supplements (nutrition in pill form); there has been a massive growth in the market for so-called 'functional foods' or nutraceuticals that are marketed on their potential health benefits; and more recently the promotion of some sometimes novel and often expensive foods as 'superfoods' because they are rich in particular nutrients, phytochemicals, antioxidants, essential fatty acids or dietary fibre.

The BSE or 'mad cow' crisis was a major nutrition-related event in the UK. When I started writing the first edition, the epidemic of this new fatal disease of cattle was reaching its peak, but there was still no evidence that the disease would directly affect people. In 1996, the British government announced the first cases in young people of a new and invariably fatal neurological disease (variant CJD) that was almost certainly caused by eating beef from cattle 'infected' with BSE. There were dire predictions in the media and by some academics that tens of thousands of young people would suffer a protracted neurological degeneration and die of this disease over the following 20 years. Both the cattle and human epidemics now seem to be all but over. Hundreds of thousands of infected cattle and millions of apparently healthy cattle have been slaughtered and burnt to try to eradicate the disease. The human epidemic may have been thankfully small (175 deaths spread over 18 years), but the disease has cost the British taxpayer billions of pounds, had a devastating effect on British farming for over a decade, and undermined consumer confidence in modern farming, food production methods and government food safety regulation.

How have developments in information technology affected the writing process and the way in which nutrition and other subjects are studied? When I started to research and write the first edition, I was just starting to use e-mail and had not yet used the internet. I had to obtain my source material by physically visiting libraries, searching the literature using huge volumes of paper indexing systems like *Index Medicus*, and then sending off scores of postal requests for hard copies of books and research papers using the Inter Library Loan system. I had to buy expensive hard copies of expert reports such as COMA reports on nutrition-related topics and statistical surveys such as the Health Survey for England and the UK National Diet and Nutrition surveys. Obtaining statistical data from other countries and making international comparisons was a difficult and frustrating process, and often the end-results of this hard work were incomplete and unsatisfactory. I now have a vast range of high-quality up-to-date statistical data, expert reports, academic reviews and research papers available to me free online. I can access this material without moving from my desk, 'at the click of a mouse'. I can search for source material using powerful search engines, for material produced by governments, international agencies, charities, professional bodies and expert groups, and use an academic search engine like Medline or PubMed to find material published in scientific journals. I can then often access this information instantly and at no direct cost to me. Most of the expensive reports that I had to buy in hard copy are now available to download without charge, and I can almost always obtain at least a free abstract of any published scientific paper and can often read the whole paper without cost because it has become open access. The references cited in this fourth edition are now supplied as an online resource and so, to facilitate the student reader's access to this vast array of free published material, I have included links to free copies of many of the sources used. Readers in many institutions, especially research-focused universities, should be able to access even more of these sources by using their institution's password-protected authentication system.

The online material includes the references, a glossary and the following resources:

- *The outline syllabus for a generic 'Introduction to Nutrition' module with indications of where to find the relevant information in the text.* This module is based on a nominal two lectures per week for 20 weeks but can be shrunk or expanded to meet the specific requirements of any particular course or group of students.
- *A series of Microsoft PowerPoint slides that give the detailed framework for each pair of lectures.* These can obviously be modified by individual tutors to meet their specific needs. These slides are designed to be used by tutors as triggers for discussion and elaboration and are not intended to be complete sets of lecture notes. I suggest to my own students that they print the slides three to a page, and use the space on the right of each slide to make additional notes.
- *A series of generic questions with plans of how they should be answered.* I have included a series of short-note questions where students would be expected to write brief accounts of well-defined topics; for my own students I am content for these answers to be a series of clear, concise bullet points. I have assumed in providing the answer plans that students would have 10–15 minutes of examination time to answer each question. I have also included a smaller number of full essay questions where students would be expected to write a structured and in-depth account of a broader topic; for higher level students there might be a requirement for critical discussion and

evaluation within the answer. These plans are intended to be used as a tool by students to guide the final stages of revision for their examinations. Note that several short notes could be combined to make an essay question, or one essay could yield several short-note questions.

This new edition together with the additional online resources is intended to be a complete learning and teaching package that individual tutors can shape and flesh out to meet the specific needs of their courses and students.

Geoffrey Webb
February 2012

ACKNOWLEDGEMENTS

With thanks to Naomi Wilkinson, Mischa Barrett, Joanna Silman and the rest of the Hodder team involved with this edition.

PART ONE

CONCEPTS AND PRINCIPLES

1 Changing priorities for nutrition education   3
2 Food selection   30
3 Methods of nutritional assessment and surveillance   64
4 Methods to establish links between diet and chronic disease   102
5 Dietary guidelines and recommendations   134
6 Cellular energetics   156

CHANGING PRIORITIES FOR NUTRITION EDUCATION

Identification of the essential nutrients 3
Adequacy: the traditional priority in nutrition 5
The current priority: diet as a means to
health promotion or disease prevention 7
Is intervention to induce dietary change
justified? 16
Effecting dietary change 23
Concluding remarks 29

IDENTIFICATION OF THE ESSENTIAL NUTRIENTS

Scientific research into food and nutrition was initially directed towards identifying the essential nutrients and quantifying our requirements for them. All of the essential nutrients must be present in our diets in certain minimum quantities if we are to remain healthy. These essential nutrients can be broadly divided into two categories.

- *The macronutrients* – carbohydrates, fats and protein, which are required in relatively large quantities and can act as dietary sources of energy.
- *The micronutrients* – vitamins and minerals which are only required in small amounts (milligram or microgram quantities) and which do not act as sources of energy.

A shortage of one of the essential micronutrients leads to adverse symptoms, often to a characteristic deficiency disease. In the first half of the twentieth century, many essential nutrients were identified and their ability to cure these deficiency diseases was recognized. Some examples are given below.

- Niacin (vitamin B_3) was shown to cure the deficiency disease *pellagra*. This often fatal disease was so prevalent in some southern states of the USA in the early decades of the twentieth century that it was thought to be an infectious disease.

Pellagra remained a problem in several southern states of America until the 1940s.

- In the late nineteenth and early twentieth centuries, up to 75 per cent of children in some British industrial cities suffered from *rickets*, which was shown to be due to lack of vitamin D. Again, it was not until the 1940s that this disease was largely eradicated in British children. Rickets can be cured either by consuming vitamin D or by exposing the skin to summer sunlight which enables us to make our own vitamin D.
- *Beriberi* exacted a heavy toll of death and misery in the rice-eating countries of the Far East well into the third quarter of the twentieth century. It is cured by thiamin (vitamin B_1), a vitamin that is largely removed from white rice during milling.

The impact of this work was such that several Nobel prizes in Physiology, Medicine or Chemistry were awarded for work on the vitamins; between 1929 and 1943 11 people shared seven Nobel prizes for vitamin-related work. It was his work on thiamin and beriberi, mentioned above, for which Christiaan Eijkman received the 1929 prize.

Such spectacular successes as these may have encouraged a 'magic bullet' image of nutrition – the expectation that simple dietary changes may be able to prevent or cure diseases other than those due to dietary inadequacy. This expectation is generally misplaced, although there is no doubt that poor nutritional status can adversely affect the course of all illnesses and some conditions do respond to restriction or extra supply of some dietary components. For example, the symptoms and/or progression of diabetes mellitus and chronic renal failure can be controlled to a degree by diet (see Chapter 17). There are even a few, relatively uncommon diseases whose symptoms are due to an inborn or acquired intolerance to a specific component of food. In these cases, while diet does not strictly cure the condition, the symptoms can be controlled by preventing or limiting intake of the offending substance; for example:

- *phenylketonuria* (intolerance to the essential amino acid phenylalanine)
- *galactosaemia* (intolerance to one of the components of milk sugar – galactose)
- *coeliac disease* (intolerance/delayed hypersensitivity to the wheat protein, gluten)
- *acute hypersensitivity* (an acute allergic response to a particular food or ingredient, such as shellfish or peanuts).

There are also a few conditions where the symptoms are alleviated by increased intake of a nutrient. For example, *pernicious anaemia* is an autoimmune condition that results in an inability to absorb vitamin B_{12} and is relieved by injections of the vitamin.

Harper (1999) gave a list of criteria for establishing that a nutrient is essential.

- The substance is essential for growth, health and survival.
- Characteristic signs of deficiency result from inadequate intakes and these are cured only by the administration of the nutrient or a known precursor.
- The severity of the deficiency symptoms is dose dependent; they get worse as the intake of nutrient decreases.
- The substance is not synthesized in the body (or only synthesized from a specific dietary precursor) and so is required throughout life. Note that a strict application of this rule would eliminate vitamin D which can be synthesized in the skin in sufficient amounts to meet our needs provided the skin is regularly exposed to summer sunlight.

Around 40 essential nutrients have now been identified, namely:

- water
- energy sources
- protein and the nine essential amino acids
- essential fatty acids
- the vitamins A, C, D, E and K
- eight substances that make up the B group of vitamins
- around 15 minerals and trace minerals.

In most cases, these nutrients have not only been identified but good estimates of average requirements have also been made. Many governments and international agencies use these estimates of requirements to publish lists of dietary standards that can be used as yardsticks to test the adequacy of diets or food supplies. These standards are variously termed 'recommended dietary/daily allowances' (RDAs) or 'dietary reference values' (DRVs) and they are discussed fully in Chapter 3.

Conditionally essential nutrients

Some substances may be required in the diet only under particular circumstances or be required only by particular groups of people, such as in premature babies, people with genetic defects or people with other pathological conditions. Harper (1999) designated these as *conditionally essential nutrients* and defined them as substances that are 'not ordinarily required in the diet but which must be supplied exogenously to specific groups that do not synthesise them in adequate amounts'. Examples are as follows.

- L-carnitine may be essential in people with rare inherited disorders of fatty acid metabolism.
- The amino acid glutamine may become essential in people with serious illness or injury because they cannot synthesize it quickly enough to meet their increased needs.
- The amino acids cysteine and tyrosine may be conditionally essential for premature babies who have not yet developed the enzymes necessary for their synthesis.
- Tyrosine becomes an essential amino acid in people with the inherited disease phenylketonuria (mentioned earlier).

Conditionally essential nutrients are discussed further in Chapter 13.

Some substances that have vitamin-like functions in the body but which are not considered to be essential are frequently taken as dietary supplements; examples are L-carnitine, creatine, glucosamine, coenzyme Q_{10} and s-adenosyl methionine. The implication underpinning their use as supplements is that endogenous synthesis may not always ensure optimal health or may become insufficient in certain pathological states. In effect it is being implied that they can become conditionally essential nutrients. Several of these substances are briefly overviewed in Chapter 13 and discussed in greater depth in Webb (2011a).

Some other substances may be desirable for health while not meeting the criteria for essentiality. Examples are fluoride for its beneficial effects on teeth, and dietary fibre for its effects on gut function. Some nutrients may also be used in doses that greatly exceed those that would be obtained from food to produce a pharmacological effect (i.e. they are used as drugs); for example, nicotinic acid (vitamin B_3) has been used as a cholesterol-lowering agent.

There are also tens of thousands of substances termed *secondary plant metabolites* that are present in the plant foods we eat. While they are not essential or even conditionally essential nutrients, many of these may have beneficial (or deleterious) effects on health. Plant preparations and extracts have been used as herbal medicines throughout human history, and many of them are now marketed and promoted as dietary supplements (or traditional herbal products within the EU) useful for maintaining or restoring health. A number of these secondary plant metabolites are popular and effective drugs and several are potent poisons. These secondary metabolites are classified and briefly overviewed in Chapter 13, and are discussed at greater length in Webb (2011a).

Key points

- In the first half of the twentieth century most of the vitamins were discovered and the ability of vitamin and mineral supplements to cure deficiency diseases was recognized.

→

Key points *continued*

- These discoveries may have encouraged the illusion that dietary change could cure many other diseases.
- A nutrient is classified as *essential* if it is needed for growth and survival, if deprivation leads to dose-dependent symptoms of deficiency, and if the substance is not synthesized in sufficient quantities to meet physiological needs.
- Some nutrients are classified as *conditionally essential* because they are essential only in some circumstances or for some people.
- Some endogenously produced substances with vitamin-like functions are promoted as dietary supplements with the implication that they may become conditionally essential under some circumstances.
- Although dietary change can rarely cure or remove the symptoms of a disease, the progress of all diseases will be affected by poor nutritional status.
- In a few fairly uncommon conditions, diet may be the sole therapy possibly because the symptoms are due to intolerance to a food or a component of food.
- Some nutrients may be used in pharmacological quantities (i.e. used as drugs).
- Intakes of some 'nutrients' may be desirable for health, while not being strictly essential.
- Plants produce thousands of so-called secondary metabolites that may have beneficial or deleterious effects on health. Some of these have been developed into effective drugs and some are potent poisons.
- Around 40 essential nutrients have been identified and estimates of average requirements have been made and published as 'recommended dietary/daily allowances' (RDAs) or 'dietary reference values' (DRVs) in the UK.

ADEQUACY: THE TRADITIONAL PRIORITY IN NUTRITION

The traditional priority in nutrition has been to ensure nutritional adequacy; that is, to ensure that diets contain adequate amounts of energy and all of the essential nutrients. Adequacy was the traditional priority in all countries and it remains the nutritional priority for the majority of the world population. Even today, dietary inadequacy is prevalent in many countries, as illustrated by the examples below.

- Large sections of the world population still suffer from overt starvation.
- Several vitamin and mineral deficiency diseases are still prevalent in many parts of the world. Vitamin A deficiency causes hundreds of thousands of children to go blind each year and is a contributory factor in the deaths of millions of infants and children in developing countries. Iodine deficiency is endemic in many parts of the world and retards the mental and physical development of tens of millions of people.
- Many more people in developing countries, especially children, suffer more subtle consequences of suboptimal nutrition (Box 1.1).

Box 1.1

Some adverse consequences of inadequate food intake

- Increased probability of suffering from a specific nutrient deficiency disease
- Reduced growth and reduced mental and physical development in children
- Wasting of muscles and essential organs; wasting of the heart muscle leads to abnormal cardiac rhythms and risk of heart failure
- Reduced capacity of the gut for digestion and absorption; an inability to digest lactose (milk sugar) and diarrhoea are both common features of malnutrition
- Impaired functioning of the immune system leading to increased risk of infection as well as more prolonged and severe symptoms of infection
- Slow healing of wounds
- Reduced strength and physical capacity that may impair the ability to earn an adequate income or cultivate food
- Changes in personality and other adverse psychological effects.

In the first half of the twentieth century, even in developed countries, the quality of a diet would

thus have been judged by its ability to supply all of the essential nutrients and to prevent nutritional inadequacy. The official priorities for improving the nutritional health of the British population during the 1930s were:

- to reduce the consumption of bread and starchy foods
- to increase the consumption of nutrient-rich, so-called 'protective foods', such as milk, cheese, eggs and green vegetables.

The following benefits were expected to result from these changes:

- a taller, more active and mentally alert population
- decreased incidence of deficiency diseases such as goitre, rickets and anaemia
- a reduced toll of death and incapacity due to infectious diseases such as pneumonia, tuberculosis and rheumatic fever.

Britons are indeed much taller now than they were in the first half of the twentieth century, and occurrences of overt deficiency diseases are rare and usually confined to particular high-risk sectors of the population. Children now mature faster and reach puberty earlier. The potential physical capability of the population has probably increased even though many of us are unfit because we are able to lead very inactive lives. Infectious diseases now account for fewer than 1 per cent of deaths in Britain.

In the affluent industrialized countries of North America, western Europe and Australasia, nutritional adequacy has in recent years been almost taken for granted. Nutrient deficiencies only become likely if total food intake is low or restricted or if the range of foods that are available or acceptable is narrowed. In these industrialized countries there is an almost limitless abundance of food and a year-round variety that would have astounded our ancestors. One would expect, therefore, that even the poor in these countries should usually be able to obtain at least their minimum needs of energy and the essential nutrients. Overt deficiency diseases are very uncommon among most sections of these populations. Over-nutrition, manifested most obviously by obesity, is far more common in such countries than all of the diseases of under-nutrition.

Overt malnutrition and deficiency diseases in the industrialized countries are usually concentrated in groups such as these:

- those who suffer chronic ill-health or some medical condition that specifically predisposes to nutrient deficiency (a high proportion of patients admitted to hospital are malnourished upon admission – see Chapter 17)
- alcoholics and drug addicts
- people at the extremes of social and economic disadvantage
- very elderly housebound people (see Chapter 16).

War or severe economic dislocation can rapidly undermine this assumption of even minimal adequacy in developed countries, as witnessed by events in parts of the former Soviet Union and former Yugoslavia during the 1980s and 1990s. Wartime mass starvation in Holland and Germany is still recent enough to be just within living memory. In Britain during the Second World War there were considerable constraints placed on the food supply by attacks on merchant shipping. This certainly led to shortages of certain foods and a more austere and less palatable diet. However, because of very effective food policy measures and strict rationing it also paradoxically led to an apparent improvement in the nutritional health of the British population.

In both the UK and USA, average energy intakes of the population have fallen substantially in recent decades – a reflection of reduced energy expenditure caused by our increasingly sedentary lifestyle. This trend towards reduced energy intake (i.e. total food intake), coupled with a high proportion of energy being obtained from nutrient-depleted sugars, fats and alcoholic drinks, may increase the likelihood of suboptimal nutrient intakes. It may even precipitate overt nutrient deficiencies in some groups such as the elderly or those on prolonged weight-reducing diets. Chapter 13 has a discussion of evidence that substantial numbers of individuals in all age groups in the UK have intakes of one or more essential nutrients that are considered to be inadequate even where average population intakes of these nutrients appear to be satisfactory, and millions of individuals show biochemical indications of a vitamin or mineral deficiency.

Key points

- Ensuring adequate intakes of energy and essential nutrients has been the traditional priority in nutrition and it remains the priority for most of the world population.
- Dietary inadequacy results in a number of adverse consequences, as listed in Box 1.1.
- In the 1930s, the dietary priorities for improving health in Britain were to reduce the consumption of starchy foods and to increase the consumption of so-called protective foods like milk, cheese, eggs and green vegetables.
- These changes to the 1930s British diet were expected to lead to a taller, more active and mentally alert population, elimination of the deficiency diseases and a reduced toll from many infectious diseases. These objectives have been largely achieved.
- In the industrialized countries, deficiency diseases are largely confined to the very elderly, the infirm, alcoholics and drug addicts, or those at the extremes of social and economic deprivation.
- War and economic disruption can lead to a rapid re-emergence of the deficiency diseases in a previously affluent country.
- UK survey data suggest that millions of individuals have less than satisfactory intake or biochemical status for one or more vitamins or minerals.

THE CURRENT PRIORITY: DIET AS A MEANS TO HEALTH PROMOTION OR DISEASE PREVENTION

The priority of health promotion and nutrition education in industrialized countries is now directed towards changing the 'Western diet and lifestyle' with the aim of reducing the toll of chronic diseases including cardiovascular disease, cancer, maturity-onset diabetes, osteoporosis and dental disease. These diseases are variously known as the *Western diseases* or the *diseases of affluence/civilization/industrialization*. As a population becomes more affluent then its life expectancy tends to increase and mortality rates, particularly among children and younger adults, fall. However, these chronic, degenerative 'diseases of industrialization' become more prevalent in middle-aged and older adults and so account for an increasing proportion of death and disability.

There is no doubt that people in industrialized countries live much longer and die of different things than they did a century ago. In 1901, average life expectancy was around 47 years in both Britain and the USA. It is now well over 75 years in both countries. In 1901, fewer than half of British people survived to reach 65 years but now the figure is around 95 per cent. In 1901, only 4 per cent of the population of Britain were aged over 65 years but now they make up 16 per cent of the population. These dramatic increases in life expectancy have been largely the result of reducing deaths, particularly in children and younger adults, from acute causes such as infection, complications of childbirth, accidents and appendicitis. Life expectancy has increased substantially for all age groups over this period; even older people have an increased expectancy of further years. This inevitably means that there have been big increases in the proportion of deaths attributable to the chronic, degenerative diseases of industrialization that affect mainly middle-aged and elderly people. Infectious diseases were the major cause of death in Britain in the nineteenth century but now it is the cardiovascular diseases (heart disease and stroke). Infectious diseases accounted for 1 in 3 deaths in Britain in 1850, about 1 in 5 deaths in 1900, but today this figure is under 1 per cent. At the turn of the twentieth century, probably fewer than a quarter of all deaths were attributed to cardiovascular disease and cancer but now the figure is three-quarters. In the period 1931 to 1991, cardiovascular diseases rose from causing 26 per cent of all deaths to 46 per cent.

There is an almost unanimous assumption that these diseases of industrialization are environmentally triggered – that is, due to the 'Western lifestyle'. This assumption leads to the widespread belief that major improvements in health and longevity can be achieved by simple modifications of lifestyle. Diet is one of the environmental variables that has received much attention in recent years, and poor diet has been blamed for contributing to the relatively poor health record of some affluent groups. Of the top 10 leading causes of death in the USA, eight have been associated with nutritional causes or excessive alcohol consumption. Numerous expert committees in the industrialized countries have suggested dietary modifications that they consider would reduce or delay mortality and morbidity from these diseases of industrialization and thus ultimately lead to increases in life expectancy and improved health. These recommendations usually include advice to reduce consumption of fats, sugar, alcohol and salt and to replace them with starchy foods and more fruits and vegetables. Consumers are being advised to eat less meat, milk, eggs and dairy produce but more bread and starchy foods and more fruits and vegetables. Compare these recommendations with the British priorities for nutrition in the 1930s when Britons were being advised to eat fewer starchy foods and more milk, cheese and eggs. A good diet today is not just one that is nutritionally adequate but one that is also considered likely to reduce morbidity and mortality from the diseases of industrialization.

Risk factors

Certain measured parameters and lifestyle characteristics partially predict an individual's likelihood of suffering from or dying of a particular disease.

- A high plasma cholesterol concentration indicates an increased risk of developing coronary heart disease.
- High blood pressure is associated with increased risk of renal failure, heart disease and stroke.
- Obesity is associated with increased likelihood of developing type 2 diabetes.

Many of these *risk markers* are thought to be a contributory cause of the disease; that is, they are not just markers for those at risk but are true risk factors that directly contribute to the development of the disease. For example, elevated plasma cholesterol concentration is generally believed to accelerate the lipid deposition and fibrosis of artery walls (atherosclerosis) that leads to increased risk of coronary heart disease. Such an assumption of cause and effect would suggest that altering the risk factor (e.g. lowering plasma cholesterol) should also reduce the risk of the disease provided such changes occur before there is irreversible damage. Much of current health promotion, nutrition education and preventive medicine is based on such assumptions. Dietary variables can be direct risk factors for disease, as in the examples below.

- A diet that is low in fruits and vegetables is associated with increased risk of several types of cancer.
- High sugar consumption is strongly implicated as a cause of tooth decay, whereas high fluoride intake seems to prevent it.

Dietary variables can also have a major influence on some of the other well-established risk factors, particularly the cardiovascular risk factors, and some examples are listed below.

- A high population salt intake is associated with high average blood pressure and increased prevalence of hypertension.
- Changes in the types of fat eaten can have readily demonstrable effects on plasma cholesterol concentration. A high proportion of saturated fat raises plasma cholesterol, but replacing saturated with unsaturated fat lowers it.

Much current nutrition research is focused on these risk factors. Individual components of the diet are related to individual diseases or even to other risk factors such as high plasma cholesterol and high blood pressure. The identification of dietary and other environmental risk factors should enable health educators to promote changes in behaviour that will lessen exposure to the risk factor, prevent the disease and so eventually improve health and longevity. However, one practical result of this approach is a profusion of papers in the medical and scientific literature cataloguing a series of suggested associations between individual dietary variables and individual diseases and risk factors. The sheer number of such reported associations is sometimes bewildering, and this bewilderment may be compounded because there are, more often than not, contradictory reports. As an extreme example, McCormick and Skrabanek (1988) suggested that a staggering 250 risk markers had been reported for coronary heart disease.

A major problem that will inevitably confront those involved in health promotion will be to decide whether and how to act on the latest reported association between a lifestyle variable and a disease.

These associations will often be relayed to the general public through brief summaries in the media that may be distorted and sensationalized. Health-conscious members of the public may then try to decide on the optimal diet and lifestyle on the basis of such snippets – this is rather like trying to work out the picture on a huge jigsaw puzzle by reading inaccurate and incomplete descriptions of some of the individual pieces. All too often the initial research on which these health stories are based is sponsored by those with commercial interests in the product, and sometimes the research seems more geared towards generating media headlines that will benefit the sponsors than advancing scientific knowledge.

Several of these individual associations are discussed and evaluated in this book. In such discussions there are two broad aims:

- to indicate not only where the current consensus of scientific opinion lies but also to give a flavour of the reasoning and evidence underpinning that position and to highlight unresolved issues and/ or alternative opinions
- to indicate diet and lifestyle patterns or modifications that are realistic, low-risk, consistent and likely to produce overall health benefits.

Are recommendations to alter diet and lifestyle offered too freely?

A drug or a food additive intended for use by vast numbers of apparently healthy people would be subject to an extremely rigorous and highly structured evaluation of both its efficacy and safety. Drugs are not licensed until the Medicines and Healthcare Products Regulatory Authority (MHRA) in the UK or Food and Drug Administration (FDA) in the USA have been satisfied that they are both safe and effective. Despite this, mistakes still occur and drugs or additives have to be withdrawn after sometimes many years of use. Compared to this rigorous approval procedure, some dietary and lifestyle interventions (including some dietary supplements and unlicensed drugs masquerading as dietary supplements) seem to be advocated on the basis of incomplete appraisal of either efficacy or safety –

perhaps, on occasion, almost recklessly. Even impartial expert committees may make premature judgements based on incomplete or incorrect evidence. There will also be a plethora of advice from those whose actions are prompted by belief in an untenable theory or myth (quackery), by political or ethical prejudice, or even by economic or other self-interest. One would not take seriously a book on brain surgery or nuclear physics by an unqualified celebrity but celebrities, self-proclaimed experts in alternative therapies and professional journalists are deemed suitable to give their advice on diet and health in the media and in diet books.

There are clear legal frameworks regulating the licensing of drugs and food additives, yet there is not, nor can there realistically be, any restriction on the offering of dietary or lifestyle advice. All that governments and professional bodies can do is to try to ensure that there is some system of registration or accreditation so that those seeking or offered advice have some means of checking the credentials of the would-be adviser. One can only hope that the responsible sections of the media will be more discerning about what they are prepared to publish and perhaps choose their diet and health contributors on the basis of their knowledge and understanding rather than solely on their celebrity status and media appeal. Regulators are being more proactive in the control and advertising of 'dietary supplements' and of health claims relating to foods.

The author's perception is thus that there is a tendency for dietary or lifestyle intervention to be advocated before rigorous appraisal has been satisfactorily completed or sometimes before it has even been really started. Dietary supplements, even plant extracts and preparations that have no significant culinary use can be sold freely and with relatively little regulation provided they do not produce obvious acute toxic effects and provided the supplier is careful with the wording of any promotional material. This is probably because of the implicit assumption that simple changes in diet and behaviour and 'natural supplements' are innocuous and that, even if they do no good, then neither will they do any harm. Intervention, rather than non-intervention, therefore becomes almost automatically regarded as the safer option: 'If dietary change cannot hurt and might help, why not make it?'. This means that even if dietary and

lifestyle advice is offered recklessly or by those with no credible expertise then it is assumed at worst to be just harmless nonsense.

Can simple changes in diet or lifestyle do any harm?

The assumption that simple dietary and lifestyle changes are innocuous seems logically inconsistent with the clear evidence that diet, lifestyle and environment are major determinants of health and longevity. This means that appropriate changes in diet and lifestyle can improve health and longevity (the theoretical justification for health promotion), but it also inevitably means that inappropriate changes can worsen health and longevity. Dietary and lifestyle changes have the potential to do harm as well as great good (see possible examples in the next section). The fact that some 'natural extracts' are potent poisons and that many nutrients and other food components are toxic in excess clearly means that they cannot be assumed to be safe by default.

Even if unjustified intervention does not do direct physiological harm, it may have important social, psychological or economic repercussions. Social and psychological factors have traditionally been the dominant influences on food selection, so any ill-conceived intervention carries the risk of causing anxiety, cultural impoverishment and social and family tensions. It has been suggested that the resources spent on unjustified health education interventions may serve only to induce a morbid preoccupation with death (McCormick and Skrabanek, 1988). Major changes in food selection practices will also have economic repercussions, perhaps disrupting the livelihoods of many people and reducing their quality of life.

Repeated changes of mind and shifts of emphasis by health educators are also liable to undermine their credibility and thereby increase public resistance to future campaigns. We saw earlier in the chapter how dietary advice changed as the nutritional priority changed away from trying to ensure adequacy and towards using diet as a means of preventing chronic disease. These changes in emphasis often reflect changing social conditions and consumption patterns, but some may be justifiably perceived as evidence of the inconsistency and thus unreliability of expert advice. The two examples below may serve to illustrate this latter point.

First, obesity was once blamed on excessive consumption of high-carbohydrate foods, like bread and potatoes. These foods would have been strictly regulated in many reducing diets (e.g. Yudkin, 1958). Nutritionists now view bread and potatoes much more positively. They are high in starch and fibre and consumers are recommended to incorporate more of them into their diet to add bulk (i.e. to reduce the energy density). This bulkier diet may in turn reduce the likelihood of excessive energy intake and obesity. These low-carbohydrate diets became fashionable again a few years ago, their popularity driven by diet books and celebrity endorsements.

Second, scientific support for nutritional guidelines aimed at lowering plasma cholesterol concentrations has now been increasing for almost 50 years. Although this cholesterol-lowering objective may have remained constant, there have been several subtle shifts of opinion as to the best dietary means to achieve this goal, as illustrated below.

- Reducing dietary cholesterol was once considered an important factor in lowering plasma cholesterol. It is now usually given low priority.
- A wholesale switch from saturated to the n-6 type of polyunsaturated fatty acids prevalent in many vegetable oils was once advocated, but very high intake of these polyunsaturated fats is now considered undesirable.
- Monounsaturated fats were once considered neutral in their effects on plasma cholesterol but are now much more positively regarded. This accounts for the current healthy image of olive oil and rapeseed (canola) oil.
- The n-3 polyunsaturated fatty acids have also been viewed much more positively in recent years, especially the long-chain acids found predominantly in fish oils.
- The current emphasis of both UK and US recommendations is to aim for a reduction in total fat intake with a proportionately greater reduction in the saturated fraction of dietary fat.

Attitudes to some individual foods could be strongly affected by such changes of emphasis. This is illustrated in Table 1.1. Certain fatty foods come

out very differently in a 'worst' to 'best' rank order when cholesterol content, total fat content, saturated fat content or ratio of polyunsaturated to saturated fatty acids (P:S ratio) is used as the criterion. Sunflower oil comes out at the 'worst' end of the rankings if total fat content is the criterion but at or near the 'best' end if cholesterol content, P:S ratio or saturated fat content is used. Eggs and liver are worst by the cholesterol criterion but around half way down by all other criteria. Prawns are at the bottom for all criteria except cholesterol content, but they are also relatively rich in the now positively regarded long-chain, n-3 polyunsaturated fatty acids.

Promoting ineffective behavioural changes will also dilute the impact of campaigns to promote effective changes. If the ineffective changes are easier to adopt than the effective ones, then they may actually inhibit effective change. Examples of this are:

- taking β-carotene supplements to lessen the damage done by cigarette smoke, rather than giving up smoking
- taking an anti-oxidant supplement, rather than eating five portions of fruit and vegetables each day
- taking supplements of milk thistle (now classified as a traditional herbal products within the EU) to protect the liver, rather than moderating alcohol consumption.

Does health promotion always promote health?

It would seem prudent to regard any dietary or lifestyle changes considered for health promotion as potentially harmful until this possibility has been actively considered and, as far as possible, eliminated. Some of the examples below may serve to demonstrate that this is a real possibility rather than just a theoretical one.

Sleeping position and cot death

Some reviewers considered this example inappropriate for a nutrition text but it does dramatically demonstrate the scale of the harm that can be caused by a simple and well-meaning promoted change in behaviour.

Table 1.1 Rank orders by different fat-related criteria of some foods*

Food	% energy as fat	% energy saturated fat	Cholesterol content	P:S ratio[1]
Liver	11	8	2	8
Lean steak	12	9=	6	4
Cheddar cheese	7	2	7	2=
Butter	1=	1	3	2=
Polyunsaturated margarine	1=	6	10=	13
Low-fat spread	1=	4	10=	10
Sunflower oil	1=	11	10=	14
Milk	9=	3	9	1
Human milk	9=	5	8	5
Chicken meat	13	12=	5	7
Avocado	5	12=	10=	9
Peanuts	6	9=	10=	11
Egg	8	7	1	6
Prawns	14	14	4	12

*Ranks are from 1 ('worst') to 14 ('best') (after Webb, 1992a).
[1] P:S ratio, ratio of polyunsaturated to saturated fatty acids.

In 1991, a campaign called 'Back to Sleep' was launched in the UK that advised parents not to lay babies down to sleep on their front (i.e. to avoid the prone sleeping position). This campaign was launched because of a substantial body of evidence suggesting that babies who slept on their front were up to eight times more likely to suffer a cot death than those laid on their back. The following year the cot death rate was halved and it has continued to decline since then and is now just a quarter of the peak rate seen in the late 1980s. The Foundation for the Study of Infant Deaths in the UK estimated that, by 2007, 15 000 babies' lives had been saved by this 'Back to Sleep' campaign. In 1993 when the cot death figures for the first year after the launch of this campaign were released, the Secretary of State for Health was quoted as saying that the sharp drop in cot deaths illustrated the benefits of health education:

> The figures on cot deaths show that behaviour change can work, can save lives.

Daily Telegraph, 30 May 1993

This campaign has been used in health promotion courses as an example of what effective health promotion can achieve.

Figure 1.1 shows the trend in cot death prevalence in England and Wales between 1971 and 2004. This graph shows that rates of cot death in 1971 were very similar to current low rates but rose steeply during the 1970s and 1980s to reach a peak of four times current levels in the late 1980s. What this chart suggests is that we had a 20-year epidemic of extra cot deaths that cost the lives of thousands of British babies, and similar epidemics were seen in many other industrialized countries which killed tens of thousands more babies. The key question, therefore, is what caused these epidemics of extra cot deaths in so many countries?

In the 1950s and 1960s, very few British babies (around 4 per cent) slept on their front. During the 1970s and much of the 1980s, health professionals and childcare writers in the UK advised parents to put babies down to sleep on their front (prone) rather than on their back (supine) as they had traditionally done. This advice to use the front sleeping position first began because premature babies were reported to suffer less respiratory distress in the prone position and babies with severe gastro-oesophageal reflux were less likely to choke on regurgitated milk. This front sleeping position then became widely used in special-care baby units

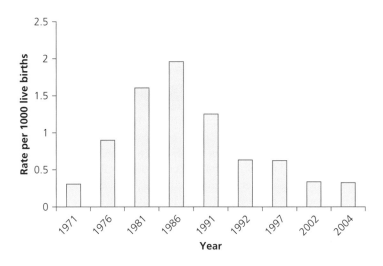

Figure 1.1 Trends in cot death rates in England & Wales.

and very soon it became usual for midwives, doctors, other healthcare professionals and babycare writers to advise all parents to use the front sleeping position. The decreased risk of choking was highlighted as being important for all babies and the back sleeping position came to be regarded as unsafe. In a survey of babycare books published before 1991, Webb (1995) found an almost unanimous recommendation to use front sleeping:

> For the first two months or so, the safest way for babies to sleep is on their fronts, head to one side, or else curled up on one side. Then if they are sick, there is no chance that they will choke.
>
> *Pregnancy Book, Health Education Council, 1984*

> A young baby is best not left alone lying on his back. Because he cannot move very much he might choke if he were sick. Lie the baby in the cot on his front with his head to one side, or on his side.
>
> *Reader's Digest, family medical adviser, 1986*

Compare the quote below which comes from the 1993 edition of the Health Education Council's *Pregnancy Book* with that from the 1984 version above:

> Babies laid to sleep on their tummies are more at risk of cot death than babies laid down to sleep on their backs or sides ... Only lay your baby down to sleep on his or her front if your doctor advises it.

Given the weight of advice from healthcare professionals and babycare writers to use the 'safer' front sleeping position, it is not surprising that the majority of parents had adopted this position by the late 1980s. This epidemic of cot deaths was therefore caused by 'experts' persuading parents to use the front sleeping position. The $c20\,000$ babies saved by 'Back to Sleep' are in fact extra babies that might have died if 'the experts' had continued to promote front sleeping. Looking back one can now see that there was never any real evidence that front sleeping would benefit more than a handful of high-risk babies, but 'what harm could a simple change of sleeping position do?'. For further discussion see Webb (1995).

As well as being an example of the benefits of effective health promotion, the foregoing example provides a quantitative demonstration of the dangers of recklessly promoting untested behaviour changes. This latter point is seldom mentioned in the media and many people including many health promotion academics are unaware of this negative aspect. It is important that we examine, analyse and fully acknowledge such 'mistakes' in order to learn not to continue to make the same mistakes.

If one is seeking to justify intervention for a whole population, then it is not enough merely to demonstrate that a specific group will benefit from the proposed change. Intervention with a small sample of 'high-risk' subjects is likely to exaggerate the benefits of intervention for the population as a whole. Such small-scale intervention will also only show up the grossest of harmful effects. It may thus fail to show up harmful effects that could be very significant for indiscriminate intervention and which might cancel out or even exceed any benefits of the intervention.

Some cholesterol-lowering interventions

As noted earlier, diets containing very large amounts of polyunsaturated fatty acids were widely advocated as a means of lowering plasma cholesterol concentrations. Short-term experiments had demonstrated very convincingly that switching from high saturated to high polyunsaturated fat diets could reduce serum cholesterol concentrations in young men (e.g. Keys *et al.*, 1959). However, there was no convincing evidence that, in the long term, such a wholesale switch from saturated to polyunsaturated fat produced any increase in life expectancy even in studies using 'high-risk' subjects. Concerns have been raised about the long-term safety of diets that are very high in polyunsaturated fat. Britons have been advised to limit their individual intakes of n-6 polyunsaturated fatty acids to no more than 10 per cent of energy with a population average of 6 per cent (COMA, 1991). Concerns have also been raised about the large rise in the ratio of n-6 to n-3 polyunsaturated fatty acids that will affect n-3 metabolism and the production of the long-chain n-3 fatty acids (see Chapter 12 for details). Some of the early cholesterol-lowering drugs like clofibrate were associated with increased mortality despite lowering blood cholesterol levels. Smith *et al.* (1993) in a review of pre-1993 cholesterol-lowering trials (about two-thirds of which involved cholesterol-lowering drugs) suggested that only those at very high risk of death from coronary heart disease showed any improved mortality risk from taking these drugs and that they should be only prescribed to very high-risk patients. (Newer statin drugs are very effective at lowering cholesterol and do lead to reduced cardiovascular and all-cause mortality – see Chapter 12.)

Reducing an asymptomatic risk factor, such as plasma cholesterol concentration, cannot, in itself, be taken as evidence of benefit. There must be evidence that it will lead to the predicted decrease in disease risk, and that there will not be an accompanying increase in some other risk.

'The world protein crisis'

In the 1950s and 1960s, protein deficiency was thought to be the most prevalent and serious form of worldwide malnutrition. It was considered likely that 'in many parts of the world the majority of young children suffer some protein malnutrition' (Trowell, 1954). Very considerable efforts and resources were committed to alleviating this perceived problem (amounting to many hundreds of millions of pounds/dollars). However, as estimates of human protein requirements were revised downwards, it then seemed probable that primary protein deficiency was likely to be uncommon and thus that the resources committed to alleviating widespread protein deficiency were largely wasted (Webb, 1989). See Chapter 11 for further discussion.

There is no compelling evidence that provision of extra protein was directly harmful. Nevertheless, scarce resources were committed to a non-beneficial measure and other, more real, problems deprived of resources. Research and teaching in nutrition were unreasonably distorted towards protein nutrition for at least a generation. In the USA (NRC, 1989a), and in the current UK dietary standards (COMA, 1991), the possibility that high intakes of protein might even be directly harmful is acknowledged and an upper limit of twice the dietary standard has been advised. There is growing evidence that high intakes of animal protein, in particular, may be associated with increased risk of some cancers.

Resources for research, development, international aid and educational programmes are always finite. If these resources are diverted into unnecessary measures or programmes based on false theories, then inevitably worthwhile projects will be deprived of funding.

Routine iron supplementation during pregnancy

Iron supplements were once routinely and almost universally prescribed for pregnant women in the UK. Many women have minor side-effects from taking these tablets – black stools, nausea, constipation or diarrhoea. These supplements were considered necessary because of the perception that the risks of anaemia in pregnancy were very high, a perception that was compounded by the misinterpretation of the normal decline in blood haemoglobin concentration during pregnancy as pathological. This decline is caused by increased plasma volume and occurs despite increased total amounts of circulating haemoglobin. In the UK, routine iron supplements in pregnancy are now thought to be unnecessary. The UK panel on dietary reference values (COMA, 1991) suggested that, for most women, the extra iron demands of pregnancy can be met by utilization of maternal stores and physiological adaptation. Note that in the USA a different view is taken and universal iron supplementation is still recommended for pregnant women. A similar natural decline in haemoglobin concentration caused by 'haemodilution' can occur in endurance athletes, and this has probably exaggerated the risk of anaemia especially in female athletes.

Use of β-carotene supplements

There is overwhelming evidence that diets high in fruits and vegetables are associated with reduced risk of several cancers; hence the current campaigns to persuade consumers to take at least five portions of fruit and vegetables per day.

β-Carotene is a plant pigment found in green and brightly coloured fruits and vegetables. It acts as a source of vitamin A and is the source of vitamin A used in many so-called ACE vitamin supplements. β-Carotene is also one of a group of anti-oxidant substances that may protect the body from oxidative damage by free radicals and perhaps lessen the risks of cancer and atherosclerosis (see Chapter 13). This means that diets high in coloured fruits and vegetables also tend to be high in β-carotene and that high carotene intakes are associated with reduced cancer risk. Low blood carotenoid levels are, as one might expect, also associated with increased cancer risk. A number of controlled trials of β-carotene supplementation have paradoxically found higher rates of cancer in the supplemented group than in the unsupplemented controls (e.g. Group, 1994; Omenn et al., 1996). Particularly in heavy smokers and asbestos workers, there is evidence that large β-carotene supplements may

increase the risk of lung cancer. Beta-carotene has traditionally been regarded as non-toxic and very large doses can be tolerated acutely without ill effects. More recently, Vivekanathan et al. (2003), in a meta-analysis of published trials, recorded a small but significant increase in both cardiovascular and all-cause mortality in those receiving the β-carotene supplements compared with those receiving a placebo. In 1998, an expert panel in the UK counselled against the taking of large β-carotene supplements (COMA, 1998) and in 2003, the Food Standards Agency (FSA, 2003) suggested a safe upper limit of 7 mg per day for supplements of β-carotene. Despite this, supplements containing at least 15 mg/day continue (late 2011) to be advertised and sold; so a dietary supplement that seems to be at best ineffective and probably does net long-term harm is still sold in amounts that are way beyond the advised safe limits. Compare this with the case of a new drug which must convince the regulators that it is both effective and safe before it is approved for sale.

Major commissioned reviews in the USA have concluded that vitamin E and vitamin C supplements (the two other so-called ACE vitamins) do not reduce heart disease, cancer or all-cause mortality, and neither do they reduce non-fatal cardiac events or have any value in the treatment of cancer (Shekelle et al., 2003; Coulter et al., 2003).

The five examples discussed above have been selected to illustrate that very popular dietary or lifestyle interventions may in later years become regarded as unnecessary or perhaps even harmful. This demonstrates how scientific opinion about the value and safety of such interventions fluctuates.

If a holistic view is taken, then it is likely that any intervention that produces no benefits will have some detrimental effects even though this may not always involve direct physiological harm. Majority support among scientists and health professionals for an intervention based on a particular theory is no guarantee that it will continue to be regarded as useful or even safe.

Those involved in health promotion and nutrition education need to be constructively critical of current fashions. They need to be receptive to criticism of current wisdom and objective in their evaluation of such criticism. They need to be cautious about advocating mass intervention, especially if there is no convincing, direct evidence of overall long-term benefit or where evidence of benefit is restricted to a relatively small 'high-risk' group. Any non-beneficial intervention should be regarded as almost inevitably detrimental in some way.

Key points

- Average life expectancy in Britain and the USA increased by more than 50 per cent during the twentieth century and this has led to a large increase in the proportion of elderly people.
- This increased life expectancy means that most deaths and much of the chronic illness and disability are now due to the chronic diseases of industrialization that affect mainly middle-aged and elderly people – cardiovascular disease, cancer, diabetes, osteoporosis.
- Reducing mortality and morbidity from these chronic diseases is now seen as the priority for nutrition education and health promotion in the industrialized nations.
- The current dietary recommendations to achieve this objective are in some ways almost the opposite of those of the 1930s (e.g. to moderate consumption of meat, eggs and dairy produce but to increase consumption of starchy foods, fruits and vegetables).
- A risk factor is some parameter that partially predicts one's risk of developing a disease and that is causally linked to the onset of the disease.
- Dietary factors can be direct risk factors or they can influence the level of others – such as plasma cholesterol, blood pressure or insulin resistance.
- Much modern health promotion is focused on identifying and reducing these risk factors, and the sheer number of such risk factors can cause confusion and increase the possibility of conflicting advice.
- Recommendations to alter diet and lifestyle are sometimes not fully underpinned by adequate supporting evidence.
- There seems to be an implicit but illogical assumption that simple changes in diet and lifestyle have the potential to do good but not harm.

→

Key points *continued*

- There are examples of dietary or lifestyle changes based on past health promotion that seem to have done net harm. For example, a recommendation to put babies to sleep in the prone position seems to have increased the risk of cot death. β-Carotene supplements have actually increased death rates in a number of controlled trials.
- Even where a non-beneficial dietary or lifestyle change does no direct physiological harm, it may have less obvious adverse consequences. An example is the resources wasted in trying to solve the illusory crisis in world protein supplies.
- Promoting ineffective behavioural change will deflect attention away from more effective measures, especially where they offer an easy alternative to making effective changes (e.g. taking an anti-oxidant pill rather than eating more fruit and vegetables).
- At the very least, recommendations that are changed or withdrawn will undermine confidence in nutrition education and increase resistance to future advice.
- It is particularly illogical to assume that 'natural supplements' are inevitably safe. Many potent poisons are natural extracts, and even some essential nutrients and other food components are very toxic in high doses.

IS INTERVENTION TO INDUCE DIETARY CHANGE JUSTIFIED?

[after Webb, 1992a]

Evidence linking diet and disease seldom materializes in complete and unequivocal form overnight. More usually, it accumulates gradually over a period of years with a high probability that some of the evidence will be conflicting. The problem of deciding when evidence is sufficient to warrant issuing advice or some other intervention is thus one that will frequently need to be faced. If action is initiated too soon then there is a risk of costly and potentially harmful errors. If action is too slow then the potential benefits of change may be unduly delayed.

There is likely to be intense pressure to take action or to issue guidelines in the light of the latest highly publicized research findings. Box 1.2 lists a set of criteria that might be used to decide whether any particular intervention is justified by available knowledge.

Box 1.2

Criteria for deciding whether an intervention is justified

- Have clear and realistic dietary objectives been set and all foreseeable aspects of their likely impact considered?
- Is there strong evidence that a large proportion of the population or target group will gain significant benefits from the proposed intervention?
- Has there been active and adequate consideration of whether the promoted action, or any consequential change, might have adverse effects on a significant number of people?
- Have the evaluations of risk and benefit been made holistically? A reduction in a disease risk marker, or even reduced incidence of a particular disease, are not ends in themselves; the ultimate criterion of success must be an increase in life expectancy or a net improvement in quality of life. Likewise the evaluation of risks should not be confined to possible direct physiological harm but should also include, for example, economic, psychological or social repercussions. It should also include the possibly harmful effects of any consequential changes and consider the damage ineffective intervention might have on the future credibility of health educators.
- Has the possibility of targeting intervention to likely gainers been fully explored so as to maximize the benefits to risks ratio?
- Has consideration been given to how the desired change can be implemented with the minimum intrusion into the chosen lifestyle and cuisine of the target group?

Intervention that precedes satisfactory consideration of the likely risks and benefits is experimentation and not health promotion.

Such criteria are probably not, in themselves, controversial. It is in deciding when these criteria have been satisfactorily fulfilled – or even properly considered – that the controversy arises.

Judging whether the intervention criteria have been fulfilled

A number of practical questions like those listed below need to be addressed and satisfactorily answered before any apparent association between a dietary variable and a disease or risk factor is translated into practical health promotion advice.

- Is the reported association likely to be genuine?
- Is the association likely to represent cause and effect?
- What change in dietary composition is realistically achievable and what magnitude of benefit is this predicted to produce?
- Is this predicted benefit sufficient to warrant intervention at the population level, or at the individual level?
- Are there any foreseeable risks from the proposed compositional change for any group within the target population?
- Are there any foreseeable non-nutritional adverse consequences of these changes?
- What changes in other nutrient intakes are likely to occur as a result of the proposed advice?
- Are there any foreseeable risks from these consequential changes?
- How can the desired compositional change be brought about?

Is the association genuine?

It is quite possible that an apparent association between diet and a disease may have arisen because of bias in the study or simply by chance. There is often a range of papers reporting conflicting findings; these need to be evaluated and weighted rather than the latest or the majority view being mechanically accepted (see section on systematic reviews and meta-analysis on p.128). It is quite possible that a common logical flaw, incorrect assumption or methodological error is present in all of the papers supporting one side of an argument.

Easterbrook *et al.* (1992) reported that, in clinical research, positive results are more likely to be published than negative ones. This means that the literature may give an unbalanced view of total research findings. This problem of publication bias is discussed further in Chapter 4 and a method for gauging its likely extent is outlined. Authors may try to highlight positive findings especially if positive findings would increase the impact of the paper and impress referees or if positive findings would be in the research sponsor's interests. In another analysis, Ravnskov (1992) reported that when citation rates were determined for papers dealing with cholesterol-lowering trials, those with positive outcomes (i.e. suggesting a beneficial effect on coronary heart disease) were cited six times more frequently than those with negative outcomes. At the author, peer review, editorial selection and citation levels there may be bias towards positive over negative findings.

Statistical significance at, or below, the 5 per cent level (i.e. $p<0.05$) is, by convention, taken as the point at which a scientist can claim that, say, a correlation or a difference between two means is 'statistically significant'. There is less than a 1 in 20 likelihood that the correlation or difference between the means has arisen simply by chance. This statistical significance may simply reflect flaws or bias in the design of the study, in the allocation of subjects, or in the measurement of variables. With numerous investigators all correlating numerous dietary variables with health indicators, it is inevitable that some statistically significant associations will arise simply by chance; authors may be tempted to highlight the one barely significant correlation in a whole battery of otherwise insignificant tests. Statistical significance is not proof of the underlying theory but an indication that any difference or association is unlikely to be due to pure chance. This should be borne in mind when evaluating isolated reports of improbable-sounding associations. Statistical significance does not always mean that a result is clinically or practically significant (see discussion on cholesterol-lowering effects of garlic later in this chapter).

Dietary guidelines often stem from qualitative reviews of the scientific literature or the conclusions of expert committees but, as already shown, even apparent consensus among experts does not guarantee that a particular opinion is correct. There was once an almost unanimous belief in a crisis of world protein supply but few would support this view today. Scientists are trained to make objective judgements based solely on scientific evidence, but they are also fallible human beings whose judgements may, perhaps unwittingly, be affected by prejudice, political or peer pressure and self-interest. Reviewers and committee members will often be selected because of their active involvement and expertise in a particular field of study. This may sometimes hamper their objectivity especially when they are required to evaluate material that may undermine or support their own work and reputation, or to evaluate material that might even jeopardize their own career or research funding. McLaren (1974) tried to identify some of the reasons for the now discredited concept of a world protein crisis or protein gap and for its persistence (see Chapter 11). He suggested that even in 1966, when this theory was still at its height, many scientists had privately expressed sympathy with his opposition to the theory and some of the measures designed to alleviate this perceived crisis. He also claims that they were unwilling to publicly support him for fear of having their research funding withdrawn. He even suggests that critical discussion of the issues was suppressed.

This book has a substantial section on nutrition research methods. Readers who are primarily interested in the practice of promoting health and healthy eating and are unlikely to participate in research projects may be tempted to disregard much of this section as superfluous to their needs. I think that this would be a narrow and short-sighted decision. Some general appreciation of the research methodology – especially the strengths, limitations and weaknesses of the various methods – is essential for any critical reading and evaluation of the literature. Anyone who wishes to keep up to date with the literature and to be able to make quality judgements about conflicting evidence, or controversial new reports, will need some basic understanding of the methodology.

Is the association causal?

Epidemiological methods produce evidence of associations between diseases and suggested causes, but even a strong association does not necessarily mean that there is a cause-and-effect relationship. It is quite probable that the statistical link between a risk marker and a disease may have arisen because both are associated with a third, confounding variable. For example, even though alcohol may not directly contribute to causing lung cancer, a statistical association between alcohol consumption and lung cancer might arise if heavy drinkers also tend to be heavy smokers. Earlier in this chapter it was noted that high fruit and vegetable consumption is associated with reduced cancer risk. This also means that high β-carotene intake is likely to be associated with lowered cancer risk but does not necessarily mean that high β-carotene intake prevents cancer. There are several other explanations for this finding such as those listed below.

- People who eat lots of fruit and vegetables may have other lifestyle characteristics that help to reduce their cancer risk – such as different smoking, drinking and exercise habits.
- High fruit and vegetable consumption may be a marker for a diet that is healthier in other respects – such as being lower in fat.
- Even if high fruit and vegetable consumption is directly protecting against cancer, it may be some component(s) other than β-carotene that is exerting the protective effect.

As we saw earlier, several controlled trials have found that β-carotene supplements appear to increase mortality rates compared to placebos.

Epidemiologists try to correct their results for the effects of confounding variables when looking for a causal link between diet and disease. There is, however, no statistical magic wand that unerringly and accurately corrects for all confounding variables; it is a matter of judgement what the likely confounders are and the process of correction itself may be imprecise, particularly if there is imprecise or limited measurement of the confounding variable (Leon, 1993). Take the examples of smoking and exercise as possible confounding variables in epidemiological studies of a relationship between diet and heart disease. Apparently reliable information on smoking habits is usually obtained in such studies and one has confidence that a reasonable correction of the results for the effects of smoking can be made. On the other hand, it is notoriously difficult to make accurate assessment of activity level, and so in many of these studies there is little or no attempt to correct for the effects of variation in activity levels. This problem of confounding variables is discussed more fully in

Chapter 4 along with criteria to help decide whether any particular association is causal.

In some cases it may be that the disease itself leads to the measured changes in diet or behaviour: an effect-and-cause relationship. It is particularly important to consider this possibility when one is comparing the current behaviour of those who have or may have the disease with those who do not. Obese people are less active than lean people; is this a cause or an effect of their obesity? A low serum vitamin A concentration may be associated with an increased risk of developing symptomatic cancer within a few years; is this a cause of the cancer or an early symptom of it?

Dietary and lifestyle changes tend not to occur in isolation; often, many changes occur simultaneously. Increasing affluence and industrialization tend to bring with them numerous changes in diet and lifestyle as well as major changes in the causes of death and disease. This means that an association between one of the 'diseases of industrialization' and one of the wealth-related environmental variables needs to be treated with extreme caution until there is substantial evidence to support this association being causal.

Realistically achievable change: magnitude of benefit?

If a cause-and-effect relationship is established between a dietary factor and a disease, one should be able to predict the magnitude of benefit that is likely to result from a given change in diet. For example, if there is a linear relationship between the average blood pressure of adult populations and their average daily salt consumption, then one can attempt to predict the reduction in average blood pressure that would result from a reduction in average salt consumption (e.g. Law *et al.*, 1991a). Then, making certain assumptions, one can go on to predict by how much the incidence of hypertension will fall and thence the beneficial effect on mortality from the hypertension-related diseases (see Chapter 15 for further discussion of this example). One must then decide what degree of change is realistically achievable and what the benefits of change on this scale are likely to be. It is unhelpful to predict the huge health gains that might result from a degree of change that is impractical or unrealistic. A reduction in average UK daily salt consumption from around 10 g to less than 1 g as seen in some populations like the Yanomamo Indians of Brazil might eradicate hypertension and produce major reductions in mortality from hypertension-related diseases. There is, however, no chance that a change of this magnitude can be achieved.

In a major commissioned review of the effects of garlic on heart disease and cancer, Mulrow *et al.* (2000) found no evidence of substantial benefit from taking garlic supplements. Trials of the effects of garlic supplements on plasma cholesterol consistently found a small but statistically significant reduction in the garlic group at 1 month and 3 months, but those that continued to 6 months found no effect. These findings suggest that garlic supplements probably have a small and transient effect on this risk factor but that this would have no clinical benefit to those taking the supplements. The effect is statistically significant but too small to have any real clinical significance, and even this small effect is probably only transient.

At what level is intervention justified?

Even when there is clear evidence of a causal association between a dietary factor and a disease, it may still be difficult to decide whether this justifies intervention at the population level. The extreme scenarios are:

- if a minor dietary change could produce a major reduction in the risk of a common fatal disease, then the case for intervention would appear strong
- if a major dietary change were only predicted to marginally reduce the risk of a relatively uncommon disease, then clearly intervention at the population level would not be justified.

In between these extremes, the significance or 'cost' of the proposed change will need to be balanced against the predicted reduction in population risk. Even where a likely benefit cannot justify intervention at the population level, if those who are particularly 'at risk' or who are particularly susceptible to the causal factor can be identified then this may justify intervention for those high-risk groups.

There are, therefore, essentially two strategies to chose from when designing a health promotion campaign aimed at risk reduction.

- *The population approach*. Advice is directed at the whole population, or large sections of it, with the aim of reducing average population exposure to the risk.
- *The individual approach*. Efforts are made to identify those most at risk from the risk factor and intervention is targeted specifically at these 'high-risk' individuals.

If one takes the example of a programme aimed at lowering plasma cholesterol in order to reduce the risk of coronary heart disease (CHD), then one could choose either of the following options.

- In the *population approach*, direct the message at the whole adult population. If successful this would be expected to lower average plasma cholesterol concentrations and shift the whole population distribution of plasma cholesterol concentrations downwards.
- In the *individual approach*, one could seek to identify those with the highest cholesterol concentrations and most 'at risk' from CHD and target the advice specifically at these 'high-risk' individuals.

Much health promotion/nutrition education in the UK has tended to use the population approach. If one is seeking to make a significant impact on population mortality/morbidity from a disease, the population approach appears to offer the greatest probability of success. Consider the example of the relationship between plasma cholesterol concentration and coronary heart disease. It is generally accepted that, at least for young and middle-aged men, high plasma cholesterol concentrations predict an increased risk of premature death from CHD. For example, Figure 1.2 shows that, for one population of American men, mortality risk for CHD approximately doubled as the plasma cholesterol concentration doubled. It is assumed that lowering of serum cholesterol will result in a corresponding reduction in CHD risk. Figure 1.3 shows that there are relatively few men in this population with very high plasma cholesterol levels (say, over 7.8 mmol/L), so restricting cholesterol-lowering efforts to these high-risk subjects can have only limited impact. Even a substantial reduction of risk in this small group will do little to affect population mortality from CHD. The majority of the population in Figures 1.2 and 1.3 (and the current population of the UK) have plasma cholesterol concentrations that are regarded as slightly or moderately elevated (say, 5.2–7.8 mmol/L). Even a small reduction in individual risks for this very large group will have a significant effect on total population mortality.

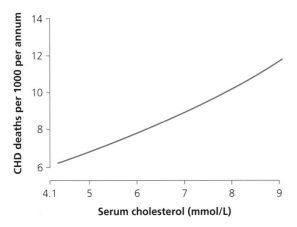

Figure 1.2 The relationship between serum cholesterol concentration and subsequent death rate from coronary heart disease (CHD) in a sample of American men. Source: Webb, GP (1992a) *Journal of Biological education* 26 (4), 270. After NACNE (1983).

Some of the advantages and disadvantages of these two approaches are listed below (after Webb and Copeman, 1996).

- If everyone is advised to change, then the promoted behaviour may become the norm and may create conditions that make it easier for any individual to change. For example, if everyone is urged to reduce their fat and saturated fat intake, then this increases the incentive for the food industry to develop and market products that are low in fat and/or saturated fat. These might be low-fat spreads, margarine and oils that are low in saturated fat, lower fat milks, and reduced-fat processed foods. The ready availability of such foods makes it easier to adopt a low-fat diet, so low-fat choices may come to be perceived as the norm.
- The population approach removes the need to identify the 'high-risk' subjects and mark them out as 'victims' of a particular condition. The individual approach may require a mass screening programme to, for example, identify those above some arbitrary cut-off point for plasma cholesterol; if screening is not universal then some 'high-risk' individuals may not be identified. Once identified, 'high-risk' individuals would probably feel threatened by their 'high-risk' classification and change might be more difficult for them to implement because the changes in product availability and social norms discussed above would be unlikely to occur.
- The population approach requires mass change and, for many, that change will offer only a small reduction in individual risk, and thus the motivation to change may be low.
- If mass change is induced, there is increased likelihood that some currently 'low-risk' individuals may be harmed by the change. It may

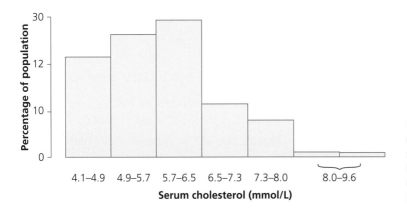

Figure 1.3 Distribution of serum cholesterol concentrations in the sample of men in figure 1.2. Source: Webb, GP (1992a) *Journal of Biological education* 26 (4), 270. After NACNE (1983).

create norms of behaviour and perhaps even changes in the range and pricing of foods that are not universally beneficial. We saw earlier that increased use of the front sleeping position for babies in the 1970s and 1980s may have helped some premature babies and some babies with particular conditions, but for the majority it increased the risk of cot death.

- The population approach may create an unhealthy preoccupation with death and disease in the whole population (McCormick and Skrabanek, 1988), so that even people at very low risk of CHD may be made extremely fearful of this condition. This would be particularly true if health promotion focused on the negative aspects of not accepting the message – if it used fear of death and disease and the threat of social isolation as the levers for effecting behavioural change.
- The population approach may lead to people being blamed for their condition and perhaps to doctors and politicians justifying the withholding of expensive treatments: 'It's your own fault that you have heart disease/cancer, because you smoke, or eat badly, or don't take enough exercise'.

The debate about whether to fortify bread with folic acid shows how difficult it can be to decide whether to adopt a population or an individual approach. Under clinical trial conditions, peri-conceptual supplements of folic acid greatly reduce the incidence of neural tube defects (NTDs) such as spina bifida. They are effective only if taken very early in pregnancy, and probably most effective if taken pre-conceptually. Since 1992, women in the UK contemplating pregnancy have been advised to take folic acid supplements, and all sexually active pre-menopausal women are now advised to take them. Supplement advice has been ineffective in reducing the incidence of NTD. Very few women take folic acid supplements routinely (those who need them least) and, as many pregnancies are not specifically planned, they are usually taken too late. Fifty countries fortify bread or flour with folic acid and this has produced sharp and immediate falls in NTD incidence. However, fortification exposes several hundred thousand people to the extra folic acid for each affected pregnancy

prevented. To justify this exposure one must be sure that the folic acid is harmless, particularly as the folic acid used to fortify foods and in supplements is not a natural form of the vitamin (conjugated folate) found in food. Several theoretical concerns about folic acid have been raised but on current evidence seem to be unfounded. Also, the case for fortification would be strengthened if it could be shown to have wider benefits. Current evidence does suggest that it could reduce the incidence of some other birth defects and improve the folate status of many elderly people currently classified as having poor folate status. Other suggested claimed benefits on heart disease risk, cognitive function and bowel cancer risk are not supported by current evidence. A detailed and referenced discussion of this example can be found in Chapter 14, and this discussion illustrates how difficult it can be to 'prove' that a proposed measure is completely safe – as discussed in the next section.

Harmful effects of intervention?

First do no harm.

Health promotion should increase life expectancy and reduce ill-health. It is illogical to assume that dietary or lifestyle changes are an inevitable 'one-way bet' and can only be beneficial. The possibility of harmful effects must be actively considered and tested. Several possible examples of simple dietary or lifestyle interventions having unexpected harmful effects have been discussed earlier in the chapter. Harmful social, psychological, economic or cultural repercussions are likely even where no direct physiological harm results from unjustified intervention. Non-beneficial intervention will, at the very least, ultimately undermine the credibility of future programmes.

What are the secondary consequences of change?

Dietary changes almost never occur in isolation. Changing the diet to produce an intended change will almost inevitably affect the intake of other nutrients. When dietary changes are to be advocated, the likely impact of the intended change on the total diet should be considered. If reduced intake of a particular food or nutrient is advised, how are the intakes of other nutrients likely to be affected, and what is likely to replace the missing food? If people are advised to increase their intake of particular foods, what will they displace from the existing diet?

For example, if food manufacturers are persuaded to use less salt in processing, what effect will this have on shelf-life and therefore on cost and availability of foods? Will it compromise the microbiological safety of some foods? Or, will it lead to increased reliance on other preservatives whose long-term safety may also be questioned? In Chapter 10 there is a brief discussion of the likely effects of using artificial sweeteners: do they reduce total energy intake by reducing sugar consumption, or is the lost sugar energy simply replaced by other foods leading to increases in total fat consumption?

Key points

- Dietary change should be recommended only if there is clear evidence that it will yield net holistic benefit.

- The possibility that change may have adverse direct or indirect effects should be considered and tested.

- Premature action based on insufficient evidence runs the risk of doing net harm, whereas undue delay means that any benefits of the intervention will also be delayed.

- Some apparent links between diet and disease may arise because of statistical freaks or reflect bias in the study design.

- Trying to obtain a consensus view from published reports will be hampered because negative results are less likely to be published and cited than studies with positive outcomes.

- Even if an intervention produces a statistically significant change in a risk factor in short-term trials, this change may not be clinically significant and/or may only be transitory.

- An association between a certain diet and a disease does not necessarily mean that there is a cause-and-effect relationship. Associations may arise because both disease risk and associated dietary factor are linked to other confounding variables.

→

Key points *continued*

- Health promotion intervention may be directed at the whole population with the aim of inducing mass change (the population approach), or it may be targeted at those individuals regarded as at higher risk of the particular disease (the individual approach).

- The population approach may create a climate and conditions that facilitate individual change and removes the need to identify and mark out those at high risk of the disease.

- Mass change may only offer many people a small likelihood of benefit and it increases the chance that some will be harmed by the change.

- The population approach may frighten even those who are at low risk of the disease, and it may foster an unhealthy preoccupation with death and disease.

- A recommended dietary change is likely to have other consequential changes on diet composition.

EFFECTING DIETARY CHANGE

It is easy to devise diets or plan menus that meet any particular set of compositional criteria, but much more difficult to make them acceptable to the clients. For example, it is easy to produce nutritionally adequate reducing diets, but the long-term dietary treatment of obesity is notoriously unsuccessful. Diets or dietary recommendations that are sympathetic to the beliefs, preferences and usual selection practices of the recipients will probably fare better than those that ignore the non-nutritional influences on food selection or try to impose the prejudices and preferences of the adviser.

Food has a host of cultural, psychological and social functions in addition to its biological function. It is these non-nutritional uses that have traditionally been the dominant influences on our food selection. If we lose sight of these functions in the perhaps fruitless pursuit of the optimal chemical diet, then any technical improvements in our nutrition may be outweighed, or at least reduced, by damage to the general emotional health of the population. Miserable, anxious people will probably suffer more illnesses and die younger than happy contented people.

Some of these non-nutritional influences on food selection are discussed in Chapter 2. If health promoters want to effect changes in eating behaviour then they must have some appreciation of the determinants of food selection practices. They can then offer practical advice that will bring about any desired changes in diet in ways that are compatible with the overall cultural milieu of the target group. Nutrition educators should try to effect compositional changes in the desired direction with the least interference in current cultural practices – a cultural conservationist approach. This is the most ethical approach as well as the most likely to succeed.

Some factors influencing the likelihood of dietary change

Fieldhouse (1998) listed certain parameters that will particularly influence the likelihood of dietary change occurring.

- *The advantage of change and the observability of that advantage.* If a relatively minor dietary change results in immediate and apparent benefits, this increases the likelihood of permanent adoption. However, if the benefits of change are not immediately apparent or are speculative, or if the change itself is seen as having a major disadvantage (e.g. restricting favoured foods, increased cost, or increased preparation time), this will decrease the chances of its adoption.
- *Its compatibility with existing beliefs, cultural values and culinary style.* Advice that is compatible with existing beliefs and behaviour is more likely to be implemented than advice that is contrary to these beliefs and behaviours. Advising a pious person to break the dietary rules of his religion, or advising a committed vegetarian to eat meat, has a low probability of success.
- *Its complexity.* The more difficult it is to implement or understand any change, the less chance there is that it will be made. Advice aimed at lowering plasma cholesterol is often perceived as requiring major reductions in the consumption of meat and dairy produce. These high-prestige and highly flavoured foods are central to the culinary practices and the food ideology of many Western consumers. Such changes may therefore be seen as requiring a complete restructuring of the diet. Promoting simple modifications of existing practices that involve relatively little 'cost' for the consumer may produce more real change than advocating much more ambitious and drastic changes that will be implemented by relatively few people. Simple suggestions are: buy leaner cuts of meat; trim off visible fat; grill (broil) rather than fry; use lower fat milk; use a spreading fat that is lower in saturated fat.

- *Its trialability.* If advice is easy to try out on a 'one-off' basis, people are more likely to try it out than if it requires more commitment – such as the learning of a new preparation method or buying new catering equipment. Getting people to try out a dietary change is the first step towards adoption of the change. Switching from butter to margarine and cooking with vegetable oil rather than animal fats seem like readily trialable changes. Fluoridation of water supplies is an example of a change that is not readily trialable. If a change requires a period of adjustment this would reduce its trialability. People may, for example, get used to food cooked without added salt, but in order to adjust to the change they may need an extended trial period. Increasing fibre intake by switching from white to wholemeal bread may seem eminently trialable. However, sudden increases in fibre intake may produce transient diarrhoea, flatulence and abdominal discomfort and it may require some time to adapt.

Advice to make a dietary change that is aimed at curing a deficiency disease has a good chance of being accepted. The major advantages of such a change are usually readily apparent within a short period and can often be observed in others who have already done it. The disadvantages of changing may be small, such as incorporation of a nutrient-rich or fortified food into the diet or even the consumption of a nutrient supplement. This sort of dietary modification is also easy to understand and implement. It can usually be tried out without any long-term commitment and the rapid and obvious benefits encourage people to continue with the change in diet.

Similarly, when a therapeutic diet gives rapid symptomatic relief, this will also act as powerful, positive reinforcement and encourage clients to stick with the diet and perhaps even to stick to it more rigorously. For example, if adoption of a low-protein diet gives symptomatic relief to patients with chronic renal failure, this may well encourage them to persevere with the diet despite its relative complexity and restrictiveness and irrespective of any possible long-term benefits on the course of the disease (see Chapter 17). Increased fibre and water intakes will often relieve constipation or give symptomatic relief from other minor bowel disorders such as diverticulosis or haemorrhoids. These benefits will act as a positive reinforcement for people suffering from these conditions.

It may be much more difficult to persuade healthy people to make changes that are aimed at reducing the long-term risk of chronic disease. The benefits of many of the health-promoting dietary changes currently recommended by expert committees are often difficult to demonstrate at the individual level and in the short term. The benefits are often expected to accrue some time after introduction of the change; they are often perceived as speculative with some expert opinion arguing against even the long-term benefits of change. These measures are designed to produce significant long-term reductions in the population risk of death and disease and the individual may only be offered a relatively small reduction in his or her individual risk of suffering from some disease at some seemingly distant date. A good part of any individual's risk of developing or dying of a particular disease is inherited. This means that anecdotal observations may often confound the predictions of the experts; there will be examples of 'healthy eaters' who nevertheless develop diet-related diseases and those who ignore dietary guidelines but remain healthy well into old age. This anecdotal tendency may be compounded by the tendency of people to adopt practices they perceive as healthful when they start to become concerned about their health so adoption of a healthy diet may apparently immediately precede the onset of overt symptoms.

The dietary changes required to meet current nutrition education guidelines may be perceived as having immediate and major disadvantages – the restriction of highly palatable sugary, salty and fatty foods and their partial replacement with bland, starchy and fibre-rich foods. Increasing fear and guilt about 'inappropriate' eating behaviours may be one way of altering the balance of advantage towards implementing change. Thus a first heart attack can persuade someone to adopt a strict cholesterol-lowering diet, or the onset of serious lung disease may persuade someone to give up smoking. However, health promotion that tries to harness such fear of death and disease as a means of inducing dietary and/or lifestyle change in healthy people serves to focus people's attention on death and disease. It may have some negative impact on quality of life. If such 'health promotion' succeeds in generating fear and guilt without changing behaviour, or results in changes that are ultimately proved not to be beneficial, then its impact will be totally negative. What is the effect of anti-smoking campaigns using graphic images and interviews of those dying from smoking-related disease on people who continue to smoke and on their children or others who care about them? Similarly, increased feedback by regular monitoring of risk factors like plasma cholesterol may improve compliance but McCormick and Skrabanek (1988) argue that such focusing on symptomless risk markers may serve only to induce an unjustified and morbid preoccupation with death. Health and wellness promotion is a very positive-sounding objective, whereas death delaying has a much more negative ring to it; nutrition education must be presented and implemented in ways that emphasize the former objectives rather than unnecessarily increasing fear of, and preoccupation with, death and disease.

Barriers to successful health promotion

Figure 1.4 summarizes some of the stages in the process of a nutrition education or health promotion message leading to changes in behaviour that benefit health. There are potential barriers or blockages to successful health promotion at each of these stages, and these blockage points are discussed below.

Blockage point 1: The receiver fails to see or hear the message

An inappropriate channel may have been chosen for the message. The channel is the vehicle for

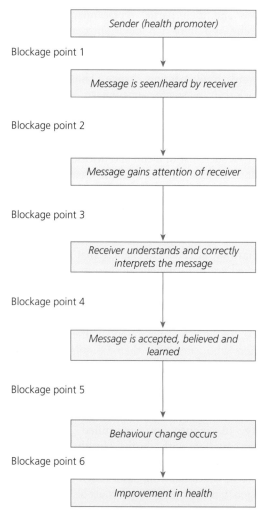

Figure 1.4 Steps in the process by which a health promotion message leads to beneficial change in behaviour and potential barriers to change (modified from Webb and Copeman, 1996).

transmitting the message – radio, television, newspaper or poster advertisements, leaflets provided at a doctor's surgery or community centre, speakers addressing groups, or one-to-one counselling. Those initiating the health promotion campaign should consider what channel is most likely to reach the target group and to influence their behaviour. They also have to consider what would be the most cost-effective vehicle for transmitting the message to the target group. One would choose different TV or radio slots and different newspapers and periodicals if targeting

teenagers than if elderly people were the primary target group. Some simple market research may need to be done to ensure that the message will reach the receiver.

Blockage point 2: The message may not gain the attention of the target group

A poster or TV advert may not attract or interest the target group – images of teenage pop stars are more likely to interest teenagers than elderly people. Programmes, posters, oral presentations and leaflets must be attractive and interesting; they must be appropriate for the target group.

Blockage point 3: The message may not be understood by the receiver

This may result in a blockage at this stage, or if the message is misinterpreted it may result in an inappropriate behaviour change. For example, a message to increase dietary fibre may result in an inappropriate behaviour change if the nature and sources of dietary fibre are misunderstood. The health promoter must ensure that their message is clear, correct, believable and realistic. They must consider the standards of education and literacy of the target group and make special provision for groups where English is not the first language. If illiteracy is common, then a written message is of little value. Ideally, any promotional material should be piloted to identify potential problems with terminology, understanding or interpretation.

Blockage point 4: The message may not be believed, or forgotten

Even if the message is believed, if it is too complex and not reinforced then it may be forgotten. The source may be seen as biased or may lack credibility with the receiver. An elderly male speaker perceived as conservative might lack credibility with an audience of streetwise teenaged girls. Promotional leaflets sponsored by a commercial company and bearing the company logo may be viewed as biased. The message may be inconsistent with existing scientific beliefs (e.g. advice to increase starchy foods may be inconsistent with the belief that they are fattening). It may be inconsistent with traditional cultural beliefs about diet, such as the need of Chinese people to balance foods classified as 'hot' and 'cold' in their cultural food classification system (see Chapter 2 for details of this example).

Blockage point 5: Behaviour change does not occur despite the message being received and understood

The required change of behaviour may be difficult or impossible for the receiver to implement. Dietary changes that increase the cost of the diet may be beyond the economic means of some groups. Some groups who are largely reliant on others to provide their food may find it impossible to implement the change – for example, children who rely on their parents to provide food or those living in residential homes for the elderly. Some people may accept and believe the message but decide to ignore it; people may continue to smoke despite being aware of its adverse effects on health.

Blockage point 6: Behaviour change occurs but does not result in improved health

The message may be wrong or inappropriately targeted (see earlier in the chapter) or it may be misunderstood and result in an inappropriate behaviour change (see blockage point 3).

In summary, those designing nutrition education or other health promotion campaigns must keep in mind the following.

- Ensure that *the source* of the message will be seen by the receivers as credible and reliable.
- Make sure that *the message* itself is clear, correct, realistic and appropriately targeted.
- Ensure that *the channel(s)* chosen for disseminating the message are likely to reach the target group, attract their attention and be likely to influence their behaviour.
- Consider the particular characteristics of *the receivers* or target group before they can design an appropriate strategy. What is their level of education and literacy? What is their first language? What are their recreational interests, cultural beliefs and media habits?

The BASNEF model (Figure 1.5)

- **B** – beliefs
- **A** – attitudes

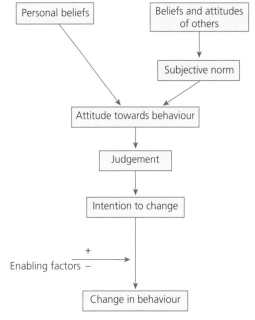

Figure 1.5 A scheme to illustrate how beliefs, attitudes, the subjective norm and enabling factors (BASNEF) interact to determine whether health promotion recommendations result in actual behaviour change (after Hubley, 1993).

- **SN** – subjective norm
- **EF** – enabling factors

An individual's beliefs about diet and health will clearly influence his or her judgement about whether a suggested change is beneficial. If one is seeking to persuade someone to modify behaviour in order to reduce the risk of a particular disease, then first the person must believe that he or she is susceptible to the disease; second that the consequences are serious; and finally that it can be prevented (Becker, 1984). Consider heart disease as a specific example. In order to make a judgement to modify her behaviour in order to avoid heart disease, a woman must believe that:

- she is at risk from heart disease (i.e. susceptible)
- heart disease can kill or disable (the consequences are serious)
- if she changes her diet and behaviour (e.g. stops smoking), her risk is reduced (prevention is possible).

It is not only the beliefs of the subjects themselves that will influence their judgements but also the influences of family, friends, colleagues, teachers, religious leaders, health workers etc. Ajzen and Fishbein (1980) described these influences from the beliefs and attitudes of others as the *perceived social pressure* or the 'subjective norm'. Health promotion has succeeded in changing several norms of behaviour.

Fifty years ago, butter would have been regarded by most UK consumers as the most natural, palatable spreading fat and margarine a cheap and inferior substitute. Those who could afford it would usually have chosen butter, and serving margarine to guests may well have been regarded as showing low esteem for them or meanness. Butter is now regarded as the least healthy of the spreading fats; it is seen as high in fat and saturated fat. The majority of UK consumers now choose either a low-fat spread or soft margarine as their everyday spreading fat and often use them for social occasions as well.

Fifty years ago almost all milk used in the UK was whole milk, but now semi-skimmed milk, which was not even widely available then, accounts for most of the milk sold in the UK.

In the 1950s, smoking was the normal behaviour in most sectors of British society and the non-smoker was often the odd one out. Now the opposite is often true; smokers are in a minority in many sectors of society and smoking is often regarded as an unacceptable or even illegal activity in many public places and social situations. Smokers are often made to feel ostracized because of their habit and required to stand outside workplaces and bars to indulge their habit.

Changing the subjective norm can encourage others to follow the change and may even make it easier for people to adopt the promoted behaviour. Consider the greater range, availability and acceptance of alternative spreading fats to butter.

There are sound health reasons for trying to reduce the number of people who are overweight and obese. Nevertheless, creating a climate (subjective norm) where fat is regarded as bad and lean good may not be a helpful health promotion approach. Most people already desperately want to become or remain lean. By focusing on body weight *per se*, health promoters may simply increase the unhappiness and discrimination already experienced by obese people. It may also encourage some normal

or even underweight young women to try to become even leaner and adopt unhealthy dietary lifestyle practices to achieve that. Health promoters will instead need to try to promote dietary and lifestyle practices that encourage better weight control (see Chapter 9 for further discussion).

Individual beliefs and the subjective norm will affect a person's judgement of any particular recommendation and thus affect his or her behaviour intentions. A host of 'enabling factors' will influence whether or not any intention or wish to change behaviour is translated into actual behaviour change. These enabling factors may come under a variety of headings such as those listed below.

- *Physical resources.* Is the change physically possible for the person? Can the person obtain the recommended foods? Are the facilities available for their preparation? For example, the range and quality of fresh fruit and vegetables available in some rural areas may be limited. If low-income groups are temporarily housed in accommodation without cooking facilities this may severely limit their dietary choices.
- *Financial resources.* Can the person afford to make the recommended changes? Fruit and vegetables provide few calories per penny and so may be uneconomic choices for those seeking to satisfy appetites on a very low income.
- *Personal resources.* Does the person have the skills and mobility necessary to implement the recommended changes? Many frail elderly people have mobility problems that restrict their shopping and cooking capabilities. Some widowed elderly men, or students living away from home for the first time, may have had very little experience of preparing food for themselves.

In Chapter 2, many of these enabling factors are discussed using the 'hierarchy of availabilities' model of food selection (see Figure 2.2 on p. 41). In this model it is assumed that a host of factors, at several levels, limit any individual's practical freedom of dietary choice and thus limit his or her ability to implement any recommended change.

People may be convinced that a health promotion message is applicable to them, the subjective norm may favour change, and the enabling factors may permit them to make the recommended change. Despite this, change may still not occur; they may make a decision (judgement) to accept the risks associated with current behaviour, perhaps because of the perceived adverse effect of change on their quality of life. In younger men, for example, the acceptance of risks associated with dangerous or unhealthy practices may be seen as an expression of their virility.

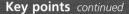

Key points

- It is relatively easy to devise diets that meet any given set of scientific criteria, but it is much more difficult to produce such a diet that will be complied with by the client.
- A dietary change is more likely to be implemented if there are clear and rapidly discernible benefits, if the change is consistent with existing beliefs and practices, and if it is easy to understand, try out and incorporate.
- A dietary change that cures a deficiency disease rapidly produces clear and apparent benefits and often involves changes that are easily understood and implemented.
- A dietary change to reduce the risk of chronic disease usually produces no immediate benefits.
  - Even the long-term benefits may be small and speculative for any individual.
  - Considerable and complex change may be required.
  - The change may be perceived as markedly reducing the desirability of the diet.
- Health promotion will be ineffective if:
  - the message is wrong
  - the message is not seen and correctly assimilated by the client
  - the message does not convince the client that change is desirable
  - the client is unable or unwilling to make the recommended changes in behaviour.

→

Key points *continued*

- The BASNEF model suggests that beliefs, attitudes, the subjective norm and a range of enabling factors are the determinants of whether a health promotion message results in actual change.
  - People must believe that the recommended change will benefit them.
  - They must be of a mind to make changes for the benefit of their long-term health.
  - The subjective norm is the beliefs and attitudes of those people who influence the client and perhaps of society as a whole.
  - Enabling factors are a range of practical things like resources, skills, mobility and knowledge that can determine the extent to which the client can change.

CONCLUDING REMARKS

If the questions posed in this chapter are fully considered by those making nutrition or other health education recommendations, then the likelihood of making changes that ultimately prove to be non-beneficial or harmful will be minimized. If a totally holistic view is taken, any intervention that is non-beneficial can probably be regarded as harmful. Observations on migrant populations show that, in general, they tend to progressively assume the mortality and morbidity patterns that are characteristic of their new homeland.

This reaffirms the belief that many of the health differences between populations are due to environment rather than genetics, and therefore also confirms that there is considerable potential for promoting health by lifestyle intervention. Paradoxically, as each population tends to have its own problem diseases, it also underlines the potential for harm from ill-considered and insufficiently tested interventions. A narrow preoccupation with changing diets to reduce the risk of one disease may simply lead to an increase in the risk of another.

2

FOOD SELECTION

Introduction and aims of the chapter	30	A model of food selection: the 'hierarchy of	
The biological model of food	31	availabilities' model	41
Dietary and cultural prejudice	32	Physical availability	42
Food classification systems	33	Economic availability	43
Non-nutritional uses of food	38	Cultural availability	56
The hierarchy of human needs	39	'Gatekeeper' limitations on food availability	62

INTRODUCTION AND AIMS OF THE CHAPTER

Most of this book focuses on food as a source of energy and nutrients – for example: which nutrients are essential and why; how much of these nutrients people need at various times of their lives; how changing the balance of nutrients eaten can affect long-term health, and so on. This chapter is in some small way intended to be an antidote to the necessary scientific reductionism of much of the rest of the book. The general aim of the chapter is to remind readers that 'people like to eat food, not nutrients', and that nutrient content has only relatively recently become a significant factor in the making of food choices. Only in the latter part of the twentieth century did our knowledge of nutrient needs and the chemical composition foods become sufficient to allow them to be major influences on food selection.

A host of seasonal, geographical, social and economic factors determine the availability of different foods to any individual or group, while cultural and preference factors affect its acceptability. Some of these influences are listed in Box 2.1.

If the promotion of health requires one to try to influence people's food choices, some understanding of the non-nutritional uses of food, and of the way non-nutritional factors interact to influence food

---

Box 2.1

Some factors affecting food choice and eating patterns (after Webb and Copeman, 1996)

- Availability of foods in the local environment; this is in turn influenced by several factors like climate, soil type, transportation links, rationing, shopping facilities
- Nutrition knowledge and/or food beliefs; this is in turn influenced by such things as cultural traditions, education, and religious/ethical beliefs
- Habit and previous food experience
- Individual likes and dislikes
- Facilities for storing, preparing and cooking
- Cooking just for oneself or eating with and/or cooking for others
- Skills in food preparation and willingness to experiment and develop new skills
- Financial resources, budgeting skills and the cost of foods; these may be affected by political decisions about taxation, subsidy and welfare payments
- Time available and the time needed to prepare and eat foods
- State of health and appetite

---

choices, is essential. It is no use devising an excellent diet plan or drawing up detailed dietary guidelines unless they are actually implemented. Diets or dietary recommendations that may seem ideal from a reductionist biological viewpoint may have little impact on actual food choices. Some people may have very limited freedom to make food choices (e.g. those living in institutions where all food is provided by a caterer). There will be some restraints on the food choices of everyone. Dietary recommendations will almost certainly be ineffective if they are culturally unacceptable to the clients, incompatible with their personal preferences or beliefs, beyond their economic means, or incompatible with what is provided by their caterer or parent.

When making dietary recommendations (or devising therapeutic diets), the advisers need to consider various questions.

- Can the clients obtain the ingredients of the recommended diet?
- Can they prepare it?
- Can they afford to implement the recommendations?
- Are the recommendations compatible with their cultural beliefs and practices?
- Will their caterer or parent provide a diet that complies with the recommendations?
- Will they find the recommended diet palatable?
- Can they tolerate the recommended foods?
- Are any population recommendations environmentally sustainable if widely implemented? (Also discussed briefly in Chapter 5.)

An appreciation of the non-nutritional roles of food and the non-nutritional influences on food selection should enable health educators to give advice that is more acceptable to clients and easier for them to act on. Dietary recommendations that are in sympathy with existing beliefs, preferences and selection practices will fare better than those that try to impose the prejudices and preferences of the adviser. This culturally sensitive approach should also reduce the likelihood that the cost of scientifically better nutrition will be increased anxiety, social tension and cultural impoverishment. Readers who wish to explore the social and cultural determinants of food choice and the non-nutritional roles of food are recommended to see Fieldhouse (1995).

Key points

- Nutrient content has not traditionally been a significant influence on food selection; 'people eat food, not nutrients'.
- Social, economic and geographical factors influence availability of food, while cultural and preference factors determine its acceptability.
- Dietary guidelines or prescribed diets are more likely to be complied with if they allow for, and are sympathetic to, the non-nutritional factors that influence or limit food choices of an individual or group.

THE BIOLOGICAL MODEL OF FOOD

The primary biological function of food is to provide the body with a sufficient supply of energy and essential nutrients to meet current physiological needs. Diet composition also influences long-term risk of chronic disease. The reductionist scientific model of food is that it is merely a complex mixture of nutrients that should be combined in optimal proportions to meet current needs and to maximize health and longevity in the longer term. Eating could then be seen simply as a flawed and inefficient behavioural mechanism used to select and consume this mixture.

Such paradigms of food and of eating might tempt one to believe that, if consumers are given extensive advice about optimal nutrient intakes coupled with full nutritional labelling of food, then they will be enabled to select the ideal diet. Increasing information about healthy eating and food composition might be expected to lead to rapid and major 'improvements' in the diet of the population (see Chapter 5 for evidence of the effect of health promotion on 'the national diet').

It is quite obvious that most people do not select their food solely according to such biological criteria. In the past, selection on this basis would not have been possible because public awareness of nutrition and food composition is comparatively recent. Even today, few people would have the skills and knowledge to select food solely on a compositional basis. It has been suggested that biological mechanisms akin to thirst or salt hunger operate for some important nutrients to enable people to intuitively select a balanced diet. There is little evidence to support such mechanisms, but there is evidence that satiation tends to be food-specific; that is, satiation for a particular food develops as that food is consumed but satiation towards other foods is less affected. Such a mechanism would tend to increase the range of foods consumed, and dietary deficiencies become less likely if energy needs are fully met and a wide variety of foods consumed. Where food supply is plentiful and varied in industrialized countries, such a mechanism might also tend to encourage overeating and obesity (see discussion of sensory-specific satiety in Chapter 9).

Much current food evangelism seems to be encouraging a trend towards the reductionist scientific models of food and eating. This could greatly impoverish human existence without necessarily extending its duration, because food has numerous social, psychological and cultural functions in addition to its biological role of supplying nutrients.

Key points

- Scientists may see food as no more than a mixture of nutrients that need to be consumed in the correct proportions and eating as merely the process by which these nutrients are selected and eaten.
- If food and eating fulfilled no other functions, one would expect scientific guidance to lead to rapid improvements in this selection process.
- But food does have many other functions and food choices are influenced by many factors which may make it difficult to persuade people to make changes in their diet that seem rational from the purely scientific viewpoint.

DIETARY AND CULTURAL PREJUDICE

There is an almost inevitable tendency to regard one's own beliefs and patterns of behaviour as the norm and so preferable to those of other cultures. Foreign or unusual cultural practices tend to be regarded as wrong, irrational or misguided. The term *ethnocentrism* has been used to describe this tendency. Ethnocentrism is apparent in reactions to alien food habits. There is a widespread tendency to

ridicule or even to abhor the food choices or eating habits of others. The intrepid explorer patronisingly accepting some revolting native delicacy to avoid offending his host is a Hollywood cliché. One manifestation of this phenomenon is in the slightly derogatory names used for other races that have their origins in food habits, such as:

- Frogs – because frog legs are a French delicacy
- Kraut – from the traditional fermented cabbage (sauerkraut) associated with German cuisine
- Limey – because of the past practice of providing lime juice to British sailors to prevent scurvy
- Eskimo – originates from a disparaging Indian term meaning 'eaters of raw flesh' (the name Inuit is now favoured).

Ethnocentric-type attitudes need not be confined to 'between culture' judgements. It is not uncommon to hear haughty disapproval and caricaturization of the dietary practices of other regions of one's own country, of other social or religious groups, or indeed of anyone who does not share a particular food ideology.

- Within England, it is not uncommon to hear disparaging comments made about the diets of 'northerners' which often implicitly blame northerners for the relatively poor health statistics of the north compared to the south.
- Vegetarianism is frequently denigrated and ridiculed by meat eaters, and conversely, some vegetarian propaganda makes very hostile comments about meat eaters.
- It is not uncommon to hear disparaging comments exchanged between those who do and those who do not consciously attempt to practise healthy eating.

Criticisms of other dietary and cultural practices are often based on prejudiced, narrow and inaccurate views of others' beliefs and behaviours. Nutritionists and dieticians are not immune to ethnocentrism but most are aware of this tendency and consciously try to avoid it when dealing with an alien culture. They might, however, be more unsuspecting and thus inclined to behave ethnocentrically when dealing with the more familiar behaviour patterns of other groups within their own culture. Although these behaviour patterns may be familiar, they may nonetheless be quite different from their own. For example, it must be very difficult for a dietician who is a committed vegetarian to give advice to a meat eater that is totally uninfluenced by her own beliefs, and vice versa, if the client is vegetarian and the dietician a meat eater.

The opposite of ethnocentrism is *cultural relativism*. The cultural relativist tries to understand and respect other cultural practices and to accept them as normal, no matter how bizarre they may at first seem or how different they are from their own. Only if practices are clearly and demonstrably dysfunctional does one try to change them. There would be little argument that such an approach was correct if one were dealing with a unique alien culture, but more familiar cultural practices may be handled with less sensitivity. The American's hamburger, the Briton's fish and chips, and even children's sweets or candies have real cultural significance. Nutrition education need not try to totally forbid or blacken the image of such foods but should rather attempt to use them within a diet that, in its entirety, complies with reasonable nutritional guidelines.

It is likely that many practices that are strongly and acutely dysfunctional to a group will have been selected out during the cultural evolution of the group. Changing social or environmental conditions, or simply increased longevity and consequent changes in health priorities, may cause traditional practices to become regarded as dysfunctional. The aim of nutrition education, under such circumstances, should be to minimize or avoid the dysfunction with the least possible cultural interference – the cultural conservationist approach. This is likely to be the most successful as well as the most ethical strategy.

Key points

- Ethnocentrism describes the tendency to regard one's own beliefs and practices as the norm and those of other cultures as wrong or abnormal.
- Ethnocentric-type attitudes can also exist within cultures. In these circumstances they may be less obvious and harder to correct.
- Cultural relativism is the acceptance of other cultural practices as normal even if they are very different from one's own.
- No matter how strange they may seem, one should try to change other dietary practices only if they are clearly dysfunctional, and then by the minimum amount to avoid the dysfunction – the cultural conservationist approach.

FOOD CLASSIFICATION SYSTEMS

Nutritionists, consumers and anthropologists all categorize foods but they use different criteria. These categorizations may be a formal and explicit classification system or a largely subconscious, practical classification.

Nutritional classification of food: food groups, plates and pyramids

Nutritionists classify foods according to the nutrients they contain, and these classifications are used to advise and guide consumers towards a healthy diet. Foods were initially classified into food groups according to their nutrient profiles, and consumers were advised to eat specified minimum amounts from each food group to ensure that their diet had adequate quantities of all the essential nutrients. As the priorities of nutrition education were widened to include the prevention of chronic diseases, so new consumer guides were developed. These new guidance systems needed to indicate not just the minimum amounts needed for adequacy but also the balance between the various food groups that would minimize the risk of a chronic disease. In the UK a tilted plate model is used, and a food guide pyramid in the USA. Food group systems and these newer food guides are discussed more fully in Chapter 5.

Key points

- Nutritionists classify foods according to their nutrient profiles.
- Food groups and food guide plates or pyramids are examples of nutritional classifications of food.

Consumer classifications of food

Consumers also classify foods but such classification systems have not traditionally had any theoretical basis in scientific nutrition. Despite this, such systems may have evolved rules that produce good practical diets even though they may have a theoretical framework that seems incompatible with scientific nutrition theory. Nutritionists and dieticians should try to understand such classification systems and to offer advice that is consistent with them.

One of the best known and most widespread of the traditional and formal classification systems is the hot and cold classification that is found in various forms in Latin America, India and China. The general principle is that good health results from a state of balance, and to maintain or restore good health there must be a balance between hot and cold. Foods are classified as hot or cold and foods should be selected and mixed to produce or maintain the balanced state. Disease results from an imbalance. Certain diseases and phases of the reproductive cycle are also regarded as hot or cold states, so certain foods will be more or less appropriate in these different circumstances. As an example, in the Chinese system a sore throat is a hot disease and might be treated by a cold food such as watermelon in order to try to restore balance. Hot foods, such as beef, dates or chilli, are considered detrimental in such hot conditions. Two surveys of Chinese families living in London (Wheeler and Tan, 1983) and Toronto (Yeung *et al.*, 1973) both found that at that time the traditional hot and cold system was still widely adhered to and practised despite Western cultural influences. Wheeler and Tan concluded that, despite the use of such a non-science-based food classification system, the dietary pattern of the London Chinese families in their survey was varied and nutritionally excellent. Any programme designed to increase the science-based nutrition and food composition knowledge of the 'gatekeepers' in these Chinese families risks undermining confidence in the traditional system and perhaps even worsening their diets. The 'gatekeepers' in English families living in the same area would probably have had more science-based nutrition knowledge, but these authors would probably have judged that, by their criteria, the English diet was inferior to that of the Chinese. Knowledge of food and nutrition is perhaps more loosely correlated with good dietetic practice than many nutritionists would like to think.

Most Western consumers do not use such a formal and overtly structured classification system, but they do classify foods. In any cultural group there is clearly a classification of potentially edible material into food and non-food. Except under conditions of extreme deprivation, any cultural group will only eat some of the substances around them that would comply with any biological definition of potential food. In the UK, there are numerous plants, animals, birds, fish and insects that are edible but are rarely if ever eaten by Britons. They are simply not viewed as potential foods and are classified as non-food. In many cases, the idea of eating such items would be repellent to most Britons. For example, cows, chickens, cabbages and crabs are seen as potential food, but not horses, dogs, crows, nettles or frogs.

The traditional main course of a British dinner (or lunch if that is the main meal of the day) consists of a meat or meat product, potatoes, one or more extra vegetables with sauce or gravy. Very few Britons would, however, consider eating such a meal or even some of the individual foods for breakfast. A 'cheeseburger and fries' is not (yet) on the breakfast menus of restaurant chains that have built their global empires on such fare. Clearly some foods are seen, or classified, as more appropriate for particular meals. These classifications of edible material into food or non-food and into foods appropriate for particular meals or occasions vary considerably even within the peoples of western Europe. In Britain, horsemeat is not classified as food and yet it has traditionally been eaten in France. Many Britons would not consider cheese and spicy cold meats as suitable breakfast foods, yet in some other European countries they would be typical breakfast fare.

Schutz *et al.* (1975) conducted a survey of 200 female, mainly white and mainly middle-class consumers distributed between four American cities. They used a questionnaire in which these consumers were asked to rate 56 different foods in terms of their appropriateness for a total of 48 food-use situations; they used a 7-point scale from 1 'never appropriate' to 7 'always appropriate'. Their aim was to allow the respondents to generate classifications of foods based on their appropriateness ratings. The authors identified five food categories based on consumer usage rather than on biological criteria, and these are listed below.

- *High-calorie treats such as wine, cakes and pies.* These were considered especially suitable for social occasions and for offering to guests. The foods in this category tended to be rated towards the inappropriate end of the scale for questions relating to healthfulness (e.g. inappropriate when 'needing to lose weight' or when 'not feeling well').

Healthy, wholesome foods seemed to be considered more suitable for everyday eating and eating alone than for parties and entertaining.

- *Speciality meal items.* These were considered suitable only for special occasions and circumstances. The authors offered liver and chilli as examples. The foods in this category were notable for the number of food-use situations for which they were rated as never appropriate.
- *Common meal items.* These were considered suitable for all occasions and all ages and would be served at main meals (e.g. meats, fish and some vegetables). They were generally rated as inappropriate 'for breakfast' and not surprisingly 'for dessert'.
- *Refreshing healthy foods such as milk, orange juice and cottage cheese.* These were considered to be nutritious but not viewed as suitable for a main course. They scored highly on the healthfulness questions 'nutritious', 'easy to digest', but were rated low as to spiciness. Perhaps spiciness/flavour and healthfulness were not seen as compatible.
- *Inexpensive filling foods.* These were considered cheap and filling as well as fattening (e.g. bread, peanut butter, potato chips (crisps) and candy bars). They were not considered appropriate for those trying to lose weight but were seen to be useful to assuage hunger between meals and appropriate for hungry teenagers.

This is, of course, just one group of investigators' interpretation of the comments expressed by one group of consumers almost 40 years ago. It does, however, highlight how even Western consumers, despite not having a formal cultural food classification system like the Chinese hot and cold system, do nonetheless have clear and, within a group, fairly consistent views on the appropriateness of different foods in different situations. They may use quite elaborate classification systems for food, even though such classification may be informal or even subconscious.

If it is to be effective, then clearly any dietary advice or any prescribed diet must recognize such views on the appropriateness of particular foods for particular occasions and situations. It will also be more likely to succeed if it uses foods that are classified as

appropriate for the individual. Many cultural groups might classify milk as a food for babies and therefore not suitable for adults, and some Western consumers might only grudgingly concede that some pulses or salads are suitable for working men.

Key points

- Consumers classify foods according to the ways in which they are used.
- The hot and cold system is an example of a formal classification system in which foods are classified as 'hot' or 'cold' and selected to maintain or restore the body's hot–cold balance.
- Even where there is no overt classification, all consumers divide potentially edible material into 'food' and 'non-food'. They also regard different foods as more or less appropriate for particular uses, occasions or people. These classifications are culture-specific.
- Dietary advisers must be aware of these cultural classifications and make sure that their recommendations are consistent with them.

Anthropological classification of foods

There have been several attempts to devise food categorization systems that could be used across cultures. These are not only useful for the anthropologist seeking to describe the diets and the uses made of foods in particular cultures, but they could also be of great use to the nutrition educator seeking to identify the most appropriate and effective ways of trying to bring about nutritional improvement.

One of the earliest and simplest of these systems is that of Passim and Bennet (1943) who divided foods up into the three categories listed below.

- *Core foods* are those that are regularly and universally consumed within the society. In developing countries, these are likely to be starchy staple foods (e.g. bread, rice, millet or cassava). In industrialized countries, including Britain and the USA, milk, potatoes, bread and meats would probably fit into this category.
- *Secondary foods* are those that have widespread but not universal use. Most fruits and vegetables

would probably be classified as secondary foods in the UK.

- *Peripheral foods* are the least widely and frequently used foods. It is in this category that the most individual variation would be expected. Most shellfish and most species of fish would probably be in this category in the UK.

Such categorization would almost certainly be easier to make in societies whose range of available foods is relatively restricted, and most difficult in societies like those in Europe and North America that have a vast array of foods available to an affluent population. Affluent consumers are able to express much more individuality in their diet structure.

Any particular food may be classified differently for different cultures, it may be classified differently for different social classes within a culture, and foods may change categories over time. Rice is clearly a core food for the Japanese but for most British groups would probably be classified as secondary. A few decades ago, rice (except pudding rice) would probably have been classified as peripheral for most social groups in Britain. Prior to 1960 many working-class Britons would almost never eat a savoury rice dish. Chinese and Indian restaurants and take-away outlets and foreign holidays have transformed this situation so that there may now be some groups, even within the indigenous population, for whom rice might be approaching the status of a core food. The growth of vegetarianism and meat-restricted diets in Britain might lead some readers to question whether meat should still be regarded as a core food.

A nutritionist trying to effect change in the diet of any community might expect to find most resistance to change in the core foods, more ready acceptance in the secondary foods, and the most flexibility in the peripheral foods.

Some foods have acquired a cultural status beyond their purely dietary and nutritional significance. They play an integral part in the cultural life of the community and they have been termed *cultural superfoods* (e.g. rice in Japan and bread in many European cultures). Rice has maintained a particular emotional and cultural status for the Japanese despite a marked fall in consumption since the Second World War, with a corresponding increase in bread consumption.

- The emperor still cultivates a symbolic crop of rice.
- In the Japanese language, the same word can mean either food or rice.
- Rice plays a part in Japanese cultural and religious rituals.
- In the past, the Japanese calendar was geared to the cycle of rice production, rice was used as a medium for taxation, and some units of measurement were based on the amount of rice necessary to feed a man for a year.

Bread has declined in its cultural significance in some European countries, but television scenes a few years ago of people in war-ravaged areas of eastern Europe queuing for bread still struck a particularly poignant chord. If the bread supply is threatened, then the situation is perceived as much more desperate than if other foods are in short supply. The arrival of bread is often seen as a symbol of hope in such circumstances. There are numerous reminders of the past importance of bread in the UK.

- Bread and dough are both used as slang terms for money.
- In Christian communion, bread is used to symbolically represent the body of Christ.
- In the Lord's Prayer, Christians pray for their daily bread.

Nutrition educators need to understand and respect the cultural significance of such foods if they want their dietary advice and guidance to be effective. Insensitive denigration of a cultural superfood may provoke incredulity or even hostility and so reduce the chances of any of the advice being taken seriously. Meat has had a particular cultural importance to many Western men, which may even have been reinforced in the past by nutrition education that presented meat as a good source of the high-quality protein that was seen as a key requirement of good nutrition. If nutrition educators now try to persuade such men that red meat and a healthy diet are incompatible, they may simply persuade them that the price for a healthy diet is too high and make them ignore all dietary advice. In an old edition of a classic British nutrition text, a passage was quoted which describes the African's craving for meat as:

> The strongest and most fraternal bond that the continent had in common. It was a dream, a longing, an aspiration that never ceased, a physiological cry of the body, stronger and more torturing than the sexual instinct.

> R. Gary, *The Roots of Heaven*, London: Michael Joseph, 1958

The speaker goes on to assume that this need for meat is a universal craving of all men. If there is even a grain of truth in this assertion then nutrition education must not suggest that the only option for healthy eating is one that would require unreasonable sacrifice. To use a slightly more recent example, chips (French fries) are a traditional and important element in British cuisine and culture. The following quotation from a serious national newspaper emphasizes the importance that some Britons attach to their chips:

> According to the Chip Census, one person in 10 would rather give up sex, alcohol and smoking than chips!

> *The Independent*, 2 March 1994

Once again, if healthy eating appears to require total avoidance of chips then the chance of acceptance by a high proportion of the British population is probably doomed. Moderate amounts of chips can be included in a diet that meets current nutritional guidelines, especially if attention is paid to advice about their method of preparation and the foods that they most appropriately complement.

Cultural superfood is just one of five food categories described by Jelliffe (1967) in a food classification system that he thought had universal application, in both developing and industrialized countries. The five categories in this system are listed below.

- *Cultural superfood* as discussed above. These were considered by Schutz *et al.* (1975) to correspond to 'common meal item' in their consumer classification.
- *Prestige foods* are reserved for important occasions or important people. According to Jelliffe, foods within this category are usually high in protein, which is often animal protein. They are also usually difficult to obtain because of their scarcity, high cost, or difficult preparation. Truffles, lobster and caviar might fall into this category in the UK. In past decades, salmon would have been in this category until the ready availability of cheaper, farmed salmon reduced its scarcity and price.
- *Body image foods* are those that are thought to promote wellness. Jelliffe lists foods that contribute to maintaining or restoring hot–cold balance as an example from developing countries. High-fibre foods or dairy products containing probiotic or good bacteria (see Chapter 19) would be an example in the UK.
- *Sympathetic magic foods* are thought to have some special properties that they impart to the consumer. An example given by Jelliffe is the avoidance of eggs by many women in East African countries because they believe that they cause infertility. As another example, he uses under-cooked steak used in the training of athletes (in 1967) because it symbolized vigour, masculinity and energy.
- *Physiologic group foods* are foods reserved for or forbidden to certain physiologic groups. Taboos against certain foods for pregnant and lactating women or for young children are examples. Breast milk, infant formula and certain cereal preparations that are normally consumed only by infants and young children are obvious examples of this category.

Key points

- Anthropologists classify foods according to their importance to a culture and the roles they play within the culture's diet.
- The simplest anthropological classification divides foods into three categories: core, secondary and peripheral.
- The same foods may be used differently and be in different categories in different cultural groups and a food may change categories within a group over time.
- A cultural superfood is one that plays an important part in the cultural life and identity of the group and has acquired a cultural significance that transcends its purely

→

Key points *continued*

nutritional one. Examples are rice in Japan, maize among the Hopi Indians, and bread in some European societies.

- Jelliffe classified foods into five categories:
  - cultural superfoods (usually the starchy staple of the group)
  - prestige foods (reserved for special occasions or important people)
  - body-image foods (thought to contribute to good health)
  - sympathetic magic foods (that impart some special property to the consumer)
  - physiologic group foods (considered suitable for particular groups).

NON-NUTRITIONAL USES OF FOOD

The primary biological role of food is to provide an adequate supply of energy and essential nutrients, but food also has many non-nutritional functions and several examples are considered below. This selection is not exhaustive but will illustrate the enormous diversity and range of potential non-nutritional uses of food.

Religion, morality and ethics

- Food and drink are used symbolically in the rituals and ceremonies of many religions. For example, bread and wine are used in Christian communion to symbolize the body and blood of Christ.
- Adherence to the dietary rules of a religion acts as a common bond for adherents and serves to differentiate them from non-believers. For example, adherence to the dietary rules and customs of the Torah helps to bond orthodox Jewish families and to set them apart from gentiles.
- Adhering to dietary rules is an outward symbol of a person's piety and self-discipline. An example is the dawn to dusk fasting undertaken by Moslems during Ramadan.
- Policing of dietary rules provides a mechanism for religious leaders to exert control over their followers and to demonstrate their authority. For example, the severe penalties for alcohol

consumption, even for non-believers, underlines the primacy of Islam and the mullahs in some countries.

- People may avoid certain foods to demonstrate their disapproval of animal cruelty or their ecological awareness. Examples are the avoidance of veal raised in crates or tuna caught in drift nets.
- People may boycott food from particular countries or companies to express their moral disapproval of human rights abuses, exploitation of workers or other perceived moral transgressions. Examples are the boycott of South African produce during the apartheid era, and boycotts of food companies that are accused of 'pushing' powdered infant formulae in developing countries.

Status and wealth

- Expensive and exotic foods can be used to demonstrate one's wealth and sophistication. An example is the serving of expensive, but essentially rather bland, caviar as a snack with champagne.
- Serving elaborate and expensive meals can be used to demonstrate esteem for guests, as in traditional feasts of welcome and the Western dinner party.
- A person's social status may be defined by whom they eat with and where they eat. For example, it was common practice for large companies to have different dining areas for workers of different status, and different Hindu castes have not traditionally eaten together.
- Unusual food choices may be used to express a person's individuality, such as serving foods associated with one's distant ethnic roots.

Interpersonal relationships

- Offerings of food and drink are commonly used to initiate and maintain personal and business relationships. Offering new neighbours a drink or food is primarily a gesture of welcome and warmth rather than an attempt to satisfy any perceived nutritional need.
- Giving of food can be a demonstration of love, and withdrawal or failure to offer food can be used to signal disapproval or even to punish. An

example is the use of bread and water punishment for prisoners. A gift of chocolate can be used as a reward, a gesture of affection or apology; any nutritional impact of the chocolate is incidental.

• Food and drink may provide a focus for social gatherings.

Political

Control of the food supply and the price of food can be a very potent method of exerting political control or of gaining political favour. Some would argue that food aid has purposes or effects beyond its obvious humanitarian one. It may salve the consciences of wealthy donor nations, foster dependence and subservience in the recipients, or help to bolster the political and diplomatic fortunes of the donor government.

Folk medicine

Diet is an element in many traditional treatments for disease. In the traditional hot and cold system, cold foods may be used to treat hot diseases. In many Western countries the boundaries between food as a source of sustenance and as a medicine are becoming increasingly blurred. There is widespread use of dietary supplements which are taken not just to ensure adequacy but also to prevent or treat diseases, and doses of nutrients consumed in this form may be much greater than that obtained from any normal diet. Some substances that should logically be classified as medicines are marketed as dietary supplements to avoid the costly process of demonstrating their safety and efficacy and obtaining a medicinal licence. In recent years there has been a huge growth in the sale of so-called functional foods (see Chapter 19) that are marketed on their potential to maintain or restore health.

Key points

• Food has many functions over and above its purely nutritional purpose.
• Dietary rules and traditions can be an important part of religious life and cultural identity.   →

Key points *continued*

• Food selection can be used to make ethical and political statements.
• Eating habits and food choices can be used to indicate a person's social status, wealth or uniqueness as an individual.
• Food can be used to initiate and foster interpersonal and business relationships.
• Control of the food supply can be used as a means of political control.
• Food can be used to reward or to punish.
• Foods can be used as medicines in traditional medicine and substances legally classified as food (dietary supplements and functional foods) are widely used for quasi-medical purposes in industrialized countries.

THE HIERARCHY OF HUMAN NEEDS

The relative importance of any particular influence on diet may be quite different in different groups, even within the same local environment. Take, for example, the influence of religion on food choice in the UK or USA. Religion would have a major influence on strictly orthodox Jews or Seventh Day Adventists but minimal influence on equally devout Anglicans or Episcopalians. The orthodox Jew would, for example:

• avoid all pig meat and meat from any animal that does not have cloven hooves and chew the cud
• not eat the hind quarters of animals or unbled meat
• not eat flightless birds, shellfish or other fish without fins and scales
• not eat meat and dairy produce together
• not prepare food on the Sabbath day.

It would be difficult to identify any specifically religious influences on the diets of the two Protestant groups, except perhaps the occasional communion bread and wine or voluntary and self-selected abstinence during Lent.

The priorities attached to the various biological and non-biological factors influencing food selection are likely to change as one moves from a situation of gross deprivation or scarcity to one of almost limitless abundance. Maslow (1943) suggested that human needs could be arranged into a hierarchy of motivation (summarized in Figure 2.1). In this very well-known theory of motivation, needs that are lower down the hierarchy must be at least partially satisfied before the higher up needs can become significant motivating factors. In Maslow's theory, the basic biological and emotional needs come at the base of the hierarchy and only once there has been reasonable satisfaction of these needs do the more aesthetic and esoteric needs become significantly motivating.

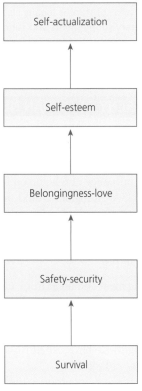

Figure 2.1 Maslow's hierarchy of human needs (after Maslow, 1943).

Maslow's hierarchy of needs can be applied to food selection. In conditions of extreme deprivation, survival is the priority, so people may resort to eating almost anything that is remotely edible, perhaps even breaking one of the strongest and most widespread of all dietary taboos, that against the consumption of human flesh. After survival, then the need to ensure future security and safety becomes motivating. Potentially edible material is classified into food and non-food and ensuring that future needs are met becomes a priority. Food hoarding, perhaps even obesity, might be outward manifestations of this desire for security. Obesity in some cultures has been sought after and admired rather than dreaded and despised as it usually is in the UK and the USA. Once security of food supply is relatively assured, then the need for love and belongingness becomes a motivating influence on food selection. This could be manifested in the extensive use of food to demonstrate group membership and affection. Then comes the need for self-esteem. This might be manifested in the selection of high-cost, prestige foods to demonstrate one's wealth and success. At the pinnacle of Maslow's hierarchy the need for self-actualization becomes motivating. Selection of food to demonstrate one's individuality or uniqueness becomes prominent, and this may be manifested in experimentation with new foods, new recipes and non-conforming patterns of selection.

The current penchant for the simple peasant foods of the East by some educated, affluent Westerners may be one manifestation of the need for self-actualization. The partial replacement of these traditional foods with a more 'Western diet' by some in the East may be symbolizing their need to demonstrate their new wealth; that is, to improve their self-esteem. In many developing countries, bottle feeds for infants are promoted as the modern and sophisticated Western alternative to 'primitive' breastfeeding. In many affluent countries, like the USA and UK, breastfeeding predominates in the upper social classes (see Chapter 16).

There may be some disagreement over the details of Maslow's hierarchy, as it has been applied to food selection, but the underlying principle seems unquestionable: that the priority attached to different influences will change with increasing affluence and food availability. The range of factors influencing selection will tend to be greater in affluent than in poor populations, and the relative prominence of these different factors will also change with increasing affluence. The more physiological, biological drives tend to become less important in the affluent.

Key points

- The importance of any influence on food selection and eating behaviour will vary from group to group.
- Religion would be a major influence on the choices of orthodox Jews but not on the choices of Protestants.
- In situations of shortage or deprivation, survival and security are dominant influences on food choices.
- In situations of abundance, prestige and aesthetic factors come into play.
- Maslow devised a theory of human motivation that envisaged a hierarchy of human needs (see Figure 2.1) which can be applied to food selection.
- In Maslow's scheme there has to be some minimum satisfaction of a need lower down in the hierarchy before the next need becomes a significant motivating influence.

A MODEL OF FOOD SELECTION: THE 'HIERARCHY OF AVAILABILITIES' MODEL

Several workers have attempted to organize and integrate the various and disparate factors influencing food selection into a unified model. Without such a model, any discussion of the vast array of factors that can influence food choices can end up being an amorphous jumble of ideas and facts. Such a model should be simple but comprehensive and provide a useful framework for consideration and discussion (e.g. in a student essay) of the factors that affect food choices. Availability of a food is clearly a prerequisite for selection. Wheeler (1992) suggested that various constraints act to limit the range of foods that are, in practice, available to the individual – in effect, that the image of the affluent Western consumer having almost limitless theoretical choice of food is partly an illusion. Practical limits on the range of foods that are really available to different individuals may greatly limit the scope of the nutrition educator for effecting change. Even if an individual understands and accepts dietary advice there may still be barriers, sometimes beyond his or her control, that prevent or limit the implementation of change.

Figure 2.2 shows a simple model for food selection. This 'hierarchy of availabilities' model assumes that many different types of factor will limit the practical availability of foods to an individual and thus the chances of different foods being eaten. As with Maslow's hierarchy of human needs, it is envisaged that some minimum availability at lower levels in the hierarchy must be achieved before the next level becomes a significant influence on selection. These influences at each level can be absolute – from complete unavailability to sole availability. More often in Western countries they will be more subtle variations in the practical availability of different foods.

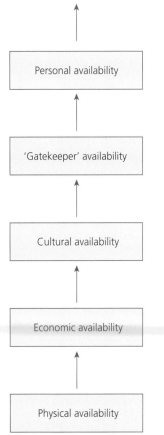

Figure 2.2 The 'Hierarchy of Availabilities Model' of food selection.

- *Physical availability.* A food can be eaten only if it is physically present in the local environment.
- *Economic availability.* People can eat only the foods that they can afford to buy. If a food is available locally but they cannot afford to buy it, then it is economically unavailable to them.

- *Cultural availability.* People will normally eat only things that they recognize as food and which are culturally acceptable to them. Foods that are present and affordable but culturally unacceptable to them are culturally unavailable.
- *'Gatekeeper' availability.* A gatekeeper is someone who controls the supply of food to others. A mother may regulate what her family eats and a catering manager may regulate what the residents of an institution eat. What the gatekeeper provides may limit the supply of particular foods even though they may be physically, economically and culturally available to the consumer.
- *Personal availability.* Even foods that have overcome all of the previous barriers to their availability may still not be consumed. Individual dislike of a food, avoidance for reasons of individual belief or because of physiological intolerance may make it personally unavailable. A man who is, or who believes that he is, allergic to fish will be effectively prevented from consuming fish. A woman revolted by the taste or texture of broccoli will not eat it, and meat will not be available to someone revolted by the idea of eating the flesh of dead animals. Someone who relies on poorly fitting dentures may be discouraged from eating foods that require a strong bite and lots of chewing.

These availabilities are not usually absolute 'all or nothing' phenomena but a continuum varying from absolute unavailability to high desirability and availability. There can be both positive and negative influences on the availability of foods at each level of the hierarchy.

- The number and locations of retail outlets stocking a food influence its physical availability.
- Subsidy increases economic availability of a food but a tax reduces it.
- Clever advertising that raises the prestige of a food might increase its cultural availability.
- Increased menu choice in an institution might lessen the impact of the gatekeeper.
- An 'acquired taste' might increase the personal availability of a food.

Much current nutrition education is geared towards partly reversing some of the dietary changes that accompany affluence. In many populations, lack of physical or economic availability limits consumption of sugars, fats and animal foods – but affluence removes these constraints. These foods often have high prestige and palatability, which increases their cultural, gatekeeper and personal availability. Nutrition education in affluent countries may be seen as trying to introduce constraints higher up the hierarchy in Figure 2.2 to compensate for the lessening of economic and physical restraints at the base of the hierarchy.

Key points

- A model of food selection should provide a framework for organizing and discussing the many disparate influences on food selection and eating.
- The 'hierarchy of availability' model is based on Maslow's hierarchy of human needs. It envisages a hierarchy of factors that will limit the practical availability of foods to any individual.
- As with Maslow's hierarchy, there must be minimum availability at a lower level in the hierarchy before influences at the next level start to come into play.
- A continuum of availability is envisaged from absolute unavailability to limitless abundance and easy access.
- The five levels of this hierarchy of availability are:
  - physical (can the food be obtained?)
  - economic (can it be afforded?)
  - cultural (is it culturally recognized as food and culturally acceptable?)
  - 'gatekeeper' (is it provided by the parent, caterer or other gatekeeper?)
  - personal (does the person like the food, can he or she eat it, and is it personally acceptable?).

PHYSICAL AVAILABILITY

There will be absolute limitations on the range of potentially edible materials that are available in any particular local environment. Physical and geographical factors are key determinants of food availability – factors such as climate, soil type, storage facilities, water supply, and quality of transportation links. The range and amounts of food available in an isolated and arid region may be severely limited by such factors. During severe famines, physical availability may be an absolute limitation on what food most people can eat.

Even within affluent countries, some foods will be available only seasonally. In fact, many seasonal foods are now imported and available all year round – although the price will often vary considerably in and out of the local season. Some foods may be unavailable locally because of lack of sufficient demand. Shops will only stock foods that they expect to sell, so kosher foods may be difficult to obtain in areas where few Jews live. Small local stores will inevitably stock a more limited range than large supermarkets, and there may even be quite marked differences in the range of products stocked by shops in poor and affluent areas.

According to Henson (1992), the number of retail food outlets in Britain fell by a third between 1976 and 1987. There was a marked trend towards fewer but larger shops. The great majority of new superstores that have opened in recent years in Britain are located on the outskirts of towns and relatively few are being opened in shopping centres and high streets. These trends inevitably meant that people on average had to travel further for their shopping. Most households in Britain now use a car to make their shopping trips. These new superstores have wider choice and lower prices than local shops, which means that they also reduce the viability of these smaller shops and may result in their closure. To take full advantage of them, consumers need good mobility (preferably access to a car), the financial resources to allow them to buy in larger quantities, and adequate storage facilities (including access to a freezer). These retailing trends may be to the disadvantage of some groups and severely affect their access to a varied and inexpensive diet; some examples are given below.

- Some people living in rural areas do not have access to a car, but local shops have all but disappeared. In some rural areas, it may be difficult to obtain a reasonable variety of fresh fruits and vegetables.
- Elderly and disabled people have limited mobility.
- Some people live in accommodation without a freezer, limited cooking facilities and no space for storing food.

In the last few years we have seen the major food retailers moving back into the high street by opening up smaller convenience-type stores, and this may improve access to affordable food for people in these disadvantaged groups who live in urban areas. Most of the large supermarket chains also have facilities for online ordering and home delivery (at a cost), which may help those with limited mobility but to make use of such facilities, consumers need computer literacy, internet access and the financial resources to afford delivery charges.

Key points

- People can eat only food that is physically accessible to them.
- During famines, physical absence of food may be an absolute limitation on food choice.
- A range of physical and geographical factors can affect what foods are available at any time and place. Many seasonal foods are, however, now available all year round – at a price.
- The trend in Britain during the latter part of the twentieth century was for fewer, larger food shops often located on the edge of town. People must therefore travel further to do their shopping.
- These large superstores offer great variety at relatively lower prices, but those with limited mobility or no car may not be able to take full advantage of them.
- There has been some move back to the high street by the larger retail chains through the opening of smaller neighbourhood supermarkets.
- Online ordering and home delivery may help those with limited mobility but only if they have internet access and can afford the delivery charges.
- People who live in rural areas without a car may have limited access to some foods, especially perishable foods like fresh fruit and vegetables.

ECONOMIC AVAILABILITY

Finance exerts a variable limiting influence on the availability of foods. In some circumstances, lack of money may have an absolute effect in limiting availability of particular foods or even of food in general. This is very clear in some developing countries where having enough money may mean the difference between relative comfort and starvation. Excepting times of acute famine, it is poverty rather than inadequate physical availability of food that is the dominant cause of malnutrition. Wealthy countries with inadequate indigenous agriculture do not go hungry, and wealthy people within poor countries do not usually go hungry either. People may go hungry even where food supplies are comparatively plentiful if they do not have the money to pay for food.

Even in affluent countries, financial constraints can have a marked effect on dietary freedom of choice. In the UK and the USA, there are quite marked differences between the food choices of the richest and poorest and this is partly due to differences in purchasing power. In these countries, health and longevity are strongly and positively correlated with higher socioeconomic status, and diet is probably one of the factors contributing to these inequalities in health. It is ironic that the chronic diseases of industrialization that are internationally strongly and positively correlated with increasing affluence are, within the industrialized countries, associated with relative poverty.

Key points

- Poverty is the major cause of malnutrition in the world. People usually go hungry because they do not have the money to buy food.
- In affluent countries there are marked differences between the diets of the richest and the poorest and there are also major inequalities in health.

International trends

If one looks worldwide at the influence of economic status on food 'selection', some very general trends emerge. Increasing affluence leads initially to increases in total energy intake, followed by a switch away from starchy staples to other higher prestige and more palatable foods, including fats, meats, dairy produce and sugars. Poleman (1975) suggested that the percentage of dietary energy that is provided by starchy staples provided a very simple economic ranking of diets. In 1875, starchy staples made up 55 per cent of total energy intake in the USA; a century later this figure had dropped to around 20 per cent. In the early decades of the twentieth century, maize was a sufficiently dominant component of the diets of poor farmers in some southern US states to trigger epidemics of pellagra (see Chapter 14).

At very low incomes, increased wealth leads to increases in energy intake, usually based on local starchy staples. Only when income level has risen beyond the point where energy needs are satisfied does increasing affluence lead to changes in the nature and quality of the diet. The local starchy staple is partly replaced by higher prestige rice or wheat. This is followed by a reduced consumption of starchy staples and replacement with foods of animal origin, fattier foods and simple sugars. In parts of some developing countries, fat accounts for less than 10 per cent of total energy intake and carbohydrate more than 75 per cent. In the UK, fat accounts for around 35 per cent of food energy and carbohydrate only 48 per cent. In the poorer areas almost all of the carbohydrate calories are likely to be starches, whereas in some richer countries a third or more of the carbohydrate calories may be in the form of simple sugars. Improved palatability, higher prestige and simple increases in physical availability all compound to persuade those with the economic means to make changes in this general direction.

Paralleling these changes in food selection practices there will be changes in the general pattern of mortality and disease. Child mortality will fall due largely to a general reduction in mortality from infectious diseases. Malnutrition and the deficiency diseases will all but disappear, life expectancy will increase, but the chronic degenerative diseases will account for an increasing proportion of deaths and will be an increasing cause of illness and disability. The nutritional guidelines aimed at reducing the prevalence of these chronic diseases (discussed in Chapter 5) would partly reverse some of these wealth-related changes in dietary habits.

- As populations become more affluent their diet changes. First there is an increase in energy consumption as starchy staples, but then the starchy food is partly replaced by animal produce, fatty foods and sugars.
- The proportion of dietary energy derived from starchy foods decreases with affluence and provides a simple economic ranking of diets.
- In some developing countries, fats account for less than 10 per cent of dietary energy and starches as much as 75 per cent.
- In some affluent countries, fats may provide 35–40 per cent of the energy and starches not much more than a quarter.
- Life expectancy increases with affluence, child mortality falls, deficiency diseases largely disappear, and deaths from acute causes such as infection fall.
- The chronic diseases of industrialization account for most deaths among affluent populations.

The problem of feeding the world

In 1798, Thomas Malthus published his now infamous *Essay on the principle of population*. In this treatise he predicted that, unless steps were taken to regulate the family size of the poor, then population growth would outstrip growth in the food supply, leading to global famine and epidemics. In the early 1960s, when world population was growing at an annual rate of around 2 per cent, a spate of Malthusian-type predictions of impending population disaster were also published.

Two hundred years ago when Malthus published his essay, the world population was less than 1 billion and in October 2011 it reached 7 billion. This rate of growth would have astounded even the most ardent Malthusian. There has, however, been a distinct slowing in the rate of population growth since the 1960s. In 1965–70, growth rate peaked at 2 per cent a year, but by 2000 it was down to 1.3 per cent (still a net addition of 76 million people each year). The deceleration in the rate of population growth has been sharper than was predicted even a few years ago. Table 2.1 shows the UN's population estimates and

projections for the period 0–2100 made in 2010 (UN, 2011). In brackets in this table are some projections made in this biennial UN publication in 1994. The projected population in 2050 has fallen from over 10 billion predicted in 1994 to the 9.20 billion predicted in 2010, and current predictions are that the world population will still be around 10 billion in 2100. Almost all of the predicted growth in population by 2050 will take place in the less developed regions, while the population of the developed regions will remain largely unchanged. In some countries, including Germany and Japan, the population is predicted to fall by 2050, but in some of the least developed countries it is expected to triple (e.g. in Chad, Liberia and Uganda).

Table 2.1 Growth in world population from year 0 to 2100*

Year	Population in billions
0	0.30
1000	0.31
1250	0.40
1500	0.50
1750	0.79
1800	0.98
1850	1.26
1900	1.65
1920	1.86
1940	2.30
1950	2.53
1960	3.04
1970	3.70
1980	4.45
1990	5.31
2000	6.12 (6.23)
2010	6.90
2020	7.58
2030	8.20
2040	8.70
2050	9.20 (10.02)
2100	10.1

*Data are from UN biennial estimates. The figures from 1950 onwards are from the 2010 estimates (UN, 2011) and in brackets are the predictions in 1994.

The projected changes in world population by 2050 are highly dependent on what happens to human fertility over this period. The projections in Table 2.1 are based on the medium variant – that it will fall from 2.65 children per woman in 2000–5 to just 2.05 children per woman by 2050. The current fertility rate is just over half that in the early 1950s when it stood at five children per woman. Although average fertility has fallen sharply over the last 50 years and is projected to continue falling slowly over the next 50 years, there is marked regional variation across the world. In the developed countries fertility is around 1.6 children per woman, but in the very least developed countries it is still five children per woman. Just eight countries are expected to account for half of the increase in world population by 2050, namely India, Pakistan, Nigeria, Democratic Republic of the Congo, Bangladesh, Uganda, the USA, Ethiopia and China.

Despite the massive increase in the world's population, calculations of worldwide production of primary foods (mainly cereals) indicate that sufficient is produced to meet the estimated nutritional needs of the world population. Yet in some poor countries there is starvation and in other richer countries there are 'mountains' and 'lakes' of surplus food. Poleman (1975) estimated that in the USA, per-capita grain consumption was 1800 pounds per year but less than 100 pounds of this was directly consumed with almost all of the rest being used as animal feed. An animal consumes between 3 and 10 pounds of grain to produce one pound of meat. In 1995, per-capita grain consumption was 250 kg per year in the developing world but 665 kg per year in the industrialized nations. The USA is the world's largest producer of surplus grain. The primary cause of worldwide malnutrition is not inadequate food production *per se* but an imbalance in the way this food is distributed between the peoples of the world. Differences in wealth are the key determinant of this uneven distribution.

The image of rapid world population growth outstripping growth in food production and being entirely responsible for creating current food shortages is not borne out by the statistics. Wortman (1976) estimated that, in developed countries, rates of food production between 1961 and 1975 rose by almost 40 per cent on a per-capita basis. Even in developing countries, population growth did not entirely negate the substantial increases in absolute food production when they were expressed on a per-capita basis. Wortman predicted that world food production was likely to keep up with population growth for some time to come. The International Food Policy Research Institute (see IFPRI, 1996) confirmed that this trend of increasing per-capita grain production also continued over the period 1970–95. In 2011, the United Nations estimated that world agriculture produces 17 per cent more calories per person than it did 30 years ago, and that, despite a 70 per cent increase in population, this is theoretically enough to provide every person with 2720 kcal per day. The IFRPI report in 1996 estimated that the number of chronically undernourished people in the world fell by 17 per cent between 1970 and 1990. Despite this overall fall the number of undernourished people in Sub-Saharan Africa almost doubled. Even though the proportion of undernourished pre-school children fell during this period, the absolute number rose because of increasing population so despite some improvements in some parts of the world, malnutrition and food insecurity still afflict the developing world on a massive scale. In an overview of the world food situation, von Braun (2005) made the following estimates of the prevalence of worldwide nutrition problems:

- 0.9 billion people suffering from hunger (i.e. a deficiency of calories and protein)
- 126 million children underweight because of inadequate food intake and frequent disease
- over 2 billion people affected by a vitamin or mineral deficiency.

Von Braun (2005) suggests that there was very little progress in reducing hunger during the 1990s, and that what little progress there had been was very uneven. China markedly reduced its number of hungry people, but rates in the rest of the developing world actually rose (e.g. by 20 per cent in Sub-Saharan Africa). Von Braun highlighted vitamin A deficiency, iron-deficiency anaemia and zinc deficiency as increasing the probability of early death in women and children, impairing the intellectual development of children and generally reducing quality of life. He estimated that vitamin A deficiency adversely affects the immune system of 40 per cent of young children in the developing countries and is responsible for an annual toll of one million child deaths. Maybe half a million children go blind each year due to vitamin A deficiency, and millions of children are stillborn, have a birth defect or are permanently mentally impaired by iodine deficiency. A recent paper in the *British Medical Journal* estimates that vitamin A supplements given to all children with vitamin A deficiency (*c*200 million) in developing countries could reduce all-cause mortality by about a quarter – potentially saving over half a million lives each year. Vitamin A supplements reduced rates of diarrhoea, measles and visual problems (Mayo-Wilson *et al.*, 2011).

In its 'Hunger notes', the United Nations (UN, 2011) suggests that 'poverty is the principal cause of hunger'. It suggests that 'harmful economic systems are the principal cause of poverty and hunger' – that is, concentration of resources and income in the hands of powerful minorities who use it to their advantage but to the detriment of the rest of the population. While conflicts do displace people and cause poverty and hunger they are not a numerically major factor. 'Hunger is a cause of poverty, and thus of hunger'; it reduces capacity to work, learn and earn. 'Climate change is increasingly viewed as a current and future cause of hunger and poverty.'

Most of the increases in cereal production since 1970 have been the result of increased yields rather than increases in the land area under cultivation. In Asia, cereal yields have doubled and those in Latin America increased by around two-thirds. The three major factors responsible for this 'Green Revolution' are listed below (from IFPRI, 1996):

- increased use of modern high-yielding crop varieties
- increased irrigation of land
- increased use of fertilizers and pesticides (use of fertilizers by farmers in developing countries quadrupled over this period).

In contrast to the other developing regions of the world, cereal production in Africa remained stagnant over the period 1970–95 largely for the reasons listed below.

- African farmers have lagged behind in the use of new crop varieties.

- Much less arable land is irrigated in Africa.
- African farmers have made less use of agricultural chemicals.

Publications from the 1970s to 2011 have all emphasized that world food production has been increasing on a per-capita basis despite continuing population growth, and nearly all the increase is still occurring in the developed countries, especially in the USA and the European Union.

The increased production of food to feed the growing world population has had a number of adverse environmental consequences. This has increased concern about whether the increases in food production are sustainable in the longer term using current approaches. Discussion of these issues is beyond the scope of this book, but some of the important points are:

- destruction of forests to increase the availability of arable land, which can increase soil erosion, affect global climate and deprive forest-dwelling people of their source of food and way of life
- adverse ecological effects of excessive use of agricultural chemicals
- over-use of irrigation, which can lower the water table, lead to salinization of land and make it agriculturally unproductive
- depletion of the world's fish stocks.

For further information and discussion, see IFPRI (1996), WRI (1997) and FAO (1996).

Key points

- Food production is sufficient to satisfy the nutritional needs of the world population but this food is unevenly distributed.
- Affluent countries have almost three times the per-capita grain consumption of developing countries. This extra grain is fed to animals to produce meat and milk.
- The rate of world population growth has fallen sharply since its peak in the 1960s. The Malthusian predictions of rapid population growth leading to worldwide famines and epidemics now look too pessimistic.
- The world population almost doubled over the period 1960–95, but per-capita grain production and energy availability increased →

Key points *continued*

and is still increasing largely because of increasing grain yields.

- The number of chronically malnourished people has fallen in recent decades, but malnutrition in children and adults, including vitamin and mineral deficiencies, remains a huge problem in much of the developing world.

- The United Nations identifies poverty as the principal cause of hunger.

- Harmful economic systems are identified by the UN as the principal cause of poverty. Income and resources are channelled disproportionately to a powerful ruling elite.

- The massive increases in grain yields seen during the 'Green Revolution' have been largely achieved by increased use of modern high-yielding varieties, greater irrigation of farmland and greater use of agricultural chemicals.

- Africa has been relatively slow to adopt these changes, and the 'Green Revolution' has largely bypassed Africa where grain production stagnated in the period 1970–95.

- Rates of malnutrition have risen sharply in Sub-Saharan Africa in recent decades.

- The increase in food availability has led to destruction of large areas of forest, salinization of land due to over-irrigation, over-use of agricultural chemicals, and depletion of the world's fish stocks.

Effects of income on food selection in industrialized countries

Even within industrialized countries, the food choices of the wealthiest and the poorest may vary quite considerably. Data presented in the previous edition of this book showed that, by the end of the millennium, most households in Britain owned a deep freeze and a microwave oven but nearly a fifth of the poor unemployed did not own a freezer and about a third did not own a microwave oven. This has implications for the economic purchasing and preparation of food, as discussed later in this section. DEFRA (2006) published a simple analysis of food expenditure according to household income; the

participating households were divided up into fifths (quintiles) according to their household income and comparisons made between the food purchases of these quintiles and its nutrient content. This analysis shows a number of interesting general trends and some of these are listed below.

- The amount of milk and cream purchased decreases progressively with increasing income but cheese purchases rise with income.
- The amount of sugar and preserves decreases markedly with increasing income and the highest income quintile purchases less than half of the amount purchased by the lowest income quintile.
- Purchases of fats and oils decrease progressively with increasing income.
- Fruit purchases increase with increasing income.
- Potato and cereal purchases decline with increasing income.
- The amount spent on eating out increases sharply with rising income, and the amount spent by the highest quintile is well over three times that spent by the lowest income group.
- Purchases of alcoholic drinks increase with increasing income, especially that consumed outside of the home.

Figure 2.3 illustrates some of these trends in household purchases across income quintiles.

While this analysis is useful for highlighting such clear trends, its usefulness is restricted by the fact that the average size and composition of the households in the different quintiles vary markedly, as does the average age of the Household Reference Person (the HRP is the person whose occupation is used to classify the socioeconomic status of the family). An alternative mode of analysis used by DEFRA was to classify households according to the occupational category of the HRP. This classification also effectively splits families into income groups but in this case household composition and average age of the HRP are similar across the groupings. This analysis has been used to construct Tables 2.2 and 2.3.

Table 2.2 shows a comparison of the food-related spending of families within these different socioeconomic groupings based on the occupation of the Household Reference Person. Groups A and B are high- and low-income groups from those where the HRP is in employment (details on the table). In

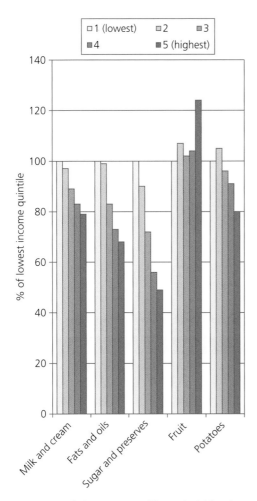

Figure 2.3 Trends in amounts of household foods purchased according to income quintile.

group C, the HRP has either never worked or is long-term unemployed.

The average household income of the highest income group is more than five times that of the unemployed group shown in the table. Spending on household food and drink (excluding alcohol) is 60 per cent higher in the high-income group compared to the unemployed group, and still 30 per cent higher than that of the group employed in routine occupations. Yet this household food spending represents over three times the proportion of household income in the unemployed group compared to the high-income group. These gaps widen still further if food and drink eaten outside the home and alcoholic drinks are included in the food spending. Despite spending much less on their food and drink, the poorer groups obtain almost as many calories per person per day and so they must inevitably obtain more calories for every penny they spend. The poorer groups are, of necessity, more economically efficient (judged on calories alone) in their food spending. This increased efficiency could be achieved in many ways, such as:

- less purchasing of unnecessary items such as bottled water or alcohol
- buying cheaper brands
- shopping in the cheapest shops
- reducing waste
- buying lower quality (or lower prestige) items that provide more calories per penny, such as cheaper types of meat and fish and cheaper meat and fish products
- taking more advantage of special offers and promotions or simply taking more advantage of seasonal fluctuations in prices of many foods
- doing more food preparation at home rather than buying relatively more expensive prepared foods or eating out
- adopting a totally different, cheaper eating pattern with much larger quantities of starchy foods, inexpensive vegetables and legumes but fewer animal foods – a dietary pattern that could be described as more 'primitive' but could also be more in line with current nutritional guidelines.

Table 2.3 compares some of the purchasing practices of our three selected economic groups. Some of the trends in this table are discussed briefly below.

- Compared to the highest income group, total meat purchases were slightly higher in the poorer employed group and markedly lower in the unemployed group. However, in the higher income group a larger proportion of the total meat purchased was fresh carcass meat. The poorer groups got considerably more meat for each penny they spent than the richer group, implying that they buy cheaper cuts and bulkier, lower quality meat products.
- As with meat, the poorer groups got more fish for each penny than the richer group, again implying higher use of cheaper varieties of fish and fish products.

Table 2.2 Differences between the food and drink expenditure of rich and poor families in the UK*

	Group A	Group B	Group C
Total household income (£/week)	1299	460	231
Household food and drink (excluding alcohol, pence per person/week)	2270	1741	1420
– Percentage of total household income	5	10.2	16.6
Eating out food and drink (excluding alcohol, pence per person/week)	1243	575	511
All food and drink (excluding alcohol, pence per person/week)	3513	2316	1931
– Percentage of total household income	7.8	13.6	22.6
All alcohol (pence per person/week)	859	538	472
– Percentage of total household income	1.9	3.2	6.0
Kcal obtained per penny (excluding alcohol)	1.5	2.5	2.6

*Data are from DEFRA (2006) and are based on the following classification using the occupation of the Household Reference Person (HRP):
Group A: employed in a higher professional or managerial capacity by a large employer
Group B: employed in routine work
Group C: never employed or long-term unemployed.

Table 2.3 Comparison of the food purchases and its nutrient content in different income groups in the UK*

	Group A	Group B	Group C
Meat and meat products (g per person/week)	1018	1091	903
Percentage carcass meat	21.7	20.3	19.4
Spending (pence per person/week)	539	459	341
Grams of meat/penny	1.89	2.38	2.65
Fish (g per person/week)	151	132	107
Spending (pence per person/week)	110	68	52
Grams of fish/penny	1.37	1.94	2.06
Fats and oils (g per person/week)	142	183	205
Sugars and preserves (g per person/week)	86	144	135
Vegetables (g per person/week) (excluding potatoes)	1127	966	774
Fruit (g per person/week)	1400	844	723
Vitamins and minerals (all % RNI)			
Calcium	124	124	108
Iron	103	98	79
Zinc	101	100	86
Vitamin A	122	114	90
Riboflavin	152	148	125
Folate	141	130	107
Vitamin C	192	142	127

*All data are from Defra (2006) and use the following classification based on the occupation of the Household Reference Person (HRP):
Group A: employed in a higher professional or managerial capacity by a large employer
Group B: employed in routine work
Group C: never employed or long-term unemployed.
RNI, reference nutrient intake.

- The poorer groups bought more sugar and preserves and more fats and oils than the richest group.
- The poorer groups bought much less fruit and vegetables (excluding potatoes) than the richer group. The unemployed bought only around half as much fruit as the richest group. People in the UK and the USA are being encouraged to eat more of these foods; at least five portions each day have been suggested. However, despite all of their nutritional merits (see Chapter 5), these foods are relatively inefficient providers of energy because of their low energy density (see Chapter 7). Fresh fruit and vegetables (excluding potatoes) accounted for only 3.5 per cent of household food energy (excluding alcohol) but over 12 per cent of expenditure whereas fats, sugars and preserves provided over 12 per cent of household food energy but only accounted for about 2.5 per cent of the expenditure.

The estimated vitamin and mineral intakes (calculated from food purchases) were generally lower in the lowest income group – those without employment. Some of these differences were large. For example, compare the intakes of groups A and C for iron, zinc, vitamin A, folate and vitamin C as shown in Table 2.3.

In an analysis from the old National Food Survey in the previous edition of this book, it was also found that poorer groups bought less of products that could be considered as non-essentials from a nutritional standpoint (e.g. they bought less than a quarter as much mineral water). There were also several examples of the poorer groups being less likely to make the healthier choice within a category, such as:

- less of the bread bought by the poorer groups was whole-grain and much more of it was standard white bread
- less of the milk bought by the poorer groups was low fat and much more of it was whole milk
- fewer of the soft drinks bought by the poorer group were low-calorie versions.

DEFRA (2006) is a household expenditure survey which measures what people buy rather than what they eat. A number of assumptions about wastage and family distribution are made in order to estimate nutrient intakes. The National Diet and Nutrition Survey (NDNS) programme has until c2006 recorded reported food consumption using weighed inventories of different age groups of the British population. The last full NDNS survey of British adults aged under 65 years (Hoare et al., 2004) compared the intakes of men and women in households that were or were not in receipt of state benefits. (Note that the more recent programme of rolling NDNS surveys of the whole population has not yet reported food and nutrient intakes broken down according to income or social class, presumably because the sample sizes are not yet sufficient to do this.) Some of the differences found between these two groups are listed below, and in general they tend to confirm the trends already discussed using the analysis from DEFRA in Tables 2.2 and 2.3.

Comparing adults in households not in receipt of state benefits with those in benefit-receiving households, in those receiving benefits:

- energy intakes were lower
- intakes of dietary fibre were lower
- added sugars made up a higher proportion of dietary energy in women
- average intakes of vitamins and minerals were generally lower, and so were average blood levels of micronutrients
- a significantly higher proportion of women had intakes of vitamin A and riboflavin that were below the lower recommended nutritional intake (LRNI, the point at which intakes are classified as inadequate – see Chapter 3), and many more had intakes of iron that were below the LRNI.

Key points

- The poorest families are less likely to own a freezer.
- Poorer families eat out much less often than richer ones and spend much less when they do eat out.
- Richer families spend more on household food than poorer ones, but this represents a much smaller proportion of their total income.
- Poorer families are much more economically efficient in their food purchasing and obtain
→

more calories per penny. For example, they tend to buy cheaper types of meat and fish and cheaper meat and fish products.

- Poorer families buy more cereals, potatoes, sugar and fats than richer families but less fruit and fresh vegetables.
- Poorer households consume fewer non-essential items like mineral water and alcoholic drinks.
- Poorer families are less likely to buy the 'healthier' option within a category, for example, bread made with less -refined flour, low-fat milk and low-calorie soft drinks.
- Recorded energy intakes are lower in adults receiving welfare payments.
- Intakes of most vitamins and minerals were lower in the lowest socioeconomic groups, as were average blood levels of micronutrients.
- Intakes of dietary fibre were lower in the lowest socioeconomic groups.
- More women in benefit-receiving households had intakes of vitamin A, riboflavin and iron that were below the LRNI.

The minimum cost of a healthy diet

Welfare payments in the UK have traditionally been calculated on the basis that enough money should be provided to allow purchase of the essentials of life but not enough to allow purchase of luxuries. The same underlying philosophy governs the welfare systems of most industrialized countries. These welfare payments should be enough to prevent claimants from going hungry or being deprived of basic shelter and clothing but not make their situation so comfortable as to discourage them from seeking employment or to encourage others to voluntarily live off the state. A more cynical Marxist interpretation of this principle would be that enough money is provided to prevent social unrest but not enough to reduce the competition for jobs and thus risk increasing the cost of labour. Pressures on public expenditure may encourage governments to economize by reducing the purchasing power of those who are dependent on welfare payments.

Calculation of a minimum subsistence level of income is far from straightforward. There are a host of factors to produce wide variations in the quality of life that different families can achieve with the same level of income. At the physiological level, people vary in their energy and nutrient requirements. Regional and individual variations in housing, transport and fuel costs make it difficult to produce a single welfare figure for a nation. Differences in cultural and personal preferences will affect the size of the required food budget. A minimally adequate income may make it difficult to live at maximum economic efficiency. For a variety of reasons such as those listed below, it is often true that 'the poor pay more'.

- The poorest may be forced to buy in small, expensive quantities; they can afford only enough to meet immediate needs.
- They may be unable to stock up when a seasonal food is cheap or when special offers are made (e.g. because they do not own a freezer, or simply lack capital).
- They may not have the transportation or personal mobility to enable them to shop at the most economical places.

Table 2.4 shows the potential magnitude of some of the differing costs of buying in small and large quantities. Webb and Copeman (1996) surveyed the differences in unit costs of the same brands of common grocery items in a large London supermarket. The general trend was for decreasing unit cost with increasing pack size – penalizing those who need to buy in minimum quantities to satisfy immediate needs. There was often a sharp decrease in unit cost between the smallest pack and the next smallest size – to the disadvantage of those living alone or buying enough for one. Special offers tended to be concentrated in the largest packs, and many special offers were in the form of discounts for multiple purchases. One would generally expect all household costs (e.g. replacement of capital items, rental charges and fuel costs) to rise on a per-capita basis as the size of the household decreases, so increasing pressure on the food budget of poor, small households.

People who are forced to shop in smaller, more accessible shops may also have to pay much more. In a survey conducted in the Reading and Oxford areas of England in 1991, the cost of a basket of 21 food items was about a quarter higher in small,

Table 2.4 Differences in costs of small and large packs of a variety of grocery items obtained from a large London supermarket in early 1995 (all comparisons are between same brands and prices are pence per unit (variable) and so are directly comparable within items)*

Item	Small size	Unit price (pence)	Large size	Unit price (pence)	Percentage price difference
Cucumber	Half	70	Whole	49	43
Mushrooms	Quarter pound	155	1 pound	115 (s.o.)	35
Peas (can)	142 g	8.3	300 g	5.4	54
Margarine	250 g	14.8	1 kg	11.9	24
Corned beef	198 g	36.4	340 g	28	30
Rice	500 g	11.8	4 kg	9.3	27
Baked beans	150 g	14	420 g	7.4	89
Chicken	Quarter	99	Whole	68 (s.o.)	46
Eggs	6	98	12	89	10
Cooking oil	500 mL	74	1 L	59	25
Weetabix	12	68	48	46	48
Tea bags	40	40.8	160	33.8	21
Milk	1 pint	28	6 pints	22.2	26
Instant coffee	50 g	212	300 g	179	18
Washing-up liquid	500 mL	126	1 L	99 (s.o.)	26
Sugar	500 g	90	1 kg	62	45
Burgers (frozen)	4	43.7	20	36	15
White bread	400 g	6	800 g	4.4	36
Flour	500 g	48	1.5 kg	27.4	75

* From Webb and Copeman (1996).
s.o., denotes special offer.

independent grocery stores than in the supermarkets owned by the large multiple chains (Henson, 1992).

Other demands on the household budget may greatly restrain food expenditure for some individuals or families. When financial resources are restricted, especially if there is a sudden decline in income (e.g. through loss of employment, retirement or long-term illness), then expenditure on food may be sacrificed in order to maintain spending on other essentials such as housing, loan repayments, clothing or fuel. Food expenditure may be sacrificed to allow purchase or retention of some prestigious item or activity that helps maintain self-esteem – such as Christmas presents for children, a car, a cable/satellite television subscription, a computer, internet access, tobacco or going to the pub. Considerable savings can often be made in the food budget without obvious acute hardship – for example by switching to cheaper brands or varieties, by reducing wastage, and by using cheaper alternatives such as margarine for butter or lower quality meat and fish products for fresh meat and fish.

Dobson et al. (1994) published a survey of the food-buying and dietary habits of low-income families living in the English Midlands. Almost all of these families were in receipt of welfare payments and half of them had mothers as lone parents. Money and the cost of food were seen as the most important factors in deciding what food could be bought. Other factors, such as taste, cultural acceptability and healthy eating, could only be considered in the light of what was economically available. These parents often saw incorporating advice about healthy eating as impractical or only partly practical in their economic circumstances.

These families all reported great difficulties in managing on their incomes. Unexpected demands for money could derail their spending plans and at these times the food budget was often reduced to cope. These families needed to adopt various strategies to cope with their restricted food budgets.

- They needed to shop around for 'best buys' and this made shopping a time-consuming activity that they ceased to enjoy.
- Parents often reported going without food themselves to minimize the impact on their children.
- The need to avoid waste of food and money meant that children's preferences were given high priority. They did not have the means to provide foods that reflected the individual tastes of family members; parents often ate what their children would eat irrespective of their own likes and dislikes. They all had to eat the same food at the same time.

The burden of coping with the money available was largely borne by the mothers who did most of the shopping and food preparation. They tried to maintain a culturally usual 'mainstream' diet. This meant that they had to eat cheaper versions of mainstream meals. Parents went to great lengths to make sure that their children were seen to be eating the same things as their peers even if it meant making sacrifices themselves. They resisted radical changes to their diets.

To subsist on a minimum income is easier for those with some degree of budget management skill. Unfortunately those with the least of these skills may often be those most likely to be required to exercise them; poor educational attainment and poor socioeconomic status are strongly correlated. Strictly theoretical calculations of minimum subsistence levels cannot allow for food choices that appear irrational or even irresponsible using strictly biological criteria. People whose self-esteem has been dented by unemployment, disability or social deprivation may buy foods to boost their spirits and self-esteem rather than out of strict scientific necessity. In *The Road to Wigan Pier*, George Orwell gives an example of an adequate but dull and low-prestige diet that in 1937 could be obtained for twenty pence (40 cents). He also gives an example of the real expenditure of an unemployed miner's family at the time. This real family spent only 4 pence each week on green vegetables and sweetened

condensed milk, nothing at all on fruit, but 9 pence on sugar (representing 4 kg of sugar), 5 pence on tea and 3 pence on jam. Clearly white bread spread with margarine and jam and washed down with sweet tea was an important part of this family's daily diet. Orwell describes this mixture as being almost devoid of nutritional value and it certainly was low in several vitamins and minerals.

> When you are unemployed, which is to say when you are underfed, harassed, bored and miserable, you don't want to eat dull wholesome food. You want something a little bit tasty. ... Unemployment is an endless misery that has got to be constantly palliated, and especially with tea, the Englishman's opium. A cup of tea or even an aspirin is much better as a temporary stimulant than a crust of brown bread.
>
> *George Orwell, The Road to Wigan Pier, London: Victor Gollancz, 1937*

Readers who would like a more scientific and detailed review of trends in the British diet between 1841 and 1994 should see Charlton and Quaife (1997). Orwell goes on to describe the poor people of a British industrial city as being small of stature and having universally bad or missing teeth – he suggests that it was rare to see a working-class person with good natural teeth. He suggests that the death rate and infant mortality rate of the poorest area of any city were always at least double those in the wealthy areas, in some cases much more than double. He was writing about mid-twentieth-century peacetime conditions in one of the wealthiest industrialized countries of the world. These few pages of Orwell's book underline how far social conditions and nutrition of most poorer people in Britain have improved over the last 75 years despite the disparity between the health and nutrition of rich and poor that still remains.

One practical consequence of the sort of effect described in the above quotation will be to make it even more difficult to persuade the less affluent to make dietary changes that they perceive as reducing either the palatability or prestige of their diet. It is important to their self-esteem that they – and especially their children – are seen to be eating like their peers (Dobson *et al.*, 1994). Diet-related disease is more prevalent in the poorer groups but they also seem to be more resistant to nutritional and other health education advice. The decline in prevalence of breastfeeding with social class is a very clear example of this (see Chapter 16). This increases the onus on those seeking to effect dietary change among all social groups to suggest changes that are simple, economically feasible and easy to incorporate permanently into usual culinary practices, and which are not overly restrictive of highly palatable and high-prestige foods. Change must not require the consumption of a diet that, although wholesome by current nutritional criteria, is perceived as dull and unpalatable, uses low-prestige ingredients or is simply different from the mainstream.

Changes must also be within any group's economic means if they are really expected to be implemented. Groom (1993) and Leather (1992) review a number of attempts to devise 'healthy' diets that comply with UK dietary guidelines and are also within the economic means of poorer families. In 1991, the UK produced a 'low-cost, healthy diet' that could be purchased for £10 ($20) per person per week at 1991 prices. However, it was suggested in Leather's review that this diet would be so different from the mainstream British diet as to be totally unrealistic. It would require, for example:

- almost total exclusion of meat and most dairy products from the diet
- a very large increase in bread consumption, and most of this bread would have to be eaten dry without butter or margarine
- large increases in consumption of tinned fruit and frozen vegetables.

It is easy to produce lists of ingredients that meet any set compositional criteria within a very small budget but it is much more expensive to purchase a collection of ingredients that can also be combined into meals that make up a culturally acceptable diet. The survey of Dobson et al. (1994) discussed earlier found that maintaining a mainstream diet was very important to low-income families. Leather (1992) reviews other work which estimates the cost of a 'modest but adequate' diet which would not only be adequate and comply with current nutrition education guidelines but also be broadly in line with the usual diet of the UK population. Using these criteria, their minimum cost for feeding an adult couple was about 70 per cent more than the minimum cost diet produced by the Ministry of Agriculture, Fisheries and Food in 1991. This modest but adequate diet cost significantly more than that spent per capita by low-income families. To stay as

close as possible to current eating patterns but to choose 'healthier' alternatives such as leaner meat, wholemeal bread and fruit leads to a substantial increase in food costs – which may be beyond the practical means of many low-income families.

Families living in 'temporary' bed and breakfast type accommodation may face yet another extra financial burden. They may have limited cooking facilities and thus be forced to rely on eating out (which is expensive) or rely largely on cold foods (which require no further cooking). Relying largely on cold foods also has its disadvantages; the diet is less varied and palatable, quite different from the diet of the culture. The minimum cost of eating a healthy diet is also likely to be higher.

Key points

- Welfare payments aim to be enough to provide sufficient money for the essentials of life but not enough to discourage people from working.
- Many factors will affect how much money any given family needs in order to provide a modest lifestyle, which makes setting the level of welfare payments a difficult and flawed process.
- Poverty may reduce the practical purchasing power of those on low incomes, for example if they:
  - cannot reach the cheapest shops
  - lack the storage facilities or capital to buy more of special offers
  - have to buy in small quantities to meet immediate needs.
- For low-income British families, financial considerations are the most important factors governing food choice. For these families, incorporating advice on healthy eating is seen as impractical.
- Poor families maximize economic efficiency by shopping around and avoiding waste. To avoid waste, children's preferences are given high priority.
- Poor families try to maintain a mainstream diet and parents make personal sacrifices to prevent their children being stigmatized by eating differently from other children.
- Poor families resist radical changes to their diets.
- During times of financial pressure, the food budget may be pared to allow spending on other essential items or bills.

Key points *continued*

- People struggling with difficult economic circumstances do not always make selections that are scientifically logical. They may buy foods that are palatable or help to maintain their self-esteem rather than those that are cheap and nutritious.

- It is possible to produce very low-cost lists of ingredients that meet particular nutritional criteria, but these may involve eating a diet that is very different from the mainstream.

- The minimum cost of a healthy diet increases markedly if the ingredients must combine to make a culturally acceptable mainstream diet.

- Lack of cooking and storage facilities will reduce the food choices of poorer people and raise the cost of a healthy diet.

CULTURAL AVAILABILITY

Beef is physically and economically available to devout Hindus in the UK but religious conviction makes it culturally unavailable. Under normal circumstances, people eat things that are culturally recognized as foods. People choose things that in their culture are considered appropriate for the particular meal or occasion and that are suitable for the lifecycle group to be fed. This has been discussed earlier in the section dealing with consumer classification of food (see p. 33). The cultural acceptability of a food may change as it becomes physically more available and more familiar. The indigenous population may initially view unfamiliar immigrant foods with suspicion and even distaste, but with time they may become more familiar and acceptable. Chinese foods and curry are now as much a part of British culture as fish and chips. Similarly, immigrants tend to gradually adopt some of the foods and dietary practices of the indigenous population. Exposure to alien foods through foreign travel may have a similar effect.

Dietary taboos

The word 'taboo' is derived from the Polynesian name for a system of religious prohibitions against the use of sacred things. It has come to mean any sacred prohibition and, with common usage, the religious connotation is no longer obligatory. One could define a *dietary taboo* as any avoidance that is maintained solely because failure to do so would generate disapproval, ostracism or punishment within one's own cultural group, or because it would compromise one's own ethical standards. A food taboo should be distinguished from a food avoidance that is based on sound empirical evidence of harm.

Many taboos are aimed at avoidance of flesh and these are often rigorously adhered to. It is said that the initial spark that ignited the Indian Mutiny against British rule in 1857 was the introduction of cartridges supposedly greased with animal fat. Hindu troops were unwilling to bite the ends off these cartridges or, indeed, even to handle them. On 6 May 1857, 85 out of 90 members of the 3rd native cavalry in Meerut refused direct orders to handle cartridges which, according to a contemporary account, they mistakenly believed to be contaminated with animal fat. They were subsequently sentenced to terms of imprisonment of between 6 and 10 years. These men would undoubtedly have been aware of the likely consequences of their disobeying a direct military order – which underlines the potential strength of such taboos.

The taboos of other cultures tend to be viewed as illogical restraints often imposed on individuals by authoritarian religious leaders. This model leads to the belief that taboos should be discouraged. This is almost certainly a misreading of the situation in most cases. Most taboos need little external compulsion to ensure adherence; people feel secure when maintaining cultural standards that have been ingrained since childhood. There are nonetheless a few examples of essentially religious taboos being incorporated into the secular law and of severe penalties being imposed on transgressors. In many Indian states the cow is legally protected, and there are severe penalties for alcohol consumption in some Moslem countries.

Most people of western European origin would not consider dietary taboos to have any significant influence on their food selection, but no society is completely free of dietary prohibitions. It is not too long ago that Roman Catholics were required to abstain from meat on Fridays and this was reintroduced in England and Wales in 2011. In the UK, cannibalism is clearly prohibited but, equally, the consumption of animals such as cats, dogs and horses would result in widespread hostility and probably ostracism by other members of society. Most British people would not recognize these as taboos because they do not classify these creatures as potential food despite their being highly regarded as foods in some other countries. In France, for example, horsemeat is eaten, sometimes even meat from British horses!

In the UK, vegetarianism would seem to be an obvious candidate for an example of a dietary taboo that may have negative nutritional implications. Certainly many omnivores would like to think so, as the vegetarian's rejection of flesh is often perceived as a threat to highly desired and high-prestige foods. There are some problems associated with a strictly vegetarian (vegan) diet (see Chapter 18). However, a well-constructed vegetarian diet can be healthy and in the current climate of nutrition opinion may even be regarded as healthier than the typical omnivorous diet. Vegetarianism must be socially inconvenient where most of the population is omnivorous and where caterers may make only nominal provision for vegetarians. These inconveniences may, however, be more than compensated for by a comradeship, akin to religious fellowship, seemingly shared by many vegetarians and by enhancement of self-actualization (see Figure 2.1).

Perhaps, taboo also played some part in the dramatic decline in breastfeeding that occurred in Britain in the decades following the Second World War or in impeding current efforts to encourage breastfeeding. The inconvenience of breastfeeding and its 'prestige' can only have been worsened by a very strong taboo against breastfeeding amongst strangers, sometimes even amongst friends and relatives. The lack of provision of a suitable environment for feeding babies in most public places increased this problem. The arrival of a modern, scientifically developed and socially acceptable alternative provided women with an ideal opportunity to free themselves of the need to continue with this 'inconvenient and embarrassing process'. A survey conducted by the Royal College of Midwives in 1993 found that more than a third of the 700 restaurants surveyed either would not permit breastfeeding at the table or would ask women to stop if another customer complained. In a second survey, half of men disagreed with women

breastfeeding 'in any place they choose'. Some reasons given for this were 'it's unnecessary', 'it's a form of exhibitionism' and 'it's disgusting behaviour'. Both of these surveys are briefly summarized by Laurent (1993). Bolling et al. (2007) reported that many UK women still said that one reason they chose not to breastfeed was because they did not like the idea or found it embarrassing. Clearly breastfeeding is seen by many men (and many women too) as a distasteful or embarrassing task that needs to be performed furtively.

Many of the best known taboos are permanent but some are only temporary. Some of the temporary ones may apply only during certain phases of the lifecycle or during illness. Some taboos may be restricted to certain groups of people. The familiar permanent religious taboos generally cause few nutritional problems. The temporary ones will also not usually give rise to adverse nutritional consequences unless they are imposed at times of rapid growth or other physiological stress. An extreme example quoted by Fieldhouse (1995) are the varied food avoidances among the women of the southern Indian state of Tamil Nadu; during lactation, for example, women should avoid meat, eggs, rice, dhal, chillies, cow's milk, sardines, fruits, potato, yam, cashew nuts and onions. These avoidances would compound with previous restrictions during pregnancy and this could have serious nutritional consequences. There is a widespread belief among various peoples that sick children should not be fed or should only be offered very restricted diets, thus potentially precipitating protein energy malnutrition. There is also a widespread belief that many adult foods, especially meat and fish, are unsuitable for young children. This leaves only the starchy staple foods with their problems of low energy and nutrient density as the major permitted food at this time of high physiological demand for energy and nutrients.

If most dietary taboos are not usually associated with any major adverse nutritional consequences, then why should nutritionists and nutrition educators study them? They provide an insight into a culture and some understanding is necessary if the general philosophy of giving advice that is culturally compatible is to be maintained. If advice is given that involves breaking an important dietary taboo then the credibility of the adviser may be damaged and their advice ignored.

If a taboo is nutritionally only marginally detrimental, neutral or perhaps even beneficial in its impact, then, no matter how bizarre or irrational it may seem, the cultural choice of the client should be respected. Some of the practices of the adviser may seem equally bizarre to the client. If a taboo is manifestly harmful, the aim of the adviser should be to eliminate the harmful impact with the minimum disruption to the cultural life of the client.

The conclusion that a taboo is harmful should be based on a wide analysis of its impact. Fieldhouse (1995) used the example of the Hindu sacred cow to make this point. There are nearly 200 million cows in India and yet their slaughter for food is generally forbidden even in times of famine. Is this illogical? Is it harmful? He points out that cows provide milk and their dead carcasses provide leather and are used as food by the lower castes. Cows provide the oxen traditionally vital for Indian agriculture; cow dung is also a major source of fuel and fertilizer in rural India. Yet they scavenge much of their food which is basically inedible to humans. The conclusion that this taboo is harmful is now less secure, and the value of the taboo in preventing destruction of these valuable and well-adapted animals in adverse conditions is, at least, arguable.

Taboos are often derived from some religious commandment, be it in the religious book of the group, the oral mythology or the edict of some historical religious leader or teacher. Many theories as to their origins exist, such as in the list below. Each can give plausible explanations of some taboos and often these different theories can be used to give equally plausible explanations of the same taboo.

- *Aesthetic.* Particular animals are rejected because of the perceived unpleasant lifestyle of the animal. For example, some people consider the flesh of the mackerel as low prestige or inferior because they regard the mackerel as a scavenger. All meat may be rejected because of the perceived cruelty involved in rearing and slaughter.
- *Health and sanitation.* There may be a belief that there is, or was, some inherent logic underlying the exclusion of particular foods on health grounds. In effect, it is suggested that taboos originate from avoiding foods that are harmful. For example, the

Jewish prohibitions against shellfish consumption may have been prompted by the risk of poisoning by the toxin produced by the plankton species *Gonyaulux tamarensis* that the shellfish may have consumed (see Chapter 19).
- *Ecology.* There is said to be some underlying environmental logic behind a particular prohibition. The exclusion of meat and fish at particular times to conserve stocks is an obvious example. The avoidance of meat by some present-day vegetarians to prevent inefficient use of grain and thus to increase world food availability would be another.
- *Religious distinction.* Taboos serve to demonstrate the separateness of a religious group from non-believers, and the self-restraint required to obey them may serve as a symbol of piety and obedience to the religious leaders.

The avoidance of pork by Jews is a very well-known taboo and each of the above theories can be used to explain its origins. Consider the following.

- *Aesthetic.* The pig is widely viewed as a dirty and scavenging animal even by people who value its flesh. Jewish dietary law states that only animals that have cloven hooves and that chew the cud are clean and therefore edible. The pig is considered unclean and therefore inedible.
- *Health and sanitation.* Pork is a source of a parasitic worm that causes the disease trichinosis. Is this the origin of the Jewish taboo against pork which is shared by other Middle Eastern peoples? Opponents of this theory argue that this is merely a later attempt at scientific rationalization. The risk of trichinosis has also been used as an argument against horsemeat consumption in France.
- *Ecology.* It is suggested that supernatural prohibitions against the consumption of pork arose because the desert conditions of the Middle East were unsuitable for efficient pig rearing. Proponents of this theory argue that taboos rarely involve abundant species that can be eaten with no threat to total food supplies.
- *Religious distinction.* It is suggested that the pork taboo was originally part of a relatively lax and general prohibition against 'imperfect' animals, including flightless birds and shellfish. Its symbolic importance was heightened when Syrian invaders forced Jews to eat pork as a

visible sign of submission; so, when Jews regained their independence, strict pork avoidance came to symbolize their Judaism and their opposition to pagan rule.

Key points

- People will normally eat only things that they recognize as food and things that they see as culturally acceptable and appropriate.
- Many religions have taboos against the consumption of particular foods, but a religious context is not always present.
- People will often go to great lengths to avoid breaking a taboo, and there is little need for external compulsion to ensure compliance.
- Some examples of taboos in western Europeans might be vegetarianism and the avoidance of horsemeat in Britain. Perhaps even the avoidance of breastfeeding in public could be classed as a taboo.
- In general, the permanent religious taboos seem to have few adverse nutritional consequences. Multiple taboos imposed at times of physiological stress – including childhood, pregnancy and illness – may have greater potential to do harm.
- Dietary advisers need to be aware of taboos and avoid giving advice that would require breaking a taboo.
- There are several theories about the origins of taboos.
  - An animal or fish becomes taboo because of its unpleasant or 'dirty' lifestyle.
  - They originate because the avoidance confers some biological or ecological benefit, such as avoidance of a foodborne disease or ecological damage.
  - They are a mechanism for binding a religious group together and distancing them from non-believers.

Effects of migration on eating habits

Migrant groups are frequently used by epidemiologists when they try to distinguish between the environmental and genetic influences on the disease patterns of populations (see Chapter 4). Migrants may also suffer from nutrition-related problems that may be much rarer both in their native homeland and among the indigenous population of their new homeland. For example, migrants to the UK from the Indian subcontinent in the 1970s suffered from mini epidemics of *rickets*, a condition that had been largely eliminated in the white population. These Britons of South Asian origin also have much higher rates of *type 2 diabetes* than the rest of the population, and partly as a consequence of this have much higher mortality from coronary heart disease (see Chapter 17). It is, therefore, useful to try to establish and understand trends and patterns to the changes in dietary habits that inevitably occur after migration, in order to answer questions like these.

- What factors influence the speed of change?
- Why is the health record of migrant groups often worse than that of the indigenous population?
- Are there any measures that might facilitate the healthful assimilation of migrant groups into their new environment?

Why should change occur at all? Culture, including food habits, is a learned phenomenon rather than something that is innate or biologically determined. Culture is transmitted between generations by the process of socialization. There is an inherent tendency of cultures to change over time. Although conflicts will inevitably arise between traditional influences and influences from the new culture, this process of change is almost inevitably greatly hastened by migration and exposure to the different cultural practices of the indigenous population. *Acculturation* is the term used to describe this acceleration of cultural change that occurs when different cultures interact. Both indigenous and migrant cultures are likely to be changed by their interaction, but migrants may feel the need to adopt aspects of the indigenous culture to facilitate their acceptance and assimilation into their new country.

Paradoxically, every culture also has a built-in resistance to change. Culture is mostly internalized – routine activities done unthinkingly in a particular way because that is the way they have always been done. After migration, however, there is repeated exposure to different culture practices, and familiarity may eventually lead to acceptance of initially strange and alien practices as normal. Dietary practices of the indigenous culture that are inconsistent with the values and beliefs of the migrants' culture may be the slowest to be adopted and also those most likely to cause social divisions within migrant communities or families. For example, migrants may be most reluctant to absorb dietary practices that would involve breaking of the food rules of their religion. The older, more conservative, migrants will probably be most resistant to such changes and may also be hostile to changes in the behaviour of younger, less ethnocentric members of their community or family. Dietary practices of migrants that are inconsistent with the values of the indigenous culture may also be a source of considerable friction between migrants and their fellow citizens. For example, Moslem and Jewish rules concerning the slaughter of animals have in the past provoked hostility in Britain from people concerned about animal welfare.

Bavly (1966) analysed changes over three generations in the diets of immigrants to Israel. She considered that the following factors had a major accelerating effect on the speed at which change occurred:

- marriage between different ethnic groups
- the homemaker working outside the home
- children receiving nutrition education at school
- children having school meals
- nutrition education via the media for immigrants of European origin.

Although this work was done some time ago, these specific influences given by Bavly may be generalized to factors that increase interaction with the indigenous population and increase familiarity with, and understanding of, indigenous dietary practices. Conversely, any factors that tend to isolate the migrant from the indigenous population and culture may be expected to slow down acculturation, such as:

- an inability to read or speak the new language, restricting interaction at the personal level and restricting access to the media
- cultural beliefs that discourage the homemaker from independent socializing outside the family
- religious beliefs and dietary rules that are at odds with the dietary practices of the indigenous majority
- living within a fairly self-contained immigrant area with shops that are run by fellow migrants and where familiar foods and even native language media are available.

Many of these isolating influences would apply to many new immigrants from the Indian subcontinent to Britain.

Migration is often prompted by the attraction of improved economic opportunities, and this encourages much migration from developing to industrialized countries. Thus large-scale migration is often accompanied by a complete change of social structure from a rural agrarian to a Western industrial type of society. In the rural agrarian community, society is likely to be based on extended and close-knit family groupings with a constant flow of food between families and individuals. In Western industrialized societies, this informal family and community support may no longer be available because they are organized into relatively isolated family groups, food is normally shared only with the immediate family, and this sharing may help to define the family. These changes in social organization may mean that, in times of hardship, the missing informal neighbourhood and family support will have to be replaced by formal charitable or state welfare support. The impact of such changes may be ameliorated where movement is into an established ethnic community.

Migrants from a rural food-orientated economy may suddenly be confronted with a cash-dominated economy. Family incomes of new immigrants are likely to be relatively low (inappropriate skills, language problems, discrimination, etc.). This combination of low income and lack of experience in cash budgeting may make them unable to cope adequately, even though the income may be technically adequate. An educational induction programme might reduce the impact of this potential problem. Food selection for migrants may be complicated by the unavailability of recognizable traditional foods and even where they are available, they may be relatively expensive because of their specialist nature. Advertising pressures may encourage the excessive consumption of foods that are high in palatability and prestige but of relatively low nutritional value. Social and cultural pressures may discourage migrant women from breastfeeding their infant although UK women of the major ethnic minorities are more likely than white British women to breastfeed (Chapter 16).

Migration from a rural agrarian society in a developing country to a Western industrialized society will probably be associated with overall trends that are similar to the worldwide changes that accompany increasing affluence. The traditional starchy and predominantly vegetarian diet is likely to diversify, become more omnivorous, and sugars and fats will progressively replace some of the starch. The diseases associated with nutritional inadequacy will decline but the chronic diseases of industrialization will almost certainly become increasingly prevalent.

Wenham and Wolff (1970) surveyed the changes in the dietary habits of Japanese immigrants to Hawaii and their descendants. Japanese migrants began arriving in Hawaii at the end of the nineteenth century to become plantation workers in Hawaii. The typical Japanese diet at this time was high in carbohydrates, and predominantly a rice and plant food diet. The major animal foods would have been fish and other seafood. Initially these migrants maintained their traditional diet; many regarded their stay in Hawaii as temporary and ate frugally in order to save for their return to Japan. After the annexation of Hawaii by the USA in 1898, these Japanese migrants started working outside of the plantations and businesses specializing in the importation of traditional Japanese foods sprang up. Initially this resulted in increased consumption of imported and high-status Japanese foods. As these Japanese foods became cheaper, their status diminished and came to be regarded as old-fashioned by many younger Japanese who preferred to eat American foods. (Note that a recent rapid influx of migrants into the UK from new EU countries in eastern Europe has similarly led to the opening of many shops specializing in the sale of eastern European foods in areas where large numbers of these migrants have settled.)

Wenham and Wolff describe how, among the Japanese migrants to Hawaii, the traditional Japanese social structure – with its strong family tradition, worship of ancestors and subordination of personal desires to the welfare of the family – was replaced by a society more fragmented and oriented to personal freedoms. The traditional Buddhist restrictions on the consumption of meat became weaker as meat was plentiful in Hawaii.

Public education seems to have been a catalyst for change among the second generation as the schools encouraged them to change their food and other habits. There also seems little doubt that the Second World War accelerated the 'Americanization' of Japanese in Hawaii. Wenham and Wolff describe a Japanese wedding in Hawaii before the war as being typically Japanese in character, with no wedding cake, but by 1945 the food at such a wedding was likely to be much more cosmopolitan but with a Western wedding cake as the highlight.

Wenham and Wolff concluded in 1970 that the Japanese in Hawaii could be classified into three groups:

- a traditional group of mainly older people who maintained a very Japanese cuisine
- a group that, despite being relatively acculturated, still consumed Japanese foods on some occasions
- an 'Americanized' group who rejected their Japanese heritage and the foods associated with it.

There may now exist a further category of Japanese–Americans who are moving back to traditional foods for health reasons and to reaffirm their ethnic identity (i.e. for reasons of self-actualization).

Williams and Qureshi (1988) suggested a similar 'four-generation' concept that could be a useful way of explaining some of the variations in food choices within any particular ethnic minority group in the UK.

- *First generation A* – made up of migrants who arrived as dependant relatives of migrant workers. They are usually retired and prefer to eat their native foods.
- *First generation B* – migrants who arrived as workers. They are usually aged 21–65 years and they accept both native and British foods.
- *Second generation* – young people who went to school in Britain and in many cases were born here. They prefer the new diet and may strongly resist attempts to force them to consume their native diet, which is alien to them.
- *Third generation* – children who were born in Britain, who feel British but who have become interested in tracing their ethnic roots. They accept both British and native foods.

Key points

- The disease patterns of migrants provide information on the relative importance of genetic and environmental factors in the aetiology of diseases.
- Migrants often have poorer health than other members of the new community.
- Migrants tend to gradually adopt elements of the diet and lifestyle of their new country – they tend to acculturate.
- The indigenous population may also adopt some elements of the migrant culture and diet.
- Changes will be slowest where the dietary practices of the indigenous population are in conflict with the values and beliefs of the migrants (e.g. where they would involve breaking a religious taboo).
- The adoption of change by some migrants may be a source of conflict with their parents and elders.
- Anything that increases interaction between the migrants and the indigenous population and familiarizes the migrants with the indigenous diet will tend to speed up the rate of change (e.g. women working outside the home and children taking school meals).
- Anything that prevents interaction will slow down the rate of acculturation. Examples are language barriers, restrictions on women working and socializing outside the home, and living within a fairly self-contained immigrant community.
- Migrants to an industrialized country from a rural area with an agricultural food-based economy may find it difficult to cope with the new cash-based economy, particularly as their incomes are likely to be relatively low.
- Several stages in the acculturation process have been recognized.
  - People who have recently migrated may initially try to stick closely to their familiar diet and people who migrate later in life may remain in this category for the rest of their lives.
  - Younger adult migrants who enter employment will become familiar with the new diet and tend to eat both the new and traditional foods.

→

Key points *continued*

- - Children of migrants who attend school in the new country may become so acculturated that they prefer the new diet and resist eating their traditional foods, perhaps to increase their sense of belonging and acceptance by their peers.
  - Descendants of migrants born or brought up in the new country may seek out their ethnic roots and eat foods associated with these roots to reaffirm their ethnic and cultural identity.

'GATEKEEPER' LIMITATIONS ON AVAILABILITY

The housewife has traditionally been regarded as the family gatekeeper regulating the availability of food to her family. If most food is eaten within formal family meals, and if food purchasing and meal construction are largely the province of the housewife, then she has the potential to impose limitations on the availability of foods to the other family members. The personal beliefs and preferences of the gatekeeper may greatly affect their choices and thus the diet of the whole family. A vegetarian gatekeeper may effectively impose vegetarianism on other family members or conversely, a non-vegetarian gatekeeper might refuse to provide a vegetarian alternative to a family member who would wish to be vegetarian. Convenience of preparation may affect the choices of the gatekeeper. Appreciation or criticisms by other family members will feed back and also be an important influence on her future choices.

A number of social changes in industrialized countries might be expected to have undermined the traditional gatekeeper role of wives and mothers.

- More food tends to be eaten outside the home or is purchased by the individual consuming it.
- Ready-made versions of dishes that have traditionally been home-made shift control over composition from the housewife to the food manufacturer.
- Other family members are more likely to participate in the shopping and food preparation.

- Within the home, there is more snacking or 'grazing' on self-selected foods available in the larder or refrigerator and fewer formal family meals.

Despite a diminution in this gatekeeper role of the mother, even within a traditional two-parent family it may still be quite considerable. Certainly much food advertising is still directed towards the gatekeeper housewife. Advertisers stress factors like the convenience of foods to a busy housewife and provide images of wives and mothers who have served the promoted food receiving acclaim from an appreciative and therefore loving family. Nicolaas (1995) conducted a survey of a representative sample of 2000 British adults on their attitudes to cooking and their cooking behaviour. This survey showed a marked divergence between attitudes and actual behaviour and suggested that the traditional gatekeeper role of the oldest adult female was still at that time largely intact in British families. Almost all the participants thought that it was important that both sexes had basic cooking skills and to teach their children how to cook. Almost all agreed with the proposition that boys should be taught how to cook. When questioned about their actual behaviour, however:

- 80 per cent of women but only 22 per cent of men claimed to prepare every meal in their household
- 3 per cent of women and 18 per cent of men admitted to never preparing a meal.

Most of the women who never prepared a meal were in the 16–24 age group, and the frequency in this age group was similar to that of young men. The complete data set strongly suggests that the majority of young people in this age group who live with their parents rely on their mothers to cook for them. In older age groups there is an even greater difference between male and female responses than those summarized above for the total sample. When adult men and women live together as partners it is usually the woman who does most of the cooking.

Catering managers may exert a considerable gatekeeper influence over those living in institutions such as hospitals, prisons, retirement homes, boarding schools and to a lesser extent those taking lunches at school or workplace. Older people living at home may have inexpensive weekday main meals delivered to them by a 'meals on wheels' service. The Caroline Walker Trust (CWT, 1995) has suggested nutritional standards and sample menu plans for 'meals on wheels' and meals provided in residential homes for the elderly.

If a person is subject to the gatekeeper influences of someone from a different cultural background, then he or she may effectively be subject to a double dose of limitation due to cultural availability. The gatekeeper may offer only foods that are personally culturally available and only some of these may be culturally available to the consumer. Unless caterers make special provision for cultural/ethnic minorities then this may severely restrict the real choices of such people (e.g. hospital patients from minority groups).

Even those people seemingly immune to the influence of gatekeepers – such as the affluent person living alone – may still use staff dining facilities in the workplace. They may have limited time available for food preparation or low incentive to cook just for themselves. They may thus rely heavily on commercially preprepared meals or restaurants.

Key points

- Wives and mothers have traditionally been the gatekeepers in western European families, but anyone who caters for someone else is acting as a gatekeeper.
- Despite major social changes, the gatekeeper role of women is largely intact in British families and women are still largely responsible for selecting and preparing the family meals.
- Gatekeepers can have almost total control over what some people eat, so their scope for making dietary changes may be dependent on the goodwill and co-operation of their gatekeeper.
- The range of food that is truly available may be considerably narrowed if a person is reliant on a gatekeeper from a different cultural background.
- Almost everyone is subject to some gatekeeper influences.

3

METHODS OF NUTRITIONAL ASSESSMENT AND SURVEILLANCE

Introduction and aims of the chapter	64	Anthropometric assessment in adults	86
Strategies for nutritional assessment	64	Anthropometric assessment in children	92
Measurement of food intake	65	Estimating fatness in animals	94
Tables of food composition	72	Biochemical assessment of nutritional status	95
Dietary standards and nutrient requirements	75		
Clinical signs for the assessment of nutritional status	85	Measurement of energy expenditure and metabolic rate	98

INTRODUCTION AND AIMS OF THE CHAPTER

This chapter deals with some of the methods used by nutritionists and dieticians to assess and monitor the nutritional status and nutritional well-being of individuals and populations. These methods range from the high-precision methods of the analytical chemist (e.g. in determining the composition of foods) to the inevitably much less precise methods used in the social and behavioural sciences (e.g. the use of questionnaires to assess physical activity levels or to qualitatively categorize individuals according to their intake of particular foods or nutrients). All of these approaches have their role to play and the full range of these methods is necessary to study all of the different aspects of nutrition.

The first aim of this chapter is to cover the range of methods available for nutritional surveillance and assessment:

- how they are conducted
- their strengths and limitations
- their general theoretical bases

- the circumstances in which different methods are more or less appropriate.

This is a first step towards successful use of these methods.

Another aim is to give readers a sufficient insight into the methods of nutritional surveillance to enable them to read and interpret the literature critically. An understanding of the relative strengths and the limitations of the methods used is essential for any critical evaluation of the conclusions drawn from data reported in scientific papers and major survey reports. Some perception of the errors inherent in methods of measurement is necessary for realistic appraisal of the results that they produce. Many of the most widely used methods in human nutrition have inevitable shortcomings that can reduce their reliability and sometimes undermine their validity.

STRATEGIES FOR NUTRITIONAL ASSESSMENT

There are two ways of approaching the assessment of dietary and nutritional status.

- *Nutrient intake.* One can try to determine whether the nutrient intake (or nutrient supply) is adequate to meet the expected needs of the individual or group under investigation. In order to make this assessment one needs three key tools:
  - a method of measuring the amounts of foods being eaten (or perhaps the available food supply)
  - a way of translating these amounts of foods into quantities of energy and essential nutrients (i.e. tables of food composition)
  - some yardstick of adequacy that can be used to determine whether the measured intakes of energy and essential nutrients are sufficient for that individual or group. These standards of dietary adequacy are called *dietary reference values* (DRVs) in the UK and the terms *recommended dietary/daily allowance* (RDA) have been widely used elsewhere, including the USA. Measured intakes may also be compared to other guidelines aimed at optimizing long-term health and reducing the risk of chronic disease, and these are also covered by the term DRV.

- *Observations and measurements.* One can study the individuals concerned to try to determine whether they have been receiving adequate amounts of energy and essential nutrients. The three types of indicator that can be used to make this assessment are as follows.
  - *Clinical signs.* One can look for clinical signs of malnutrition or the symptoms of a nutrient deficiency.
  - *Anthropometry.* One can make anthropometric measurements such as body weight and height and then either compare these measurements to appropriate standards or monitor changes within the individual or group over time.
  - *Biochemical assessment.* One can make biochemical measurements, usually on blood or urine samples, that indicate either general nutritional status of the donor or the status with regard to any specific nutrient.

MEASUREMENT OF FOOD INTAKE

Measures of food intake have a variety of purposes, such as:

- to assess the adequacy of the diets of populations, groups or individuals and to identify any problem nutrients
- to relate dietary factors in populations or individuals to disease incidence or risk factors (e.g. plasma cholesterol concentration)
- to compare the diets of different countries, regions and socioeconomic groups and different age and ethnic groups
- to monitor changes in the diets of populations, groups or individuals over time and thus, for example, monitor the effectiveness of nutrition education programmes.

Population or group methods

Food balance sheets

These are used to estimate the average per-capita food and nutrient consumption of nations (see Figure 3.1 for a summary). Food balance sheets usually yield no information about distribution within the population. They will not show up, for example, regional differences in nutrient intakes, socioeconomic influences on nutrient intakes, or age and sex differences in nutrient intakes.

Domestic food production is first estimated. Governments and international agencies (e.g. the Food and Agriculture Organization of the United Nations, FAO) routinely make estimates of total crop yields and total agricultural production of countries. Any food imports are added to this total and any exports are subtracted from it. Allowance is made for any change in food stocks within the country during the period. This estimate of food available for human consumption must then be corrected for wastage and any food not consumed by humans, such as animal fodder and pet foods. Such methods allow crude estimates of population adequacy and allow crude comparisons of actual intakes with nutrition education guidelines to be made. They also enable international comparisons to be made. For example, one could compare the average per-capita energy intake of different populations or relate average per-capita sugar consumption to rates of dental caries in different populations.

Home-produced food and small-scale production sites will be one potentially large source of error in

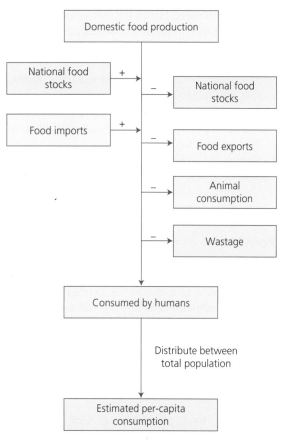

Figure 3.1 Schematic diagram to illustrate how food balance sheets can be used to estimate per-capita food consumption in a country.

these estimates. Wastage will be difficult to estimate accurately and is likely to depend on the affluence of the population – the rich are expected to waste more than the poor. Within the European Union, construction of national food balance sheets has been complicated by the introduction of the single market with the consequent reduction in checks on movements of food between member states.

The average intakes of residents of an institution can similarly be estimated from the amount of food entering the institution over a period of time.

Household budget surveys

The National Food Survey (NFS) of the UK is an example of a national household survey that was undertaken annually for about 60 years. This survey ended in 2001 when it was replaced by the Expenditure and Food Survey (EFS) – which was an amalgamation of the NFS and another national survey that had been running since 1957, the Family Expenditure Survey (FES). The EFS ran from 2001 to 2007 when it was slightly modified again and renamed the *Living Costs and Food* (LCF) *module* of a wider Integrated Household Survey. The nutrition and food-related data of both the EFS and the latest version of this survey, the LCF module, are published by the Department for Environment, Food and Rural Affairs (DEFRA) under the title Family Food. These surveys provide an important historical record of changes in the British diet over more than 70 years; MAFF (1991) reviewed the changes recorded in the first 50 years of the National Food Survey. Data from the earlier surveys are still available from the DEFRA website.

In the National Food Survey, one member of a nationally representative survey of 7000–8000 households was asked to record in a diary all food entering the household for human consumption during one week; both amounts of food and expenditure on it were recorded. Records were collected at different times throughout the year and home-grown food was included in the log. Up to 1992 no information was collected about alcoholic drinks, soft drinks (soda) or confectionery (candies) as these are often purchased by individual family members. From 1992 onwards those purchased for home consumption were recorded and the nutritional analyses presented both including (total household food and drink) and excluding these products (household food excluding soft drinks, alcohol and confectionery); this enabled comparisons to still be made with results from earlier years. For most of its existence no detailed information was collected in the NFS on meals eaten outside the home; merely the number of such meals consumed by each family member was recorded. In the later years of the survey some information on meals eaten outside the home was recorded and reported separately from household food and drink.

The Family Expenditure Survey which also finished in 2001 used a similar sized representative sample to that of the NFS. In this survey, every household member aged over 16 years was issued with a diary and recorded all expenditure including food expenditure, but amounts of food were not recorded. The recording period was 14 days and once again the sampling was spread throughout the year.

The Expenditure and Food Survey used similar representative samples of UK households to those used in the two surveys it replaced. The recording period in this survey was 14 days and all household members aged 7 years or over completed a diary. Each person's expenditure on all items including food and drink was recorded and where possible amounts of food purchased also recorded; where this was not possible (e.g. food eaten out) amounts were estimated using standard portion sizes. Information was also recorded concerning the composition of the household, the ages and sexes of the family members and their ethnic origin, the family's income and socioeconomic status, and the region of the country in which they lived.

The latest version of all these surveys, the LCF module, contains the following three elements.

- *A household questionnaire.* This collects details of the family relationships, ethnicity, employment details and ownership of household durable items. It also records regular payments made by all households, including housing costs and utility bills, as well as large amounts spent on infrequently purchased items like cars, holidays and home improvements.
- *An individual survey for each household member over 16 years of age.* This records details of their income from employment, welfare payments and assets. When combined this also gives an overview of the household income.
- *A diary like that described for the EFS.* Details of expenditure over a 2-week period are recorded, including food expenditure.

When data from the old National Food Survey and Family Expenditure Survey were compared, substantial differences in estimates of food expenditure between the two surveys were found (Paterakis and Nelson, 2003). The data from the EFS were considered by DEFRA in 2003 to be more comparable with the older FES than the NFS. Complex adjustments were applied to the results of the EFS to make them comparable to those obtained from the NFS and so enable historical comparisons to be made and trends followed; details of this adjustment procedure can be found in DEFRA (2003).

The results of the Living Costs and Food survey and its antecedents can be used for many purposes such as those listed below. Many other countries also conduct household budget surveys which can be used for some or all of these functions depending on exactly how they are conducted.

- The UK household budget surveys can be used to monitor changes in UK food purchasing practices over time. They can thus, for example, be used to monitor the effects of health promotion campaigns, price changes, the effects of 'food scares' (like the BSE crisis in the UK) and to correlate changes in diet with changes in measures of health and disease. In Chapter 5, these surveys are used to quantify some of the major changes in the British diet over recent decades, such as the massive switch from animal-derived cooking and spreading fats to those made from vegetable oils. Changes in the scope and execution of these surveys over time have to be borne in mind and allowed for when making historical comparisons.
- These surveys provide information about regional differences in dietary habits within the UK. These data may be of use in trying to explain some of the regional differences in the health and disease patterns within the UK.
- They provide information on differences in food purchasing practices of different ethnic groups within the UK.
- They provide information on seasonal patterns of food purchasing.
- They provide information about differences in the diets of different socioeconomic groups. One can compare the diets of rich and poor, the diets of young and old, the diets of the employed, unemployed and retired. One can compare diets of households with their 'reference adults' in different occupational categories.
- These household budget surveys give information about how food purchasing and eating habits differ according to family structure. One can compare the diets of single-adult or two-adult families with those that have varying numbers of children.
- It is possible to make crude estimations of the supply of energy and essential nutrients in UK diets and thus the probable levels of dietary

adequacy and highlight nutrients whose intakes may be less than satisfactory. One can also make crude estimations of the degree to which current diets comply with current dietary guidelines. One can monitor how intakes of nutrients are changing with respect to both standards of adequacy and dietary guidelines for the prevention of chronic disease.

There are a number of errors and uncertainties when these household budget surveys are used to quantify what people eat, and some of these are considered below.

• These surveys do not measure what people eat, they measure what they buy. Differences in wastage rates and preparation practices will not show up. For example, if a family buys 500 g of meat but trims the fat off before they eat it, this will give the same record as another family that buys this meat and eats all of the fat. Similar temporal changes in food preparation practices may also occur but not show up in these surveys.
• Families may change their purchasing behaviour during the survey period. They might buy more food than usual, and this tendency may be proportionately greater in lower income groups.
• A survey may not be truly representative of the whole population. Some groups are excluded from these surveys, such as the single homeless and those low-income families housed 'temporarily' in bed and breakfast type accommodation. Some poorer groups may be deterred from participating in the survey because of embarrassment about the diet they can afford. According to DEFRA (2004), only 60 per cent of those families selected for the Expenditure and Food Survey responded – which was a lower response than for previous such surveys.
• No attempt is made to record distribution of the purchased food between family members, although assumptions about wastage, distribution and losses of nutrients during cooking and preparation are made in order to estimate individual intakes of food and nutrients. These surveys can only estimate average consumption per person. One consequence of this is that, for example, the average per-capita expenditure on food decreases with increasing family size, partly

because children tend to eat less than adults do (it may also be more economic to buy in bulk).
• When the recording is done by a single family member, as with the old National Food Survey, then other family members may buy snacks, drinks and sweets that they consume outside the home and which go unrecorded in the household log. This should be less likely with the replacements because all family members keep an expenditure diary.

Finally, Paterakis and Nelson (2003) noted marked differences in the food expenditure data provided by the old National Food Survey and the Family Expenditure Survey. They noted that there were also substantial differences in time trends between the two surveys which could lead to different conclusions regarding changes in consumption patterns. This means that the absolute values recorded by any household budget survey will certainly be affected by differences in methodology, making comparisons between surveys problematic (e.g. comparing results from countries within the EU). Even within countries, conclusions about temporal changes in food purchasing, one of the major strengths of these surveys, may also vary according to the precise methodology.

Individual methods

Individual methods of assessing food intake may either involve prospective recording of food as it is eaten or may assess intake retrospectively by the use of interviews or questionnaires. These methods, almost inevitably, rely to a large extent on the honesty of the subjects.

Retrospective methods

Twenty-four hour recall has frequently been used to retrospectively assess the food and nutrient intakes of subjects. An interviewer asks subjects to recount the types and amounts of all food and drink consumed during the previous day. This recalled list is then translated into estimates of energy and nutrient intakes by the use of food tables. The method has been used in large-scale epidemiological surveys where large numbers of subjects need to be dealt with quickly and cheaply and where precision in assessing the intake of any individual is deemed not to be essential. The method requires relatively little commitment from the subject, so co-operation rates tend to be good. As the assessment is retrospective, subjects do not alter their intakes in response to monitoring. Some of the limitations and sources of error in this method are listed below.

- *Memory errors.* Subjects are likely to forget some of the items that have been consumed. This method tends to significantly underestimate total calorie intake and seems to particularly underestimate, for example, alcohol intake. This method, even when used with probing to try to improve memory, probably under-records energy and most nutrients by at least 20 per cent. This makes any assessment of the prevalence of dietary inadequacy using this method highly suspect.
- *Quantification errors.* It is difficult to quantify portions in retrospect. It may be particularly difficult for the very young and the very old to conceptualize amounts. Several lists of standard portion sizes have been published. An example is the standard guide to UK food portion sizes by Crawley (1994), with lists of weights of individual items (like chocolate bars) and average UK portion sizes for many foods. The Food Standards Agency in the UK has sponsored research to produce up-to-date information on average food portion sizes and a preliminary report was published in 2008 (www.food.gov.uk/multimedia/pdfs/reviewportions.pdf). Food models or photographs are sometimes used to aid this quantification process; subjects are shown photographs of various portions and asked to indicate which is closest to the one they ate, and a weight for this portion is given. Nelson *et al.* (1997) have published a photographic atlas of food portion sizes.
- *Intra-individual variation.* Intake may not be representative of the subject's usual intake. The day chosen for the record may not be typical of the subject's usual daily intake. Weekend and weekday intakes may be very different in some subjects. Illness or stress may affect the appetite of a subject. Some social occasion or event may exaggerate the subject's usual intake. Even where subjects are of regular habits and no particular

factors have distorted that day's intake, the intake of many nutrients tends to fluctuate quite markedly from day to day, so one day's intake cannot be taken to represent the subject's habitual intake.
- *Interviewer bias.* Any interview-based survey is susceptible to bias. The interviewer may encourage subjects to remember particular dietary items more than others and thus may obtain a distorted picture of the real diet. If the interviewer indicates approval or disapproval of certain foods or drinks this may also encourage distorted recall. It requires skill and training to take a proper diet history.

It might seem logical to extend the recall period if one wishes to get a more representative picture of a subject's usual dietary pattern but one would, of course, expect memory errors to increase exponentially as the recall period is extended. It is possible to use a succession of 24-hour recalls to get a more representative picture of an individual's habitual intake. To try to get a more representative picture of a dietary pattern, detailed *dietary histories* may be taken by interview or more frequently food frequency *questionnaires* may be used. The investigators may be interested in the intakes of particular nutrients, so the frequency of consumption of the types of food that contain these nutrients may give a useful indication of the usual intake of that nutrient. For example, assessing the frequency, types and amounts of fruit and vegetables consumed would be a useful guide to vitamin C or β-carotene intakes. Food frequency questionnaires are not suitable for assessing actual intakes of nutrients but are useful for categorizing individuals into low, medium and high intakes for any selected nutrient.

Prospective methods

The *weighed inventory* requires that the subjects weigh and record all items of food and drink consumed over a predetermined period (a week is often used). The operator must then translate this food inventory into nutrient intakes using food tables. Household measures (cup, spoon, slice, etc.) can be recorded in a *food diary* rather than subjects being required to weigh everything. This would clearly involve some loss of accuracy in determining the size of portions of many food items. These prospective methods have the advantage of being direct, accurate, current and of variable length, enabling more representative assessments of average intakes to be made. Some disadvantages of these methods are listed below.

- Subjects may still forget to record some items they consume, especially snacks.
- The methods are labour-intensive for both subject and operator, and considerable motivation and skill on the part of the subject are required for accurate and complete recording. Participation rates may therefore be low and this may make the population sampled unrepresentative of that being surveyed.
- This type of recording usually requires that subjects be numerate and literate. In order to obtain records from subjects who do not have these skills, a variety of methods have been tried. For example, subjects can photograph their food and drink; subjects have been given balances that have a tape recorder incorporated so that the subject's oral description of the weighed food can be recorded.
- Prospective methods may be invalidated if subjects modify their behaviour in response to monitoring, in an attempt to impress the operator, or to simplify the recording process, or simply because their awareness of their food and drink intake has been heightened by the recording process. There is evidence, for example, that subjects involved in clinical trials may conform to the recommended diet more closely on recording days.

Discussion

All of the methods of recording food intake so far described require that the estimated amounts of food eaten be translated into amounts of energy and nutrients by the use of some food composition database – paper-based food tables or a computerized version of the database. With *duplicate sample analysis*, a duplicate sample of all food eaten is prepared and may be subject to direct chemical analysis. This method does not therefore have to depend on the use of a food composition database. Use of food tables may, for example, overestimate the intake of labile vitamins such as vitamin C in people relying on hospital or other institutional food

that has been kept hot for extended periods. For example, Jones *et al.* (1988) found very low vitamin C intakes among a group of long-stay hospital patients when assessed by analysis of representative samples of the food eaten. These intakes were much lower than would have been obtained using conventional food tables. The study indicated that prolonged warm holding of food was an important factor in this low intake and suggested it might also apply to other heat-labile nutrients. This method is obviously labour-intensive, expensive and requires good analytical facilities. It is most appropriately used in a metabolic research setting.

Box 3.1 gives a summary of the relative advantages and disadvantages of retrospective and prospective methods of dietary assessment.

Box 3.1

Relative merits of retrospective and prospective methods of measuring food intake

Problems with all methods

- *Honesty.* Most methods rely on the honesty of subjects. Records that are clearly invalid may need to be identified and excluded, e.g. recorded energy intakes that are below 1.2 times the basal metabolic rate in non-dieting subjects.
- *Under-recording.* For one reason or another, most methods tend to under-record energy intakes and there is considerable evidence that this under-recording is more pronounced in the obese.
- *Intra-individual variation.* One assumes that the intake of nutrients during the monitored period is representative of habitual intakes. It will require several days of monitoring to get a reasonable assessment of habitual intakes for most nutrients. For some nutrients (e.g. vitamin A) where intra-individual variation is particularly great, it may require longer.
- *Population sampling bias.* When sampling populations one assumes that the sampled group is representative of the total test population. The more commitment and skill a method requires, the less likely this is to be

→

true. Some groups may be difficult to access (e.g. homeless people, disabled people). When sampling some groups (e.g. young children or the very elderly) one may need a proxy to carry out the recording.

- *Food table errors.* All methods except duplicate sample analysis rely on the use of food tables. This may be a particular problem in determining intakes of residents in hospitals and care institutions where prolonged warm holding may destroy much of the heat-labile vitamin content.
- *Coding errors.* When subject records are analysed, some entries may be ambiguous and misclassified.

Retrospective methods

Advantages

- Tend to be quick and cheap.
- Require little commitment from subjects so tend to get high participation rates.
- Honest subjects cannot change their habits in response to monitoring because the food has already been eaten.

Disadvantages

- Very prone to memory errors.
- Retrospective quantification can be difficult.
- Interviewer may influence the subject.

Prospective methods

Advantages

- Greater accuracy because less prone to memory and quantification errors.

Disadvantages

- Require commitment and competent record-keeping by subjects and this can reduce participation rates.
- Subjects may deliberately or unwittingly modify their eating in response to monitoring, e.g. to simplify recording, to deceive/impress the recorder, or simply because of heightened awareness.

Even though the weighed inventory method of assessing food and nutrient intake is very labour-intensive, it has been used to periodically assess the diets and nutritional status of large representative samples in various age groups of the UK population. Since 1986 there has been a series of National Dietary and Nutritional Surveys (the NDNS programme). These surveys aim to provide comprehensive information of the dietary habits and nutritional status of Britons in all age groups and to monitor changes in these over time. This programme began in 1986–7 with the collection of data for the first NDNS survey of British adults aged 16–64 years (Gregory *et al.*, 1990) and this has been followed up by a series of other reports on other age groups:

- the NDNS survey of children aged 1.5–4.5 years (Gregory *et al.*, 1995)
- the NDNS survey of people aged over 65 years (Finch *et al.*, 1998)
- the NDNS survey of young people aged 4–18 years (Gregory *et al.*, 2000).

A second NDNS survey of adults aged 19–64 years was published in five volumes between 2003 and 2004 with the fifth being a summary volume (Hoare *et al.*, 2004). The first survey of Gregory *et al.* (1990) was jointly commissioned by the then Ministry of Agriculture, Fisheries and Food (MAFF) and the Department of Health. The Food Standards Agency took over responsibility for the NDNS programme and all five volumes of the second adult survey can be accessed free online. These surveys have other elements that are relevant to diet, health and nutritional status as well as the results of the weighed inventory. For example, the second survey of adults (summarized by Hoare *et al.*, 2004) consists of the following elements:

- a dietary interview that determines information on the eating and drinking habits and sociodemographic information such as age, marital status, social class, etc.
- a 7-day weighed inventory of all food and drink consumed
- a 24-hour urine collection with analysis
- physical measurements such as height, weight (for calculation of body mass index, BMI), waist and hip circumference and blood pressure
- a 7-day activity diary
- a blood sample which was analysed for biochemical indicators of nutritional status and plasma cholesterol levels.

In 2006, the Food Standards Agency and the Department of Health decided to move to a rolling programme of surveys and they commissioned phase 1 of this programme to run from 2008 to 2012. This programme uses representative samples of the British population aged over 18 months (annual sample size 1000–1500 people). The nature of the data collected is similar to that recorded in earlier NDNS reports, although the food intake is now recorded using a 4-day estimated food diary rather than a weighed intake as used previously, and information on oral health is also recorded. The first results from this rolling programme were published in early 2010; these can be found in Bates *et al.* (2010), which also includes details of the methodology and intended purposes of the programme.

Key points

- Measurements of food intake can be used to assess dietary adequacy, to monitor the degree of compliance with nutritional guidelines, to make comparisons between groups or populations, and to relate dietary variables to disease risk.

- The food intakes of populations can be determined by the use of food balance sheets, by representative surveys of household food purchases, or even by assessing the individual diets of representative population samples.

- Individual methods of assessing food intake can be retrospective or prospective. One can either ask subjects to provide information about what they have already eaten (e.g. 24-hour recall or a food frequency questionnaire) or ask subjects to record what they eat over a period (e.g. 7-day weighed inventory).

- Choice of method of measuring food intake will depend on the time and resources available and on the purpose of the measurement.

- The advantages and disadvantages of the various methods are listed in Box 3.1.

- Up to 2006, the NDNS programme in the UK used a weighed inventory together with blood and urine analysis and physical measurements to periodically assess the dietary practices and nutritional status of the different age groups of Britons.   →

Key points *continued*

- In 2006, a rolling programme of NDNS surveys was started using representative samples of the British population aged over 18 months. This rolling programme uses a 4-day estimated food diary rather than the 7-day weighed intake of earlier NDNS reports from specific age groups.

TABLES OF FOOD COMPOSITION

Food tables are an essential tool of both nutritional surveillance and research. Printed food tables contain lists of thousands of foods and the amounts of each nutrient in a standard amount (100–g) of each food are given. They are based on standard databases such as that maintained by the US Department of Agriculture (USDA) or the UK Nutrient Databank that has been maintained by the Food Standards Agency and is published in book form as McCance and Widdowson's *The Composition of Foods* (a sixth summary edition published in 2002 plus 10 supplemental publications). To translate food intakes into nutrient intakes with such printed tables is very tedious and time-consuming. The content of each nutrient in the consumed portion of each food has to be calculated from the tables and eventually the total consumption of each nutrient determined.

Nowadays, the information contained within these printed tables is available on computer software, requiring the investigator merely to key in the foods and portion sizes and the computer will then automatically translate these into nutrient intakes. The program will not only accept weights of foods but will translate household measures or descriptive portions into estimated weights of food or use a database of standard portion sizes that have been incorporated into the software. These programs will also calculate the nutrient intakes as proportions of the standard reference values appropriate for a subject whose size, age, sex, activity level and reproductive status have also been entered.

Both forms of these tables are the result of thousands of hours of meticulous analytical work. To give the nutrient contents of 1000 foods requires more than 30000 individual determinations and many more if individual amino acids and fatty acids are included. Discussion of these analytical methods would be inappropriate for a book of this type. A few of these methods are discussed in other sections of the book; for example, determination of the energy content of foods is outlined in Chapter 6 and the protein content of foods in Chapter 10.

The analytical methods used to determine the nutrient content of foods are often extremely precise with a very low level of measurement error. However, several sources of error are inherent in the use of food tables and these may produce errors and uncertainties that are orders of magnitude greater than the errors in the analytical methods. Food tables can give only an indication of the typical or average composition of a food, and that may in some cases be very different from the actual composition of the sample of food that has been eaten. Some of these errors are considered below.

Food tables: problems and errors

Limited range of foods covered by the tables

The major databases mentioned above each contain several thousand different food items including many menu items from the major restaurant chains. Despite this, there will inevitably be foods eaten that are not specifically listed in the printed tables or computer software that uses them. In such circumstances the operator either has to find alternative sources of information (such as nutritional information on the food label) or has to judge what food is the nearest equivalent in the food tables. For example, British tables do not specifically list goat meat which is frequently used as an ingredient in curries, so one would use the composition of generic curried meat. Continued innovation on the part of food manufacturers and increased availability of foods from different parts of the world mean that this will be an ongoing problem. In fairness, it must be said that it is now quite difficult to find gaps in the British database; the range of foods listed has increased very substantially over the last couple of decades and includes many foods traditionally eaten by Britain's long-established minority ethnic communities. However, the recent influx of migrants from eastern Europe may not yet have been fully catered for in the existing database.

Recipe variations

Many dishes are extensive mixtures of foods, but it is often not practicable in diet records or histories to obtain the precise mixture of ingredients used in the preparation of a particular dish. Even though the food tables may list this dish, the recipe used for the analysis in the tables may be quite different from that consumed. Thus, for example, bolognese sauce is something that will be listed in the tables but will vary markedly in its composition from cook to cook. The range and proportions of the main ingredients used, leanness of the meat, the amount of thickening agent (e.g. flour) and salt, and the proportion of water may all vary considerably. When estimating the nutrients in something like a slice of pie, the proportions of crust and filling used by the analyst may be very different from those actually eaten.

Brand variations

Different brands of the same commercially prepared foods will vary, and the composition of any single brand may vary significantly from batch to batch. There are several brands of 'baked beans canned in tomato sauce'; food tables can only give an average or typical composition.

Nutrient supplementation

Some foods may be supplemented with nutrients. This could be a source of considerable error if the supplementation in the analysed and eaten foods is different.

Biological variations

Just as different brands and recipes of prepared foods will vary in their composition, so different varieties of natural foods will vary in their composition. There may even be marked variation, particularly seasonal variation, within the same variety. Rump (buttock) steak from different cattle may have markedly different proportions of fat and lean. The vitamin C content of apples varies greatly between different varieties. The vitamin D content of milk varies between summer and winter. Once again, food tables can only indicate an average or a typical composition.

Method and duration of storage

The nutrient content of foods changes during storage. Milk left in strong sunlight loses much of its riboflavin (vitamin B$_2$). The vitamin C content of main crop potatoes after 8–9 months of storage will be only about a quarter of that when they were freshly dug. Stale vegetables generally may have lost much of their original vitamin C. Foods on which mould has grown may acquire dietetically significant amounts of vitamin B$_{12}$. Warm holding of food prior to its being eaten may lead to destruction of most of the heat-labile vitamins in it.

Vitamin precursors and variants

Some vitamins may have several different chemical forms or may be present in the form of a precursor. When the vitamin activity of foods is assessed, the activity contributed by the different chemical forms must be estimated and added together. Vitamin A activity in food is due to vitamin A itself (retinol), the plant-derived pigment β-carotene and other plant pigments that have vitamin A activity, such as cryptoxanthine and α-carotene (see Chapter 12). The niacin (vitamin B$_3$) derived from food may come either directly from vitamin in the food or indirectly by conversion of the amino acid tryptophan to niacin.

Bioavailability of vitamins and minerals

Food tables can give a precise estimate of the amount of a chemical in a food but they give no indication of its bioavailability; that is, how much of it is absorbed in the gut. Iron from meat is much better absorbed than that from vegetable sources, and iron absorption is increased by vitamin C and alcohol but decreased by fibre and tannin. The calcium in milk is much better absorbed than that in most other foods. There may also be uncertainty about the biological activity of some forms of a vitamin in foods (e.g. some of the conjugated forms of folic acid).

Use of table and cooking salt

Salt is frequently added to food during cooking and at the table. Use of a weighed inventory and standard food tables is therefore regarded as an unreliable means of estimating an individual's total salt intake.

Calcium from bone

Pieces of bone in meat and fish may greatly increase the calcium content. With canned fish, the bones are softened and made more readily edible. Cutting meat with a saw produces powdered bone that sticks to the meat and is eaten.

Contamination from utensils and cooking vessels

Contact of foods with processing machines or with cooking utensils may significantly affect the content of metallic elements. Cooking or brewing in iron pots may enhance the iron content of foods very considerably.

Minerals from cooking water

Cooking food in hard tapwater may significantly increase the content of calcium and other minerals. Variation in the content of drinking water may greatly affect the intake of some minerals, such as fluoride.

Minerals from adhered soil

Contamination of food with small amounts of soil may affect its mineral content.

Key points

- Food tables contain lists of the nutrient contents of thousands of foods.
- They can be used to convert amounts of food into amounts of energy and nutrients.
- They can give only a typical or average composition and are prone to many limitations and sources of error.
  - Some foods may be missing from the database.
  - There are biological variations in the composition of plants and animals and brand and recipe variations in the composition of prepared foods.
  - Variation in the method and duration of food storage will affect its composition.
  - The tables take no account of variations in the bioavailability of nutrients.
  - The mineral content of foods may be affected by the addition of salt, the presence of adhered bone, mineral content of the cooking water, or leeching of minerals into food from utensils and storage vessels.

DIETARY STANDARDS AND NUTRIENT REQUIREMENTS

Origins of dietary standards

In 1941, the National Research Council in the USA established a committee whose brief was to produce a comprehensive set of dietary standards. These standards were intended to be a yardstick against which diets or food supplies could be assessed to determine their likely adequacy. The first printed version of the standards appeared in 1943 and they were called *recommended dietary allowances* (RDAs). These were the first official and comprehensive set of dietary standards. Many other governments and international agencies now regularly publish their own dietary standards and the American RDAs have been revised and re-published regularly since 1943. The 1943 edition of the American RDAs covered just six pages and dealt with only ten nutrients; the current British version of these standards (COMA, 1991) covers more than 200 pages and deals with more than 30 nutrients.

The first British RDAs were published by the British Medical Association in 1950. In 1969 the first truly official set of UK standards was published by the then Department of Health and Social Security (see Webb, 1994).

Definitions and explanations

For the purposes of setting dietary standards, the population is divided up into subgroups. Children are divided up into bands according to their age and sex. Adults are subdivided according to their age and sex with separate standards for pregnant and lactating women. Then standards are set for energy and each nutrient for each of these population subgroups; see Table 3.1 for a plan of the layout of these tables. These standards are intended for use with healthy people and they make no allowance for the effects of illness and injury on nutrient needs.

The RDA in the USA is the suggested average daily intake of a nutrient that is sufficient to meet the needs of nearly all healthy people in that age and sex grouping. It represents the best estimate of the requirement of those people in the population with a particularly high need for that nutrient. The RDA does *not* represent the minimum requirement when it is used to assess the diets of individuals. Rather, it should be thought of as lying within a 'zone of safety'; the further intake is below the RDA then the greater is the risk of deficiency, and the further above the RDA then the greater is the risk of toxicity.

Until 1991, the British standards were also termed RDAs and this term is still to be found on British food labels where it refers to the RDA set by the European Union. However, in the current version of the British standards (COMA, 1991), the general term *dietary reference values* (DRVs) is used to cover a range of differently defined values. The word 'recommended' has been specifically avoided as it was felt to wrongly imply that the RDA represented the minimum desirable intake for health and thus that intakes below the RDA represented inadequacy. Instead of a single RDA, three reference values are offered for protein, vitamins and minerals in these new British standards. The highest of these

Table 3.1 Plan of the layout of tables of dietary standards (e.g. RDA or RNI)

Age group (examples)	Nutrient 1	Nutrient 2	Nutrient 3	Nutrient 4, etc.
0–3 months				
7–10 years				
11–14 years (female)				
19–50 years (male)				
50+ years (female)				
Pregnant				
Lactating				

RDA, recommended daily allowence; RNI, reference nutrient intake.

three values is called the *reference nutrient intake* (RNI). It is essentially equivalent to the old RDA as it also represents the estimated requirement of those people with the highest need for the nutrient. In practice it is still the value that is used in most circumstances. The other two DRVs offered for these nutrients are the *estimated average requirement* (EAR), which is self-explanatory, and the *lower reference nutrient intake* (LRNI). The LRNI is the best estimate of the requirement of those individuals with a low need for the nutrient. The requirement of almost everyone should lie within the range covered by the LRNI and the RNI.

COMA (1991) assumed that the variation in nutrient requirements of individuals follows a normal distribution (Figure 3.2). Approximately half of the population should require more and half less than the estimated average requirement. The standard deviation is a precisely defined statistical measure of the variation of individual values around the mean or average in a normal distribution. The RNI is set at a notional two of these standard deviations above the mean and the LRNI a notional two standard deviations below the mean.

The characteristics of a normal distribution mean that the requirements of all but 5 per cent of the population should lie within the range covered by

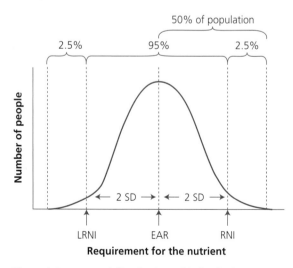

Figure 3.2 A normal distribution of individual nutrient needs within a population with the theoretical positions of the UK dietary reference values. EAR, estimated average requirement; LRNI, lower reference nutrient intake; RNI, reference nutrient intake.

two standard deviations on either side of the mean. Thus the RNI and LRNI should theoretically satisfy the needs of 97.5 per cent and 2.5 per cent of the population respectively. The RNI should represent an amount sufficient, or more than sufficient, to satisfy the needs of practically all healthy people (essentially the same definition as the American RDA). The panel considered that the RNI would be sufficient for everyone despite the theoretical risk that 2.5 per cent of the population are not provided for. There is considerable lack of precision in most of the estimations used to set dietary standards and so they tend to be set generously.

COMA (1991) suggested that this system of standards allows for more meaningful interpretation of measured or predicted intakes that fall below the RNI (i.e. the old RDA). At the extremes, if an individual's habitual intake is below the LRNI then the diet is almost certainly not able to maintain adequacy as it has been defined for that nutrient. If intake is above the RNI then it is safe to assume that the individual is receiving an adequate supply. In between these two extremes the chances of adequacy fall, to a statistically predictable extent, as the intake approaches the LRNI; for example, an individual consuming the EAR has a 50 per cent chance of adequacy. Note that the iron requirements of women are an example where requirements for a nutrient are known not to be normally distributed; high iron losses in menstrual blood in some women skew or distort the distribution. Note that when interpreting the results of nutrition surveys (e.g. in Chapters 12 and 15), individuals with intakes below the LRNI are classified as having inadequate intakes and this definition is used to estimate the prevalence of dietary inadequacy for vitamins and minerals. While the LRNI is theoretically sufficient for 2.5 per cent of the population, it is unlikely that all of those with the lowest intakes will have the lowest needs.

The RDAs for energy have traditionally been set at the best estimate of average requirement, rather than at the upper extremity of estimated requirement. Whereas for most nutrients, a modest surplus over requirement is not considered likely to be detrimental, this is not so with excessive energy intake that may lead to obesity. Consistent with this traditional practice, the latest UK standards give only an EAR for energy. Any individual's energy requirement will depend on many factors, particularly his or her size and activity level, and appetite should ensure that adequate intakes of energy are consumed by healthy non-dieting subjects. The EAR for energy is set for a person of average weight and with a specified (low) level of physical activity.

The COMA panel considered that, for eight nutrients, they did not have sufficient information to estimate the rather precisely defined set of values discussed above. In these cases they merely suggested a safe intake: 'a level or range of intakes at which there is little risk of either deficiency or toxic effects'.

The 1991 UK standards also, for the first time, set reference values for the various fat and carbohydrate fractions, including dietary fibre. These values are clearly directed towards reducing the risk of chronic disease. At the time, this broke new ground for these standards because their traditional function has been solely to set standards of nutritional adequacy. COMA (1991) attempted to integrate the functions of standards of adequacy and that of nutritional guidelines aimed at reducing the risk of chronic disease. The reference values for fat and carbohydrate fractions are discussed in Chapter 4.

The formal and precise statistical definitions used by COMA should not be allowed to obscure the fact that judgement plays a major part in the setting of these values. The criterion that any dietary standards committee uses to define adequacy is almost inevitably a matter of judgement and opinion. There may also be considerable errors and uncertainties in estimating the average amount required to satisfy this criterion and in estimating the standard deviation of requirement. Any particular reference value is the consensus view of one panel of experts based on the information available to them and in the prevailing social, political and economic climate. There may be genuine differences of opinion between different panels of experts and probably even between the experts within any given panel. Any particular panel's reference values are likely to be the result of compromises between the differing views of its individual members. Some non-scientific considerations may also influence different committees to differing extents. Thus, the dairy industry might lobby for the calcium standard to be high, fruit growers lobby for a high vitamin C standard and meat and fish suppliers may be keen to keep the protein standard high. Where fruit is cheap

and plentiful a committee may be generous with vitamin C allowances because the cost of erring on the high side is perceived as minimal. However, where fruit is, for much of the year, an expensive imported luxury then a panel may be more conservative in their vitamin C standard.

In the USA, the recommended dietary allowances have been revised and republished nine times since the original 1943 issue; the last single-volume of RDAs was published in 1989 (NRC, 1989a). Since 1994, American and Canadian scientists have collaborated in updating and expanding the concept of the RDA and have issued a series of publications that have set a series of values in addition to the RDAs and given a detailed account of the evidence and rationale for the values for each nutrient. The term *dietary reference intakes* (DRIs) has been used to collectively cover this expanded set of dietary standards, as briefly defined below.

- The RDA is as defined previously.
- The *estimated average requirement* (EAR) is as used in Britain since 1991 and the term *estimated energy requirement* (EER) is the equivalent value used for energy.
- *Adequate intake* (AI) is the value used when an accurate RDA cannot be set and it is essentially the same as the 'safe intake' used in the British standards.
- The tolerable *upper intake level* (UL) is the highest average daily intake that is likely to pose no adverse risk to health to almost all individuals within the general population. This value was seen as a necessary addition because of the increased use of fortified foods and nutrient supplements.
- The *acceptable macronutrient distribution range* (AMDR) is the range of intakes of energy-yielding nutrients like carbohydrates and fats that are associated with reduced risk of chronic disease while still providing adequate intakes of essential nutrients. These values are the American equivalent of the dietary reference values (DRVs) for the energy-yielding nutrients set by COMA in 1991, and in both cases they are set as percentages of energy intake.

There have been some very significant variations in these dietary standards over the years and there are still quite marked variations in the dietary standards used in different countries. Historical differences can be partly explained by the differences in scientific information available to panels, but current international differences are largely due to variations in the way the same information has been interpreted by panels of experts. There are several quite marked differences between the American RDA and the British RNI even though they are essentially equivalent in their definitions. In general, American RDAs are higher than UK RNIs, and Table 3.2 lists many examples of standards in Britain and the USA for adults aged under 50 years. The table shows, for example, that the American RDA for vitamin C is more than double the British RNI.

In Chapter 11, the huge historical variations in protein standards for children are reviewed and discussed. In Chapter 16, the differences in the current UK and US standards for pregnant women are highlighted and discussed. Table 3.3 shows the

European Union's RDAs used for food labelling purposes within the EU and thus found on many British food labels.

Uses of dietary standards

A set of dietary standards enables nutritionists to predict the nutritional requirements of groups of people or of nations. Governments and food aid agencies can use them to identify the needs of populations, to decide whether available supplies are adequate for the population to be fed, and to identify nutrients whose supply is deficient or only marginally adequate. They thus provide the means to make informed food policy decisions, for example decisions about:

- the amount and type of food aid required by a population or group

Table 3.2 The reference nutrient intake (RNI), lower reference nutrient intake (LRNI) and American recommended daily allowance (RDA) for selected micronutrients for adults aged 19–50 years

Nutrient	Male			Female		
	RNI	LRNI	RDA	RNI	LRNI	RDA
Vitamin A (µgRE/day)	700	300	900	600	250	700
Thiamin (mg/day)	1.0	0.6	1.2	0.8	0.45	1.1
Riboflavin (mg/day)	1.3	0.8	1.3	1.1	0.8	1.1
Niacin (mgNE/day)	17	11	16	13	9	14
Vitamin B_6 (mg/day)	1.4	1.0	1.3	1.2	0.9	1.3
Folate[1] (µg/day)	200	100	400	200	100	400
Vitamin B_{12} (µg/day)	1.5	1.0	2.4	1.5	1.0	2.4
Vitamin C (mg/day)	40	10	90	40	10	75
Vitamin D[2] (µg/day)	–	–	15	–	–	15
Vitamin E (mg/day)	> 4[3]	15	–	> 3[3]	15	–
Calcium (mg/day)	700	400	1000	700	400	1000
Chromium (µg/day)	> 25[3]	35	–	> 25[3]	25	–
Iron (mg/day)	8.7	4.7	8	14.8	8	18
Iodine (µg/day)	140	70	150	140	70	150
Magnesium (mg/day)	300	190	400	270	150	310
Potassium (mg/day)	3500	2000	4700	3500	2000	4700
Selenium (µg/day)	75	40	55	60	40	55
Zinc (mg/day)	9.5	5.5	11	7	4	8

[1] It is now recommended that women of child-bearing age should take 400µg/day supplement of folic acid.
[2] For vitamin D, in the UK it is assumed that most adults can make sufficient vitamin D when their skin is exposed to summer sunlight; the US value has recently been raised.
[3] Safe intake, used where the panel felt that they did not have enough information to set formal RNI and LRNI.

Table 3.3 Recommended daily allowances (RDAs) used for food labelling within the European Union

Nutrient	'Labelling' RDA
Vitamin A (μgRE)	800
Thiamin (mg)	1.4
Riboflavin (mg)	1.6
Niacin (mgNE)	18
Vitamin B_6 (mg)	2
Folate (μg)	200
Vitamin B_{12} (μg)	1
Biotin (μg)	150
Pantothenic acid (mg)	6
Vitamin C (mg)	60
Vitamin D (μg)	5
Vitamin E (mg)	10
Calcium (mg)	800
Iodine (μg)	150
Iron (mg)	14
Magnesium (mg)	300
Phosphorus (mg)	800
Zinc (mg)	15

- the priorities for agricultural production and food imports
- which foods might be beneficially subsidized or, if foods need to be rationed, the size of rations needed
- whether to fortify foods with added vitamins or minerals.

Similarly, they are used by institutional caterers (e.g. in prisons or schools), and those catering for the armed forces to assess the food requirements of their client population and to check proposed menus for their nutritional adequacy. Those devising therapeutic or reducing diets can check any proposed diets for adequacy using these standards.

These standards provide the means to assess nutritional adequacy after an intake survey. They can be used as a yardstick for assessing the adequacy of groups or individuals. In the UK, the LRNI is regarded as the cut-off point below which an individual intake is classified as inadequate, and the RNI would indicate that intake is certainly adequate. In the USA, the RDA is set such that if

the average intake of a group is above the RDA then this should ensure that practically all members of the group are obtaining an adequate amount for their needs; and in the UK the RNI is regarded as a similar ideal minimum for the group average. When individuals are being assessed, it must be borne in mind that intakes below the RDA (and RNI in the UK) do not necessarily represent inadequacy. When assessing the nutritional adequacy of individuals, it should also be remembered that there are very substantial fluctuations in the intakes of some nutrients from day to day. The habitual intake of the individual over a period of some days should ideally be the one that is compared to the standard.

Most consumers will be exposed to these standards when they are used on food labels to give a meaningful indication of nutrient content. Absolute numerical amounts of nutrients will be meaningless to most consumers, but when they are expressed as a percentage of the RDA they become more meaningful. COMA (1991) suggested that the EAR was the most appropriate reference value to use for food labelling in Britain. As Britain is a member of the EU, the RDAs seen on British food labels are actually set by the European Directive on food labelling and these differ slightly from the recommendations in the UK DRV (see Table 3.3 for a list of these labelling RDAs). In the USA, a *reference daily intake* (RDI) is used to indicate essential nutrient content on food labels. It is set at the higher of the two adult RDA values and referred to on the label as simply the 'daily value'.

Inaccurate standards

Setting dietary standards too low will negate their purpose. A yardstick of adequacy that does not meet the criterion of adequacy is of no use – and is probably worse than no standard at all because it will tend to induce a false sense of security and complacency. A serious underestimate of the standards for a nutrient could result in a nutrient deficiency being falsely ruled out as the cause of some pathology. Perhaps more probably, it could result in a suboptimally nourished group being reassured as to their dietary adequacy.

Such arguments about the obvious hazards of setting standards too low mean that there will be a strong temptation to err on the side of generosity when setting them. This may be especially true in affluent countries where the need to avoid waste of resources is less acute. There are, however, potentially adverse consequences that may result if these standards are set too high.

- Some nutrients (e.g. iron and some fat-soluble vitamins) are toxic in excess. An unrealistically high standard value might encourage sensitive individuals to consume hazardous amounts.
- High standard values may encourage the production or supply of unnecessary excesses, which will result in wasteful use of resources.
- High standard values may create the illusion of widespread deficiency and result in unnecessary and wasteful measures to combat an illusory problem.
- Unreasonably high 'target' values for particular nutrients may lead to distortion of the diet, with deleterious effects on the intake of other nutrients.
- If an unreasonably high standard results in the classification of large numbers of people as deficient, but there are no other manifestations of deficiency, then this may discredit the standards and may, in the longer term, undermine the credibility of nutrition education in general.

Some of the consequences of earlier exaggeration of human protein requirements are discussed in Chapter 11, which might serve as a case study to illustrate most of these points.

Defining requirements

The first problem that has to be confronted when devising a set of dietary standards is to decide on the criteria that will be used to define adequacy. Ideally one would like to determine the intake that maximizes growth, health and longevity, but these are not a readily measurable set of parameters. *Overt deficiency* of a nutrient will often produce a well-defined deficiency syndrome so that the minimum requirement will be an intake that prevents clinical signs of deficiency. *Optimal intakes* are assumed to be some way above this minimum requirement. Subclinical indications of impairment or depletion of nutrient stores may occur long before overt clinical signs of deficiency. COMA (1991) decided

that the estimated average requirement (EAR) should allow for 'a degree of storage of the nutrient to allow for periods of low intake or high demand without detriment to health'. This is actually a rather loose (vague) definition and the committee had to translate it into a quantitative and measurable criterion case by case.

This problem of defining an adequate intake is well illustrated by the example of vitamin C. It is generally agreed that, in adults, around 10 mg per day of this vitamin is sufficient to prevent the deficiency disease *scurvy*. Below 30 mg/day, negligible levels of the vitamin are detectable in plasma. At intakes of between 30 and 70 mg/day, plasma vitamin levels rise steeply, and they start to plateau at intakes of between 70 and 100 mg/day. COMA chose an adult RNI of 40 mg/day because, at this intake, most individuals would have measurable amounts of vitamin C in their plasma that is available for transfer to sites of depletion. Essentially the same available data have resulted in an American RDA of 90 mg/day for men and 75 mg/day for women. Some people advocate daily intakes of gram quantities of this vitamin in order to maximize resistance to infection. COMA (1991) listed numerous suggested benefits of very high vitamin C intakes, yet none of these influenced their DRVs. The underlying criterion in setting the DRVs is dietary adequacy, even though the additional requirement for adequate stores represents a large safety margin over that required for minimal adequacy (i.e. prevention of scurvy).

The following sections cover the various methods that have been used to assess nutrient requirements and to set dietary standards for these nutrients. Examples of the use of each approach are also explained. Many readers may find it sufficient to select a small number of nutrients to use as illustrative case studies of how standards are set. Note that the method used to set the EAR for energy is explained in Chapter 7.

Deprivation studies

The most obvious and direct way of assessing the minimum requirement for a nutrient is to use an experimental diet that lacks the nutrient and see how much of it needs to be added to this diet to prevent or cure the signs of deficiency. Experiments in Sheffield, England, during the Second World War demonstrated that volunteers started to develop signs of the deficiency disease scurvy after a couple of months on a diet free of vitamin C. Intakes of around 10 mg/day were shown to prevent the development of scurvy and to cure the clinical signs. Thus 10 mg/day is the minimum requirement for vitamin C and COMA chose this as the LRNI for vitamin C.

Deprivation studies of this type may require the consumption of very restricted diets for long periods before clinical signs of deficiency develop in previously well-nourished adults. For example, it takes up to 2 years of depletion before such adults develop even limited signs of vitamin A deficiency. This is because the liver contains large amounts of stored vitamin A. The volunteers need to consume a very restricted and unpalatable diet for a long time and this may also have some adverse consequences on their long-term health. It would be ethically unacceptable to deliberately subject vulnerable groups, including children and pregnant or lactating women, to this type of deprivation. This means that the extra requirements of these groups usually have to be inferred from less direct methods.

As an alternative to controlled experiments it is possible to use epidemiological data relating average intakes of a nutrient to the presence or absence of clinical signs of deficiency in populations. For example, it has been observed that the deficiency disease *beriberi* occurs when average population intake of thiamin falls below 0.2 mg/1000 kcal (4.2 MJ) but when average intake is above this level beriberi does not occur.

Radioactive tracer studies

If a known amount of radioactively labelled vitamin, or other nutrient, is administered to a volunteer then, assuming that this labelled vitamin disperses evenly in the body pool of that vitamin, the dilution of the radioactivity can be used to estimate the total size of that body pool. A sample of plasma is taken and the amount of vitamin and the amount of radioactivity in the sample measured. The specific activity of vitamin in the plasma sample (i.e. the radioactivity per unit weight of vitamin) can be used to calculate the total pool size provided that

the amount of radioactivity administered is known. For example:

- administer 1 million units of radioactivity
- specific activity in sample is measured as 1000 units of radioactivity per mg of vitamin
- so radioactivity has been diluted in 1000 mg of vitamin (i.e. in a 1000 mg body pool of the vitamin).

If, after administration of a radioactive vitamin load, the body losses of radioactivity are monitored this will enable the rate of vitamin loss or depletion to be determined.

Using this approach, Baker *et al.* (1971) found that the average body pool of vitamin C in a group of healthy, well-nourished American men was around 1500 mg. On a diet without vitamin C, this pool depleted at a rate of around 3 per cent per day. This 3 per cent depletion rate is termed the *fractional catabolic rate* and was found to be independent of the pool size; that is, 3 per cent of whatever is in the body is lost no matter how much or how little is present in the body. When the body pool fell below 300 mg then symptoms of scurvy started to appear. The team estimated that, in order to maintain the body pool above 300 mg and thus prevent scurvy, their subjects needed to take in 9 mg/day (i.e. 3 per cent of 300 mg). This agrees very well with the *c*10 mg/day to prevent scurvy found in the much earlier depletion study in Sheffield.

Balance studies

These methods rely on the assumption that, in healthy, well-nourished adults of stable body weight, the body pool size of some nutrients remains constant. Healthy adults are, for example, in approximate daily balance for nitrogen (i.e. protein), calcium and sodium. Over a wide range of intakes and suitable measurement periods, the intake is approximately equal to the output. Any variations in intake are compensated for by changes in the rate of absorption from the gut, changes in the rate of excretion, or changes in the rate of metabolism. If, say, calcium intake is progressively reduced then initially losses of calcium in urine and faeces will also decline and balance will be maintained. Eventually, however, a point will be reached when balance can no longer be maintained and output starts to exceed input. It would seem reasonable to propose that the minimum intake at which balance can be maintained represents the subject's minimum requirement for calcium. Such short-term experiments do not exclude the very real possibility that long-term adaptation to chronically low calcium intakes will occur.

COMA (1991) assumed that the average daily loss of calcium via urine and skin in British adults was 160 mg/day. In order to replace this daily loss they estimated that an intake of 525 mg/day would be required, assuming that around 30 per cent of dietary calcium is absorbed. They chose this as the adult EAR for calcium. They added or subtracted 30 per cent to allow for individual variation and therefore came up with 700 mg/day and 400 mg/day as the RNI and LRNI respectively.

Factorial methods

Factorial calculations are essentially predictions of the requirements of particular groups or individuals taking into account a number of measured variables (or factors) and making a number of apparently logical assumptions. For example, during growth or pregnancy certain nutrients will be retained and accumulate in the growing body or pregnant woman. Knowing the rate at which these nutrients accumulate during pregnancy or growth, one can then make predictions of the amount required. For example:

Estimated requirement for pregnancy
= amount to achieve balance (from value for non-pregnant women)
plus
daily accumulation rate of nutrient during pregnancy × factor to allow for assumed efficiency of absorption and assimilation.

COMA (1991) predicted the increase in EAR for energy of women during lactation using the following factorial calculation:

Increase in EAR for energy during lactation
= average energy content of daily milk production × 100/80
(assuming 80% conversion of dietary energy to milk energy)
minus

an allowance for the contribution from the extra maternal fat stores laid down during pregnancy.

It should always be borne in mind that, no matter how logical they may seem, such values are theoretical predictions and they may not represent actual physiological need. Physiological adaptations may occur that will reduce the predicted requirement. For example, the efficiency of calcium and iron absorption from the gut increases during pregnancy (see Chapter 16).

Measurement of blood or tissue levels

COMA (1991) defined some reference values according to the intake required to maintain a particular circulating level or tissue level of the nutrient. As we have already seen, the LRNI for vitamin C is set at the intake that prevents scurvy (10 mg/day in adults). The RNI is set at a level that maintains a measurable amount of vitamin C in plasma in most adults (40 mg/day) and the EAR (25 mg/day) is set half way between the LRNI and the RNI.

The reference values for vitamin A in the UK are based on the intake that is estimated as necessary to maintain a liver concentration of 20 μg of vitamin A per gram of liver. To estimate the intake of vitamin required in order to maintain this target liver concentration, the panel had to perform quite an elaborate factorial calculation (summarized in Figure 3.3).

First they had to predict the size of the body pool required to achieve this liver concentration. They thus had to make assumptions about what proportion of the body is liver and about how the total body pool of vitamin A partitions between the liver and other tissues. The fractional catabolic rate of vitamin A has been measured at 0.5 per cent of the body pool lost per day, so an amount equivalent to 0.5 per cent of this estimated pool would have to be replaced each day. Finally, assumptions had to be made about the efficiency with which ingested vitamin A is stored in the liver in order to convert this replacement requirement into an intake requirement.

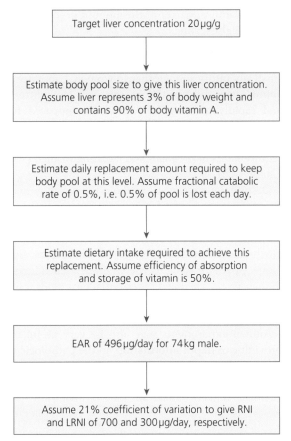

Figure 3.3 A scheme to illustrate the calculations and assumptions required to estimate the vitamin A intake required to maintain a designated liver concentration and thus to set the dietary reference values for vitamin A (after COMA, 1991). EAR, estimated average requirements; LRNI, lower reference nutrient intake; RNI, reference nutrient intake.

Biochemical markers

COMA (1991) used the intake required to 'maintain a given degree of enzyme saturation' as another criterion for determining reference values. An example of this is the use of the erythrocyte glutathione reductase activation test to assess and define nutritional status for riboflavin (vitamin B_2).

Glutathione reductase is an enzyme present in red blood cells whose activity is dependent on the presence of a cofactor (FAD) that is derived from riboflavin. The enzyme cannot function in the absence of the cofactor. In *riboflavin deficiency* the activity of this enzyme is low because of reduced availability of the cofactor. In red blood cells taken from well-nourished subjects, the activity of this enzyme will be higher because it is not limited by the availability of the cofactor. To perform the activation test, the activity of glutathione reductase is measured in two samples of red cells from the subject – one has had excess FAD added while the other has not. The ratio of these two activities is called the 'erythrocyte glutathione reductase activation coefficient' (EGRAC). It is a measure of the extent to which enzyme activity has been limited by riboflavin availability in the unsupplemented sample, and thus is a measure of the subject's riboflavin status. The RNI is set at the intake that maintains the EGRAC at 1.3 or less in almost all people. (See later in this chapter and in Chapter 13 for critical discussion of this cut-off value.)

Similar enzyme activation tests are used to assess status for thiamin (vitamin B_1) and vitamin B_6.

- Activation of the enzyme transketolase in red cells is used to determine thiamin status (a thiamin-derived cofactor is necessary for transketolase to function).
- Activation of the enzyme glutamic oxaloacetic transaminase in erythrocytes can be used to assess vitamin B_6 status.

Biological markers

Blood haemoglobin concentration has been widely used in the past as a measure of nutritional status for iron. It is now regarded as an insensitive and unreliable indicator of iron status for reasons such as those listed below.

- Haemoglobin concentration changes in response to a number of physiological factors such as training, altitude and pregnancy.
- Iron stores may be depleted without any change in blood haemoglobin concentration (see under 'biochemical assessment' later in this chapter for further discussion of iron status assessment).

Vitamin K status is frequently assessed by functional tests of prothrombin levels in blood. Prothrombin is one of several clotting factors whose synthesis in the liver depends on vitamin K as an essential cofactor. Thus in *vitamin K deficiency*, prothrombin levels fall and blood clotting is impaired. To measure the prothrombin time, excess calcium and tissue thromboplastin are added to fresh plasma that has been previously depleted of calcium to prevent clotting. The time taken for the plasma to clot under these conditions is dependent on the amount of prothrombin present, and thus on the vitamin K status of the donor. Anticoagulant drugs, like warfarin, work by blocking the effect of vitamin K. Prothrombin time is thus a useful way of monitoring vitamin K status, and thus of regulating drug dosage during anticoagulant therapy.

Animal experiments

Animal experiments are of limited value in quantifying the nutrient needs of human beings. They may even encourage widely erroneous estimates to be made. It is extremely difficult to allow for species differences in nutrient requirements and to scale between species as different in size as rats and people. The examples below illustrate some of the difficulties of predicting human nutrient needs from those of laboratory animals.

Most rapidly growing young animals need a relatively high proportion of their dietary energy as protein, but human babies grow more slowly and thus are likely to need proportionally less than most other young mammals. Rat milk has around 25 per cent of its energy as protein compared to only around 6–7 per cent in human milk. Predicting the protein needs of human children from those of young rats is likely to exaggerate the needs of children.

Pauling (1972) used the measured rate of vitamin C synthesis in the rat (which does not require dietary vitamin C) to support his highly controversial view that gram quantities of the vitamin are required for optimal human health. He scaled up the rat's rate of production on a simple weight-to-weight basis and estimated that rats of human size would make 2–4 g/day of the vitamin. He suggested that this gave an indication of human requirements. This procedure seems extremely dubious on several grounds. Consider the decision to scale up the rat's rate of vitamin C synthesis on a simple weight-to-weight basis. Vitamin needs may be more related to metabolic needs than simple body weight, and if one scales according to relative metabolic rate then one might predict that the human-size rat would only

make around a quarter of the amount predicted by body-weight scaling.

The expected nutritional burdens of pregnancy and lactation are also relatively much greater in small laboratory animals than in women. Laboratory animals have short gestations, relatively larger litters and rapidly growing infants when compared to human beings. Extrapolating from laboratory animals is likely to exaggerate any extra nutritional requirements of pregnant and lactating women (see Chapter 16).

Despite these reservations about the use of animal experiments to quantify human needs, they have played a vital role in the identification of the essential nutrients and their physiological and biochemical functions. Several of those awarded Nobel prizes for work on the vitamins used animals in their work. The need for essential fatty acids was, for example, demonstrated in the rat 40 years before unequivocal confirmation in an adult human being.

Animal experiments may also be very useful in providing in-depth information on the pathological changes that accompany prolonged deficiency and in determining whether prolonged marginal adequacy is likely to have any long-term detrimental effects.

> ### Key points
>
> - Dietary standards are yardsticks of nutritional adequacy, called 'dietary reference intakes' in the USA and 'dietary reference values' in the UK.
> - Reference values are set for each nutrient for each of the various age and sex groups within the population.
> - The RDA in the USA and the RNI (reference nutrient intake) in the UK represent an estimate of the requirements of those healthy people in the age group with the highest need.
> - The RNI is set at a notional two standard deviations above the estimated average requirement (EAR).
> - The LRNI (lower reference nutrient intake) is set at two standard deviations below the EAR.
> - The LRNI is the estimated requirement of those with the lowest need for the nutrient and thus is assumed to be insufficient to meet most people's needs.
>
> →

- The standards for energy are set at the estimated average requirement.
- The setting of dietary standards depends on the judgement of panels of experts and so they vary from country to country and vary over time.
- Reference values are very dependent on the definition of *adequacy* used.
- COMA (1991) defined the EAR as an amount that would prevent deficiency and allow some degree of storage. These standards can be used to:
  - assess whether food supplies or nutrient intakes are adequate
  - estimate the needs of groups or populations
  - check whether menus or prescribed diets are adequate.
- Use of RDAs on food labels makes nutrient contents more meaningful to consumers.
- On labels in the USA, the higher of the two adult RDAs is present as the 'reference daily intake', whereas in the UK the RDA set by the European Union is used.
- Standards that are set too low are obviously of no use, but setting values too high may also produce other more subtle problems.
- Many different methods can be used to define and determine what is an adequate intake of a particular nutrient, such as:
  - direct measurement of the amount needed to cure or prevent deficiency
  - use of radioactively labelled nutrient to measure body pool size and fractional catabolic rate or rate of excretion
  - estimation of the minimum amount necessary to maintain balance between input and losses of the nutrient
  - factorial estimates of the amount of nutrient required (e.g. to produce milk in lactation to support growth or growth of the products of conception in pregnancy)
  - estimates of the amount necessary to achieve a particular blood or tissue level, a specified level of enzyme activity, or some biological marker.
- Animal studies have been invaluable in *identifying* essential nutrients and the effects of deficiency but are of little value in *quantifying* human nutrient requirements.

CLINICAL SIGNS FOR THE ASSESSMENT OF NUTRITIONAL STATUS

Nutrient deficiencies ultimately lead to clinically recognizable deficiency diseases. Identification of the clinical signs usually requires little or no specialized equipment and is cheap, simple and quick, thus enabling assessment surveys to be conducted even in the most inaccessible places. Non-medical personnel can be trained to conduct clinical surveys of nutritional status by recording the presence or absence of various clinical signs from appropriate checklists. Some clinical signs that may indicate a nutritional deficiency are listed in Box 3.2.

Box 3.2

Clinical signs that may indicate a nutritional deficiency (one possible dietary cause is given in parenthesis)

Note that several of these symptoms can be indicative of more than one nutritional deficiency or they may indicate other non-nutritional conditions. They can be profitably used to construct screening checklists, which can be used to identify individuals in need of further investigation or to assess the level of nutrient deficiency in a population.

- Loose, hanging clothes or a wasted appearance (energy/protein deficit and weight loss)
- Loss of hair pigment and easy 'pluckability' (energy/protein deficit in children? – kwashiorkor)
- White foamy spots on the cornea (Bitot's spots – vitamin A)
- Dry and infected cornea (vitamin A)
- Oedema (thiamin, B_1 – beriberi)
- Several types of dermatitis (in skin exposed to sunlight, niacin – pellagra)
- Enlargement of the liver (energy/protein deficit – kwashiorkor)
- Loss of peripheral sensation (thiamin)
- Spongy, bleeding gums (vitamin C – scurvy)
- Angular stomatitis – spongy lesions at the corners of the mouth (riboflavin)
- Pale conjunctiva (iron-deficiency anaemia)
- Red inflamed tongue (riboflavin)
- Spontaneous bruising (vitamin C)

Box 3.2 *continued*

- Tiny subdermal haemorrhages or petechiae (vitamin C)
- Swelling of the thyroid gland in the neck or goitre (iodine)
- Bowed legs (vitamin D – rickets)
- Mental confusion (water – dehydration)
- Confusion or dementia (niacin)

The potential problem of population sampling bias as mentioned in Box 3.1 is one that can affect any type of dietary or nutritional survey. Those conducting the survey must take steps to actively ensure that the people assessed are representative of the whole population under investigation. Those most badly affected by deficiency diseases may well be those least accessible to the survey team – the weak, the frail, the elderly, pregnant and lactating women and babies are the least likely to be out and about. Sampling people in the street or those who are mobile enough to attend a centre may well overestimate the nutritional status of the population. This may be particularly important when clinical signs are used because they are often present only in people most severely affected by dietary deprivation.

The clinical signs of deficiency usually become recognizable only after severe and prolonged deficiency, so they are relatively insensitive indicators of nutritional status. It is generally assumed that suboptimal intakes of nutrients produce subclinical impairment of physiological functioning that occur long before disease becomes apparent. In surveys in affluent countries, very few cases of clinical deficiency would be found in most sectors of the population. Surveys that use clinical signs would therefore tend to provide only limited information about the nutrient status of the population – for example, that there are no deficiencies severe or persistent enough to induce overt clinical deficiency. Clinical signs are therefore not useful as early indicators of nutritional problems that can warn of the need to implement preventative measures. They may be much more useful in providing a quick guide to the extent of nutritional deficiency in less affluent countries, during famine, and even in high-risk groups in affluent countries – the homeless,

alcoholics, underprivileged children and the frail elderly.

Clinical signs tend to be qualitative and subjective. Any attempt to grade or quantify clinical signs is likely to depend on subjective judgements. For example, grading the severity of goitre (swelling of the thyroid gland due to iodine deficiency) depends on the judgement of the assessor about the degree of thyroid enlargement, so clinicians may produce considerably different grades for the same population.

Clinical signs are not very specific indicators of nutrient deficiencies. Some symptoms are common to several deficiency diseases and also to non-nutritional causes. Some form of dermatitis is, for example, common to several deficiency diseases and may also be induced by a variety of non-nutritional causes. Oedema may be a symptom of beriberi, protein-energy malnutrition, heart failure, kidney disease, etc.

ANTHROPOMETRIC ASSESSMENT IN ADULTS

Box 3.3 lists some of the anthropometric measures that may be used to assess nutritional status.

Box 3.3

Anthropometric measures used for nutritional assessment

Unintentional weight loss over 3 months

- Up to 5%: mild depletion
- 5–10%: moderate depletion
- Over 10%: severe depletion

Useful for screening new admissions to hospital or residential care homes.

Body mass index (BMI)

- Under 18.5 kg/m^2: underweight*
- 18.5–25 kg/m^2: ideal
- 25–30 kg/m^2: overweight
- 30+ kg/m^2: obese
- 40+ kg/m^2: severely obese

The standard way of classifying people on the basis of their height and weight.

→

Box 3.3 *continued*

* Note that until recently 20 kg/m² was used as the lower limit for normal and has recently been lowered to 18.5, but some of the sources used later in this book continue to use 20 kg/m² as the cut-off point for normal.

Demiquet index

An alternative to BMI in people who cannot stand erect, such as the elderly. Alternatively, demi-span or knee height can be used in regression equations to predict height and then BMI can be estimated.

Measures of mid or upper arm circumference

Mid-arm circumference (MAC)

Useful as a simple indicator of nutritional status when compared to standards or as an indicator of weight change when measured sequentially. Can be used in those confined to bed.

Mid-arm muscle circumference (MAMC)

MAC × (π × triceps skinfold)
Indicator of lean body mass or to monitor changes in it.

Arm muscle area

(MAMC)²/4π

Skinfold calipers

Measure skinfold thickness at several sites to indicate the amount of fat stored subcutaneously in these sites and then translate into an estimate of percentage body fat with a calibration chart or table. A more direct assessment of body fat than weight; particularly useful for athletes who have unusually high amounts of muscle for their weight.

Bioelectrical impedance

Pass a weak alternating current between two points on the body and the impedance (resistance) depends on the relative amounts of fat and lean in the body. Not strictly an anthropometric method but included here for convenience. Gives a rapid and direct estimate of body fat using an internal calibration with little technical skill required.

Body density

Fat is less dense than lean tissue. If one assumes that fat has a density of 0.9 kg/L and lean tissue 1.10 kg/L, then it is possible to estimate the percentage of body fat from the body density.

→

Box 3.3 *continued*

Not suitable for routine use. Traditionally the method used for calibration of other methods of measuring fatness (e.g. skinfold measurements and bioelectrical impedance). Volume is usually measured by underwater weighing which is technically difficult and requires specialist facilities.

Uses of anthropometric assessment

Anthropometry is the scientific study of the measurement of the human body. Anthropometric assessment means making nutritional assessment by means of physical measurements of body weight and dimensions. Body composition may be estimated from anthropometric measurements and this can have a variety of uses.

- It allows one to make an assessment of nutritional status. Anthropometric measurements can be used to detect undernutrition or obesity in adults and children and to indicate whether the growth of children has been satisfactory.
- It enables one to make more useful comparisons of metabolic rate between individuals or groups. Adipose tissue has a low metabolic rate, and so expressing metabolic rate per unit of lean body mass is more meaningful than simply expressing it per unit of total weight.
- Certain drug dosages may be calculated per unit of lean body weight.

Changes in body weight may be due to gain or loss of water, lean tissue and/or fat. Longitudinal measurements of body composition may help to decide the composition of any weight change. Most of the measures currently available for assessing body composition are relatively insensitive and thus could only be reliably used for this purpose if the weight change were substantial.

Height and weight

Body weight alone can only be a useful indicator of nutritional status in adults if it is measured repeatedly over a period. It can then, for example, be used to monitor changes in the nutritional status of patients in hospital or those living in residential homes for the elderly. Unintentional weight loss can be an indicator of disease or deteriorating nutritional status as a result of adverse socioeconomic status. Many hospital admission forms have a question about weight change in the previous 3 months (see Box 3.3) designed to help identify patients who are nutritionally 'at risk'.

An individual's 'ideal' weight will be very dependent on his or her height. In the past, weight-for-height tables were the most common way of assessing people's weight status. These tables list the desirable weight ranges for men and women of any particular height and age. Three desirable ranges would usually be given for each height for each sex depending on frame size – whether the person is of light, medium or heavy build. Obesity was then defined as more than 20 per cent over the person's ideal weight range and underweight defined as more than 10 per cent below the ideal weight range. The tables produced by the Metropolitan Life Insurance Company have been widely used for this purpose. Note that the original purpose of the tables was for commercial use in assessing actuarial risk in people taking out life insurance policies. They were produced by recording the heights and weights of large numbers of life insurance applicants and then relating initial weight to risk of dying (and thus claiming on the policy) in the succeeding years. These ideal ranges were those associated with the lowest death rates. People above or below these ranges (i.e. underweight or overweight) had higher death rates.

These tables are relatively cumbersome and inconvenient to use, especially as they require some assessment of frame size to be made. There are objective measures of frame size such as wrist circumference and elbow breadth which are not difficult to measure in a clinic or laboratory, but they add to the inconvenience of weight-for-height tables particularly for studies with large groups or populations.

The body mass index

The body mass index (BMI) has become the standard way of classifying adults using their heights and weights. This measure has been shown

empirically to be the best simple and quantitative anthropometric indicator of body composition and thus of nutritional status.

BMI = body weight (kg) *divided by* height squared (m^2).

Note that the BMI can be calculated from heights and weights in Imperial units using the following approximation:

BMI = 750 × weight (pounds) *divided by* height squared (in^2).

The normal range for the BMI was for many years set at 20–25 kg/m^2. Any value significantly below this range was taken to indicate underweight and values above would be considered to indicate varying degrees of overweight or obesity (see Box 3.3). This classification was still used in the NDNS survey of British adults (Hoare *et al.*, 2004) and in some other sources of population data (e.g. the NDNS survey of older adults of Finch *et al.*, 1998). In recent years there has been some reconsideration of where the lower level of normality should lie. Many people with a BMI slightly below 20 are perfectly well and healthy and have good appetites and apparently healthy diets. The range of normality has thus been extended to be from 18.5 to 25 kg/m^2.

The following is a system for classifying varying degrees of underweight using the BMI, after Heymsfield and Baumgartner (2006):

- <16 kg/m^2 – grade III protein-energy malnutrition
- 16–17 kg/m^2 – grade II protein-energy malnutrition
- 17–18.5 kg/m^2 – underweight
- 18.5–25 kg/m^2 – normal.

When the BMI is being used to classify people as underweight or too fat, then it is being implicitly assumed that variations in weight for a given height are primarily due to variations in adiposity – that heavy means fat and light means lean. This assumption generally holds reasonably well, but there are some circumstances where it clearly does not hold. Examples are given below.

- *Body builders*. People with very well-developed musculature will be heavy but have very low fat content. In this case their BMI may falsely indicate obesity. In the past, some very muscular American footballers were rejected for military service because they were heavy and so mistakenly classified as obese.

- *The elderly*. As people age, so the mass of muscle and bone in the body tends to fall and is replaced by fat. A group of elderly people will have a higher average body fat content than a group of young adults of the same height and weight. In elderly women, in particular, loss of lean tissue and bone mass may mean that the BMI remains within the normal range even though more direct measures of fatness may indicate excess adiposity.
- *Oedema and dehydration*. Changes in body fluid content can produce major changes in body weight without any change in body fat content. Excess accumulation of tissue fluid (oedema) can lead to a substantial increase in body weight and may obscure the person's malnourished state. Oedema is a common symptom of malnutrition and of many other conditions such as heart failure, kidney disease, liver disease and pregnancy. Oedema may be a major hindrance to the anthropometric assessment of nutritional status in hospital patients and malnourished children in developing countries.

Alternatives to height measurements

Accurate measurement of height requires that the subject be able to stand erect. In subjects who cannot stand erect, some alternative measure of skeletal size is needed. *Demi-span* is one such measure, being the distance from the web of the fingers (between the middle and ring fingers) and the sternal notch when the subject's arm is held horizontally to the side (with support if necessary). Some disabled people and many very elderly people are unable to stand upright for height to be accurately measured, so COMA (1992) recommended that demi-span measurements should be included in all nutritional surveys of older people.

The following equations are for estimating height (cm) from demi-span (cm) measurements in people aged over 55 years:

Height for men = (1.2 × demi-span) + 71
Height for women = (1.2 × demi-span) + 67.

This enables the BMI to be estimated from measurements of weight and demi-span. The Royal College of Nursing published a set of nutritional standards for elderly people (RCN, 1993). Webb

and Copeman (1996) have also compiled a list of anthropometric norms for elderly people. Demi-span measurements can also be used to derive indices with body weight, which are analogous to the BMI – the Mindex and the Demiquet index:

Mindex = weight (kg) *divided by* demi-span (m)
Demiquet index = weight (kg) *divided by* demi-span squared (m²).

Knee height is another way of estimating skeletal size but is used less frequently than demi-span. Knee height is measured in a seated position and is the height from the floor to the knee joint space. The following equations can be used to estimate full height (cm) from knee height (cm):

Height for men = 64.19 + (knee height × 2.03) − (0.04 × age)
Height for women = 84.88 + (knee height × 1.83) − (0.24 × age).

Skinfold calipers

The traditional method for more direct estimation of fatness in people is measurement of skinfold thickness using skinfold calipers. Spring-loaded calipers are used which exert a constant pressure on a fold of skin and the thickness of the skinfold is indicated on a meter. The thickness of the skinfold will be largely dependent on the amount of fat stored subcutaneously in the region of the skinfold. Skinfold thicknesses are measured at several sites and the assumption is made that the amount of fat stored subcutaneously at these sites (as measured by the skinfold thickness) will be representative of the total amount of body fat. Using the method of Durnin and Womersley (1974), skinfold thickness in millimetres is determined at four sites: over the triceps muscle; over the biceps; in the subscapular region; and in the suprailiac region. The total of these four skinfolds is then translated into an estimate of percentage body fat using a calibration table or formula. Figure 3.4 shows the relationship between the sum of these four skinfolds and percentage body fat (estimated by body density) in 17- to 29-year-old men and women, and Table 3.4 can be used to estimate percentage fatness from these four skinfolds. The single triceps skinfold thickness is sometimes used in nutritional surveys. It has the obvious advantage, in such circumstances, that it can be measured quickly and without the need for subjects to undress.

Some of the problems associated with use of skinfold calipers are summarized below.

- It is relatively time-consuming and subjects need to undress to have their skinfolds measured.
- It requires a great deal of skill and care to obtain accurate and reliable skinfold measurements.
- The process of translating skinfold measurements into estimates of fatness relies on calibration tables derived from body density measurements and so any errors in the use of density are also inherent in this method.
- There are considerable variations between individuals in the distribution of body fat, as well as pronounced inter-racial differences. Standards need to be appropriate for the racial group being assessed.

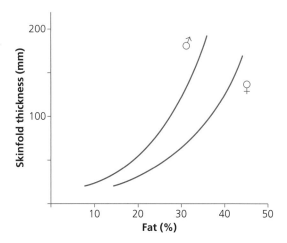

Figure 3.4 Relationship between caliper measurements of skinfold thickness at four sites and body fat content estimated from body density in young adults. Data from Durnin and Womersley (1974).

Table 3.4 Chart for converting the sum of four skinfolds into estimates of percentage body fat*

Skinfolds (mm)	Males (age in years)				Females (age in years)			
	17–29	30–39	40–49	50+	16–29	30–39	40–49	50+
20	8.1	12.2	12.2	12.6	14.1	17.0	19.8	21.4
30	12.9	16.2	17.7	18.6	19.5	21.8	24.5	26.6
40	16.4	19.2	21.4	22.9	23.4	25.5	28.2	30.3
50	19.0	21.5	24.6	26.5	26.5	28.2	31.0	33.4
60	21.2	23.5	27.1	29.2	29.1	30.6	33.2	35.7
70	23.1	25.1	29.3	31.6	31.2	32.5	35.0	37.7
80	24.8	26.6	31.2	33.8	33.1	34.3	36.7	39.6
90	26.2	27.8	33.0	35.8	34.8	35.8	38.3	41.2
100	27.6	29.0	34.4	37.4	36.4	37.2	39.7	42.6
110	28.8	30.1	35.8	39.0	37.8	38.6	41.0	43.9
120	30.0	31.1	37.0	40.4	39.0	39.6	42.0	45.1
130	31.0	31.9	38.2	41.8	40.2	40.6	43.0	46.2
140	32.0	32.7	39.2	43.0	41.3	41.6	44.0	47.2
150	32.9	33.5	40.2	44.1	42.3	42.6	45.0	48.2
160	33.7	34.3	41.2	45.1	43.3	43.6	45.8	49.2
170	34.5		42.0	46.1	44.1	44.4	46.6	50.0
180	35.3					45.2	47.4	50.8
190	35.9					45.9	48.2	51.6
200						46.5	48.8	52.4
210							49.4	53.0

*Data of Durnin and Womersley (1974), who used density measured by underwater weighing to estimate fatness in a sample of Scottish people.

Bioelectrical impedance

Bioelectrical impedance (BIA) is a method of measuring body composition now being used in many health centres and fitness clubs. It is included here in the anthropometry section for convenience. The devices that use this principle are becoming much cheaper and their operation is fairly simple. These devices give an almost instant estimate of the amount of fat and lean in the body and so their use is likely to grow.

The method relies on the fact that fatty tissue is a much poorer conductor of electricity than is lean tissue. Electrodes are placed on one of the subject's hands and feet, a current is generated by the machine's battery in one limb, passes through the body and is picked up by the electrode on the other limb. Newer machines may simply require the subject to stand on metal plates and these measure weight as well as impedance. The machine uses the resistance to the current – or the 'impedance' (because it is alternating current) – to estimate lean body mass and body fat. If the subject's age, sex, height and weight are keyed in, this machine gives a rapid figure for the amount and percentage of fat in the body.

Estimation of fatness from body density

The calibration of the skinfold method of determining fatness (see Table 3.4) has been obtained by using body density as a reference method. The density of fat (0.9 kg/L) is less than that of lean tissue (1.1 kg/L), so measurement of whole body density enables one to estimate the proportion of fat in the body:

Density = mass *divided by* volume.

Mass may be determined by simple weighing. Volume is measured by comparing the weight of the body in air and its weight when fully immersed in water. The difference between these two values is the weight of water displaced by the body (Archimedes' principle). Knowing the density of water (1 kg/L), one can thus calculate the volume of water displaced (i.e. the volume of the body). The principle is very simple but the technical procedures required to obtain accurate and valid values are quite elaborate.

- Subjects wear a weighted belt to ensure that they are fully immersed and correction has to be made for this.
- Corrections will need to be made for the residual air in the lungs during the immersion, which will greatly distort density measurements.

This method requires sentient and co-operative subjects. It is not suitable for routine use or for use with young children. It has traditionally been used as the reference method against which other methods are calibrated and validated (e.g. skinfold calipers and bioelectrical impedance).

An alternative method of measuring body volume is air displacement plethysmography (use of the Bod Pod). The subject is seated inside a plastic chamber of known volume and breathes through a mouthpiece connected to the atmosphere. The presence of the subject inside the chamber displaces air and this difference in the volume of air in the chamber and with the subject inside is the volume of the subject's body. The volume of air inside the chamber can be estimated by injecting a known amount of air into the chamber and measuring the pressure change. As with underwater weighing, an allowance has to be made for residual air in the lungs. When inside the chamber the subject must wear a minimum amount of close-fitting clothing and a tight cap to cover the hair. Fields *et al.* (2004) have written a review of this method and images of the apparatus can be found by typing the term 'Bod Pod' into an internet search engine.

Body water content as a predictor of body fat content

Measurement of body water content should enable good estimates of body fatness to be made as there is an almost perfect inverse correlation between percentage body water and percentage body fat (see Figure 3.6 later in this chapter). The body can be seen as consisting of two compartments: lean tissue with a constant proportion of water (around 73 per cent) and water-free fat. A measure of body water allows one to estimate proportions of lean and fat in the body. In order to estimate body water content in a living person or animal, one needs some chemical substance that is non-toxic, will readily and evenly disperse in all of the body water and is readily measurable. Water that is labelled with the deuterium isotope of hydrogen (heavy water) or the radioactive isotope of hydrogen (tritiated water) seems to fulfil these criteria. The degree of dilution of this labelled water has been used to calculate the total volume of body water. After allowing time for dispersal of a measured dose, the concentration of the chemical in a sample of body fluid is measured. Knowing the amount of the substance introduced and the final concentration, one can estimate the amount of diluting fluid (i.e. the body water).

Mid-arm circumference measures

In immobile adults who cannot be weighed (e.g. unconscious hospital patients), mid-arm circumference (MAC) of the upper arm can be a useful anthropometric indicator of nutritional status. A single measurement needs standards for interpretation, but longitudinal changes in this measure are a reasonably sensitive indicator of changes in body weight. Mid-arm circumference has been widely used as a simple and rapid means of assessing nutritional status in children. A piece of previously calibrated and colour-coded tape can be used. If the circumference lies within the green region then this can be taken to indicate normality; the yellow region suggests mild malnutrition, and a circumference within the red region indicates frank malnutrition.

Mid-arm muscle circumference (MAMC) has been widely used as a simple measure of lean body mass. The circumference of the mid arm is measured with a tape and the triceps skinfold measured with calipers. Then:

$$MAMC = MAC - (\pi \times triceps\ skinfold).$$

Changes in MAMC are taken to indicate changes in lean body mass and once again may be a useful longitudinal measure of nutritional status in hospital patients.

ANTHROPOMETRIC ASSESSMENT IN CHILDREN

Anthropometric measurements are cumulative indicators of the nutritional status and general health of children. A low value for height or length provides evidence of the chronic effects of malnutrition; weight-for-height is a more acute measure and indicates current nutritional status. These simple measures require little equipment or professional training and so even non-specialists can easily and cheaply produce reliable results. Interpretation of the results requires that they be compared with standards. The need for reliable standards is a recurrent problem when interpreting anthropometric measurements. If standards of height and weight for children are derived from children in affluent countries, then poor children in developing countries may not correspond well with such standards. These differences between rich and poor are largely a reflection of chronic adaptation to undernutrition by the poor, which may make interpretation of results and deciding on appropriate responses difficult.

For example, an anthropometric survey of children in rural Bangladesh is likely to show that their average heights and weights are some way below those of typical American children of the same age but they may be typical of children living in rural Bangladesh and thus they are not specifically 'at risk'.

This point is well illustrated by considering some of the changes that have occurred in the anthropometric characteristics of affluent populations during the twentieth century.

- Britons are on average several inches taller than they were at the start of that century and they mature quicker. Britons in the higher socioeconomic groups have always been taller than those in the lower groups but this gap narrowed considerably during the twentieth century.
- Sexual maturation occurs earlier now than at the start of that century (e.g. girls start menstruating 2–3 years earlier and boys reach their adult stature at 19 years rather than their mid-twenties).
- The normal or average values of height and weight of British children thus changed very significantly during the course of that century.

Note that large cross-sectional measurements of height in British adults have found a decrease in average height with increasing age. Part of this is a real tendency for people to decrease in height as they grow older, but most of it is due to the tendency for younger generations to be taller than their parents and grandparents.

Body size is not only dependent on environmental factors, like diet, but is also genetically determined. Some races of people may be genetically smaller than others and this is another factor that makes the use of non-local standards problematic. Within races there is a natural biological variation in the genetic component of height. This will obviously create difficulties in assessing the nutritional status of an individual child from a single set of anthropometric measurements. Is a child short because it is genetically small or because it is chronically malnourished? Growth curves are more useful ways of monitoring the nutritional status of individual children. Provided the child remains on its predicted growth curve, whether the absolute values are low or high is in most cases unimportant. If a child on a high growth curve dips significantly below that curve then this may indicate a nutrition or health problem even though it may be close to average for its age. A child who remains on a low growth curve will be assessed as growing satisfactorily even though it may be below average size for its age.

Centiles are frequently used to interpret anthropometric measures in children. If the growth curves of a population are plotted, then one can produce growth curves that are typical of each per cent (or centile) of the population – the largest 1 per cent through to the smallest 1 per cent. If, for example, point measurements on a group indicate an average height for age that is substantially below the 50th centile, this would suggest impaired growth in the sample group. If a point measurement on an individual shows a value at the extremes of the range (e.g. below the 5th centile), this indicates a probability that growth has been unsatisfactory. Figure 3.5 shows the WHO standards of height for age in girls up to 5 years; the 3rd, 10th, 50th, 90th and 97th centiles are given. If a girl has a height for age below the 3rd centile then there is a less than 3 per cent probability that she has been growing satisfactorily.

Body mass index in children

Although the BMI is the single most widely used anthropometric measure in adults, its use in

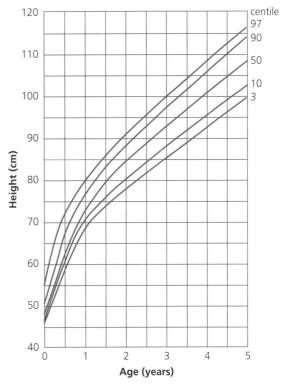

Figure 3.5 WHO standards of height (length) for age, in girls aged up to 5 years. The 97th, 90th, 50th, 10th, and 3rd centiles are shown.

children has been hindered by a lack of universally agreed standards and 'cut-off' points like those that exist for adults. If such standards could be established then, as in adults, BMI could be used in children to assess and classify them, to monitor changes in levels of adiposity over time, and to make regional or international comparisons. The main difficulty is that BMI changes markedly with age and the examples of median BMI at different ages are listed below to illustrate this (Cole *et al.*, 2000):

- birth – $13\,\mathrm{kg/m^2}$
- 1 year – $17\,\mathrm{kg/m^2}$
- 6 years – $15.5\,\mathrm{kg/m^2}$
- 20 years – $21\,\mathrm{kg/m^2}$.

Two main systems of standards have been used in the UK. First, values have been compared to a 1990 reference sample of British children (Cole *et al.*, 1995) . This large representative sample was used to construct centile curves of BMI with age from birth until adulthood, and values falling above the 95th centile are taken to indicate obesity and those above the 85th centile are classified as overweight. (A similar set of reference data for American children has been used in the USA.) Such a system is useful for monitoring changes over time in a given population, but it is rather arbitrary in its classification and of limited value for making international comparisons. Cole *et al.* (2000) therefore devised a set of international standards based on the adult 'cut-off' points for obesity (BMI >30) and overweight (BMI <25). They used a sample of almost 100 000 children drawn from six different countries and plotted centile curves of BMI against age for these children, and used the centile curves that at 18 years went through the adult 'cut-off' for obesity and overweight. Selected values from this set of 'cut-off' points are shown in Table 3.5. In the original source, which can be accessed freely online (http://bmj.com/cgi/pmidlookup?view=long &pmid=10797032), a more extensive list is given at half-yearly intervals from 2 years of age onwards.

Table 3.5 Selected values for the estimated equivalent of an adult body mass index (BMI, kg/m^2) of 25 (overweight) and a BMI of 30 (obese) at various ages*

Age (years)	BMI indicating overweight		BMI indicating obese	
	Boys	**Girls**	**Boys**	**Girls**
2	18.41	18.02	20.09	19.81
4	17.55	17.28	19.29	19.15
6	17.55	17.34	19.78	19.65
8	18.44	18.35	21.60	21.57
10	19.84	19.85	24.00	24.11
12	21.22	21.68	26.02	26.67
14	22.62	23.34	27.63	28.57
16	23.90	24.37	28.88	29.43
18	25	25	30	30

*The data are taken from Cole *et al.* (2000) and are based upon a sample of almost 100 000 children from six different countries.

Key points

- Weight-for-height is a measure of acute nutritional status in children but oedema may distort weight measurements.
- Height-for-age (or weight-for-age) is a cumulative or chronic measure of past status.
- Failure to grow and gain weight may be directly due to nutritional inadequacy or be a secondary consequence of ill-health.
- Genetic variation in size hinders the interpretation of height and/or weight measurements in children.
- Centiles (hundredths) are one way of allowing for genetic differences in size.
  - If an individual value is below the appropriate 5th centile, this means that there is only a 5 per cent chance that that child has been growing satisfactorily.
  - The average for a well-nourished population of children should be close to the 50th centile.
  - If serial measurements are made, a child should approximately follow its centile line.
- The BMI changes with age in children and so its use has been hindered by a lack of accepted standards.
- In one classification system for BMI in children, values are compared to an historical representative national data set and values above the 85th centile for age classified as overweight and those above the 95th centile classified as obese.
- A less arbitrary and more internationally useful system determines from the centile lines for a large international sample of children the lines that correspond to a BMI of 25 or 30 at age 18 years.
- These centile lines allow values for each age that correspond to these adult values to be calculated and tabulated, and examples are shown in Table 3.5.

ESTIMATING FATNESS IN ANIMALS

The fat content of dead animals can be measured directly by extracting the fat with a suitable solvent such as chloroform. Animal experimenters thus have the option of using this precise analytical method at the end of their experiment. This analytical method also provides an absolute standard against which other methods of estimating fatness can be calibrated and validated. In humans, of course, any method of estimating fatness can be validated and calibrated only against another estimate.

Experimental animals can be used to show that there is an almost perfect negative correlation between the percentage of body water and the percentage of body fat (Figure 3.6). This validates the use of body water measurements to predict body fatness. In the mice used to derive Figure 3.6, when body water was expressed as a percentage of the fat-free weight, then all values were within the range 74–76 per cent. This validates the earlier assumption that the body is made up of lean tissue with a constant proportion of water plus water-free fat. Other methods, similar to those described for people, are also available to estimate the fatness of animals: weight/length indices; density; and, in animals that store fat subcutaneously (e.g. pigs), skinfold thickness. Rodents do not store much of their fat subcutaneously but dissection and weighing of one fat storage organ may be used to predict total fat content in dead animals (Webb and Jakobson, 1980).

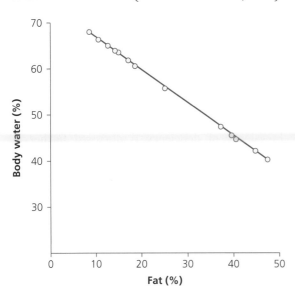

Figure 3.6 The relationship between percentage body fat and percentage body water in mice. To illustrate the value of body water measurements in predicting body fat content. Data from Webb and Jakobson (1980).

Key points

- Body composition of animals can be measured accurately and directly by chemical analysis of the carcass.
- Carcass analysis can be used to calibrate and validate other less direct methods of estimating body composition. In humans, any method of estimating body composition can be calibrated and validated only by comparison with other estimates.
- Chemical analyses of animal carcasses show that percentage body water is highly negatively correlated with percentage fat and that the water content of the fat-free mass is constant.

BIOCHEMICAL ASSESSMENT OF NUTRITIONAL STATUS

Biochemical measures of nutrient status yield objective and quantitative measures and are the most sensitive indicators of nutritional status. They can usually be measured with great precision as is common with such analytical procedures. A number of these biochemical measures of nutrient status were discussed in the section dealing with the methods used to assess nutrient requirements; for example:

- measures of blood and tissue levels of nutrients or metabolites
- measures of nutrient excretion rates
- enzyme activation tests
- functional biochemical tests such as prothrombin time.

Table 3.6 gives a short list of some commonly used biochemical tests of nutritional status and the values that indicate normality and/or deficiency.

Biochemical measurements need laboratory facilities and they are relatively expensive and time-consuming to perform. Interpretation of the values obtained will depend on the limits of normality that have been set, and this will often be a matter of judgement. For example, blood haemoglobin concentration can be measured with considerable precision but deciding on the level that should be taken to indicate anaemia will be a matter of judgement. Thus translating surveys of haemoglobin

Table 3.6 Examples of biochemical tests of nutritional status*

Nutrient	Test	Deficiency	Adequacy
Protein/energy	Serum albumin		35–45 g/L
Protein/energy	Serum transferrin		2.5–3.0 g/L
Vitamin C	Plasma vitamin C	<11 μmol/L	
Thiamin (B$_1$)	Erythrocyte transketolase activation coefficient (ETKAC)	>1.25	
Riboflavin (B$_2$)	Erythrocyte glutathione reductase activation coefficient (EGRAC)	>1.3	
Vitamin B$_6$	Erythrocyte aspartate transaminase activation coefficient (EAATAC)	>2.00	
Niacin	Urinary N′ methyl nicotinamide excretion (mg nicotinamide/g creatinine)	<0.5	>1.6
Folic acid	Serum folate (acute status)	<6.3 nmol/L	>7 nmol/L
	Red cell folate (long-term status)	<337 nmol/L	>422 nmol/L
Vitamin B$_{12}$	Serum B$_{12}$		>118 pmol/L
Vitamin A	Plasma retinol used for long-term status (clinical tests are often used)	<0.35 μmol/L	>0.7 μmol/L
Vitamin D	Plasma 25-OH cholecalciferol (D$_3$)		>25 nmol/L
Vitamin E	Total tocopherol in serum	<11.6 μmol/L	
	Plasma tocopherol to cholesterol ratio	<2.25 μmol/mmol	
Iron	Blood haemoglobin (men)	<13 g/dL	
	Blood haemoglobin (women)	<12 g/dL	
	Serum ferritin (men)	<20 μg/L	
	Serum ferritin (women)	<15 μg/L	
Zinc	Serum zinc	<10 μmol/L	>18 μmol/L

*Critical values for micronutrients in adults are largely taken from Ruston *et al.* (2004).

measurements into assessments of the prevalence of anaemia will depend very much on the limits of normality that are used. A figure of 12 g of haemoglobin per 100 mL of blood (12 g/dL) at sea level has traditionally been taken as the level below which there is a progressively increasing risk of anaemia in women (13 g/dL for men). If this value is taken as the lower limit of normality, the prevalence of iron-deficiency anaemia in pre-menopausal women is high even in industrialized countries (10–20 per cent). However, clinical symptoms of anaemia may not become apparent until haemoglobin level falls well below 12 g/dL. Conversely, substantial depletion of iron stores (as measured by serum ferritin concentration) and some symptoms of iron deficiency may occur without any decrease in blood haemoglobin concentration. Assessment of iron status and prevalence of deficiency is discussed further in Chapter 15.

Perhaps the most striking recent illustration of the difficulties in setting realistic and useful thresholds for adequacy with biochemical methods of assessment is that of riboflavin. Riboflavin status is assessed biochemically by measuring the erythrocyte glutathione reductase activation coefficient (EGRAC) as described earlier in the chapter, and an EGRAC >1.3 is taken to indicate riboflavin inadequacy. Hoare *et al.* (2004) reported that around two-thirds of British adults were classified as deficient in riboflavin using this criterion, rising to around 80 per cent in those under 25 years (details in Chapter 13). The average intake of riboflavin recorded in this survey was around 1.5 times the RNI. It is difficult to reconcile these two values. If one takes the biochemical classification at face value, it suggests that the RNI is set too low and that riboflavin inadequacy is a major problem in the UK and perhaps that food fortification with this vitamin needs to be considered. It seems more probable, as suggested by Hoare's team, that the biochemical assay is very sensitive and considerably overstates the real prevalence of riboflavin deficiency, and that consideration should be given to adjusting the biochemical criterion for riboflavin deficiency. Note that Finch *et al.* (1998) also found a high prevalence of riboflavin deficiency in their NDNS survey of older adults using this same criterion (see Chapter 16).

Measurements made on urine samples have the obvious advantage of requiring no invasive procedures and of giving relatively large samples, thus avoiding the need for special micro-analytical techniques. They can be useful if the excretion rate of an intact nutrient or readily identifiable derivative can be related to nutritional status. Rates of urine flow, and thus the concentration of solutes in urine samples, are very variable and greatly influenced by, for example:

- recent fluid consumption
- physical activity
- consumption of substances that have diuretic or anti-diuretic activity (e.g. caffeine or nicotine).

Twenty-four hour samples may give more meaningful results but their collection will be impracticable in many survey situations. Even where they are feasible, checks will be required to ensure that the samples are complete in non-captive subjects. As an example, it is generally agreed that the best method of assessing salt intake on any particular day is to measure the sodium excreted in the urine in a 24-hour period (see Chapter 15). In order to ensure that the 24-h urine sample is complete, subjects may be asked to take doses of a marker substance (para-amino benzoic acid) with their meals. Only where there is practically complete recovery of the marker in the urine sample will the sample be accepted as complete. Note that the sodium excreted in a single 24-h sample may not be a reliable indication of habitual salt intake (see Chapter 15).

Urinary levels of the B vitamins have traditionally been used as measures of nutritional status for these vitamins. The values are often expressed as amount of nutrient (or nutrient derivative) per gram of creatinine in the urine sample – as seen for niacin in Table 3.6. It is assumed that the excretion of creatinine is approximately constant, so this gives a more meaningful value than the amount of nutrient per unit volume of urine because the latter is so dependent on the rate of urine flow.

Blood samples give much greater scope for assessing nutrient status. Plasma, serum or blood cell concentrations of nutrients are extensively used as specific measures of nutritional status. Enzyme activation tests using red blood cell enzymes (as discussed earlier in the chapter) are also used. Plasma albumin concentration drops in severe protein-energy malnutrition and it has been widely used as a general biochemical indicator of nutritional status. Many medical conditions also result in a reduced plasma albumin concentration – examples are liver and kidney disease, some cancers and infection. Albumin has a relatively long half-life in plasma and so it is now regarded as too insensitive and non-specific to be a good biochemical indicator of nutritional status. Other plasma proteins with shorter half-lives in plasma may give a more sensitive indicator of protein energy status – examples are transferrin (which transports iron in plasma) and retinol-binding protein (which transports vitamin A or retinol)

Blood tests require facilities and personnel capable of taking and safely handling, transporting and storing blood samples. Analysis of blood samples often requires special micro-analytical techniques because of the limited volumes that can be taken for analysis.

Key points

- Clinical signs, anthropometric measurements and biochemical analyses of body fluid samples can all be used to assess nutritional status. Examples are given in Boxes 3.1, 3.2 and 3.3.
- With any nutritional assessment of groups or populations, steps must be taken to ensure that the sampled group is representative of the whole population under investigation.

→

Key points *continued*

- Clinical signs can be incorporated into checklists that can be used for screening and assessment by non-specialists and without the need for specialist equipment. They have the following merits and disadvantages.
  - They are quick, simple, and cheap to record.
  - They are insensitive indicators of malnutrition and do not give early warning of an impending nutritional problem.
  - Some signs are common to several nutrient deficiencies and to non-nutritional problems and so they are not specific.
  - They are qualitative and subjective because they depend on the opinion of the assessor and often yield just a yes/no response or a descriptive grading of severity.
- Anthropometric methods of assessment have the following merits and disadvantages.
  - They are quantitative and objective.
  - Many are quick and simple to perform, require only simple equipment and do not require specialist personnel.
  - Accurate assessment of fatness with skinfold calipers does require care and technical expertise.
  - They often need reliable standards to interpret their results. Some are more useful if measured sequentially to monitor changes in nutritional status.
  - Previous obesity can reduce their sensitivity in detecting deteriorating nutritional status.
  - Oedema can substantially distort body weight and undermine any of the methods that rely on accurate body weight measurement.
- Biochemical methods have the following merits and disadvantages.
  - They are quantitative and objective.
  - They are the most sensitive methods of nutritional assessment.
  - In many cases, they are highly specific indicators of the status for a particular nutrient.
  - They are time-consuming, expensive and they need specialist laboratory facilities and personnel.
  - Standards of normality may be difficult to set in some cases.

→

Key points *continued*

  - If concentration of a nutrient or metabolite in urine is measured, either some mechanism has to be found to correct for the wide variation in rates of urine flow or a complete 24-hour sample should be collected.
  - If blood analyses are used, this requires an invasive collection procedure and often requires a micro-analytical technique because of the small volumes that are available for the analysis.

MEASUREMENT OF ENERGY EXPENDITURE AND METABOLIC RATE

Metabolic rate is the rate at which energy is expended by the body. Energy expenditure may be rather crudely and indirectly assessed from measurements of energy intake. As energy can neither be created nor destroyed, then energy expenditure over any given period must be equal to the intake plus or minus any change in body energy stores.

$$\text{Energy expenditure} = \text{energy intake} \pm \text{change in body energy.}$$

If expenditure is measured in this way then the errors in measuring intake and changes in body energy will compound. The methods of measuring changes in body energy are insensitive, making this method unreliable for measurement of expenditure over short periods. Tens of thousands of calories may be added to or lost from body energy without their being quantifiable by the simple routine methods of measuring body composition. This error is minimized if the time period is long, but this also means that subjects will be required to monitor intakes for extended periods.

All of the energy expended by the body is ultimately lost as heat. It is theoretically possible to measure this directly in a whole-body calorimeter. This is a chamber surrounded by a water jacket in which the heat released by the subject in the chamber is measured by a rise in temperature in the surrounding water. It is more usual to predict energy expenditure from measures of oxygen consumption and/or carbon dioxide evolution. Foodstuffs are metabolically oxidized to carbon dioxide, water and, in the case of protein, nitrogenous waste products like urea. This oxidation process consumes atmospheric oxygen and produces carbon dioxide. The chemical equations for the oxidation of the various foodstuffs can be used to predict the energy equivalent of oxygen, which is the amount of energy released when a litre of oxygen is used to metabolically oxidize food. For example, the chemical equation for the oxidation of glucose is:

$$C_6H_{12}O_6 + 6O_2 = 6CO_2 + 6H_2O.$$

In real terms this means that 180 g of glucose with 6×22.4 L of oxygen yields 6×22.4 L of carbon dioxide and 6×18 g of water. Oxidation of 180 g of glucose yields around 665 kcal (2800 kJ). Thus one litre of oxygen yields approximately 4.95 kcal (20.8 kJ) when it is being used to metabolize glucose (i.e. 665 divided by 6×22.4). Similar calculations can be performed using the other substrates and they yield energy equivalents for oxygen that are not very different from that for glucose. If a mixture of substrates is being oxidized, then a figure of 4.86 kcal (20.4 kJ) per litre of oxygen can be used as the approximate energy equivalent of oxygen. If more precise estimation is required then the ratio of carbon dioxide evolution to oxygen consumption, the *respiratory quotient* (RQ), gives an indication of the balance of substrates being metabolized. The RQ is 1.0 if carbohydrate is being oxidized but only 0.71 if fat is being oxidized. Tables that list the energy equivalent of oxygen at various RQs are available.

The simplest way of measuring oxygen consumption (and carbon dioxide evolution) is to use a Douglas bag. This is a large plastic bag fitted with a two-way valve so that the subject, who breathes through a mouthpiece attached to the valve, sucks in air from the atmosphere and then blows it out into the bag. All the expired air can be collected over a period and then the volume and composition of this expired air can be measured. Knowing the composition of the inspired atmospheric air means that the subject's oxygen consumption and carbon dioxide evolution can be calculated. Note that the collection period is limited to a few minutes even if the capacity of the bag is large (100 L).

The static spirometer is essentially a metal bell that is filled with oxygen and is suspended with its open end under water. The subject breathes through a tube connected to the oxygen-containing chamber of the bell. The bell rises and falls as the volume of gas inside the bell changes, so it will fall and rise with each inspiration and expiration. If the system contains a carbon dioxide absorber then the bell will gradually sink as the subject uses up the oxygen in the bell. This change in volume of oxygen inside the bell can be recorded on a calibrated chart and the rate of oxygen consumption determined. This is a standard undergraduate practical exercise. It is limited to a few minutes of measurement of resting oxygen consumption or very short periods of consumption with static exercise (e.g. on an exercise bicycle).

Portable respirometers have been developed that can be strapped on the back and thus used and worn while performing everyday domestic, leisure or employment tasks. These respirometers, such as the Max Planck respirometer, monitor the volume of gas expired by the wearer and divert a small proportion of the expired gas to a collection bag for later analysis. They are once again only suitable for relatively short-term recording but they can be used to quantify the energy costs of a variety of tasks.

If subjects keep a detailed record of their 5 minute by 5 minute activities over a day (activity diary) then total energy expenditure can be roughly estimated using the measured energy costs of the various activities.

A number of research units have respiration chambers that allow relatively long-term measurement of energy expenditure of subjects performing any routine tasks that may be done within the chamber. The respiration chamber is essentially a small room, which has a controlled and measured flow of air through it. Oxygen consumption and carbon dioxide production by the subject can be measured by the difference in the composition of air as it enters and leaves the chamber. These pieces of equipment are, in practice, complex and expensive and thus restricted to well-funded research units. They can be used to monitor long-term energy expenditure of subjects who can live in the chamber for several days and perform tasks that simulate normal daily activity.

The doubly labelled water method has more recently been used to determine the long-term energy expenditure of free-living subjects going about their normal daily activities. Subjects are given a dose of doubly labelled water ($^2H_2{}^{18}O$), which contains the heavy isotopes of hydrogen (^2H) and oxygen (^{18}O). The subjects lose the labelled oxygen more rapidly than the labelled hydrogen because the hydrogen is lost only as water whereas the oxygen is lost as both water and carbon dioxide. This is due to the action of the enzyme carbonic anhydrase that promotes the exchange of oxygen between water and carbon dioxide. The difference between the rates of loss of labelled hydrogen and labelled oxygen is a measure of the rate of carbon dioxide evolution and thus it can be used to estimate long-term rate of carbon dioxide evolution and thus long-term energy expenditure. Comparisons of total energy expenditure measurements by respiration chamber and by the doubly labelled water method suggest that this method gives an accurate measure of energy expenditure. Using this method, investigators now have an acceptably accurate means of estimating the long-term energy expenditure of free-living people.

Comparisons of metabolic rates between individuals

Basal metabolic rate (BMR) is the minimum rate of energy expenditure in a conscious, resting animal or person. It is the metabolic rate measured in a rested, fasted individual who has been lying in a room at thermoneutral temperature for half an hour. Absolute BMR obviously tends to increase with increasing body size. Large animals have higher absolute BMRs than small ones. Fully grown adults have larger BMRs than small children. However, relative BMR (i.e. per unit body mass) declines with increasing body size. Small animals have larger relative metabolic rates than large ones. Small children have higher relative metabolic rates than adults. The equation given below is found to approximately predict the BMR of mammals of different sizes both within and between species:

$$\text{Basal metabolic rate (kcal/day)} = 70 \times \text{weight (kg)}^{3/4}.$$

There are regression equations that can be used to estimate the BMR of an individual from his or her body weight, and more information on BMR and its prediction from body weight can be found in Chapter 7. Human metabolic rates have traditionally been expressed per unit of body surface area: kcal (or kJ) per hour per m^2. Even in human adults, if BMR is expressed per unit of body weight, then large variations between individuals are found, particularly between fat and thin individuals. Adipose tissue has a much lower metabolic rate than lean tissue, so increasing adipose tissue mass has relatively much less effect in increasing whole body metabolic rate than increasing lean tissue mass. Increasing adipose tissue mass also has less effect on body surface area, so expressing BMR per unit surface area (m^2) tends to reduce the individual variation and has been a useful way of comparing BMRs in different individuals. Nomograms are available that enable surface area to be predicted from measurements of height and weight.

Nowadays, it is considered that the best way of comparing and expressing BMRs of people is to express it per unit weight of lean tissue: kcal (or kJ) per hour per kilogram of lean tissue. When expressed in this way the BMRs of men and women are not different, whereas when expressed per unit surface area then those of women are about 10 per cent less than those of men. This is an artefact due to the much higher body fat content of women.

Key points

- Metabolic rate is the rate of energy expenditure of the body. Basal metabolic rate (BMR) is the minimum metabolic rate measured in a conscious person who is rested, warm and fasted.
- Metabolic rate can be measured directly by measuring heat output, but it is usually calculated from the rates of oxygen consumption and/or carbon dioxide production.
- Conventional methods of measuring metabolic rate by oxygen consumption only allow it to be monitored for a few minutes at a time. Even in a respiration chamber, subjects are restricted to

→

Key points *continued*

the activities that can be carried out in a small room.

- The doubly labelled water method allows long-term energy expenditure to be measured in free-living subjects.

- Absolute BMR increases with body size whereas relative BMR (i.e. per unit body weight) decreases with size. Small animals or people have smaller absolute but larger relative BMRs than larger subjects.

- BMR (in kcal/day) can be roughly predicted by multiplying the body weight (in kg) raised to the power 0.75 by a constant (70).

- Metabolic rates of people have traditionally been expressed per unit of body surface area. If this method is used, then men have higher relative BMRs than women.

- It is better to express relative metabolic rate per unit of lean tissue mass and then the sex difference in relative BMR disappears because it is an artefact caused by the higher body fat content of females.

METHODS TO ESTABLISH LINKS BETWEEN DIET AND CHRONIC DISEASE

Introduction and aims of the chapter	102	Cohort studies	112
Strategic approaches: observational versus experimental	102	Case–control studies	115
		Cross-sectional studies	117
Features and problems of epidemiological methods	104	'Experiments' of nature	118
		Animal experiments	118
Cross-cultural comparisons	107	Human experimental studies	121
Time trends	110	In-vitro studies	132
Migration studies	112	Scientific honesty	133

INTRODUCTION AND AIMS OF THE CHAPTER

The first aim of this chapter is to make readers aware of the wide variety of methods available for investigating possible links between diet and well-being, and in particular the risks of chronic disease. This encompasses the ways in which the methods are used, their theoretical bases, their strengths and limitations, and how the data generated can be interpreted. This is the first stage in preparing to use these methods. Although the focus of this book is the link between diet and disease risk, these are the same methods that would be used to assess the influence of other environmental and lifestyle variables on health and disease, such as:

- the effects of smoking
- the effects of exercise
- the impact of exposure to occupational or environmental hazards
- the effects of sunlight exposure.

Another aim is to give readers sufficient understanding of these methods and their relative strengths and weaknesses to enable them to read the scientific literature critically. For example:

- to recognize the difference between an association found in an epidemiological study and the demonstration of 'cause and effect'
- to understand why a demonstration that something causes an apparently favourable change in a risk factor, or reduces the incidence of one disease, does not guarantee that it will yield holistic benefits on health and longevity.

STRATEGIC APPROACHES: OBSERVATIONAL VERSUS EXPERIMENTAL

There are two major approaches that can be used to investigate possible links between dietary or other lifestyle variables and diseases or disease risk factors such as high blood pressure or high plasma cholesterol concentration.

- *The observational approach.* Observational, epidemiological methods are used to relate differences in the diets or lifestyle characteristics of populations or individuals to their risk of developing a disease or their measured level of a disease risk factor. *Descriptive* epidemiological methods rely on looking at the occurrence and distribution of diseases in groups or populations, whereas with *analytical* epidemiological methods data are collected from individuals with the aim of testing a hypothesis. Analytical studies may involve the use of a *control group*.

- *The experimental approach.* In the experimental approach, investigators try to produce a controlled change in the diet or other behaviour of individuals or populations to determine the effect that this has on the disease/mortality risk or the measured level of a risk factor such as blood pressure or plasma cholesterol. This approach almost invariably involves comparison between test and control *groups*, or sometimes between test and control *periods*.

Box 4.1 outlines some methods available to investigate possible links between diet and disease. The methods are classified under three headings: descriptive epidemiology, analytical epidemiology and experimental. In the following sections, the principles and problems of these methods are discussed using illustrative examples. The examples have been chosen to illustrate methodology and problems. Well-known classical studies and older studies have often been chosen for illustrative purposes. Several of these classical papers were very influential on the later direction that research took and greatly influenced scientific opinion of their time. Some studies have been chosen because they illustrate weaknesses of methodology.

Box 4.1

Research methods to investigate links between diet and disease

Observational methods

Descriptive epidemiology

- *Cross-cultural comparisons.* Correlation is made between the level of a dietary factor and the frequency of a disease in different populations. These may be comparisons between nations or between special groups within a nation (e.g. between Seventh Day Adventists and the rest of the population in the USA).

→

Box 4.1 *continued*

- *Time trends.* Changes in the dietary habits of populations are correlated with changes in disease frequency.
- *Migration studies.* The changes in dietary habits that follow migration are correlated with changes in disease frequency in the migrant population.
- *'Experiments of nature'.* This involves the use of people with some genetic mutation or other accident of nature that increases (or decreases) their exposure to some suggested disease risk factor. Does the increased exposure to the risk factor result in increased rate of disease?

Analytical epidemiology

- *Cohort studies.* The dietary characteristics of a large sample of individuals are measured. The samples are selected and the measurements made in order to test a hypothesis. The deaths and the causes of mortality and/or morbidity of individuals within the sample are then monitored over the succeeding years. Disease risk is then correlated with the level of exposure to possible dietary risk factors.
- *Case–control studies.* Established cases of the disease are identified and matched to a sample of non-sufferers – the controls. The past diet (or other exposure) of the cases and controls is then compared to see if this provides evidence of greater exposure to the suggested risk factor in the case group (or greater exposure to a possible protective factor in the control group).

Experimental methods

- *Animal experiments.* Dietary changes are tested in short- or long-term controlled experiments with laboratory animals to see if they result in the postulated change in risk factor or disease frequency.
- *Short-term human experiments.* Dietary changes are tested in short-term controlled experiments to see if they result in the postulated change in risk factor measurement.
- *Clinical trials.* A dietary change that is expected to lead to improved prognosis in patients is tested under controlled conditions to see if it yields the expected benefits. Ideally the treatment is compared to the effects of a dummy treatment (placebo), and neither the investigators nor the patient know who has

→

Box 4.1 *continued*

received the real and dummy treatments until after the study is completed (double-blind trial).

- *Intervention trial.* This is a population-level trial. An attempt is made to change the exposure of a test population to the postulated dietary factor, for example by encouragement or possibly by a nutrient fortification programme. The change in disease frequency is compared to that in a control population that has not received the intervention.

- *Systematic reviews and meta-analyses.* All trials of a particular intervention that meet set quality criteria are identified. These are then weighted according to sample size and used to do a combined statistical analysis. This allows several smaller studies to be combined together to produce a single study of much greater statistical power.

FEATURES AND PROBLEMS OF EPIDEMIOLOGICAL METHODS

Does association prove 'cause and effect'?

Epidemiological methods can produce evidence of an association between two variables. However, although there can be evidence of an association between a measured dietary variable and a disease, for example, that does not mean necessarily that there is a cause-and-effect relationship between the dietary factor and the disease. The association may be coincidental and dependent on a relationship between both tested variables and a third unconsidered or confounding variable (or many confounding variables). It is even possible that in some cases there may be an 'effect-and-cause' relationship, if the disease results in a change in the dietary variable. This very important distinction is discussed in Chapter 1 and several examples are described there.

The problem of confounding variables pervades all types of epidemiological investigations. Epidemiologists use various means and statistical devices to correct for variables they suspect to be confounding, but this is an imperfect process and the quality of this correction is likely to vary considerably from study to study.

Consider coronary heart disease. There are scores of risk markers for this disease, so the task of identifying any one of them as independent of all the others is formidable. An apparent protective effect of moderate doses of alcohol against coronary heart disease has been reported many times (see Chapter 5), but how many authors will have considered or corrected for level of physical activity as a potential confounding variable? One large English survey reported a strong positive association between alcohol consumption and level of physical activity (White *et al.*, 1993). Barker *et al.* (1998) list six characteristics that would make it more likely that a demonstrated association was causal.

- *Strength of the association.* The stronger the association, the less the likelihood that it is due to some unforeseen confounding factor.
- *Is it graded or dose dependent?* There is usually a graded effect of true causes rather than a threshold effect.
- *Independence of the association.* The relationship remains significant even after correction for potentially confounding variables.
- *Consistency of the finding.* If the association is found in a variety of studies using different investigative approaches, this makes it more likely that it is due to cause and effect.
- *Reversibility.* If reduced exposure to the suspected cause leads to reduced incidence of the disease, this increases the likelihood of it being a true cause.
- *Plausibility.* The association is more likely to be cause and effect if there is a believable mechanism to explain the causality of the association, which can be supported by laboratory studies. A plausible mechanism unsupported by corroborating laboratory studies probably adds little weight to the argument. It is quite possible to devise plausible mechanisms for most observations, and often equally plausible mechanisms for opposing findings. The most plausible and intellectually satisfying mechanism may not be the one that ultimately proves to be correct.

Sources and quality of data

Information about the diets of individuals and populations is derived from the methods discussed in Chapter 3. Food balance sheets or household expenditure surveys are often the basis for international dietary comparisons. Methods that correlate dietary factors with disease risk in individuals clearly require individual methods of dietary assessment. When dietary surveys of large representative samples are made, these can be properly used for international comparisons; an example is the rolling programme of NDNS surveys in the UK. If small, unrepresentative survey results are extrapolated and taken to represent whole populations then this can be major source of error. The many sources of error and uncertainty in estimating dietary intakes are discussed in Chapter 3. Acceptably accurate and representative measures of habitual dietary intake are clearly a prerequisite for detecting associations between diet and disease risk.

Information about rates of mortality from specific diseases is usually obtained through some analysis of information recorded on death certificates. Death certificates have now been internationally standardized, as have the nomenclature and diagnostic criteria for the various causes of death. The World Health Organization publishes an International Classification of Diseases, Injuries and Causes of Death (ICD) which is regularly revised. Death certificates in the UK list both the underlying (main) cause and contributory causes of death. There will, however, still be differences between individual physicians and this variation is likely to be even greater between those in different regions or nations. There may be straightforward errors of diagnosis, different diagnostic criteria or terminology may be used at different times or in different centres, even the accuracy of the age recording on death certificates may vary. When autopsies have been used to confirm the accuracy of previously recorded causes of death, they show that errors in diagnosing the causes of death in individual patients may be frequent. Both false positives (i.e. people falsely diagnosed as dying of the disease) and false negatives (i.e. people dying of the disease but not recognized as such) tend to occur. If individuals are the unit of comparison then these two errors compound, but they do tend to cancel out if population mortality is calculated. Even though the number of individual errors of diagnosis may be quite large, provided false negatives and false positives occur at similar rates then the accuracy of the estimate of population mortality may be little affected. If there is systematic over- or under-recording of deaths from any cause, this will seriously distort population comparisons – for example, any attempt to play down the prevalence of a disease to protect the tourist industry or for other commercial or political reasons.

Accurate and representative measures of morbidity in populations are likely to be more difficult to obtain than mortality data. Investigators will almost certainly have to rely on less rigorous and uniform methods of collecting data than death certificates. Some sources of information about disease frequency in populations are:

- notification or registration of particular diseases – any variations in the efficiency of these collection procedures in different areas will distort the estimates of disease frequency
- analysis of reasons for hospital admission or general practitioner consultation – multiple recordings of the same individuals due to re-admissions is one source of error here
- social security data on reasons for absences from work
- extrapolation from relatively small-scale and possibly unrepresentative survey samples.

Incidence and prevalence are terms used to indicate disease frequency.

- *Incidence* is the number of new cases of the disease occurring within a specified period.
- *Prevalence* is the number of cases of the disease existing at any particular point in time.

Prevalence is dependent both on the incidence and the duration of the disease. A chronic disease will have a much greater prevalence than an acute one of similar incidence. As an example, the incidence of cystic fibrosis in the UK remained fairly constant for many years at around 300–400 per year but the prevalence has increased in recent years because the survival time of sufferers has increased. The chronic diseases of industrialization, almost by definition, therefore have high prevalence. Not only do they cause reduced quality of life for large numbers of people but they also exert a considerable drain on health and social care budgets.

If an asymptomatic risk factor, like plasma cholesterol level or blood pressure, is being related to diet, then investigators will have to rely on data obtained from their own or published surveys. If these surveys are used to make international comparisons, they may have been conducted in the various countries by investigators using different protocols. Since the start of the 1990s there have been annual health surveys of representative samples of English adults that have included anthropometric measurements and measurements of major risk factors as a result of the 1990 Health of the Nation White Paper (also similar Welsh and Scottish surveys). The rolling programme of NDNS surveys also includes anthropometric measurements and measurements of some key diet-related risk factors such as blood pressure and blood lipoprotein concentrations.

Age standardization

Whenever comparisons of the death (or disease) rates between different populations or groups are made, some allowance has to be made for any differences in their age structures. For example, the simplest measure of mortality is the crude death rate for the specified cause (per thousand):

(Deaths in one year *divided by* number of people in the population) × 1000.

This ratio is often of limited value because (a) mortality from many causes is so highly age dependent, and (b) some populations have widely varying age structures. Higher birth rates and shorter life expectancies mean, for example, that populations in developing countries tend to have a lower average age than in the Western industrialized countries. A more useful measure for international or regional comparisons would be the age-specific death rate; for example:

(Annual number of deaths in males aged 45–54 years *divided by* number of men in this age group in the population) × 1000.

To make more complete comparisons, the *standard mortality ratio* (SMR) is a useful and widely used measure. To calculate the SMR it is necessary to use a standard or reference population, in which all the various age-specific mortality rates for the cause under investigation have been established. Then, for each age band of the test population, one must calculate how many deaths would be expected or predicted:

- given the number of people of that age in the test population
- assuming the same age-specific death rate as in the reference population.

For example, the number of males aged 45–49 years in the test population *multiplied by* the death rate from the particular cause for males aged 45–49 years in the reference population *equals* the number of predicted deaths in 45- to 49-year-old males in the test population. This calculation is made for each relevant age group in the population and the total number of predicted deaths in the test population is thus calculated. The total number of *actual* deaths in the test population is then expressed as a percentage (or ratio) of the predicted number of deaths from that cause in that test population:

SMR = (actual number of deaths in test population *divided by* predicted number of deaths)
(× 100 to express as percentage)

The SMR can be used for international comparisons, to make regional comparisons within any given country, or to make comparisons between other groups. When used for regional comparisons within a country, the whole national population can be used as a reference population. For example, comparisons of the SMR for gastric cancer in different regions of the UK in the early 1980s showed that the SMR was over 115 per cent in Wales but less than 85 per cent in parts of East Anglia. People in Wales therefore had a 1.15 times greater risk of dying of this disease than the national population, whereas those in East Anglia had less than 85 per cent of the risk of the whole population. Regional differences in diet, lifestyle and environment within the UK can be compared to see if any are associated with this variation in gastric cancer mortality. This might provide important clues about the aetiology of gastric cancer.

Key points

- Epidemiological methods provide evidence of association between dietary variables and disease risk.
- Epidemiological association between two variables does not necessarily mean that they are causally related. Association may arise because both of the tested variables are linked to other confounding variables.

→

Key points *continued*

- An association is more likely to be causal if it is strong, consistent between studies, dose dependent, independent of likely confounding variables and reversible, and can be explained by a plausible mechanism that can be supported by experiment.
- Information about causes of death is usually obtained directly or indirectly from death certificates.
- There is an international classification system for causes of death (ICD) and a standardization of the format of death certificates.
- Errors do occur in the diagnosis of cause of death – both false negatives and false positives. These tend to compound when individuals are the unit of study but tend to cancel out when population mortality rates are calculated.
- Accurate information on frequency of non-fatal diseases or disease risk factors is likely to be more problematic than calculation of mortality rates.
- Information on non-fatal disease frequency is obtained from the following sources:
  - disease notifications or registers
  - analysis of reasons for hospital admission, physician consultations or absences from work
  - surveys.
- Incidence is the number of new cases of a disease that occur within a specified time period.
- Prevalence is the number of cases of a disease that exist at any point in time. It is a product of the incidence and duration of the disease.
- Comparisons of crude death rates between groups or populations may be of little value if they are not age (and sex) standardized, because the age and sex structures of different populations may be very different.
- Age-specific death rate is the rate of death from a disease within a specified age and sex group.
- The standard mortality ratio (SMR) is the ratio of predicted deaths to actual deaths in test populations.
- The predicted number of deaths is calculated as those that would occur in a population of this age structure if the age-specific death rates were the same as those in a reference population.

CROSS-CULTURAL COMPARISONS

An early indication that diet may be implicated in the aetiology of a disease often comes from cross-cultural associations between a population measure of the dietary variable and population mortality or morbidity rates from the disease. Some examples are given below.

- A positive association between the average saturated fat intakes of populations and their mortality rates from coronary heart disease points towards high saturated fat intakes as a possible causal factor in coronary heart disease.
- A positive association between per-capita sugar consumption in different countries and the average number of decayed, missing and filled teeth in young people implicates sugar in the aetiology of dental caries.
- A positive association between per-capita salt consumption and blood pressure in various adult populations implicates high salt intake in the aetiology of hypertension.
- A negative association between per-capita fibre consumption and bowel cancer mortality in various populations has been used to implicate the fibre depletion of Western diets in the aetiology of bowel cancer.

There are large variations between nations in mortality and morbidity rates from the diet-related diseases of industrialization. It is, therefore, common to see cross-population associations between a dietary variable and one of these diseases used to implicate diet as a major cause of the disease – as in the four examples listed above. It is, of course, very premature to then assume a cause-and-effect relationship between that dietary factor and the disease. As populations become more affluent, numerous changes in diet, lifestyle and environmental conditions tend to occur simultaneously, opening up the likelihood that there will be many confounding variables. For example, all of the following changes may accompany increasing affluence and industrialization:

- increased fat and saturated fat consumption
- lower consumption of starches and fibre
- increased use of simple sugars, salt and perhaps alcohol and tobacco

- increased consumption of animal protein
- reduced incidence of nutritional deficiencies
- reduced physical activity
- increased proportions of overweight and obese people
- improved medical care
- many other changes in diet, lifestyle and environment.

Accompanying these trends for change in diet and lifestyle there will be general trends in patterns of mortality and morbidity. Life expectancy increases, mortality from infectious diseases and other acute causes declines, but there will be increased prevalence of and mortality from the various chronic diseases of industrialization. Cross-cultural studies tend to focus on individual associations between one of these lifestyle or dietary changes and one of these chronic diseases. Thus the association between saturated fat intake and coronary heart disease mortality is used to support the proposition that high saturated fat intake causes heart disease, and the negative association between fibre intake and bowel cancer is used to support the proposition that low fibre intake causes bowel cancer. As high-fat diets tend to be low in fibre, and vice versa, it would certainly be possible to produce equally convincing correlations between fibre intake and coronary heart disease (negatively correlated) and between saturated fat intake and bowel cancer.

The classic paper of Gleibermann (1973) on the relationship between the average salt intake and blood pressure of adult populations illustrates several of these problems of cross-cultural studies. She gleaned, from the literature, estimates of the salt intakes and blood pressures of middle-aged people in 27 populations from various parts of the world. The data for the male populations have been used to construct a simple scatter diagram (Figure 4.1). The correlation coefficient and line of best fit have also been calculated. There is a highly significant, positive and apparently linear relationship between the average salt intake and the mean blood pressure of these populations, consistent with the hypothesis that high salt intake is causally linked to the development of hypertension.

The two variables in Figure 4.1 were measured by numerous investigators. The methods, conditions of measurement and quality of measurement are

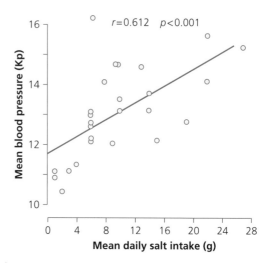

Figure 4.1 Simple scatter diagram showing the relationship between estimated salt intake and mean blood pressure in 27 male populations. Data from Gleibermann (1973).

therefore not consistent across the groups. As noted in Chapter 3, salt intake is a particularly problematic measurement. The methods used to determine salt intakes in these 27 populations are variable and in some cases unspecified, ranging from the high-precision 24-hour sodium excretion method to 'educated guesses' made by Gleibermann herself. Recorded blood pressure may be very much influenced by the method used and the care taken by the measurer to standardize the conditions (blood pressure may be affected by how long the subjects are allowed to relax before measurement, and it may be raised if measured in anxious subjects).

Although the correlation shown by Figure 4.1 is highly statistically significant, there is a considerable scatter of points around the line of best fit. The correlation coefficient (r) is 0.61, suggesting that only about 37 per cent (r^2) of the variation in population blood pressures is accounted for by variation in their salt intake. It is possible that this association is due to some confounding variable or variables. For example, the populations with the lowest blood pressures and lowest salt intakes would also tend to be active, have low levels of obesity, have relatively low alcohol intakes, have high potassium intakes, etc. All these factors are thought to favour lower blood pressure. Subsequent investigators have suggested that the inclusion of different races may have increased the scatter with Gleibermamnn's data because black populations might be genetically more sensitive to the hypertensive effects of salt (e.g. Law *et al.*, 1991a).

The range of daily salt intakes shown in Figure 4.1 is huge, from around 1 g to well over 25 g. The average salt intakes in the UK and USA are some way below the middle of this range. If one takes the linear relationship at face value, then one could predict that specified falls in any population's average salt intake would be associated with specified falls in average blood pressure. One could then go on to make predictions about the expected benefits for that population (reductions in the prevalence of hypertension and hypertension-related diseases). It would be hard to demonstrate conclusively that this association was linear over the whole range. This is what one is assuming when predicting that small or moderate reductions in salt intakes of the populations around the centre of the range will have predictable effects on average blood pressure.

Numerous studies conducted in Western industrialized countries have measured blood pressure and salt intakes in large samples of individuals living in particular towns or regions. In many of these studies no association is found between individual salt intake and individual blood pressure. One explanation for this disparity is that the gold-standard method for measuring salt intake (24 h sodium excretion) is probably a poor measure of an individual's habitual salt intake. This fact alone would make it improbable that one would find a correlation between individual salt intake measured in this way and blood pressure even if habitual salt intake is a major determinant of individual blood pressure (see Chapter 15 for further discussion).

Such disparities between cross-cultural and within-population studies are common in epidemiological studies and also tend to be found, for example, when dietary saturated fat intake and plasma cholesterol are correlated. Taking these results at face value, one might conclude that while average salt intake is an important determinant of average population blood pressure, individual differences in salt intake are not a major factor in producing the differences in blood pressure within a single population. This may initially seem like a

contradiction because, of course, the influence of salt on population blood pressure would have to be a summation of its effects on the blood pressure of individuals. However, numerous other factors may also affect an individual's blood pressure, such as:

- individual genetic variation
- levels of activity and obesity
- alcohol consumption
- genetic variation in susceptibility to the hypertensive effects of salt.

These other influences on blood pressure may mask any effect of salt on an individual's blood pressure. Some people may have high blood pressure because they are overweight, inactive and consume large amounts of alcohol, yet their salt consumption may be low. Other people may have low blood pressure despite high salt intake because they are fit, abstemious, and relatively salt insensitive due to their genetic make-up. Significant numbers of such people would, of course, make it difficult to find a statistically significant association between salt intake and blood pressure, especially as most people within any given population will be concentrated around the mean value and the total range of salt intakes may be relatively narrow. This problem is discussed further in the section dealing with short-term human experiments later in this chapter.

Anomalous populations

Cross-cultural studies may highlight anomalous populations who deviate very significantly from the general trend. These anomalous populations may provide useful information that can lead to modification of existing theories or to additional areas of investigation. Observations that Greenland Eskimos had low rates of heart disease despite a diet high in fats of animal origin were important in focusing attention on the potential dietary and therapeutic benefits of fish oils (Dyerberg and Bang, 1979; see Chapter 12 for further discussion).

McKeigue *et al.* (1985) found that the South Asian population living in one area of London had much higher rates of coronary heart disease than the white population living in the same area. This was despite their apparently lower exposure to many of the traditional risk markers for coronary heart disease; they had lower serum cholesterol levels, smoked less, drank less alcohol, consumed less saturated fat and cholesterol, and many were lacto-vegetarian (see Chapter 18 for further discussion).

Special groups

There are 'special groups' within populations who, because of their religion or occupation, behave differently from the majority of the people around them. Such groups are often intensively studied because there should be fewer confounding variables between these groups and the rest of their own population than are seen in other cross-cultural studies. For example, Seventh Day Adventists in the USA are a religious group who abstain from alcohol and tobacco and around half of them are ovolacto-vegetarian. They have lower rates of coronary heart disease and many types of cancer (including bowel cancer) than the US population as a whole (see under vegetarianism in Chapter 18).

Despite the use of such groups because of better matching than in most cross-cultural studies, there may still be numerous differences in the diet and lifestyle of these groups compared to 'the average American'. Picking out one dietary or other lifestyle difference between such groups and the rest of population may still produce false assumptions about cause and effect. A religion may 'impose' numerous lifestyle and dietary constraints on its adherents, religious groups may be socially, intellectually or even genetically unrepresentative of the population as a whole, and of course their religious faith may provide emotional comfort that lessens the impact of stresses on mental and physical health. It has, for example, even been suggested that being religious may in itself protect against the development of bowel cancer (Kune *et al.*, 1993).

Key points

- Use of cross-cultural comparisons to identify associations between diet and disease risk is particularly prone to confounding effects.
- Increasing affluence and industrialization bring with them multiple changes in diet composition and lifestyle as well as major changes in life expectancy and disease frequencies.

→

Key points *continued*

- Several associations between diet and disease risk factors that are consistently found in between-population studies are not apparent in samples of individuals from within the same population (e.g. the association between daily salt intake and blood pressure). Some of the possible reasons for this dichotomy are:
  - measures of the average nutrient intakes of populations may be much more valid than measures of the habitual intakes of individuals
  - within populations there is likely to be a much narrower range of nutrient intakes and probably risk factor levels
  - many factors other than the dietary variable may influence an individual's risk factor level and so obscure the relationship.
- In cross-cultural studies, anomalous populations who deviate markedly from the general trend may open up new areas of investigation or generate new hypotheses.
- Special groups within populations whose diet and behaviour differ markedly from the bulk of the population are of special interest. There are likely to be fewer confounding variables than with other cross-cultural comparisons.

TIME TRENDS

Populations' diets and lifestyles tend to change over time, and the changes may be particularly rapid and pronounced if there has been rapid economic development and industrialization. Epidemiologists may look for associations between the changes in a population's diet and its mortality and morbidity rates for particular diseases. Seasonal changes may also be important if an acute event is being studied.

During the twentieth century, salt consumption declined in the USA and western Europe as salting of foods was largely replaced by refrigeration and other preservation methods. This was associated with reduced mortality rates for stroke and gastric cancer (high blood pressure being a risk factor for stroke). These observations have been used to support the proposition that salt is an aetiological influence for both of these diseases (Joossens and Geboers, 1981). Figure 4.2 shows a very strong correlation between average death rates from stroke and gastric cancer in 12 industrialized countries between 1955 and 1972. This is consistent with the hypothesis that a change in exposure to a common causal influence (i.e. reduced intake of dietary salt) was responsible for the decline in mortality from both diseases. The apparent, relative acceleration in the rate of stroke mortality after 1972 is attributed to the population impact of anti-hypertensive drugs, which would be expected to reduce mortality from stroke but not gastric cancer. MacGregor and de Wardener (1998) give several further examples of associations between falling salt consumption and falling blood pressure, but the decline in salt intake in these studies was partly induced by active publicity campaigns rather than being wholly spontaneous – so they cannot be classified as descriptive epidemiological studies.

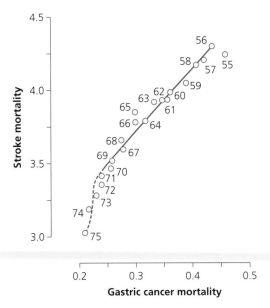

Figure 4.2 Time trends in mortality rates from gastric cancer and stroke over 20 years. Each point represents average death rates from these diseases in 12 industrialized countries for that year, e.g. 55 represents rates in 1955. *Source*: Webb, GP (1992a) *Journal of Biological Education*, 26 (4) 266. Simplified from Joossens, JV and Geboers, J (1981) *Proceedings of the Nutrition Society* 40, 40.

Chapter 9 presents data that show a marked increase in the prevalence of obesity in England over 25 years. Later in the same chapter (see Figure 9.13), data are presented showing that the average per-capita calorie intake has declined markedly in

recent decades; that is, we are eating less but getting fatter. These paradoxical time trends are used to support the hypothesis that declining physical activity is a major underlying cause of the rising levels of overweight and obesity.

Figure 1.1 in Chapter 1 shows trends in the rates of cot deaths in England and Wales between 1971 and 2004. The rising prevalence between 1971 and its peak rate in 1986 is linked in the text to an increasing use of the front or prone sleeping position. The decline in cot death rates after 1986 is linked to a switch back to the supine or back-sleeping position; the halving of the rate between 1991 and 1992 is linked to the 1991 start of an active campaign aimed at encouraging the back-sleeping position – the 'Back to Sleep' campaign.

The Japanese are frequently used by those investigating links between diet and disease as an example of a nation that, though affluent and industrialized, has a diet very different from the typical American and western European diet. The Japanese diet has much less meat and dairy produce but much more vegetable matter and seafood. Since the Second World War, however, the Japanese diet has undergone considerable 'westernization'. For example, between 1950 and 1986, total fat intake trebled, the ratio of animal to vegetable fat doubled, and the number of US-style fast-food outlets mushroomed. Mortality patterns of the Japanese also changed dramatically over this time scale. By 1986, two-thirds of deaths in Japan were due to cardiovascular diseases, cancer and diabetes, whereas in 1950 only one-third had been due to these causes. Deaths from cancer also increased two and a half times over this period, as did deaths from heart disease. In Chapter 10 it is noted that, in 1960, age-standardized rates of bowel cancer in Japan were only about a third of UK levels but are now similar to UK rates.

These changes in Japanese mortality patterns are consistent with our views on the causal influences of diet on particular chronic diseases. Note, however, that the average height of Japanese boys increased by more than 20 per cent over this period, and there were also very big increases in the total life expectancy of the Japanese – making them now one of the most long-lived populations in the world. Fujita (1992) reviewed these changes in the Japanese diet and he concluded that 'they have greatly improved the nutritional status of the

Japanese people'. He further suggested that the rise in crude mortality rates from the diseases of industrialization was 'mainly due to increases in the actual numbers of elderly people, rather than to westernising effects in dietary habits'.

Key points

- Temporal changes in disease frequency can be associated with corresponding changes in diet in genetically stable populations.
- These changes may take place rapidly if there is rapid industrialization in a country.
- Many of the problems of cross-cultural studies also apply to the analysis of time trends.
- Increases in the proportion of deaths due to chronic age-related diseases are inevitable when the life expectancy of a population rises.

MIGRATION STUDIES

One possible explanation of the differences between the morbidity and mortality patterns of different nations is that they are due to genetic differences between the populations. Studies on migrants are a useful means of distinguishing between environmental and genetic influences on disease frequency. People who migrate are immediately exposed to the new environmental conditions and they tend to progressively adopt aspects of the dietary and lifestyle habits of the indigenous population. However, unless widespread intermarriage occurs, migrants retain the genetic characteristics of their country of origin. Migrant populations generally also tend to progressively acquire the morbidity and mortality characteristics of their new homeland (Barker *et al.*, 1998). These trends indicate that, although there are undoubtedly variations in genetic susceptibility to different diseases both within and between populations, environmental factors have a predominant influence on disease rates in populations. The differences in the mortality and morbidity patterns in different nations are predominantly due to differences in environment, lifestyle and diet rather than to the genetic differences between populations. In some instances where the change in risk exposure occurs at the time of migration, the time lag between migration and change in disease frequency may suggest the length of the latent period between the initiating event and the appearance of symptoms.

In Chapter 19 it is suggested that when women from areas like China and Japan, where consumption of soy products is high and rates of breast cancer comparatively low, migrate to countries where soy consumption is low, then rates of breast cancer remain low in the migrants themselves but rise in subsequent generations. This observation has been used to support the hypothesis that exposure to the phyto-oestrogens in soy products in early life (or even in the womb) has a lifelong effect in reducing the risk of breast cancer.

Mortality rate for stroke has for a long time been much higher in Japan than in the USA, whereas mortality from coronary heart disease has been much higher in the USA than in Japan. In Japanese migrants to the USA and their descendants, mortality rates for these diseases move over time towards those typical of other Americans. This would indicate that these differences in mortality rates in the two countries are due to diet or other lifestyle factors, and thus that they are potentially alterable by intervention. McKay *et al.* (2004) have published a review of the effects of migration on health.

Key points

- Migration is accompanied by immediate changes in the environment and usually more gradual changes in diet as migrants acculturate to their new surroundings.
- Unless there is extensive intermarriage, migrant populations remain genetically similar to those in their country of origin.
- Migration is usually accompanied by a gradual shift in disease frequencies away from that in the country of origin and towards that typical of the new country.
- Migration studies suggest that many of the differences in disease frequencies seen between populations are due to environmental and lifestyle factors rather than to genetic differences between races.

COHORT STUDIES

In a cohort study, a sample of people (or cohort) is selected either from within the same population or, less commonly, from several populations. Details of the individual diets, lifestyles and other characteristics of all members of the cohort are then recorded and their subsequent health and mortality monitored for a period of years or even decades. The sample is selected and the data are collected with the aim of testing a hypothesis about the cause of a disease. The investigators then look for associations between the measured characteristics and the subsequent risks of mortality or morbidity. They look for dietary, lifestyle or other characteristics that are predictive of increased risk of a particular disease. To use a simple non-health example, a university could record the entry qualifications of its new students and see whether these predict the eventual level of achievement of students at the end of their courses: is there a significant association between entry-level scores and final level of attainment?

Cohort studies usually require large sample groups and long follow-up times in order to get enough cases of a disease for meaningful statistical analysis. For example, a sample of 100 000 middle-aged northern Europeans would be required to get 150 cases of colon cancer within a 5-year follow-up. Cohort studies therefore inevitably require major commitments of time, effort and money and are generally not suitable to study uncommon diseases. A number of famous cohort studies have been conducted using tens or even hundreds of thousands of subjects and some of these are still ongoing after several decades. Such studies are not limited to investigating any one diet–disease relationship, but can be used to provide data on dozens of such relationships. For example, data from the American Nurses' Health Study has been used to investigate several relationships between environmental factors and diseases:

- obesity and coronary heart disease (Manson *et al.*, 1990)
- vitamin E and coronary heart disease (Stampfer *et al.*, 1993)
- meat, fat, fibre and colon or breast cancer (Willett *et al.*, 1990)
- *trans*-fatty acids and coronary heart disease (Willett *et al.*, 1993).

Many problems of such studies are common to other areas of epidemiology, such as:

- the accuracy of the end-point diagnosis
- the reliability, range and validity of the original measurements (several long-running, sophisticated cohort studies have made repeat measurements on surviving members of the cohort at regular intervals)
- the problem of confounding variables.

Large and well-conducted cohort studies are considered to be the most powerful and robust of the epidemiological methods. A number of large and sometimes ongoing cohort studies have had major influences on our current views about the ways in which diet and lifestyle influence health and disease risk. Some examples of the better known of these are described briefly below, along with web links where further details of these studies can be found.

- The European Prospective Investigation into Cancer and Nutrition (EPIC) is one of the largest studies of diet and lifestyle ever undertaken. It is made up of a cohort of over half a million people from 23 centres in 10 European countries. The study was started in 1992 and between 1993 and 1999 it recruited a sample of 520 000 European adults aged over 20 years. Detailed information was collected about diet and lifestyle using a questionnaire, and anthropometric measurements and blood samples were collected at the time of recruitment. The aim of this study was to investigate the relationship between diet and other lifestyle factors and the incidence of chronic diseases, particularly cancer. Some of the results from this study are discussed in Chapter 10 in the section dealing with dietary influences on bowel cancer risk. See http://epic.iarc.fr/index.php for further details.
- The Framingham study was started in 1948 when a cohort of just over 5000 men and women resident in the town of Framingham in Massachusetts in the USA were recruited. Detailed physical examinations and lifestyle questionnaires were completed on each of these subjects with the aim of identifying common factors and characteristics that related to cardiovascular disease risk. Detailed medical histories and physical examinations were carried out at 2-yearly intervals. In 1971, a second, similar sized cohort was recruited and it was

made up of the adult children of the original cohort along with their spouses. In 2002, a third generation made up of grandchildren of the original cohort was recruited. In 1994, in order to reflect the changing ethnic make-up of people of Framingham and its surrounding towns, a so-called Omni cohort made up of people of African-American, Hispanic, Asian, Indian Pacific Islander and Native American origins was recruited (a second Omni cohort was recruited in 2003). See www.nhlbi.nih.gov/about/framingham for more details.

- The Nurses' Health Study was started in 1976 when around 120 000 married American nurses were recruited and asked to fill in health-related questionnaires. The primary motivation with this first cohort of participants (aged 30–55 years in 1976) was to assess the long-term consequences of oral contraceptive use. The participants were sent follow-up questionnaires at 2-yearly intervals and, in 1980, food frequency and diet questionnaires were first included. In 1989, a second slightly younger cohort was recruited with the aim of looking not just at the effects of oral contraceptive use but also at diet and lifestyle as risk factors for subsequent disease. In 2008, recruitment began for a Nurses' Health Study III. See www.channing.harvard.edu/nhs/index.php/history for more details.

As a practical example of a cohort study, Morris *et al.* (1980) asked 18 000 middle-aged British civil servants to complete a questionnaire on a Monday morning detailing, among other things, a 5-minute by 5-minute record of how they spent the previous Friday and Saturday. They found that over the next 8 years, those who had reported engaging in vigorous leisure time activity had only half the incidence of coronary heart disease of those who reported no such vigorous activity (even allowing for differences in smoking of the two groups). This finding is consistent with the hypothesis that exercise reduces the risk of coronary heart disease. It does not prove that the differences in heart disease rates were caused by differences in exercise levels. There are several other possible explanations, such as those listed below.

- Perhaps those best equipped for vigorous physical activity, and thus more inclined to

participate, are also less prone to coronary heart disease.
- Perhaps a reluctance to participate in vigorous leisure time activity is an early indication of existing but undiagnosed coronary heart disease.
- Perhaps participation in leisure-time activity is a marker for those who are most health conscious and who eat healthier diets and generally lead healthier lifestyles.

When cohort studies are used to assess the relationships between exposure to an environmental factor and disease, the term *relative risk* is widely used:

Relative risk = incidence in exposed group *divided by* incidence in unexposed group.

In the example of Morris *et al.* (1980), the relative risk of coronary heart disease in the inactive smokers could be compared to that of the active non-smokers:

Relative risk = CHD incidence in inactive smokers *divided by* CHD incidence in active non-smokers.

In many dietary studies the population is divided into fifths or quintiles according to their level of consumption of a particular nutrient; that is, the fifth with the lowest consumption (or exposure) through to the fifth with the highest consumption. The relative risk in each quintile can then be expressed in relation to that of the lowest quintile; for example:

Relative risk = incidence of disease in any other quintile *divided by* incidence in lowest quintile.

Figure 4.3 shows the relative risk of developing colon cancer in differing quintiles of a cohort of almost 90 000 American nurses (i.e. using data from the Nurses' Health Study) divided according to their consumption of animal fat (Willett *et al.*, 1990). The results indicate that there is a progressive increase in risk of colon cancer associated with increased animal fat consumption; the effect was statistically significant.

Positive results from an apparently rigorous cohort study are usually given particular weight when conclusions are made about relationships between lifestyle factors and disease.

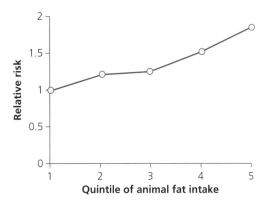

Figure 4.3 Relative risk of colon cancer according to quintile of animal fat intake. A cohort of almost 90 000 American nurses was followed for 6 years and there were 150 recorded cases. *Source:* Simplified after Willett, WC *et al.* (1990) *New England Journal of Medicine* 323, 1669.

Key points

- Cohort studies are expensive and time-consuming because they require large samples of subjects to be followed for long periods.

- Cohort studies are usually impracticable for investigating the causes of uncommon diseases but can be used to investigate the causes of several diseases simultaneously.

- Deaths in the first few years of the study may represent those with existing disease at the start of the study and may need to be excluded from the analysis.

- Relative risk is the ratio of the incidence of disease in the exposed group to that in the unexposed group.

- Relative risk can be calculated in quintiles of the population divided according to their level of exposure to the independent variable (e.g. the dietary factor). The incidence in each quintile is expressed as a ratio of that in the lowest quintile of exposure.

CASE–CONTROL STUDIES

In case–control studies, investigators try to identify differences in the diet, lifestyle or other characteristics of matched groups of disease sufferers and controls. Often such studies are retrospective. A group of those suffering from, or dying of, a particular disease is matched with a group who can act as controls. The investigators then try to retrospectively identify differences in the past diets, behaviours or occupations of the two groups that might account for the presence of the disease in the case group. Returning to the example of predicting final-degree results from entry qualifications (see p. 113), a case–control study could be used to identify the characteristics of students who have attained first-class degrees. One could take a group of students attaining first-class degrees (*cases*) and match them with some obtaining lower grades (*controls*) and see whether the entry or other characteristics of the two groups were different.

Matching of cases and controls is clearly a critical factor in such investigations. Sample sizes are usually small, which means that testing and correction for the effects of confounding variables cannot be undertaken in the final analysis of the results. Ideally one would match only for confounding variables; that is, those independently linked to both the suspected cause and the disease under investigation. Matching for factors that are linked to the cause but not independently to the disease will actually tend to obscure any relationship between the suspected cause and the disease. Barker *et al.* (1998) use the example of a suspected link between taking the oral contraceptive and deep vein thrombosis (DVT). Religious belief may be linked to the use of a contraceptive but is unlikely to be causally linked to the disease. They make the point that 'perfect matching of influences which determine exposure to the suspected cause will result in the frequency of exposure in cases and controls becoming identical'.

In addition to the problem of control selection, it may be extremely difficult to obtain reliable information about past behaviour, especially past dietary practices. Present behaviour may be an unreliable guide to past behaviour because the disease or awareness of it may modify current behaviour; differences between controls and cases may be as a result of the disease rather than its cause. Some diseases, like cancer, are probably initiated many years before overt clinical symptoms appear. This may make it desirable to compare the behaviours of the two groups many years previously.

If one tries to assess things like past smoking habits or the position in which a baby was laid down to sleep, one could expect reasonably accurate responses. If one wants to assess habitual salt intake 5 years ago then this will present a much greater challenge.

Case–control studies helped to highlight the apparently causal link between prone (front) sleeping and risk of cot death. More than 20 case–control studies were published over a 20-year period from the early 1970s. Each of these found that babies who had died 'from cot death' were more likely to have slept on their fronts than those who did not die (Webb, 1995; DH, 1992a).

Cramer *et al.* (1989) tried to test the hypothesis that high dietary galactose consumption (from lactose or milk sugar) was implicated in the aetiology of ovarian cancer. Approximately equal numbers of sufferers and non-sufferers from the disease were asked to fill in a food frequency questionnaire, focusing on the dietary patterns in the previous 5 years but asking the 'cases' to ignore changes in food preferences since their diagnosis of cancer. Lactose consumption was not significantly different in the cases and controls, neither were there any significant differences when several other specific dairy foods were considered separately. However, eating yoghurt (which is depleted of lactose) at least once a month was associated with significantly increased relative risk of ovarian cancer. The implication was that yoghurt consumption is causally linked to the development of ovarian cancer; but, as explained below, there are many other explanations for these results.

- Yoghurt is a food with a 'healthy image' and ovarian cancer is sometimes called the 'silent cancer' because the disease has often progressed to an advanced stage before its clinical recognition. Perhaps minor subclinical effects of the disease persuaded the cases to include more healthy foods in their diets prior to the onset of clinically overt symptoms.
- The more associations one tests, the more likely it is that one of them will be statistically significant simply by chance. Lactose consumption *per se* was not associated with risk of ovarian cancer, so

these authors then looked for a link with several individual dairy foods.
- The sufferers also differed from the controls in several other respects. The cases were more likely to be Jewish, college educated, never married, no children, and never having used oral contraceptives. It is not unreasonable to suggest that women with such characteristics might also be more likely to eat yoghurt. The differences in yoghurt consumption may be due to some other characteristic of women who develop ovarian cancer, rather than yoghurt consumption being directly, causally linked to the development of ovarian cancer.

Case–control studies may be prospective. Clinical records or stored samples may be used to yield information that is more reliable or at least less subject to bias than asking questions about past behaviour. For example, levels of carotenoids in stored blood samples can be used as an objective marker for fruit and vegetable consumption around the time of the blood collection. On occasion, such information may be recorded or stored with the specific intention of referring back to it when cases have become apparent. Wald *et al.* (1980) investigated the possibility of a link between vitamin A status and risk of cancer. Serum samples were collected and frozen from 16 000 men over a 3-year period. From this large sample, 86 men subsequently developed cancer and were matched with 172 men who did not develop cancer. They were matched for age, smoking habits and time at which the samples were collected. The serum retinol (vitamin A) concentrations were then measured in the stored samples from both groups of men. Serum retinol concentrations were found to be lower in the cases than in the controls, consistent with the hypothesis that poor dietary vitamin A status increases cancer risk. There are several reasons (see below) why these results and those of other similar studies need to be interpreted cautiously.

- The time between sample collection and clinical diagnosis was short (1–4 years). It is quite likely that an existing undiagnosed cancerous condition might have resulted in reduced serum retinol concentration. The difference in serum retinol concentrations of cases and controls may be a product of early cancer rather than its cause.

- Serum retinol concentration is an insensitive measure of dietary status for vitamin A in individuals. Serum retinol concentrations start to fall only when liver stores are seriously depleted. Other factors, including infection, may influence plasma retinol concentrations.

In cohort studies, relative risk can be calculated directly, but in case–control studies an indirect measure of relative risk, the *odds ratio*, has to be used. This is defined as:

Odds ratio = odds of exposure to the suspected cause among the cases *divided by* odds of exposure among the controls.

In most case–control studies this is calculated using the equation:

Odds ratio = (number of exposed cases × number of unexposed controls) *divided by* (number of unexposed cases × number of exposed controls).

If the experiment has been designed using matched pairs of cases and controls, then:

Odds ratio = number of pairs with case exposed but control unexposed *divided by* number of pairs with case unexposed but control exposed.

As with the relative risk in cohort studies, the odds ratio can be calculated at each of several different levels of exposure, such as with quintiles of exposure as was seen in Figure 4.3.

Case–control studies of some type account for many of the putative links between diet or lifestyle and disease that fleetingly attract the attention of the health correspondents of the media. They can be conducted cheaply and quickly and so are available even to those with very limited research facilities. This type of study is clearly an important tool for the epidemiologist seeking to identify causes of many diseases. However, many of these studies relating to diet have major methodological difficulties and are open to several interpretations. Often these studies do no more than point to the possibility of a causative link that is worthy of further investigation.

Key points

- In case–control studies, the matching of cases to controls is of paramount importance. Ideally they need to be matched only for likely confounding variables that are independently linked to both the suspected cause and the outcome measure.
- Ideally one should compare diets of cases and controls at the time of disease initiation.
- It may be very difficult to obtain reliable measures of past diet. The current diet of a disease sufferer may be a *result* of having the disease rather than its cause.
- Stored blood or other samples may be used to give more objective measures of past nutritional status.
- Odds ratio is the measure of relative risk used in case–control studies. In most studies it is the product of the number of exposed cases and unexposed controls divided by the product of the unexposed cases and the exposed controls.

CROSS-SECTIONAL STUDIES

If one is using a risk marker or a symptom as the measure of outcome, it is possible to get 'immediate' results using a survey of a cross-section of the population. If one assessed the diet and nutritional status of a large sample of people and then measured a disease risk marker or symptom, one could look for correlations between consumption of a particular substance and the measured outcome. Thus one could look at the relationship between measured saturated fat intake and blood cholesterol concentration or between habitual salt intake and blood pressure. The ongoing programme of NDNS surveys provides an opportunity for such cross-sectional analysis. Thus in the first survey of adults, Gregory *et al.* (1990) found no significant correlation between dietary saturated fat intake and serum low-density lipoprotein (LDL) cholesterol concentration in men (see Chapter 12).

Chapter 9 has a discussion of the link between reported levels of physical activity and the risk of being overweight or obese. When a representative sample of English adults were classified on the basis of a questionnaire into high-, medium- and low-activity groups, rates of obesity and being overweight were inversely related to activity category; that is, the most active were the least likely to be overweight or obese.

'EXPERIMENTS' OF NATURE

Observations made on victims of some congenital or acquired disorder may provide useful evidence about the relationships between diet and disease. For example, the observation that people with familial hypercholesteraemia (an inherited tendency to very high plasma cholesterol concentration) are very prone to premature coronary heart disease supports the belief that plasma cholesterol levels and CHD risk are positively associated. The Nobel prize-winning work of Brown and Goldstein (1984) indicates that the high plasma cholesterol in these people is a primary consequence of their genetic defect, and this supports the proposition that the association is causal (discussed further in Chapter 12).

ANIMAL EXPERIMENTS

This topic has been the subject of two critical reviews by the author (Webb, 1990, 1992b). Animal experiments allow researchers to perform high-precision, well-controlled and, if necessary, long-term experiments to directly test hypotheses. Technical, ethical or financial constraints would often make it difficult or impossible to undertake such experiments using human subjects. The reliability of well-designed and competently executed animal experiments should be high. The researcher can thus have confidence that a statistically significant difference between, say, an experimental group and a control group is due to the treatment. It should be repeatable if the experimental circumstances are replicated. Epidemiologists, on the other hand, have to rely on finding statistical associations between naturalistic observations of diseases or disease markers and potential causes. These observational human studies cannot be properly controlled. Confounding variables may lead to a false assumption that two associated variables are causally linked and, conversely, other influences on the dependent variable (the disease) may obscure a causative association.

Animal experiments are thus likely to be much more reliable than human epidemiology and even many human experiments. The problem with animal experiments is their questionable validity. It may be difficult to decide to what extent hypotheses generated or supported solely by the results of animal experiments may be applied to people. Strictly speaking, animal experiments can be used only to generate hypotheses about humans. The hypotheses should then be tested by direct experiments with humans or, if that is not possible, then the extent to which human observations are consistent with the animal-generated hypotheses can be assessed. In practice, however, results from animal experiments may be extrapolated to people with little experimental confirmation in people and sometimes with little consideration of biological factors that might make such projections unsafe. It is a measure of the robustness of animal experimentation that often, despite such lack of rigour, essentially correct conclusions about humans are drawn from these experiments.

Animal experiments have played a key role in progressing our knowledge of human biology. They have also, therefore, made an important contribution to producing the practical medical, surgical and nutritional benefits that have resulted from the application of that knowledge. Only around 20 per cent of the Nobel prize winners in Physiology and Medicine up to 1985 used human subjects for their research, and only around 10 per cent did not use some non-human species (Webb, 1992b). These Nobel prizes represent a yardstick to assess the contribution of animal experiments because they acknowledge landmark achievements in advancing physiological and medical knowledge. Almost all prize winners have made use of non-human species in their research.

There is also clear evidence that animal experiments have sometimes misled those doing research in human biology and medicine. Two examples are given below.

- Dietary cholesterol was once widely regarded as the dominant influence on plasma cholesterol concentration. Frantz and Moore (1969) in a review of 'the sterol hypothesis of atherogenesis' concluded that, although saturated fat was an important influence on plasma cholesterol, its effect was probably to potentiate the effects of dietary cholesterol. Dietary cholesterol is now considered to be a relatively minor influence on plasma cholesterol concentration for most people. According to Frantz and Moore, experiments with herbivorous, laboratory rabbits were the major evidence directly supporting their view of dietary cholesterol as the dominant influence on blood cholesterol concentration.

- In Chapter 11 it is argued that experiments with laboratory rats were an important factor in exaggerating the protein requirements of children and thus in falsely indicating a huge deficit in world protein supplies.

Animal experiments are an important research tool in the study of human nutrition and they have made major contributions to advancing understanding of all aspects of human biology. Animal experiments also have a considerable potential to mislead the human nutritionist, especially if results generated in experiments with small laboratory animals are extrapolated to people with little consideration of the factors that might invalidate such projections and with little attempt to corroborate the animal-generated hypothesis with studies in people.

The sections below consider several problems that may make it difficult to extrapolate the results of nutrition experiments with laboratory animals to people.

Species differences in nutrient requirements

There may be both qualitative and quantitative differences in the nutritional requirements of species. Most mammals, unlike primates and guinea-pigs, make their own vitamin C and therefore do not require a dietary supply. All mammals require an exogenous source of protein, but the requirements of children and other young primates are low compared to other mammals because of their slow growth rate. The milk of most mammals has 20–25 per cent of the energy as protein, whereas in humans and chimpanzees this figure is only around 6 per cent (see Chapter 11).

Species differences in feeding pattern and diet character

Animals may be exposed to a type of diet or a mode of feeding that is totally different from their natural one. Their response in such an experiment may not be a good guide to the response of people, especially if the experimental diet or feeding pattern is much more akin to the natural one in humans. For example, rabbits are herbivores and would not normally encounter cholesterol in their diets because cholesterol is found exclusively in foods of animal origin. Rabbits may be metabolically ill-equipped to handle large dietary loads of cholesterol. They certainly seem to be much more sensitive to the atherogenic effects of cholesterol than many other laboratory species. Omnivorous and carnivorous species should be better adapted to handling dietary loads of cholesterol and thus less susceptible to its atherogenic effects. With the benefit of hindsight, the assumption that the rabbit's response to dietary cholesterol would predict the human response seems unsafe. This partly explains why dietary cholesterol was regarded as a much greater influence on plasma cholesterol and atherogenesis than it is now.

Controlled experimental conditions versus real life

Animal experiments are usually performed under highly controlled conditions. Experimental and control groups are matched and treated identically except for imposed differences in the experimental variables. Strictly speaking one is then only able to assume that the test treatment produces the results obtained under the specified conditions of the experiment. In practice, one tends to assume that essentially similar effects would result from the treatment even if some of the background conditions were changed (e.g. in free-living, genetically diverse, wild animals of the same species). Changes in background conditions might sometimes substantially alter the response of even the experimental species to the experimental treatment. For example, controlled experiments with laboratory animals might sometimes not even predict the response of free-living wild animals of the same species, let alone the response of human beings.

Take as an example the key role that animal experiments play in the toxicological testing of food additives (see Chapter 19 for further discussion of this topic). Such tests often involve exposing experimental animals to huge doses of single additives over their whole lifespan under laboratory conditions. If additives show no adverse effects under these test conditions it is then assumed that they are generally non-toxic to that species in those doses. Under different conditions, however, the additive might have harmful effects. There might be interactions between the additive and some other factor. The additive might, for example, become harmful in one of the following circumstances:

- in the presence of other additives, drugs or chemicals
- when there is a particular nutrient inadequacy or the diet is low in anti-oxidants
- when there is exposure to cigarette smoke or alcohol
- if animals with differing genotypes are exposed.

There is, for example, a well-known interaction between certain older antidepressant drugs (monoamine oxidase inhibitors, MAOIs) and certain foods containing tyramine (e.g. cheese). The tyramine causes a dangerous rise in blood pressure in people taking these drugs.

Differences in species sizes

One of the major advantages of using laboratory animals for experiments is their small size, which greatly reduces research costs. Home Office data indicate that over 80 per cent of animals used for experiments in the UK are rodents, and mice make up almost 70 per cent of the total (Table 4.1). This small size also leaves experimenters with the difficulty of how to allow for differences in size when projecting results from animal experiments to humans. It is usual to scale dosages and requirements according to body weight, but this is more because of convention and convenience than because there is convincing evidence of its validity. In Chapter 3, four-fold differences were obtained when projecting the rat's rate of vitamin C synthesis to human size depending on whether relative body weight or relative metabolic rate was used as the basis for the scaling.

Let us assume that one might wish to model, in a mouse experiment, the sugar consumption of two human populations, one consuming around 40 kg

Table 4.1 Breakdown of species used for animal experiments in the UK (Home Office data)

Species	Proportion of total
Mice	69%
Rats	12%
Other rodents	1%
Other mammals	3%
Fish	10%
Birds	4%
Reptiles and amphibians	1%

per person per year and one consuming around half this amount. These amounts represent something close to 20 and 10 per cent, respectively, of total energy intake for the human populations. If one scales this human consumption according to relative body weight to set the experimental consumption in the mice, then sugar would represent only around 2.5 and 1.3 per cent of total calories in the two groups of mice.

As discussed earlier in this chapter, the relative metabolic rate (i.e. energy expenditure per unit weight) declines with increasing body size in mammals. Small animals like mice have much faster metabolic rates than larger species like man. This accounts for the large differences produced when the scaling is by relative body weight or relative metabolic rate in the two examples above.

Rodents are widely used in studies on energy balance that are directed towards increasing understanding of human energy balance regulation (see Chapter 9). The size difference in relative metabolic rate is just one of several factors that greatly complicate the human nutritionist's interpretation of energy balance studies conducted with small mammals. It is sometimes difficult to project even qualitatively the results from energy balance studies on rodents to humans. Two examples are given below.

- The relative energy costs of locomotion (i.e. energy required to move a specific mass a specific distance) decline with increasing body size. There is also the added complication that, in humans, bipedal locomotion seems to double the energy cost of walking compared to that of a similarly sized quadruped. This makes it difficult to assess the impact of activity level on overall human energy expenditure from small animal studies.

- Small animals rely on heat generation as their principal physiological response to cold, whereas large animals and people rely much more on heat conservation to maintain body temperature in the cold. When mice are used then the situation may be still further complicated because mice have been shown to become torpid when fasted; they allow substantial and prolonged falls in body temperature in order to conserve energy (e.g. Webb *et al.*, 1982). Most investigators, in the past, have assumed that mice are always homeothermic. Such factors would clearly make it difficult to predict the effects of environmental temperature on human energy needs from experiments with mice. They may also complicate more fundamental decisions about the relative importance of variations in energy intake or expenditure to overall energy balance, and thus to the development of obesity. In Chapter 9 it is argued that experiments with rodents were largely responsible for encouraging the belief that much human obesity might be triggered by a reduced metabolic or thermogenic (heat-generating) response to overfeeding – that some thermogenic defect was an important cause of human obesity.

Key points

- Use of laboratory animals for experiments extends the range of experiments that are ethically and technically feasible.
- Well-designed animal experiments should yield reliable and repeatable results.
- The results from experiments with laboratory animals may not validly predict the responses of free-living people.
- Animal experiments have made a major contribution to understanding of human biology and to the practical benefits that have resulted from the application of that knowledge.
- Animal experiments also have the potential to mislead human biologists, particularly if the results are simply extrapolated to humans.

→

Key points *continued*

- There are species differences in the quantitative requirements for nutrients and even some differences in the range of nutrients that are essential to different mammals.
- Different species have different types of diet. The response of a species to a foreign dietary component may be a poor guide to the response of a species for which it is normal.
- The effects of a dietary alteration under a set of controlled conditions may not predict what would happen under a different set of background conditions and thus that of free-living animals or people.
- It is very difficult to scale doses or nutrient requirements between species of vastly different sizes. Scaling according to body weight may be misleading.
- It can also be difficult to scale the energy costs of exercise and homeothermy between large and small species. This is a particular problem if small animals like mice are used as models for humans in energy balance studies.

HUMAN EXPERIMENTAL STUDIES

Human experimental studies are divided in this section into three categories for ease of discussion: short-term experiments, clinical trials and intervention trials. The overall design strategy is similar in the three types, the differences being to do with the scale and duration of the study, the nature of the experimental constraints and outcome measurements, and whether or not the subject is expected to gain therapeutic benefit from the experimental treatment. The issues listed below are discussed at various points within this section but they apply to most human experiments and in many cases to animal experiments as well.

- *Subject selection.* If the control and test groups are not matched at the start of an experiment for factors that can affect the outcome (e.g. age or initial disease severity) then this can bias the outcome. If healthy subjects are used in a trial of a preventive change then this is called primary intervention. In a secondary trial the intervention is tested in those with previous disease history.

- *Measures of outcome.* Outcomes may be long term and holistic, such as the effect on disease prevalence or mortality or even total mortality. Often they are more acute and/or reductionist, such as changes in subjective measures of symptom severity, risk factor level (e.g. plasma cholesterol concentration), or some objective measure of disease progression like narrowing of the joint space in arthritis.
- *The placebo effect.* A placebo is a dummy treatment that should be indistinguishable from the real treatment. Its purpose is to allow researchers to differentiate between the physiological benefits of treatment and psychological benefits due to the subject's expectation of benefit. The more subjective the measure of outcome, the more important it is to account for any psychological effects of an intervention. For example, in trials of therapies for depression it is common for the placebo to result in benefits for more than 25 per cent of subjects; and in studies of the treatment of menopausal hot flushes placebos may produce benefits in up to 50 per cent of subjects. In his popular book *Bad Science*, Goldacre (2008) devotes a whole chapter to the placebo effect and he discusses studies (the scientific references are given) which, for example, suggest that placebos have a bigger effect if (a) multiple pills are given, (b) certain colours of pills are used, (c) capsules rather than pills are used, (d) placebos are given by injection, or (e) patients are told by the doctor how effective they are likely to be.
- *Operator bias.* The person conducting an experiment may influence the outcome. If the outcome is subjective, the researcher may be affected if he or she knows which subjects are being treated and inadvertently affect the responses of the subjects. In a double-blind trial, neither subject nor researcher knows whether they are receiving the real or placebo treatment until after the data collection has been completed.
- *Treatment compliance.* In animal experiments and with human subjects in a controlled environment (e.g. a hospital ward) one can ensure that each subject complies with the experimental protocol. In free-living human subjects one cannot ensure compliance (e.g. that they take a vitamin pill as expected, or follow a dietary change as requested). Often one cannot even reliably assess the degree of compliance in different subjects.

Short-term human experiments

Most of the hypotheses relating diet to the risk of chronic disease suggest that prolonged exposure to the dietary risk factor eventually leads to increased risk of developing clinical disease. Clearly such hypotheses are not directly testable in acute experiments. However, these diet–disease hypotheses often involve hypothetical chains of apparently reversible steps between exposure to the initial dietary risk factor and the onset of clinical disease. The diet–heart hypothesis, for example, envisages changes in plasma cholesterol resulting from high intake of dietary saturated fats leading to lipid deposition in artery walls, atherosclerosis, and ultimately increased risk of coronary heart disease (see Chapter 12 for details). In the 'oxidant theory of disease' (see Chapter 13 for details), unquenched free radicals can cause oxidative damage to cellular components which may cumulatively increase risk of chronic disease; anti-oxidants quench free radicals and reduce measures of oxidative damage to cellular components and thus ultimately reduce chronic disease risk. It may be possible to test individual steps in such hypotheses in short-term experiments without exposing the experimental subjects to any significant long-term risks.

Keys *et al.* (1959) began a classical series of studies that have had a tremendous influence on thinking about the relationship between diet and heart disease. They were able to demonstrate that changing the ratio of polyunsaturated to saturated fats in the diet had predictable acute effects on plasma cholesterol concentration. When subjects switched from diets high in saturated fat and low in polyunsaturated fat to diets low in saturated fat and high in polyunsaturated fat (i.e. from low to high P:S ratio), their plasma cholesterol concentration fell (Figure 4.4). All the subjects showed some decline in plasma cholesterol even though the degree of responsiveness varied. The total fat content of the two diets was matched. Two particular problems with this type of experiment are considered below.

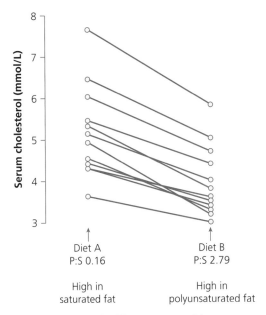

Figure 4.4 Effects of different types of fat on serum cholesterol in 12 men. Total fat in the two diets was matched. Data of Keys *et al.* (1959). *Source:* Webb, GP (1992a) *Journal of Biological Education* 26 (4), 266. After NACNE (1983).

- The results of such acute experiments may not necessarily predict the chronic response. The subjects may adapt to any change in the longer term.
- Support for one element of any hypothesis does not confirm the whole hypothesis. In the example above, even if diets high in polyunsaturated fat and low in saturated fat reduce plasma cholesterol, it does not necessarily follow that this will lead to improved health and longevity or even necessarily to a reduced risk of CHD. All one has actually demonstrated is a short-term decline in an asymptomatic risk marker.

Further consideration of the data in Figure 4.4 may help to explain the apparent contradiction between the results of between-population and within-population epidemiological studies of the relationship between saturated fat intake and plasma cholesterol concentration. Saturated fat intake appears to be a major determinant of average population plasma cholesterol despite the fact that, within populations, there appears to be no significant association between serum cholesterol concentration and saturated fat intake. In this experiment, the dietary change in P:S ratio has had a cholesterol-lowering effect in these individuals and the appropriate statistical test (a paired *t*-test) would show that this effect was highly statistically significant. This dietary change appears to have shifted the whole distribution of individual serum cholesterol concentrations downwards. If the sample were large enough, one would expect this would significantly reduce average plasma cholesterol of the sample population. Yet, the range of cholesterol concentrations of subjects consuming a matched diet, say diet A, is huge and the average reduction in cholesterol resulting from the dietary change to diet B is relatively small in comparison. The difference between the two means is less than a third of the difference between the highest and lowest values on diet A. This is despite the fact that the magnitude of this experimental dietary change was enormous; it is probably towards the extreme ends of the range of practical feasibility with regard to P:S ratio on a high-fat diet. Although the ratio of polyunsaturated to saturated fat clearly affects individual plasma cholesterol levels, and therefore average population levels, it is not the primary factor determining where any individual lies within the population range of plasma cholesterol concentrations.

Key points

- A dietary factor may contribute to the cause of a disease by initiating a reversible chain of events that eventually results in clinical disease.
- It may be possible to test elements of this chain of events in short-term human experiments without exposing the subjects to significant risk.
- In the diet–heart hypothesis, high saturated fat intake is postulated to raise plasma cholesterol concentration, which ultimately can lead to increased risk of coronary heart disease. This element of the hypothesis can be tested experimentally.
- The experimental confirmation of one step in the hypothetical chain does not prove the whole hypothesis.
- Acute responses to dietary change may not always be the same as chronic responses.

Clinical trials

Clinical trials are usually used to test the effectiveness of a treatment on the course or severity of a disease or symptom or its effectiveness as a preventative measure. The aim of such trials is to isolate and quantify the effect of the treatment under test. It is therefore necessary to eliminate, minimize or allow for other influences on the disease progression or severity such as those listed below.

- There may be variation in disease progression or severity that is unrelated to the intervention. This requires that there be a matched control group or control period.
- There may be considerable variation in the initial disease severity. This could be a source of bias if the control and experimental groups are not initially well matched. If the sample is large enough, simply allocating subjects randomly to control and experimental groups will make it likely that groups will be initially well matched. In some studies, particularly small ones, there may need to be more formal matching for disease severity.
- A placebo effect of treatment may occur – a psychologically based improvement that results from the patient's *expectation* that treatment will yield benefits. If the outcome measure involves any subjective grading of symptom severity, this placebo effect is likely to be particularly important. Ideally the control subjects would be given a dummy treatment which they cannot distinguish from the real treatment – the placebo. Note that in clinical trials of 'treatments' for a disease it may be considered unethical to offer a placebo to subjects when effective treatments are already established; see Goldacre (2008) for further discussion of this.
- There may be unconscious bias on the part of the operator who measures outcomes and who administers the real and dummy treatments. Ideally the experimenter should also be unaware of which patients are receiving real and dummy treatments until after the data collection has been completed. This is particularly important if the outcome measure involves any subjective judgements. If the operator knows which are the real and the dummy treatments, this could affect

how he or she interacts with the subjects and thus partly undermine the effects of the placebo control.

When dealing with clinical trials of dietary interventions, there may be particular problems such as those listed below that may make it impossible to achieve the design aims listed above.

- A dietary intervention aimed at varying intake of a particular nutrient will usually involve consequential changes in the intakes of other nutrients.
- If the intervention is a special diet, it may be difficult or impossible to allow for the placebo effect and to eliminate operator bias. This will be easier if the dietary change can be accomplished by the use of a supplement in pill form.
- If the intervention is a special diet, there are likely to be variations in the degree of compliance and it may be difficult or impossible to objectively assess the level of compliance.

One ideal model of a clinical trial is the double-blind random-crossover type. Patients are given indistinguishable real or dummy treatments during two consecutive trial periods and some measure of treatment success is made at the end of both treatment periods. Patients would be randomly assigned to receive either real or dummy treatment first. Neither patient nor experimenter knows whether real or dummy treatment is being given at any particular time. It may even be possible to ensure uniform compliance by administering treatment (e.g. a tablet) in the presence of the experimenter. Below is an example to illustrate this type of experimental design.

MacGregor *et al.* (1982) prescribed patients with mild to moderate hypertension a diet designed to be low in sodium. All subjects were required to remain on this experimental diet throughout the 10 weeks of the experiment. After a 2-week adjustment period, the subjects then received either slow-release sodium tablets or placebos during two consecutive monthly periods. The sodium tablets raised salt intake and negated the effects of the low-salt diet. The real and dummy tablets were identical and were administered using the double-blind random-crossover model; see Figure 4.5 for a summary of the experimental protocol. Blood pressure was found to be significantly lower at the end of the placebo period compared to the salt supplementation period. This supports the hypothesis that moderate salt restriction can have at least some short-term effect of lowering blood pressure in this category of patient.

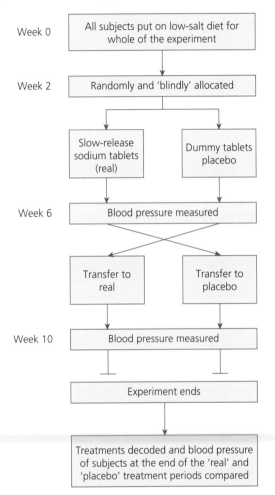

Figure 4.5 Plan of the experimental protocol of MacGregor *et al.* (1982) to illustrate a double-blind, random-crossover trial.

In Chapter 16, a large double-blind clinical trial is described that was set up to test whether folic acid supplements given to high-risk pregnant women reduced the risk of babies being born with neural tube defects. The subjects were almost 2000 women, from seven countries and 33 centres, who were at high risk of having babies with neural tube defects (because of a previously affected pregnancy). They were randomly assigned to receive one of four

treatments starting when they planned to become pregnant again:

- folic acid supplements
- other vitamin supplements
- both of these
- neither of these, just a placebo.

There were many fewer affected babies in the two folic-acid supplemented groups compared to the two groups not receiving folic acid supplements (MRC, 1991). It has since been demonstrated that folic acid supplements are also effective in preventing first occurrence of neural tube defects in random samples of women (see Chapter 16).

Clinical trials vary in the quality of their design and execution. In a good clinical trial there will be:

- effective double-blinding so that neither the subjects nor the experimenters can tell who is receiving real or placebo treatments at any given time
- unbiased allocation of subjects to control and test groups so that groups are well matched at the start
- detailed records of number of subjects who drop out during the course of the trial and the reasons why they drop out (subjects may drop out in large numbers if they find a treatment ineffective or if they suffer side-effects).

Where clinical trials are being assessed for quality, especially if they are being judged on their suitability for inclusion in a meta-analysis (see later in this chapter), then a quantitative grading system for quality assessment may be used. One of the best known and most widely used of these quality grading schemes is the *Jadad score* (Jadad *et al.*, 1996). In this system, clinical trials are allocated points according to the following criteria.

- If a trial is described as double-blind it is given one point, and a second point if a satisfactory method of achieving that double-blinding is described. If the method is described and deemed unsatisfactory then no points are given.
- If there is said to be random allocation of subjects to different groups, then one point is given and a second point is given if a satisfactory mechanism for that random allocation is described. If the method of allocation is deemed unsatisfactory then no points are given.

- One point is given if the report has details of numbers of dropouts and their reasons for dropping out.

This means that the best designed and reported trials will receive a Jadad score of 5 and the worst a score of 0.

Key points

- Clinical trials aim to isolate and quantify the effects of a treatment on the course, onset or severity of a disease.
- With large samples it may be sufficient to randomly allocate subjects to control and test groups, but in small studies there often needs to be more direct matching of subjects for initial severity.
- The use of a dummy treatment (placebo) in the control group can allow for any psychological effects of treatment.
- In the double-blind design, neither patient nor researchers know who has been allocated to the treatment and control groups until the end of the study.
- Clinical trials of dietary interventions have particular difficulties, such as:
  - it may be difficult to produce isolated changes in diet
  - it may be difficult to design a placebo treatment that is not easily recognizable by either subjects or researchers
  - there can be variation in compliance with the prescribed diet that may be difficult to quantify.
- Clinical trials vary in the quality of their design and execution. The Jadad score is a quantitative assessment of their quality. Trials are given a score of 0 (worst) to 5 (best) depending on: how well they are double-blinded (0–2 points), how subjects are allocated in an unbiased way to control and test groups (0–2 points), and whether clear records are kept of dropouts and their reasons for dropping out (0–1 points).

Intervention trials

These are essentially long-term experiments at the population level. The design aim is to make the intended variable or variables the only difference between matched control and experimental groups. The scale and duration of most intervention trials, and perhaps also the nature of the intervention itself, may make it impossible to impose the level of rigour in design that can be accomplished with small, short-term experiments or clinical trials. Some of the problems that may be encountered are given below.

- *Selection of subjects.* In some intervention trials, a 'high-risk' group may be used as subjects. Even if an intervention is convincingly shown to benefit such subjects, this does not necessarily mean that the intervention will yield net benefit to the population as a whole.
- *Ethics of withholding treatment or information from the control group.* When such high-risk subjects are used, there may be an ethical dilemma about how to treat the control group. If they are made aware of their high-risk status, control groups may significantly alter their behaviour during the course of the experiment.
- *Multiple intervention.* Most of the chronic diseases of industrialization are assumed to have a multifactorial aetiology. Multiple risk factor interventions may be used to maximize the likely benefit. In some cases, the experimental aspects of the trial may be given low priority because the primary purpose is to promote health within a population rather than to test the efficacy of the intervention. Using such multiple interventions may make it impossible to quantify the contribution of any particular intervention to the overall benefits (or harm) demonstrated for the experimental group. Factorial design of experiments can aid in this respect but may not be practicable in many trials. Note that the previously discussed clinical trial of folic acid supplementation in pregnant women is an example of a factorial design. With such a design it is possible to statistically test the effects of several interventions and also to test for any possible interaction between interventions.
- *Measure of outcome.* An intervention trial may be designed to test the effect of the intervention on a particular disease risk marker or on morbidity or mortality from a particular disease. Even if the intervention produces the expected beneficial effect in such cases, the ultimate holistic test of the benefit of the intervention is whether such

narrow benefits result in a reduction in total morbidity or mortality. Statistically significant reductions in these holistic measures may require impossibly large subject groups and long periods of study.

Some early studies of the effects of water fluoridation on the dental health of UK children come closer to an 'ideal' design than most intervention trials. In 1956, three trial areas of the UK started to fluoridate their water supplies while three neighbouring areas were used as controls. Prevalence of caries in the teeth of the children in the control and trial areas was similar prior to fluoridation, but by 1961 the trial areas had shown a considerable relative improvement. One of the trial areas later discontinued fluoridation, and within 5 years caries prevalence had risen back up to the level in the control areas. This trial provided very convincing evidence of the benefit of fluoridation to the dental health of children. The controversy that has prevented widespread fluoridation of water supplies in the UK revolves around its long-term safety rather than its efficacy in preventing dental caries. Absolute long-term safety is, of course, much more difficult to demonstrate convincingly.

In the Multiple Risk Factor Intervention Trial (MRFIT, 1982), a third of a million American men were screened to identify 13 000 who were classified as at 'high risk' of coronary heart disease (often referred to as the MR FIT study). These high-risk men were then randomly assigned to experimental and control groups. The experimental group received intensive dietary counselling aimed at both normalization of plasma cholesterol concentration and body weight; they received aggressive treatment for hypertension and intensive counselling to help them reduce their use of tobacco. The control group received no counselling but they, and their personal physicians, were advised of their high-risk status and the results of annual physical examinations sent to their physicians. They were classified as 'usual care'. The intervention was apparently very successful in modifying behaviour and in producing measurable reductions in the objective risk markers (e.g. plasma cholesterol concentration). However, the study failed to show any beneficial effects of intervention; that is, there was no difference in either total mortality or even CHD disease mortality between the two groups after 7 years of follow-up.

This failure has been partly explained by the behaviour of the control group, who also appeared to modify their behaviour once they became aware of their high-risk status. It has also been suggested that harmful effects of the anti-hypertensive therapy may have cancelled out and obscured the beneficial effects of other aspects of the intervention. This trial is now 30 years old, but a recent meta-analysis of multiple risk factor intervention trials that used counselling and education aimed at behaviour change did not reduce CHD mortality or clinical events in the general population but did achieve some reduction in mortality in high-risk groups including hypertensives and diabetics (Ebrahim *et al.*, 2011).

Both of these trials could be described as *primary intervention trials* because they aimed to prevent the onset of disease in asymptomatic subjects. Rarely have such trials produced significant reductions in total mortality when dietary interventions have been used. Other trials are described as *secondary intervention trials* because they use subjects who have already experienced a disease event such as a myocardial infarction (MI). These are an extreme example of a high-risk group and one would need to be particularly cautious about assuming that any benefit demonstrated in such a group would have net beneficial effects on the population as a whole. Burr *et al.* (1991) tested the effects of three dietary interventions on total 2-year mortality in 2000 men who had recovered from an MI. The three dietary interventions were advice to:

- increase cereal fibre consumption
- reduce total fat intake
- eat oily fish or take fish oil capsules twice weekly.

The subjects were randomly allocated to receive or not to receive advice on each of these three interventions, and the allocations were made independently of allocations for the other two interventions. Thus there were eight possible combinations of interventions or non-interventions, including a group who received no intervention at all. The fish oil intervention almost uniquely, for a dietary intervention, did produce a significant reduction in total all-cause mortality. One suggestion as to why this trial alone has produced a statistically significant fall in total mortality is because there appeared to be almost no tendency for the non-fish-advised men to increase their fish consumption. At the time, the potential therapeutic effects of fish oils were not widely known in the UK. In many other intervention trials, control subjects have also tended to modify their behaviour in the direction of that counselled for the intervention group.

Key points

- Intervention trials are long-term population-level experiments.
- The scale and duration of these studies and the nature of the interventions may pose considerable design problems.
- If high-risk subjects are used then it cannot be assumed that any net benefit demonstrated in the study will translate to a net benefit for the general population.
- It may pose ethical problems if high-risk control subjects are denied the intervention that is expected to be beneficial.
- It will undermine the study if control subjects alter their behaviour in the direction of that suggested for the experimental groups.
- If multiple interventions are used, it may be difficult to decide which intervention has produced any study benefits.
- A reduction in mortality for a particular disease or disease risk factor does not necessarily mean that the intervention has produced a net benefit.
- Statistically significant reductions in total mortality may require impossibly large groups and long periods of study. Primary dietary interventions have rarely produced statistically significant reductions in total mortality.
- A secondary intervention trial uses subjects who have already experienced a disease event.

Systematic reviews and meta-analyses

The costs and difficulties of conducting a controlled trial increase with the size and duration of the study. For this reason many clinical trials have used relatively small numbers of subjects. This means that even well-designed and executed studies may not have the statistical power to provide a definitive judgement of the value of the intervention. This means that even though the scientific literature might contain many individual studies of a particular intervention it may still be difficult to make a clear judgement of its effectiveness. These studies will vary in size and quality and in the details of their design, so simply counting how many studies are for, against or inconclusive is not a helpful or valid procedure.

A systematic review aims to identify, using preset and objective search methodology, as many as possible of the studies that have addressed a particular topic. One or more electronic databases of published papers will be used to identify all papers that use the key search words. Additional preset and systematic search methods may be used to find additional studies, such as the reference lists of papers from the primary search and perhaps some method for trying to get data from studies that have not been formally published.

A meta-analysis of studies identified from a systematic review involves a statistical pooling of all studies that meet predetermined quality and eligibility criteria. In this way, the data from a number of small studies of limited statistical power can be combined and treated as if they were from a single study of much greater statistical power. Individual component studies in the meta-analysis are weighted according to the sample size used. In theory, a well-conducted systematic review and meta-analysis should give a much better indication of the true answer to a question than a simple for-and-against count or a qualitative and subjective interpretation by the reviewer.

When studies are combined in a meta-analysis, it is assumed that they are all essentially homogeneous and that any differences between them in terms of outcome are due to chance. This is often not the case. For example, differences in outcome may be due to 'real' differences in the nature of the subjects; that is, a treatment may have different effects in different categories of subject. The reviewers will set general eligibility criteria for inclusion in the meta-analysis, such as:

- the characteristics of the subjects (e.g. their age and sex)
- the diagnostic criteria used to select subjects for the trial and the severity level of medical condition being investigated
- the minimum duration of the trial

- the minimum 'dose' level of the intervention being tested
- the outcome measures used.

In addition to these general eligibility criteria, reviewers might set a minimum quality level for inclusion in the meta-analysis, such as a minimum Jadad score (see above). If reviewers use different eligibility criteria for inclusion of trials in their meta-analysis, they might come to different conclusions about the efficacy of any intervention or treatment despite apparently reviewing the same body of scientific literature. Alternatively, reviewers might analyse the data before and after exclusion of some trials on quality or other grounds, so they might show an analysis with all trials included and then another for those with a minimum quality score, a minimum duration or a minimum dose level. Webb (2007, 2011b) has noted that, in meta-analyses of the efficacy of supplements, reviewers frequently note that the apparent efficacy of these supplements tends to decrease when only the larger and better designed studies are included (e.g. McAlindon *et al.*, 2000; Bjelakovic *et al.*, 2008).

These selected examples seem to be part of a general trend in which trials of lower methodological quality produce a higher estimate of benefit from the intervention than higher quality trials.

These anecdotal observations are supported by a more systematic study by Moher *et al.* (1998). They randomly selected 11 meta-analyses of various medical interventions for treatment of a variety of conditions. They repeated these meta-analyses but divided up the studies according to quality. They found that many of the trials were of low quality and that lower quality trials were associated with a 34 per cent increase in estimated treatment benefit compared to the better conducted trials. This finding was consistent when two different methods were used for quality classification.

One might expect some reduction in level of statistical significance when reviewers reduce the number of studies in a meta-analysis by setting higher quality criteria (because sample size has been reduced). However, if there is also a substantial drop in the size of the treatment effect then this would indicate that the lower quality trials were biasing results in favour of the treatment.

Some of the other pitfalls of this approach are summarized below (after Naylor, 1997).

Publication bias

It is a general observation that studies with positive outcomes are more likely to be published than those with negative or inconclusive outcomes (e.g. Easterbrook *et al.*, 1991). If studies are funded by organizations or companies who have a commercial interest in the outcome of a trial, this might lead to lack of publication of trials with negative outcomes and perhaps selective publication or highlighting of positive findings. This is seen as a major problem in the area of dietary supplements because of the high level of involvement of manufacturing companies in the funding of trials. It is now common to see authors of scientific papers and clinical trials acknowledge sources of funding and any 'conflicting interests'. This may also be a problem with drug trials as the following example shows.

Turner *et al.* (2008) identified 74 trials of antidepressant drugs registered with the Food and Drugs Administration (FDA) in the USA. Only one of 38 trials with positive outcomes was not published, whereas 22 of the 36 studies with negative or questionable results were not published and 11 were published in a way that, in the opinion of Turner's team, conveyed a positive outcome.

It is possible to detect whether substantial publication bias has occurred, and one of the simplest and most widely used of these methods is the *funnel plot*. The assumption is made that small trials will give more variable results than larger trials of the same quality. In a funnel plot the effect estimate of each trial is plotted against the sample size. In the absence of bias one would expect to see a symmetrical (funnel-shaped) scattering of trials around the true effect estimate. The larger and more consistent trials should be closely grouped at the top of the funnel and then, as trial sizes get smaller and more inconsistent in their results, the scattering around the true result should get larger but still remain broadly symmetrical. If there is a lack of symmetry (usually a lack of small trials showing a negative effect) then this would suggest publication bias – that some of the small negative trials have not been published. This is illustrated in Figure 4.6 where a funnel plot of 35 simulated studies is shown and this plot is then redrawn as if five small trials with negative outcomes had not been published. See Sutton *et al.* (2000) and Egger *et al.* (1997) for further details and discussion.

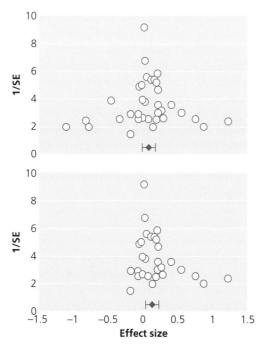

Figure 4.6 Typical funnel plot generated using 35 simulated studies in the top graph and the same plot at the bottom after removing 5 smaller trials with negative outcomes, to illustrate the typical manifestation of publication bias. Reproduced from Sutton *et al.* (2000) *British Medical Journal* 320, 1574.

Multiple publishing

Some trials are published more than once. If these are all included in a meta-analysis then this can bias its outcome. Naylor (1997) quotes the example of a single study being the source for seven different publications. These reports of the same trial had different authorships – which makes it more difficult to identify that they all related to the same study.

Selection bias

Unless the selection of papers for inclusion in the meta-analysis is done strictly using preset objective criteria, this may be a source of bias. It is usual for at least two people to independently assess whether individual trials meet the reviewers' eligibility criteria. Note the earlier comments about how changing eligibility criteria can affect the outcome of a meta-analysis.

The results of a meta-analysis are frequently presented visually in the form of a *forest plot*, an example of which is shown in Figure 4.7 (Linde *et al.*, 2008). Each of the 18 horizontal lines represents one clinical trial of the herbal product St John's wort versus a placebo in the treatment of major depression; St John's wort has been widely sold as a dietary supplement, and still is outside of the European Union. The bullet in the middle of the line represents the mean treatment effect and the limits of the lines represent the 95 per cent confidence limits. The size of the bullet gives an indication of the weighting applied to that study. Any bullet to the left of the vertical zero line favours the placebo and any to the right favours St John's wort. The trials have been divided by precision (i.e. size) and the more precise trial results favour the effect of St John's wort over the placebo more than the lower higher precision trials, as is generally the case. Interestingly, when the trials were divided according to whether they originated from a German-speaking country or not, the studies from German-speaking countries produced results that were more favourable to St John's wort than those from other countries which found no significant benefit from the herbal extract. Linde *et al.* (2008) speculate on some possible reasons for this difference.

Several examples of meta-analyses will be found in later chapters of this book. For example, in Chapter 13 there is discussion of a meta-analysis by Vivekanathan *et al.* (2003). These authors used seven large randomized trials of the effects of vitamin E supplements on long-term mortality and morbidity from cardiovascular disease and eight trials of β-carotene supplements. This analysis found no suggestion of any benefits for vitamin E supplements and evidence that β-carotene supplements caused a small but statistically significant increase in both all-cause and cardiovascular mortality. They concluded that their analysis provided no support for routine supplementation with vitamin E and that supplements of β-carotene were contraindicated.

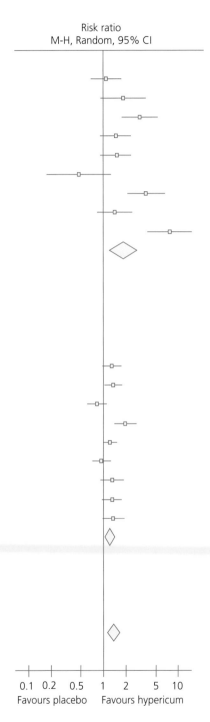

Risk ratio
M-H, Random, 95% CI

0.1 0.2   0.5   1   2   5   10
Favours placebo   Favours hypericum

Figure 4.7 Typical forest-plot presentation of the data from a meta-analysis. The plot shows results (risk ratio with 95 per cent confidence intervals (CI)) from 18 clinical trials of St John's wort (Hypericum) against a placebo for the treatment of depression. The top nine trials were the lowest quality while the bottom nine were the highest quality. The three diamonds represent (from top to bottom) the combined weighted result of: the eight lowest quality trials, the eight highest quality trials, and all 16 trials. Reproduced with permission from Linde *et al.* (2008) *Cochrane Database of Systematic Reviews)* Oct 8;(4): CD000448.

The *Cochrane Library* contains a large electronically searchable database of systematic reviews that can be accessed freely by most readers of this book (see www.thecochranelibrary.com/view/0/index.html). The Cochrane Collaboration is a non-profit organization that aims to improve healthcare decision-making by increasing the availability of systematic reviews of healthcare interventions.

Key points

- A systematic review aims to identify all trials of a particular hypothesis using predetermined and systematic searching of the literature.
- In addition to electronic searching of the literature, other methods may be used to identify clinical trials including those that may not have been formally published.
- In a meta-analysis, studies that meet set quality and other eligibility criteria are weighted according to sample size and then combined into a single study of greater statistical power.
- Factors that may distort the outcome of a meta-analysis are selection bias, publication bias and multiple publishing of the same data set.
- Publication bias means that trials with positive outcomes are more likely to be published than those with negative outcomes. This leads to distortion of the meta-analysis in favour of the intervention.
- Funnel plots (e.g. Figure 4.6) are used as a simple means of trying to detect publication bias.
- In order to minimize selection bias, formal quality and eligibility criteria are set and several assessors independently decide which trials meet these criteria.
- In general, smaller trials and lower quality trials tend to give a higher estimate of the benefit of any intervention than larger and higher quality trials.
- Forest plots (e.g. Figure 4.7) are a common way of visually presenting the results of a meta-analysis.
- The Cochrane Library contains a searchable electronic database of high-quality systematic reviews of the efficacy and safety of healthcare interventions.

IN-VITRO STUDIES

In-vitro studies are literally studies that have been done 'in glass', and this contrasts with studies using animals or people which are termed in-vivo or 'in life'. In-vitro studies would include:

- simple analytical studies measuring the level of a substance presumed to be beneficial in a food (e.g. measuring levels of anti-oxidants in berries)
- experiments with isolated cells including tumour cells (e.g. what effect does a food component have on growth of tumour cells?)
- experiments using micro-organisms (e.g. the mutagenicity of a substance in bacteria may be a guide to its likely carcinogenicity)
- the effect of a food component on a receptor or enzyme system (e.g. phyto-oestrogens in soya beans bind to and weakly stimulate mammalian oestrogen receptors).

As an example, the dietary supplement gluocosamine is widely used to prevent or alleviate the symptoms of arthritis. There is evidence that it can stimulate the production of cartilage in cultured chondrocytes, and this has been used as support for the view that it may help in joint repair and maintenance even though the concentrations required are high in relation to those found *in vivo* after glucosamine supplementation (Bassleer *et al.*, 1998).

The results of such experiments must be interpreted conservatively until there is collaboration from more holistic studies. Extravagant media claims like the following are often made about specific foods or supplements on the basis of such studies:

- a substance with high levels of potential anti-oxidants may be claimed as being able to prevent cancer
- a substance that reduces the growth of isolated tumour cells may be claimed to have value in treating cancer
- a food substance able to kill bacteria in culture may be claimed to have potential anti-infective properties when eaten.

Key points

- In-vitro studies are those done not with whole animals or people; they are done 'in glass'. They might include:
  - analysing for the presence of a particular chemical constituent
  - measuring effects on micro-organisms or isolated cells
  - measuring the effects on an enzyme's activity or the ability to bind with a receptor.
- The results of in-vitro studies need to be interpreted with caution. They should not be used to make extravagant claims about the curative or disease-preventing potential of a food or food component.

SCIENTIFIC HONESTY

It is generally assumed by those reviewing and reading scientific papers that the researchers have been honest, honourable and unbiased in the conduct, analysis and reporting of their research. Reviewers look for flaws in the study, errors in the analysis of the results or for errors of logic in the interpretation of the results. There are, however, some occasions where authors have been accused of knowingly publishing false research results in order to advance their careers or for commercial gain. It is almost impossible for non-specialists to spot such fraudulent data that have already deceived specialist reviewers and editors. Sometimes papers are retracted when evidence of fraud is found, but non-specialists might not be aware of the retraction of a paper that they have already read and maybe have a hard copy of. If one paper by an author is retracted as the result of alleged scientific fraud, then this must call into question other papers written by the same author. Reference to five papers which were discussed in previous editions of this book have been excluded because of present doubts about their veracity.

A paper published in the journal *Nutrition* by the Canadian researcher R. K. Chandra in 2001 was retracted in 2005. This paper described a placebo-controlled trial that seemed to show that moderate doses of vitamins and minerals taken as supplements improved cognitive functioning in elderly people. The author has published more than 200 articles, and four of these were cited in the previous edition of this book as study evidence that vitamin and mineral supplements might have beneficial effects on immune function in elderly people. Much of the published work of the author must now be reconsidered, especially as it is claimed that he benefitted handsomely from sales of his multivitamin mixture sold as an 'evidence-based' (his own published trials) nutrition supplement for the elderly. Readers are referred to Smith (2005) and Hamblin (2006) for further details.

In the previous edition of this book, a paper in the influential journal *Nature* by Ahluwalia *et al.* (published 2004) was cited in the section on anti-oxidants and the oxidant theory of disease. This paper suggested neutrophils did not, as generally believed, kill ingested bacteria by generating an oxidative pulse of free radicals but that an influx of potassium ions through a key ion channel was the key event leading to microbial destruction. This paper raised quite fundamental doubts about the role of free radicals in the aetiology of chronic disease and ageing. Other research groups have been unable to reproduce these results, and it was reported that the ion conductance channel said by Ahluwalia's report to be essential in innate immunity (i.e. in the killing of ingested bacteria in neutrophils) is not even present on neutrophils; see DeCoursey (2007) for a detailed discussion of this work. In November 2010, Ahluwalia's seven co-authors retracted their paper and he was accused of multiple counts of scientific fraud.

Key points

- On rare occasions authors may display scientific dishonesty by publishing results that they know to be false. This may be very difficult for reviewers and readers to detect.
- Even when a suspect paper is retracted, non-specialists who have already read the paper may take some time to become aware of the retraction, and the other work of the accused author must also become dubious.

DIETARY GUIDELINES AND RECOMMENDATIONS

5

The range of 'expert reports' and their
consistency   134
Variations in the presentation of guidelines
and recommendations   136
'Food' recommendations   137
Energy and body weight   139
Recommendations for fats, carbohydrates,
protein and salt   140
Alcohol   143
How current UK diets compare with 'ideal'
intakes   146
Other nutrients   147
Willingness to change   147
Some barriers to dietary change   149
Aids to food selection   150
Concluding remarks   154

THE RANGE OF 'EXPERT REPORTS' AND THEIR CONSISTENCY

Over the past several decades there have been dozens of expert reports published in the industrialized countries that have produced sets of dietary guidelines or recommended changes in national diets. These guidelines and recommendations have been aimed at reducing morbidity and mortality from the diseases of industrialization and so ultimately at promoting health and longevity. Prior to this, most published dietary recommendations and guidelines were geared towards assuring adequate intakes of the essential nutrients and preventing the consequences of deficiency. The first fairly comprehensive standards of adequacy were published as early as 1943 in the USA. Truswell (1999) reviewed dietary guidelines around the world at the end of the millennium.

Some of these sets of dietary guidelines have focused on one aspect of diet and health. For example, in the UK, COMA (1994a) focused on 'nutritional aspects of cardiovascular disease' whereas COMA (1998) was concerned with 'nutritional aspects of the development of cancer'.

Other reports have attempted to synthesize current ideas on the relationship between diet and individual diseases and produced more general and comprehensive guidelines aimed at 'reducing chronic disease risk' and promoting health; examples are NRC (1989b) in the USA and COMA (1991) in the UK.

These many reports from around the world inevitably vary somewhat in the way the recommendations are framed, the scope of their recommendations, the precise quantitative targets and the priority attached to the various recommendations. Nevertheless, in general qualitative terms, there is a striking level of agreement and consistency between almost all of these reports; examples of fundamental disagreement are rare. This certainly adds a cumulative weight to the recommendations and guidelines. Most of these reports directly or indirectly recommend the changes listed below, or at least make recommendations that are consistent with them.

- Maintain your *body mass index* (BMI) within the ideal range (i.e. avoid excessive weight gain), by restricting energy intake and/or increasing energy expenditure (exercise).

- Eat a variety of foods with ample amounts of starchy, fibre-rich foods and plenty of fruits and vegetables.
- Reduce the proportion of fat (especially the saturated type) in your diet and perhaps reduce or not increase cholesterol intake.
- Reduce salt consumption.
- Reduce or not increase the consumption of added sugars (i.e. those not naturally present in fruit, vegetables and milk).
- Limit your consumption of alcohol.

In the UK, the report of the National Advisory Committee on Nutrition Education (NACNE, 1983) had a great influence on nutrition education. This committee, for the first time in the UK, attempted to offer a comprehensive set of quantitative dietary targets for the UK population. Its publication generated considerable debate and controversy in the UK, and this debate helped focus attention on the relationships between diet and chronic degenerative diseases. NACNE suggested that its full recommendations could be implemented 'within 15 years' (i.e. by 1998) and that a third of the recommended changes could be achieved 'within 5 years' (by around 1988).

In retrospect, several of the NACNE targets now look unrealistic to try and achieve within a 15-year period, such as the aim to reduce total fat intake by almost a quarter and almost halve intakes of saturated fat and added sugars. NACNE's short-term target for total dietary fat (i.e. to reduce total fat to no more than about 35 per cent of food energy by 1988) appeared in the Department of Health report on *The Health of the Nation* (DH, 1992) as a target for the year 2005! Data from the National Dietary and Nutrition Survey in 2009 indicate that adults have now just about achieved this goal. The COMA reports on *Dietary Reference Values*, *Nutritional Aspects of Cardiovascular Disease* and *Nutritional Aspects of the Development of Cancer* (COMA, 1991, 1994a, 1998 respectively) are still currently regarded as the authoritative sources of UK dietary recommendations and guidelines. This chapter will use a synthesis of the recommendations in these three reports as the current UK position.

In the USA, *Dietary Goals for the United States* published in 1977 was the first report to focus specifically on reducing the risk of chronic degenerative disease. It also aroused considerable critical comment and discussion at the time. According to Truswell (1999), one collection of commentaries on this report contains almost 900 pages. Some of the criticisms of this report seem very familiar and many of them are still commonly made about all reports of this type. Some examples of these criticisms are listed below (after Truswell).

- Some of the recommendations are wrong or too extreme, or some important issues are not adequately covered. In this particular report, there were criticisms that the target for salt was too ambitious and that there were no targets for obesity.
- The report is premature and based on inadequate scientific evidence.
- The recommendations might not be appropriate for the whole population. In particular, the guidelines might be more appropriate for overweight middle-aged males than for active, rapidly growing children and perhaps even for women.
- The report is unnecessary because health and life expectancy are already improving.
- The recommended changes might have serious negative impact on important industries like the sugar industry and the dairy industry.
- A general resentment was expressed that governments and their experts were trying to instruct people on what to eat.

The National Research Council report of 1989 (NRC, 1989b) offered a comprehensive set of dietary recommendations and goals and, while there have been several sets of guidelines offered since then, these still represent a very concise set of targets that would be regarded as consistent with current more complex and lengthy advice. *Dietary Guidelines for Americans* is published every 5 years and the latest edition was published in 2010 jointly by the Departments of Health and Human Services and Agriculture (DHHS/USDA, 2010). These new guidelines offer tailored recommendations to different lifecycle and racial groups within the US population and these issues are discussed in Chapters 16 and 18. The general recommendations are consistent with the international consensus summary offered at the start of this chapter. These latest guidelines are summarized under four headings.

- *Balancing calories to manage weight.* Americans are advised to increase physical activity, to reduce the time they spend in sedentary activities, and to control their calorie intake to manage body weight – which will mean eating less for those who are overweight or obese.
- *Foods and food components to reduce.* In this section guidelines are set for reducing or limiting intakes of salt, saturated fatty acids, cholesterol, *trans*-fatty acids, solid fats, added sugars, refined cereal grains and alcohol.
- *Foods and nutrients to increase.* These include fruits and vegetables, whole grains, low-fat milk and milk products, oils (to replace solid fats), seafood, dietary fibre, potassium, calcium and vitamin D.
- *Building healthy eating patterns.* Americans are advised to select an eating pattern that meets nutrient needs over time at an appropriate energy level (see the section on adopting a 'low-risk' lifestyle in Chapter 9) and to follow food safety recommendations to reduce the risk of food poisoning (see microbiological safety of food in Chapter 19).

The World Health Organization (WHO, 1990) published a set of nutritional goals in the form of suggested minimum-to-maximum ranges for selected nutrients. The minimum suggested intake of the nutrient should be sufficient to prevent deficiency, while the maximum should be consistent with the aim of reducing the risk of chronic degenerative disease. These goals were intended to have worldwide application and are summarized below.

- Total fat should make up 15–30 per cent of energy intake, and countries consuming high amounts of fat should ultimately work towards the lower end of this range.
- Saturated fatty acids should not exceed 10 per cent of total energy, with no lower limit.
- Polyunsaturated fatty acids should make up 3–7 per cent of energy intake.
- Cholesterol intake should be below 300 mg/day, with no lower limit.
- Carbohydrate should provide 55–75 per cent of dietary energy and complex carbohydrate (starch) 50–75 per cent.
- Dietary fibre intake should be 27–40 g/day (which corresponds to approximately 20–25 g of non-starch polysaccharide, NSP).

- Added sugars should contribute no more than 10 per cent of dietary energy, with no lower limit.
- Protein from mixed sources should provide 10–15 per cent of dietary energy.
- Salt intake should be less than 6 g/day, with no lower limit specified (although some small amount of salt intake is essential).

Key points

- In recent decades the focus of nutrition education has been on preventing chronic diseases rather than simply ensuring dietary adequacy.
- Many sets of recommendations and guidelines have been produced in the last few decades and there is a remarkable consistency about the general qualitative changes that they recommend for industrialized countries.
- Consumers should eat more starch, fibre and fruits and vegetables but less fat, saturated fat, added sugar and salt. Excessive alcohol consumption should be avoided.
- Most of these reports also encourage increased levels of physical activity and physical fitness.
- Criticisms of these reports, particularly the earlier ones, have been on the following grounds:
  - a recommendation is wrong or impractical
  - a recommendation is premature and there is insufficient evidence to justify it
  - a recommendation may be inappropriate for some sectors of the population
  - implementing the recommendation(s) will have adverse economic consequences
  - governments should not try to control what people eat.
- The World Health Organization has published a set of nutritional goals that are intended to have worldwide application.

VARIATIONS IN THE PRESENTATION OF GUIDELINES AND RECOMMENDATIONS

Some reports on diet and health frame their advice in the form of simple qualitative or semi-quantitative recommendations that are easy to understand by the general public: 'Eat five portions of fruits and vegetables each day', 'Reduce consumption of fatty foods, especially those rich in saturated fat', and so on. Other more technical reports aimed at scientists and health professionals usually frame their recommendations in a more quantitative way like the WHO goals listed earlier. It is expected that health professionals and health promoters will interpret these quantitative ideals and translate them into practical dietary recommendations for their clients.

Some quantitative recommendations such as those for salt and fibre are given simply as grams per day. However, for the energy-yielding nutrients (fats, carbohydrates and proteins) these recommendations are often framed as a percentage of the dietary energy as seen in some of the WHO recommendations listed earlier. This method of presentation allows the amount of the nutrient to be expressed in a single number that does not have to be adjusted as energy intake varies, or be qualified by a statement of the energy intake at which it applies. It effectively represents the concentration of the nutrient in the diet. Further discussion of this procedure and the calculations involved may be found in Chapter 7. A recommendation that carbohydrates should be 50 per cent of total energy means that carbohydrates should provide 50 per cent of the total energy consumed. Sometimes recommendations are expressed as a percentage of the food energy rather than total energy, to eliminate the distorting effects of alcohol. The recommendation that Britons should reduce fat to 33 per cent of their total average energy intake is approximately equivalent to 35 per cent of their average food energy excluding alcohol. Alcohol normally has a diluting effect on the proportion of energy derived from the other macronutrients.

In the UK, dietary recommendations have usually been framed as targets for average population consumption, such as (DH, 1992):

> reduce the average percentage of food energy from about 40 per cent in 1990 to no more than 35 per cent by 2005.

Earlier than that, the NRC (1989b) gave its recommendations in the form of individual minimum or maximum intakes:

> fat should make up no more than 30 per cent of an individual's energy intake.

If a 'percentage of energy' target is set as an individual maximum or minimum, this requires a much greater change than if the same target is set as an ideal population average.

Current dietary reference values (DRVs) for macronutrients in the USA (summarized in NAS, 2004) are presented in a much more detailed format with specific amounts (g/day) offered for each age group for carbohydrate, dietary fibre, total fat and n-6 and n-3 polyunsaturated fatty acids, just as they are for vitamins and minerals.

Some recommendations may be targeted at specific groups (e.g. guidelines for pregnant women), or they may exclude particular groups (e.g. children under 5 years). This chapter will generally consider recommendations intended for all healthy people aged over 5 years. Recommendations for specific lifecycle groups are dealt with in Chapter 16.

Key points

- Some reports frame their recommendations in simple qualitative terms that can be interpreted by the general public.

- Others reports offer quantitative targets that health professionals and health promoters need to translate into practical terms for their clients.

- Quantitative fat, carbohydrate and protein targets are sometimes expressed as a percentage of total energy or food energy (excluding alcohol). This method of expression means that the numerical recommendation does not need to be qualified by the energy intake at which it applies and effectively represents the concentration of fat, carbohydrate or protein in the diet.

- In Britain, targets are usually expressed as population averages whereas in the past US targets were given as individual maxima and minima.

- Current US dietary standards give numerical values in grams per day for each life-stage group for carbohydrates, dietary fibre, total fat and n-6 and n-3 polyunsaturated fatty acids.

'FOOD' RECOMMENDATIONS

Consumers in the UK, the USA and elsewhere are encouraged to eat a variety of foods each day. Foods have different profiles of essential nutrients and different profiles of potentially toxic substances in them. Eating a variety of foods makes it more likely that adequate amounts of all the essential nutrients will be consumed and less likely that any toxins in food will be consumed in hazardous amounts. Consumers in most countries are encouraged to eat foods from different categories or food groups to ensure the adequacy of their diets (see later). Japanese consumers are advised to eat at least 30 foods each day!

In both the UK and the USA, consumers are being advised to increase their consumption of fruits and vegetables. More specifically, there is an active campaign in the UK that urges consumers to eat a minimum of five portions of fruit and vegetable each day with only one of this five being fruit juice. A portion of fruit and vegetables is nominally 80 g and this translates approximately into the following practical amounts for different fruits and vegetables (after Ogunbadejo and Nicholson, 2010):

- 3 tablespoons of: fresh, raw, tinned or frozen vegetables or mixed vegetables dishes like vegetable curry or ratatouille; or pulses; or tinned, frozen or stewed fruit dishes
- 1 tablespoon of dried fruit
- a handful of very small fruits such as cherries, grapes or berries
- 2 small fruits such as plums or apricots
- 1 medium fruit such as an apple or pear
- half a large fruit such as a grapefruit
- an average slice of melon or similar very large fruit
- a small glass (150 mL) of fruit juice
- a cereal bowl of salad.

Diets low in fruits and vegetables have been associated in numerous epidemiological studies with elevated rates of cancer and cardiovascular disease. There are several possible reasons why fruits and vegetables might exert a protective effect against these diseases, such as those listed below.

- They are major sources of dietary fibre including the soluble components of dietary fibre.
- They are low in energy and so they make the diet bulky and less energy dense, which may help in weight control.
- They increase the proportion of dietary energy that is derived from carbohydrate and so reduce the proportion from fat, and they also alter the balance of dietary proteins, increasing the proportion of total protein that is of vegetable origin.

- They are the major sources of vitamin C and other anti-oxidants such as β-carotene and the other carotenoids and non-nutrient anti-oxidants. These anti-oxidants inhibit the oxidative damage to cells caused by free radicals that may be important in the aetiology of both cancer and cardiovascular disease (see Chapter 13 for further critical discussion).
- They are important sources of potassium, and high potassium intake may help in the prevention of high blood pressure.

Some nutritionists might be sceptical about the putative health benefits of any one of these compositional changes, but almost all would support the recommendation to increase consumption of fruits and vegetables. The cumulative evidence supporting this food change is overwhelming – although there is a real possibility that other non-nutritional differences may contribute to the association between high fruit and vegetable intake and reduced risk of chronic disease. People consuming more fruits and vegetables may be more health conscious or more affluent and thus have other lifestyle characteristics favourable to long-term health. For example, those who eat more fruits and vegetables may be:

- more physically active and leaner
- less likely to smoke or consume excessive amounts of alcohol.

Ogunbadejo and Nicholson (2010) give a detailed analysis of fruit and vegetable consumption patterns in English adults. Table 5.1 shows the percentage of adults in different age and sex groupings who consumed specified numbers of portions of fruits and vegetables, and the mean number of daily portions consumed by these groupings. Around three-quarters of all adults failed to consume the recommended five or more portions, and around 10 per cent consumed less than one portion a day. In general, women consumed slightly more fruit and vegetables than men, and both men's and women's fruit and vegetable consumption tended to increase with age up until 75 years and then fell back slightly. The 16- to 24-year age group seem to be consistently worse than the rest of the adult population in their consumption of fruits and vegetables. Consumption was positively associated with income: 32 per cent of men and 37 per cent of women in the highest income quintile consumed five or more daily

Table 5.1 Fruit and vegetable consumption in age and sex groupings of English adults*

Daily consumption	Men		Women	
	16–24 years	All	16–24 years	All
<1 portion daily	11%	10%	12%	9%
<3 portions	56%	47%	49%	40%
5 or more	17%	25%	18%	28%
Mean daily portions	2.9	3.4	3.1	3.7

*Data from Ogunbadejo and Nicholson (2010).

portions, but only 18 per cent of men and 19 per cent of women in the lowest income quintile did so.

It is recommended in both the UK and the USA that starchy foods like cereals and potatoes should be more prominent in the diet. This would increase the amount of dietary fibre and the proportion of dietary energy coming from starch. This would almost inevitably lead to a reduction in the proportion being derived from fat and/or sugar because there is not much variation in protein intake. It would also lower the energy density of the diet.

Britons and Americans are encouraged to increase their consumption of oily fish (e.g. mackerel, herring, salmon, trout and sardines). These oily fish are the only rich sources of the long-chain n-3 (ω-3) polyunsaturated fatty acids. These fatty acids may have a number of effects that would be regarded as beneficial for many people, such as:

- an anti-inflammatory effect
- an anti-aggregating effect on blood platelets that reduces the tendency of blood to clot and increases bleeding time
- beneficial effects on blood lipoprotein profiles.

Adults in the UK are recommended to eat two portions of fish per week, of which at least one portion (140 g) should be oily fish. Bates *et al.* (2010) estimated that the average adult consumption of oily fish was less than half this recommended level at 56 g/week. The n-3 polyunsaturated fatty acids represent around 1 per cent of food energy and the lowest 2.5 percentile is about half this value, which is still above the individual minimum of 0.2 per cent set by COMA (1991) as the minimum necessary to prevent essential fatty acid deficiency; it is half what is regarded as the optimal level.

There is a more detailed discussion of the actions of fish oils in Chapter 12. Concentrated fish oil supplements have not been overtly recommended for the general population, although they may be useful for some individuals, and some preparations have medicinal licences in the UK for the treatment of high blood triacylglycerol levels and for use in people with existing cardiac disease.

Key points

- People should eat a variety of foods selected from each of the major food groups.
- Dietary variety helps to ensure adequacy and reduces the risk of toxins being consumed in hazardous amounts.
- Five daily portions of fruits and vegetables are recommended in the UK. Five portions are defined as 400 g (80 g per portion).
- Only a quarter of English adults eat five or more daily portions of fruit and vegetables.
- Fruits and vegetables are good sources of dietary fibre, potassium and anti-oxidants. High fruit and vegetable diets tend to be bulky and low in fat, which may assist in weight control.
- High fruit and vegetable intake may be a marker for people who are generally more health conscious and have other healthy lifestyle characteristics.
- Starchy cereals and potatoes should be more prominent in UK and US diets.
- An increased consumption of oily fish is recommended, but English adults eat less than half the recommended amount.

ENERGY AND BODY WEIGHT

Most dietary guidelines emphasize the importance of maintaining an ideal body weight (BMI in the range 18.5–25) by matching energy intake to expenditure. Details of current activity levels and targets for increasing activity are given in Chapter 18. Over 60 per cent of British and American adults are either overweight or obese and these figures have been rising alarmingly during the past few decades. Obesity and being overweight are associated with reduced life expectancy and increased illness and disability, as well as having social and psychological consequences that further reduce the quality of life. In particular, obesity is associated with increased risk of type 2 diabetes, hypertension, cardiovascular diseases and several types of cancer (see Chapter 9 for details on the prevalence and consequences of obesity).

In both the UK and the USA, sufficient physical activity is recognized as a key factor in the maintenance of an ideal body weight. Both the US and UK populations have become increasingly sedentary in recent decades. There is clear evidence in the UK that average energy intakes have fallen substantially in the last few decades (e.g. Prentice and Jebb, 1995), but over the same period average BMI has increased and the numbers of overweight and obese adults have also increased sharply. National surveys of activity and physical fitness of British adults have found very high levels of inactivity and low levels of aerobic fitness among the majority of the adult population (Chapter 18 has further details). In Chapter 9 it is argued that inactivity is a major cause of the epidemic of obesity sweeping through most industrialized and many developing countries. Increased activity should ultimately lead to a reduction in average BMI and some moderation in the numbers of obese and overweight people in these countries. Concentrating on reducing energy intake still further does not seem to be the solution to this persistent problem of obesity. Increased activity and fitness have many other health benefits that are discussed in Chapter 18.

> **Key points**
>
> - Body mass index should be kept within the ideal 18.5–25 kg/m^2 range.
> - Inactivity is an important cause of obesity and increased activity is important in the control of body weight.
>
>   →

> **Key points** *continued*
>
> - Dietary guidelines around the world generally recommend increased levels of physical activity to prevent excessive weight gain.
> - Britons eat less than 60 years ago but are now much fatter.
> - Activity and fitness are associated with numerous other health benefits.

RECOMMENDATIONS FOR FATS, CARBOHYDRATES, PROTEIN AND SALT

UK targets

- The contribution of fat to total energy should be reduced. In the UK the aim is to get fat consumption down to a population average of 35 per cent of food energy (33 per cent of total energy).
- The contribution of saturated fatty acids should be reduced to an average 11 per cent of food energy (10 per cent of total energy).
- Polyunsaturated n-6 (ω-6) fatty acid intake should not increase any further. COMA (1991) suggested a population average of 6 per cent of total energy from these fatty acids with no individual's intake exceeding 10 per cent.
- Cholesterol intakes in the UK should not increase. Cholesterol is generally regarded, at least in the UK, as a relatively minor influence on plasma cholesterol. If saturated fat intake is reduced, this may well also cause a drop in cholesterol intake as some foods are important contributors of both cholesterol and saturated fat to the diet. Average cholesterol intakes are probably less than a third of the amounts consumed in the 1960s.
- COMA (1994a) recommended increasing intake of long chain n-3 (ω-3) polyunsaturated fatty acids from an average of 0.1 g/day to 0.2 g/day. This is effectively a recommendation to eat twice as much oily fish.
- COMA (1991) recommended that carbohydrates should provide an average 50 per cent of food energy (47 per cent of total energy).

- Added sugars or non-milk extrinsic sugars should make up less than 11 per cent of food energy (10 per cent of total energy intake). The term *non-milk extrinsic sugars* covers all of the sugars that are not present in milk or within the cell walls of fruits and vegetables; it is almost synonymous with *added sugars* except that it would include the sugar in extracted fruit juices. The intrinsic sugars are those found naturally in fruits and vegetables, and Britons are encouraged to eat more of these along with the complex carbohydrates.
- If Britons are to obtain 50 per cent of their food energy from carbohydrate and only 11 per cent from added sugars, it follows that 39 per cent should come from starches and intrinsic sugars combined.
- COMA (1991) recommended a 50 per cent increase in the intakes of dietary fibre or non-starch polysaccharide; that is, to aim for a daily intake of about 18 g of non-starch polysaccharide (equivalent to around 25 g of dietary fibre).
- Current protein intakes should be maintained. Both COMA (1991) and NRC (1989a) specifically counselled against taking in more than double the RNI (RDA) of protein.
- An upper limit of 6 g/day for salt intake has been suggested. This amounts to a reduction of around a third for Britons.

In Table 5.2 these varied recommendations and targets have been synthesized into a British diet of 'ideal' composition.

As noted earlier, in the USA there are detailed guidelines given for each life-stage group, but the following are some more general recommendations.

- Less than 10 per cent of calories should come from saturated fat.
- Total fat intake should represent between 20 and 35 per cent of calories, with most coming from polyunsaturated and monounsaturated fatty acids.
- Cholesterol intake should be less than 300 mg/day.
- Adequate intakes of dietary fibre are set at 14 g per 1000 kcal of the energy requirement.
- A maximum intake for sodium is suggested which translates to just under 6 g/day of salt, with a lower target of under 4 g/day for African-Americans, adults aged over 51 years, and those with hypertension, diabetes or chronic renal disease.
- Adults are recommended to consume 4.7 g/day of potassium.

Rationale

Overall, the recommended changes would be expected to make the diet more bulky and to reduce the amount of energy derived from each gram of food (the *energy density* of the diet). Reducing the content of fat and sugar and replacing it with foods rich in starch, fibre and higher water content (fruits

Table 5.2 The composition of a diet that would meet current UK guidelines*

Nutrient	'Ideal' intake
Total fat	≤33% of total energy
Saturated fatty acids	≤10% of total energy
n-6 (ω-6) polyunsaturated fatty acids	7% of total energy
n-3 (ω-3) polyunsaturated fatty acids	≥0.2% of total energy
Total carbohydrate	≥47% of total energy
Added sugars	≤10% of total energy
Starch and intrinsic sugars	≥37% of total energy
Alcohol	≤5% of total energy
Protein	15% of total energy
Non-starch polysaccharide	>18 g/day
Salt	<6 g/day

*These recommendations would be generally consistent with US guidelines.

and vegetables) would all contribute to reducing the energy density of the diet. This bulky and less energy-dense diet should aid weight control and lessen the risks of excessive weight gain and obesity. Such a diet would also have more nutrients per unit of energy (higher *nutrient density*) because fats and sugars (and alcohol) add a lot of energy but few nutrients.

The changes in fat consumption would be expected to lead to the following benefits.

- *Better weight control.* Fat is palatable, a concentrated source of energy, less satiating than carbohydrate and very efficiently converted to body storage fat, so it encourages overeating and fat storage.
- *Reduced plasma (LDL) cholesterol concentration* and a corresponding reduction in atherosclerosis and risk of cardiovascular diseases. High intakes of saturated fat raise plasma cholesterol, and replacing saturated fat with unsaturated fat reduces the level. An elevated plasma cholesterol level is causally linked to increased risk of coronary heart disease. These changes may also reduce the tendency of blood to clot and form thromboses.
- *Reduced risk of some cancers such as bowel cancer* which are associated with a diet that is high in animal fat and low in carbohydrate.

A reduced consumption of added sugars should lead to improved dental health. Both dental decay (caries) and gum disease are strongly linked to high sugar consumption, especially frequent consumption of sugary snacks and drinks between main meals. The priority should therefore be to concentrate on reducing this between-meal sugar and reducing the frequency of consumption of sugary drinks and snacks.

Increased intakes of complex carbohydrate are an inevitable requirement if fat and sugar intakes are to be reduced. Non-starch polysaccharide should additionally lead to improved bowel function, less constipation and reduced incidence of minor bowel conditions like haemorrhoids (piles) and diverticulosis. High-fibre diets are also associated with reduced risk of bowel cancer and improved glycaemic control. Some forms of fibre have a plasma cholesterol-lowering effect.

A reduction in salt intake is expected to lead to a reduction in average population blood pressure and a reduced rate of rise of blood pressure with age. This should lead to reduced incidence of hypertension and ultimately to reduced incidence of strokes, CHD and renal failure. High salt intake may also be a factor in the aetiology of stomach cancer, so a reduction in salt intake should further decrease the prevalence of this. High intakes of potassium may also have beneficial effects on blood pressure.

Key points

- Dietary targets for the average person in the UK are as follows.
  - Fat should provide no more than 35 per cent of food energy.
  - Saturated fat should provide no more 11 per cent of food energy.
  - Cholesterol intake should not increase.
  - Long-chain n-3 (ω-3) polyunsaturated fatty acid intake should be doubled.
  - There should be no increase in n-6 (ω-6) polyunsaturated fatty acids, with a maximum of 10 per cent of energy.
  - Carbohydrates should make up at least 50 per cent of food energy.
  - Added sugars should be less than 11 per cent of food energy.
  - Non-starch polysaccharide intakes should be over 18 g/day.
  - Salt intake should be cut to 6 g/day.
- Similar recommendations have been made in the USA.
- These changes should:
  - produce a diet that is less energy-dense but more nutrient-dense
  - improve body weight control
  - reduce plasma cholesterol concentrations and so reduce the risk of cardiovascular diseases
  - reduce the risk of bowel and some other cancers
  - improve dental health
  - reduce constipation and other bowel disorders such as haemorrhoids and diverticulosis
  - reduce average blood pressure and the prevalence of hypertension and so lead to reduced incidence of strokes, renal failure and coronary heart disease.

ALCOHOL

There is general agreement that excessive alcohol intake is damaging to health, and so alcohol should be used only in moderation or not at all. Alcohol misuse also leads to a range of social problems such as increased crime (e.g. drunken driving, criminal disorder and violence), absenteeism and family breakdown. What constitutes an acceptable and healthy alcohol intake is a rather more contentious issue. There is persuasive evidence that small amounts of alcohol may have some beneficial effects on health but excessive alcohol consumption has severe health and social consequences. High alcohol consumption leads to an increased risk of liver disease, stroke, fatal accident, birth defects, hypertension, and several forms of cancer. In the UK it has been estimated that excessive alcohol consumption accounted for 5 per cent of all deaths in 2005.

In 2011, the Centers for Disease Control estimated that excessive alcohol consumption costs Americans more than $200 billion a year in medical, law enforcement and employment costs (CDC, 2011). The British Medical Association has produced a very detailed report on the effects of alcohol misuse in the UK (BMA, 2008). It quotes other sources which suggest that in 2004 the annual cost of alcohol-related harm in England was £20 billion, including:

- £1.7 billion in healthcare costs
- £7.3 billion costs of alcohol-related crime and public disorder
- £6.4 billion from loss of productivity and profitability in the workplace.

Many studies have reported higher mortality in those who abstain from alcohol completely as compared to those consuming moderate amounts of alcohol. High alcohol intakes are, on the other hand, associated with sharply increasing mortality rates – the so-called 'J-curve' (or U-curve) of mortality. It has been argued that this J-curve is merely an artefact due to the inclusion of reformed alcoholics in the abstaining group. However, there are many reports supporting the idea of a protective association between moderate alcohol consumption and, in particular, coronary heart disease and that this remains even after correcting for this effect (e.g.

Rimm *et al.*, 1993). Doll *et al.* (2005) conducted a large 23-year cohort study of 12 000 male doctors who were aged between 48 and 78 years at the start of the study. They found that mortality was highly significantly lower (RR = 0.81) in drinkers with an average intake of 2–3 units/day than in non-drinkers, owing to reduced numbers of deaths from heart and respiratory disease. This difference narrowed slightly (RR = 0.88) but remained statistically significant even when the ex-drinkers, who did have raised mortality, were combined with the drinkers. The study team concluded that some of the apparent protective effects of alcohol in this older male population were real effects.

A 10- to 12-year cohort study conducted in Denmark (Gronbaek *et al.*, 1994) confirmed the J-shaped relationship between total mortality and alcohol consumption, with lowest relative mortality risk in those consuming between 1 and 6 units of alcohol weekly. This study also reported that only with weekly alcohol consumption in excess of 42 units was total mortality significantly higher than in those consuming low amounts of alcohol. This study found that age did not change the relationship between mortality risk and alcohol consumption and that the apparent benefits of small amounts of alcohol applied to all adults. Some other studies – for example Klatsky *et al.* (1992) in the USA – have reported that the relative risk of dying as a result of alcohol consumption is higher in younger people than older people because of the alcohol-related increase in deaths from violence and traffic accidents in younger adults. Gronbaek *et al.* (1994) suggest that this difference in findings between the American and Danish studies may be because accidents and violence are less prominent as causes of death among young Danes than among young Americans. White *et al.* (2002) also reported age differences in the level of alcohol consumption associated with lowest mortality. They found that in men aged under 35 years, and in women under 55 years, there was a direct dose–response relationship between alcohol consumption and mortality with no apparent J- or U-curve. In those aged over 65 years they found that lowest mortality was found in women consuming 3 units of alcohol per week and men consuming 8 units per week.

There is quite consistent evidence that consumption of small amounts of alcohol (1–3 units/day) is associated with reduced total mortality in elderly men, partly because of reduced numbers of deaths from heart disease. In younger men and in women the findings are less consistent but are generally less favourable towards alcohol having a protective effect, or only at lower doses than in older men.

With alcohol, the priority has been to moderate the intakes of high consumers rather than to aim for a more universal reduction. Despite a substantial body of evidence that alcohol in moderation may have some beneficial effects, expert committees have generally shied away from recommending people, even elderly men, to drink alcohol. Many people find it difficult to gauge and to regulate their intake of alcohol, and this explains the general reluctance of expert committees to recommend that people should consume alcohol. Back in 1983, NACNE recommended a reduction in alcohol consumption from an average 6 per cent to 4 per cent of total energy (current figures are 8 per cent for men and 5 per cent for women). They suggested that this should be achieved by curtailing the consumption of high consumers rather than shifting the whole distribution of intakes as with their other recommendations.

Current US guidelines recommend that if people do drink alcohol then they should limit their consumption to no more than about 2 units of alcohol in any one day for men and just 1 unit for women. They further suggest that alcoholic beverages should not be consumed at all by those who cannot control their alcohol intake, by women who are or might become pregnant, by lactating women and by adolescents.

A unit of alcohol is defined as 8 g of pure alcohol, which is equivalent to half a pint of ordinary beer (284 mL), a small glass of wine (75 mL) or a single measure of spirits. In the UK, the recommended maximum weekly intake of alcohol was for some time 21 units for men and 14 units for women. In 1995 the Department of Health rather controversially raised these safe drinking limits to 28 units for men and 21 units for women. This alcohol should be spread fairly evenly throughout the week and high consumption on particular days (binge drinking) should be avoided. Given this need to avoid binge drinking, the recommended maximum alcohol intakes are now usually presented

as daily maxima of 4 units for men and 3 for women. This 1995 DH statement also contained some positive encouragement for older people who do not drink to consider taking one or two units per day. It is generally recommended on both sides of the Atlantic that pregnant women should avoid alcohol. Alcohol impairs judgement and coordination and slows down reflexes so should be avoided when driving or participating in any other activity where such impairments could be hazardous (e.g. operating machinery).

Table 5.3 shows the distribution of reported alcohol intakes in British men and women in 2000–1. This shows that 60 per cent of men and 43 per cent of women in this survey reported that they exceeded the recommended maximum number of daily units on at least one day in the sampled week. The proportions exceeding these daily maxima were substantially higher in the youngest age group. Half of young men and a third of young women consumed more than double the recommended levels on at

Table 5.3 Distribution of alcohol use in British men and women based on maximum number of units consumed during a 7-day dietary record of adults aged 19–64 years*

	All (% recording)	19–24 years (% recording)
Men		
Nothing in 7 days	20	20
Up to 4 units[1]	20	14
4–8 units	21	15
8+ units	39	50
Mean daily units	7.8	9.4
Women		
Nothing	33	29
Up to 3 units[1]	23	14
3–6 units	21	23
6+ units	22	34
Mean daily units	3.6	5.3

*Data from Hoare et al. (2004).
[1] Note that UK recommendations are that men should consume a maximum of 4 units in any one day and women a maximum of 3, i.e. 60% of men (43% of women) and 65% of the younger men (57% of younger women) exceeded these maxima on at least one day.

least one day in the sample week. Figures from the 2009 NDNS survey (Bates *et al.*, 2010) cannot be directly compared to those in Table 5.3 because they included people aged 16–18 and those aged over 65 years, and heavy drinking is less prevalent in these two age groups. Bates *et al.* (2011) reported that 43 per cent of men aged over 16 years (including the over-65s) had drunk more than 4 units on at least one day in the reporting week and 28 per cent more than 8 units. For women, 30 per cent drank more than 3 units and 15 per cent more than 6 units. These figures from Bates' team are very similar to those reported by Craig and Hirani (2010) in the *Health Survey for England 2009*. This survey also reported that when those not drinking at all were excluded then 60 per cent of male drinkers and 55 per cent of female drinkers exceeded their recommended maximum on at least one day, and 35 per cent of men and 27 per cent of women drank more than twice the recommended maximum number of units on at least one day.

Mechanisms by which alcohol may reduce risk of coronary heart disease

Low to moderate alcohol intake seems to be associated with reduced total mortality, largely as a result of reduced mortality from coronary heart disease. Even though heavy drinkers have higher total mortality this is largely due to causes other than CHD. Below are listed several suggested mechanisms by which alcohol may protect against CHD. Consult COMA (1998) for primary sources.

- Alcohol intake is associated with increased levels of high-density lipoproteins (HDL) in plasma. This is the cholesterol-containing lipoprotein fraction in plasma that removes excess cholesterol to the liver and affords protection against atherosclerosis and CHD (see Chapter 12 for further details on HDL).
- Some alcoholic drinks (especially red wine) may contain substances that act as anti-oxidants that help to prevent the free radical damage that is implicated in the aetiology of atherosclerosis. Polyphenols in red wine (particularly a substance called *trans*-resveratrol) have been the subject of much study and, on the basis of in-vitro studies with vascular endothelium and short-term studies with animals, are claimed to be cardio-protective. One widely publicized study found that wines from two particular regions had the highest concentrations of these polyphenols and it was widely implied, on the basis of this very limited evidence, that these wines were the healthiest and this was a factor in the longevity of the people living in these particular wine-producing regions (Corder *et al.*, 2006).

- Alcohol may reduce the tendency of blood to clot and for thromboses to form. Alcohol consumption is associated with reduced plasma fibrinogen levels and reduced activity of platelets. (Fibrinogen is a key protein in blood clotting and platelet activation is also a key step in blood coagulation.)

Key points

- Alcohol should be consumed in moderation or not at all. Alcohol should be avoided during pregnancy and when driving or operating machinery.
- High alcohol consumption has serious health and social consequences and is associated with steeply increasing mortality.
- At least in older people and especially older men, low alcohol consumption is associated with lower mortality than complete abstention and seems to afford some protection against coronary heart disease.
- The relationship between alcohol consumption and mortality risk is often described as a J- or U-shaped curve.
- Alcohol consumption raises the HDL-cholesterol concentration in blood and reduces the tendency of blood to clot.
- Some alcoholic drinks contain anti-oxidants that may afford protection against damage by free radicals.
- Recommendations for alcohol in the UK are a maximum of 3 units per day for women and 4 units per day for men.
- American men are advised to drink up to two drinks per day and women only one per day.
- A unit of alcohol is a small glass of wine, a half-pint of ordinary beer or a standard measure of spirits (*c*8 g of pure alcohol).
- Around 60 per cent of male drinkers and 55 per cent of female drinkers in the UK exceed the UK guidelines on at least one day in a week.

HOW CURRENT UK DIETS COMPARE WITH 'IDEAL' INTAKES

Table 5.4 shows a summary of the macronutrient composition of the British adult diet as determined by the NDNS survey (Bates *et al.*, 2010). These values were very similar to those recorded in 2000–1 (Hoare *et al.*, 2004) and small differences could be simply due to differences in the protocols of the two surveys. One apparent change was the rise in the food energy derived from protein from 16.1 to 17.6 per cent. These values in Table 5.4 generally represent substantial improvements on those recorded in 1986–7 by Gregory *et al.* (1990). The percentage of food energy from fat in this survey is around the DRV (35 per cent) when the average of the two sexes is used; this is compared to just over 40 per cent in 1986–7. Although the values for saturated fat are still somewhat higher than the DRV, they are nonetheless a substantial improvement on the almost 17 per cent recorded in 1986–7. There has been a reduction in the energy derived from non-milk extrinsic sugars towards the target DRV and a substantial increase in the proportion of energy that comes from all carbohydrates.

Average salt intakes recorded in Table 5.4 are around 60 per cent higher than the DRV and three-quarters of the adult population exceeded the recommended maximum; note that these are figures from 2000–1 because data in Bates *et al.* (2009) give values for the amount of food salt excluding discretionary salt used in home cooking and at the table. While there has been some small increase in average recorded intakes of NSP in this latest NDNS survey compared to 1986–7, most adults still do not consume the recommended ≥18 g per day.

Key points

- According to the 2009 NDNS adult survey, the average British diet when compared to current UK guidelines:
  - was close to the target of 35 per cent of dietary energy as fat
  - was just 1.8 per cent over the target of 11 per cent of food energy as saturated fat
  - was about 3 per cent below the target of 50 per cent of food energy from carbohydrate
  - was 2.5 per cent over the target of 11 per cent of food energy as non-milk extrinsic sugars
  - was 60 per cent higher than the target of no more than 6 g of salt/day
  - had 4 g/day too little NSP and most adults failed to consume the recommended ≥18 g of NSP per day.
- These values, which are detailed in Table 5.4, represent significant movements towards the target values since those recorded in 1986–7, with the exception of those for salt.

Table 5.4 Macronutrient composition of the typical adult British diet (values are percentage of food energy unless otherwise stated)*

	Nutrient as % of food energy			
	Men	Women	All	Target (DRV)
Fat	35.5	34.7	35.1	35
Saturated fatty acids	13.0	12.6	12.8	11
Protein	17.8	17.5	17.6	–
Total carbohydrate	46.8	47.8	47.3	50
Non-milk extrinsic sugars	13.0	12.1	12.5	11
Salt (g/day)[1]	11.0	8.1	9.5	<6
NSP (g/day)[2]	15.1	13.0	14.0	18+

*Data from Bates *et al.* (2010).
  DRV, dietary reference value; NSP, non-starch polysaccharide.
[1] 15% of men and 31% of women met the target for salt (these are 2000–1 values as Bates' team were unable to estimate total salt intakes).
[2] Most adults did not meet the target for NSP.

OTHER NUTRIENTS

The importance of obtaining intakes of all the essential nutrients in line with current dietary standards is generally acknowledged; that is, ensuring the diet contains adequate amounts of energy and all of the essential nutrients.

Calcium and iron

Milk and milk products are the most important sources of calcium in UK and US diets. Meat is a major source of dietary iron in its most readily absorbed form as haem. There has been concern that calcium and iron intakes might fall along with any fall in saturated fat consumption. Iron and calcium intakes can be maintained despite cuts in fat and saturated fat if low-fat dairy products, fish, lean meat and poultry are substituted for fatty meats, full-fat dairy products and other fried and fatty foods. Back in 1983, NACNE recognized the importance of milk in maintaining adequate calcium intakes. They suggested that the wider availability of lower fat milk would allow calcium intakes to be maintained despite the recommended cuts in saturated fat intake. Low-fat milk has indeed become more available in the UK and semi-skimmed milk now accounts for the majority of milk drunk in Britain. The issue of calcium and its importance in bone health is discussed at length in Chapter 15.

Fluoride

NAS (2004) recommend optimal intakes of fluoride especially in children whose teeth are developing. COMA (1991) endorsed the more widespread fluoridation of public water supplies up to a level of 1 part per million (ppm) and set a safe daily intake of fluoride for infants of 0.05 mg per kilogram of body weight. The effects of fluoride on dental health are discussed in Chapter 10.

Potassium

Increased consumption of fruits and vegetables would lead to an increase in potassium intake. COMA (1994a) specifically recommended an increase in average potassium intake to about 3.5 g/day in adults (4.7 g/day in the USA). There is evidence that high potassium intake protects against the hypertensive effects of salt. Bates *et al.* (2010) found that average potassium intakes were below the 3.5 g/day RNI for both men and women with an average of only 2.6 g/day in women; 20 per cent of women recorded intakes that were below the LRNI of only 2 g/day.

Key points

- It is important that adequate amounts of all essential nutrients be consumed.
- Calcium and iron intakes can be maintained despite reductions in saturated fat if lean meat, poultry and low-fat milk replace fatty meats, full-fat dairy products and other fatty foods.
- In both the UK and the USA, minimum intakes of fluoride are recommended, especially in young children, in order to protect against dental decay.
- High potassium intake may help to prevent high blood pressure. Increased fruit and vegetable consumption would lead to increased potassium intakes, and British adults have been recommended to increase potassium intake to 3.5 g/day (4.7 g/day in the USA).
- Twenty per cent of British women recorded potassium intakes of less than 2 g/day.

WILLINGNESS TO CHANGE

It is sometimes argued that health promotion and nutrition education in particular are doomed to be ineffective because consumers are unwilling to make changes to their diets on health grounds. For example, in a short article that was largely critical of health promotion, Watts (1998) suggested that 'no one has yet fathomed out how to persuade anyone to live more healthily'. It is quite clear, however, that health advice and health promotion can produce major shifts in national behaviour. In the 1970s and early 1980s, many parents in the UK and elsewhere were persuaded to use a front-sleeping position for their babies rather than the traditional back-sleeping position. In the early 1990s many were then persuaded to revert to the traditional back position to reduce the risk of cot death (see Chapter 1 and Webb, 1995). Smoking is much less prevalent now than it was when the links between smoking and lung cancer were first established and publicized, so in several sectors of British society smoking has gone from being accepted as the social norm to being a minority, anti-social activity.

There is also ample evidence that Britons and Americans made huge changes to their diets in the last quarter of the twentieth century. These changes were largely driven by the desire to control body weight and the publicity about the links between diet and health. Table 5.5 shows a comparison of fat purchases for home consumption in the UK in 1975 and 1996 with some indication of changes since 1996; the scale of the changes in the table in just a 20-year period is quite dramatic. Some other health-driven changes to British diets are listed below.

- Low-fat milks became readily available in the early 1980s in the UK. Before this almost all the fresh liquid milk sold was whole-fat. Between 1986 and 2005, low-fat milk increased from 19 per cent of liquid milk sales to around 70 per cent.
- In 1986, about 7 per cent of the soft drinks purchased for home consumption were low-calorie versions. By 2005 this had risen to 30 per cent.
- In the late 1960s, sales of sugar amounted to around half a kilogram per person per week. By

2005 this had fallen to 35 g/week. (Note that total added sugar consumption has not dropped by anything like this amount because it has to some extent been offset by greater consumption of sugar in manufactured products.)

- In 1976, sales of wholemeal bread made up a negligible proportion of total bread sales. Improvements in the texture of wholemeal bread coupled with health messages about dietary fibre have caused it to rise so that, in 2005, just under a quarter of loaves of bread sold were wholemeal.

Many of these changes that have occurred in recent decades are the result of simple replacement of a traditional product with another of similar or better utilitarian value – so they have been easy to understand and implement. Butter and hard margarine have been replaced by soft margarine and low-fat spreads in most British homes (see Table 5.5). Semi-skimmed (1.7 per cent) and skimmed milk have largely replaced whole milk. Even though the new 'healthier product' is sometimes considered slightly less palatable than the traditional product, people have been prepared in large numbers to make this relatively small sacrifice for their health or to try to lose weight. Table 5.5 shows that, despite the dramatic changes in the types of cooking

Table 5.5 Comparison of fats purchased for home consumption in the UK in 1975 and 1996*

	1975	1996
'Yellow' fats (as % of yellow-fat sales)		
Butter	68	25
Soft margarine	14	21+
Other margarine	18	<3
Low-fat spreads	–	51[1]
Cooking fats (as % of cooking-fat sales)		
Vegetable oils	22	77[2]
Other fats (mainly lard)	78	23
Fats as percentage of food energy[3]		
Total fat	41.3	39.7
Saturated fatty acids	20.3	15.4
Polyunsaturated fatty acids	4.6	7.2
P:S ratio	0.19	0.46

*Data source: National Food Survey.
[1] In 2004–5, low- and reduced-fat spreads accounted for 60% of the spreading-fat market.
[2] Vegetable oils in 2004–5 had a market share of 81% of cooking-fat sales.
[3] More recent data and dietary fats as a percentage of food energy can be seen in Table 5.4.

and spreading fats used in British homes, there was little change in the overall prominence of fat in British diets between 1975 and 1996 (although as seen in Table 5.4 the contribution of fat to food energy has declined since 1996 and is now close to the DRV of 35 per cent). Health promoters and nutrition educators should consider this when framing their dietary advice or devising their campaigns. People need to be offered simple, realistic and relatively painless ways of achieving or moving towards the desired nutritional goals.

Key points

- Despite assertions to the contrary, consumers have made substantial dietary changes as a result of health information and heath promotion.
- Since 1975, the following changes to the British diet have occurred:
  - a massive switch from the use of butter and hard margarine initially to soft margarine and more recently to low-fat spreads
  - a huge switch from the use of animal-derived cooking fats like lard to use of vegetable oils for cooking
  - replacement of whole milk with low-fat milks which now account for most liquid milk sales
  - large increases in the sales of low-calorie soft drinks and wholemeal bread.
- Many of these dietary changes involved the simple replacement of a traditional product by an alternative that, although possibly less palatable, has similar utilitarian characteristics and is perceived as healthier or less fattening.
- Past experience thus suggests that if consumers are offered simple, realistic and relatively painless ways of improving their diets then many will make such changes.

SOME BARRIERS TO DIETARY CHANGE

Figure 1.4 in Chapter 1 summarizes the pathway by which a health promotion message is transmitted to the public and successfully results in improvements in health. At each step on this pathway there are potential barriers that may prevent effective change being made. Below are listed a number of factors that may discourage consumers from changing their diets in the direction suggested in this chapter – a number of *potential barriers to change*.

Palatability

Fat and sugar are major contributors to the palatability of Western diets. Starch and fibre are bland, so high-fibre high-starch diets are often perceived as deficient in taste, smell and an appealing texture. As populations become more affluent their natural inclination is to replace much of the starchy food that makes up the bulk of peasant diets with foods that are much higher in fat and sugar.

The sugar–fat seesaw

It may prove particularly difficult to reduce simultaneously the contribution of both fats and sugars to the diet. This would inevitably involve a substantial increase in starch consumption. In a free-living affluent population there tends to be an inverse relationship between sugar and fat consumption. People who get a low proportion of their energy from fat tend to get a high proportion from sugar, and vice versa; this is the so-called 'sugar–fat seesaw'. Survey data quoted by McColl (1988) suggested that people who consumed less than 35 per cent of their calories as fat derived, on average, more than 25 per cent of their calories from sugars. Back in 1986–7, Gregory *et al.* (1990) found that, while 13 per cent of their sample of British adults met the target of no more than 33 per cent of total energy from fat, only 1 per cent met both this fat target and that for added sugars. Those men and women who met the fat targets and sugar targets had higher alcohol intakes than those who did not; that is, alcohol tended to dilute the fat and sugar and so help some individuals to meet sugar or fat targets. This sugar–fat seesaw might, in practice, increase the difficulty for individuals of meeting both fat and sugar targets. Since 1990 there have been substantial movements towards the DRV for both fats and added sugars in the UK (see Table 5.4).

Availability of healthy alternatives

We saw in the previous section that many of the most striking changes in the British diet in recent decades have resulted from the substitution of a traditional food by one perceived as healthier or less fattening. If people are to continue to make these substitutions then the healthy alternatives must be readily available, affordable and acceptable in terms of their palatability.

The massive switch from whole to low-fat milk coincided with the much greater availability of low-fat milks, especially semi-skimmed, in the early 1980s. The increase in sales of wholemeal bread was partly the result of improved texture of these products. Low-fat spreads were unavailable 25 years ago but now account for the bulk of the 'yellow-fat' market in Britain.

It may be argued that public demand will be sufficient to ensure increasing availability of these 'healthier' alternatives. However, in order to demonstrate that demand, the public must be given reasonable access to a product. Will a perceived future demand always be sufficient incentive for manufacturers and retailers to provide healthy options, particularly for a product likely to yield no increase in – or perhaps lower – profit margins? While the ranges of these low-fat, low-sugar and low-salt products are increasing all the time, some of them may be relatively expensive or perceived as poor value for money by low-income families trying to satisfy their appetites with strictly limited funds. For example:

- extra-lean mincemeat (for hamburgers) is often considerably more expensive than the standard version
- low-fat milk costs the same as whole milk but provides fewer calories, so the healthier version provides far fewer calories per penny. This applies to most low-fat and sugar products
- fruits and vegetables are an expensive source of energy, especially the more exotic and appealing varieties
- the cheapest white bread in British supermarkets costs much less than a wholemeal loaf.

Skills and knowledge

It is easier for people to reduce their fat intake or increase their fibre intake if they have a reasonable idea of the relative amounts of these in different foods. Have people got the skills and knowledge to prepare meals that are both appetising and more in tune with current guidelines? Are food, nutrition and food preparation given sufficient weighting in our schools?

Traditional nutritional beliefs

Some older consumers may be reluctant to increase their consumption of starchy foods because they still perceive then as fattening. A reduction in consumption of meat and cheese may be hindered by their perception as valuable sources of first-class protein.

Key points

- A number of factors may act as barriers or hindrances to the implementation of current nutritional guidelines.
- Sugar and fat add palatability to the diet whereas starch and fibre are bland. This may discourage the replacement of substantial amounts of fatty and sugary foods by starchy foods.
- In affluent diets there is often a sugar–fat seesaw, which makes it more difficult to simultaneously reduce the proportions of energy derived from both fat and sugar.
- Substitution of traditional foods by 'healthier' alternatives requires that the healthier options be readily available, affordable and palatable.
- Many of the 'healthier' options are more expensive than the traditional product, particularly when costed as calories per penny. This may hinder dietary improvement in low-income groups.
- People may lack the knowledge and skills to implement the guidelines.
- Some outdated beliefs may discourage beneficial dietary change, e.g. 'starchy foods are fattening', and 'high intakes of meat and cheese are necessary to meet protein needs'. They may simply provide some people who are reluctant to change with an excuse for not changing.

AIDS TO FOOD SELECTION

Selecting food solely according to biological criteria requires considerable knowledge of nutrition and food composition. It takes some skill to routinely translate current views on optimal intakes into meals and diets. Dieticians and nutrition educators therefore need ways of translating complex technical guidelines into advice that is easy to understand, remember and implement. When 'adequacy' was the nutritional priority, *food groups* were a simple and effective means of helping people to select on a constituent basis. Foods were grouped according to the nutrients they provided, so people could be advised that, if they consumed specified minimum numbers of portions from each of the groups, nutritional adequacy would probably be assured.

The most widely used of these systems was the *four food group plan*. Foods were placed into four basic food groups and minimum numbers of servings from each group were recommended. These groups and an outline of their essential nutrient profiles are listed below.

- *The milk group* (milk, cheese, yoghurt and other milk products). These provide good amounts of energy, good-quality protein, vitamin A, calcium and riboflavin.
- *The meat group* (meat, fish, eggs and meat substitutes such as pulses and nuts). These provide protein, B vitamins, vitamin A and iron.
- *The fruit and vegetable group* (fruits and those vegetables not classified as meat substitutes). These provide carotene, vitamin C, folate, riboflavin, potassium and fibre.
- *The bread and cereals group* (bread, rice, pasta, breakfast cereals and products made from flour). Whole-grain cereals are good sources of B vitamins, some minerals and fibre. White flour still provides reasonable amounts of fibre and it is often fortified with vitamins and minerals (in the UK, with iron, calcium and some B vitamins).

People were advised to eat a minimum of two portions each day from the meat and milk groups and a minimum of four portions from the other two groups. As the foods in the groups have differing profiles of essential nutrients, then provided consumers ate enough to satisfy their appetite and ate these minimum numbers of portions, nutritional adequacy was practically assured.

A number of foods are not covered in any of these categories, examples being butter, oil and other fats, sugar and alcoholic drinks. This is because they are largely sources of energy and provide few nutrients, so no minimum portions were recommended. They were to be used sparingly because of their low nutrient density.

Several generations of American schoolchildren and college students have been taught the basic four food group plan since its development in 1955. This classification system will still be familiar to many American adults although less familiar to most British adults.

Food group schemes were designed to ensure nutritional adequacy rather than to guide consumers towards a diet that helped to prevent chronic diseases. Many foods in the milk and meat groups are now seen as rich sources of dietary fat and cholesterol as well as nutrients (e.g. whole milk, cheese, fatty meat). Many foods in the cereals group are seen as low in fat and sugar and high in fibre and starch in addition to being sources of some nutrients. Many foods in the fruit and vegetable group are very low in energy density and practically fat-free in their natural unprocessed state. In order to comply with the compositional guidelines discussed in this chapter, consumers need to be encouraged to:

- increase their consumption of cereals, vegetables and fruits
- moderate their consumption of meats and dairy foods
- minimise their consumption of fatty and sugary foods that do not fit into any of the four groups
- choose foods within the food groups that are low in fat and added sugars but high in fibre.

For some time, nutrition educators tried to adapt this four food group guide to modern nutritional priorities, for example highlighting the low-fat/low-sugar options within each group. However, a food guide that merely suggested minimum quantities from the food groups was unsuited to modern dietary guidelines with their emphasis on moderating intakes of some foods and food groups and increasing the prominence of other food groups in the diet.

In 1992, the US Department of Agriculture (USDA, 1992) published a new guide to food selection intended to update and replace the basic four food group plan: the *food guide pyramid* (Figure 5.1). This was a development of the food groups and was designed to reflect the dual aims of selecting a diet that is not only adequate but meets nutritional guidelines aimed at reducing the risk of chronic diseases.

At the base of the food pyramid are the starchy grain foods that should contribute more servings than any other single group to the ideal diet: between 6 and 11 servings depending on total energy intake (in the range 1600–2800 kcal or 6.7–11.8 MJ). On the next tier of the pyramid are the fruit and vegetable groups: a total of between 5 and 9 servings from these groups depending on energy intake. At the third level are the foods of animal origin (including the vegetarian alternatives to meat and milk such as pulses, nuts, soya milk and modern meat substitutes). There should be 2 or 3 servings from each group on this tier (i.e. from the meat and milk groups). At the top of the pyramid are the fats, oils and sweets – foods such as salad dressings, cream, butter, margarine, soft drinks, sweets (candies), sweet desserts and alcoholic drinks. These provide few nutrients but are high in energy, sugars and fats, so they should be used sparingly in the ideal diet, especially for those seeking to lose weight. In the figure a triangle symbol is distributed lightly within the cereal, fruit and milk groups to show that

some foods from these categories may contain added sugars; examples are sweetened breakfast cereals, fruit canned in syrup, some flavoured yoghurts, milk shake and ice cream. Also in the figure, a circle symbol is distributed lightly throughout the cereal and vegetable groups to show that these may contain added fats. The same symbol appears more densely in the meat and milk groups to show that many of the foods here contain substantial amounts of naturally occurring fat. The top layer of the pyramid contains a high density of both triangles and circles to emphasize its role as a major contributor of fats and added sugar to the diet.

The food pyramid thus indicates a general dietary structure that should ensure adequacy and yet at the same time make it more likely that other nutrition education guidelines aimed at reducing chronic diseases will also be met. Highlighting the likely sources of fat and added sugars in the diet with the circle and triangle symbols should aid

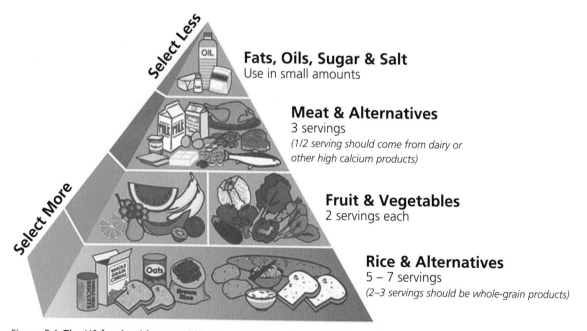

Figure 5.1 The US food guide pyramid and, on the right, the real intakes of Americans presented in pyramid format.

consumers in making choices that reduce intakes of fat and added sugars.

Figure 5.1 also shows, on the right, an estimate of what the average American really eats. This 'real' pyramid is much more top-heavy than the ideal one, with foods from the fats and sugars group providing 41 per cent of the calories. The milk and meat group provides around 3.5 servings compared with the 4 to 6 suggested, and fruits and vegetables provide 3.6 servings (including a large contribution from potatoes) compared with the suggested 5 to 9 servings. The bread and cereals group provide 6.8 servings, which is just within the 6 to 11 servings suggested. This shows just how large are the dietary changes required by the US food guide pyramid.

Following the launch of the food guide pyramid in the USA, a British version appeared in 1993. This was an unofficial attempt to provide Britons with some form of nationally accepted food guide for the first time. It was produced jointly by the Flour Advisory Bureau and the Dunn Nutrition Laboratory in Cambridge. The British *healthy eating pyramid* was in most of its essentials identical to the US version except that potatoes were included with the cereals at the base of the pyramid (rather than with the other vegetables). The fruits and vegetables were represented as a single group on the second tier of the pyramid with a recommended 5 to 9 daily servings.

In early 1994, the Nutrition Task Force had identified the need for a national pictorial food guide as a priority for implementing the dietary and nutritional targets set out in 1992 in *The Health of the Nation*. Research on the best form that this food guide should take was undertaken on behalf of the Health Education Authority. A variety of different formats were tested with both the general public and with health professionals. This research showed that such pictorial guides could improve people's understanding of nutritional concepts. A plate shape was found to be more effective at conveying those nutritional concepts than the pyramid, and a tilted plate model proved most appealing to members of the public (Hunt *et al.*, 1995). The Health Education Authority in the UK published the first official national food guide in mid-1994. It used the image of a tilted plate with five food groups occupying segments (Figure 5.2).

Two large segments occupy about 30 per cent of the plate each:

- starchy foods – the bread, cereals and potatoes group
- the fruit and vegetable group.

Two medium-sized segments occupy about 15 per cent of the plate each:

- meat, fish, eggs and pulses
- milk and milk products like cheese and yoghurt.

The smallest sector of the plate represents less than 10 per cent of the area and contains:

- fatty and sugary foods.

The general dietary structure indicated in the tilted plate model is essentially the same as that suggested

The eatwell plate

Use the eatwell plate to help you get the balance right. It shows how much of what you eat should come from each food group.

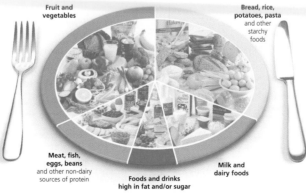

Fruit and vegetables

Bread, rice, potatoes, pasta and other starchy foods

Meat, fish, eggs, beans and other non-dairy sources of protein

Foods and drinks high in fat and/or sugar

Milk and dairy foods

© Crown copyright 2011

Department of Health in association with the Welsh Assembly Government, the Scottish Government and the Food Standards Agency in Northern Ireland

Figure 5.2 The tilted plate model used as the national food guide in the UK.

by the American pyramid. The diet should contain large amounts of starchy foods and fruits and vegetables, more moderate amounts of foods from the meat and milk groups, and strictly limited amounts of fatty and sugary foods. In the form that is used for general display (e.g. in supermarkets and for general guidance to the public) it contains no recommended numbers of portions. It is felt that the wide variation in individual energy intakes – and thus the wide variation in numbers of recommended portions – would make this information difficult for the general lay person to interpret. The tilted plate on general release does contain additional advice for selection within each food group.

- Choose low-fat options from the meat and milk groups where possible.
- Eat a variety of fruits and vegetables.
- Eat all types of starchy foods and choose high-fibre varieties where possible.

There is a version of this tilted plate model that does contain recommended numbers of portions. It is intended for use by health professionals in one-to-one counselling, where they can interpret this quantitative information in a way that is appropriate to the individual client. The portion guides are similar to those suggested on the US pyramid guide:

- 5–9 measures of fruits and vegetables
- 5–14 measures of bread, cereals and potatoes
- 2–3 measures of meat, fish and alternatives
- 2–3 measures of milk and dairy foods
- 0–4 measures of fatty and sugary foods.

Key points

- Nutrition educators have used a variety of guidance tools to translate technical nutritional guidelines into practical and comprehensible dietary advice.
- Food groups helped to guide consumers towards a nutritionally adequate diet. Foods were grouped into four or more categories with differing nutrient profiles and consumers advised to eat a minimum number of portions from each category daily.
- Milk, meat, cereals, and fruits and vegetables were the four groups of the basic plan. Sugary and fatty foods were in a separate category outside the main food groups.

→

Key points *continued*

- New food guides became necessary when 'preventing chronic disease' became a major nutritional priority and when guidelines often stressed reducing or moderating intakes of certain dietary components.
- The USA now has a food guide pyramid (see Figure 5.1). Foods are arranged on the pyramid to indicate their ideal prominence in the diet. Circular and triangular symbols indicate the likely sources of fat and added sugar.
- In the UK a tilted plate model is used (see Figure 5.2). Text messages on the plate urge consumers to choose low-fat and high-fibre options from within the appropriate groups.
- The US pyramid has suggested ranges for ideal numbers of daily portions from each of the food groups. Only the version of the British guide intended for use by health professionals has these portion guidelines.

CONCLUDING REMARKS

Although many nutritionists would argue over specific diet/disease issues, few would disagree with the proposition that significant health benefits are likely to accrue if Americans and Britons were leaner, more active, consumed alcohol moderately, ate less fat, sugar and salt but more fruits, vegetables and cereals. The basic qualitative message transmitted by the US food guide pyramid and the British tilted plate enjoys consensus support of nutritionists and dieticians.

In this chapter, recommendations have been considered in terms of their effects on the health of people eating them. Dietary changes will also inevitably have social, economic and environmental consequences. Some dietary changes that might be deemed nutritionally desirable may not be sustainable by everyone who adopts them. If those in the wealthy industrialized countries make dietary changes that soak up more of the world's resources, will health promotion in wealthy countries be at the expense of still greater deprivation in poorer ones? Some examples of these issues are listed below.

- The world's oceans are already suffering depletion of fish stocks due to over-fishing. If people are encouraged to eat more fish, will this situation worsen? Is fish farming a realistic alternative to wild fish? Is it capable of producing fish on a huge scale without heavy inputs of energy and other negative ecological repercussions?

- If all Western consumers start eating many more fruits and vegetables each day, will many of these be transported into Northern countries with all the resultant fuel costs? What effects will their growth have on groundwater resources in the producing country? Will they be grown as cash crops for export at the expense of the staple crops needed to feed the local population?
- If Western consumers reduce their consumption of meat and dairy foods and replace them with starchy cereals and roots, this should have a positive impact on sustainability. It takes 3–10 kilos of grain to produce one kilo of meat or poultry. However, what if these Western consumers are encouraged to waste many of the expensively produced calories in animal foods? If they eat only the leaner cuts of meat and discard much of the fat in animal carcasses, if skimmed milk and lean meat are seen as healthy nutrient-rich products, will the market for butterfat, lard and beef fat shrink still further? How many millions of severely undernourished children in developing countries could have been fed with the millions of tons of grain used to produce the beef burnt in Britain since 1988 in order to protect British consumers from BSE ('mad cow disease' – see Chapter 19 for details of BSE).

- The dietary changes brought about by health promotion have already had a noticeable effect on the nature of farming and the countryside. In the UK, huge yellow swathes of land devoted to the growth of oilseed rape have become a feature of many parts of the countryside. Can the hill land in the more mountainous parts be used productively for purposes other than grazing animals?
- Some of the recommended dietary changes seem to be encouraging a more artificial and less natural diet, such as the use of low-fat spreads, low-calorie drinks and some meat substitutes.

Detailed discussion of such issues is beyond the scope of a book such as this, and beyond the capabilities of its author but they are issues that need to be considered by those advocating dietary change.

Key points

- Most nutritionists would agree with the broad thrust of current nutritional guidelines despite questioning particular elements of them.
- The environmental, economic and cultural impacts of recommended dietary changes need to be considered as well as simply their nutritional desirability for residents of the home country.
- Expert committees must ensure that any recommendations they make are sustainable if implemented on a mass scale by many populations.

6

CELLULAR ENERGETICS

Introduction and aims of the chapter	156	Metabolism of fatty acids and glycerol	160
Overview of metabolism	156	Metabolism of amino acids	161
Metabolism of glucose and the		The pentose phosphate pathway	161
monosaccharides	158	Overview of macronutrient handling in the gut	162

INTRODUCTION AND AIMS OF THE CHAPTER

This very brief and greatly simplified outline of the energy conversions within the cell is not intended to be an introduction to the study of biochemistry. Only the minimum of factual biochemistry to allow illustration of the broad principles and concepts has been included. The purpose is to give readers with no biochemical background enough perception of the biochemical processes of the cell to help their understanding of nutrition. This short summary may also provide a useful overview for readers who have studied biochemistry. Certain nutritionally important observations should be clarified by this discussion, such as those listed below.

- Fatty acids cannot be converted to glucose but glucose can be converted to fat.
- The human brain cannot use fatty acids as substrates, but during starvation it obtains more than half of its energy from the metabolism of ketone bodies that are derived from fatty acids.
- Many vitamins are essential as precursors of the coenzymes that are necessary to allow enzyme-mediated reactions to occur.
- Amino acids can serve as energy sources and can be used to generate glucose during fasting.
- Certain substances can 'uncouple' the link between oxidation (energy production) and phosphorylation (ATP synthesis) and thus cause this energy to be released as heat. This is how brown fat in some animals generates heat for maintaining body temperature in the cold.

OVERVIEW OF METABOLISM

The catabolism (breakdown) of carbohydrates, fats and proteins within cells releases chemical energy. This energy is used to drive all the energy-requiring processes of the cell, including synthetic processes, muscle contraction, transport of materials across cell membranes, and nerve conduction. *Adenosine triphosphate* (ATP) plays a pivotal role as a short-term energy store within the cell. The chemical energy released during the catabolic metabolism of foodstuffs is stored as high-energy ATP and then the breakdown of ATP is used to drive the other energy-requiring processes. Each cell produces its own ATP; it is not transported between cells.

Although they will not discussed in the following outline, it should be borne in mind that every cellular reaction is catalysed (speeded up) by a specific *enzyme*. The reactions would not occur to any significant extent in the absence of the specific enzyme – it is the enzymes within the cell that determine what reactions can occur within the cell and thus determine the nature of the cell. Enzymes are proteins and the genetic code (contained within the DNA molecule) codes for the proteins of the cell. It is the proteins an organism produces that determine its characteristics. Genetic diseases are the result of an error in one of the proteins produced by that individual. Many enzymes require non-protein moieties known as *coenzymes* or *cofactors* in order to function. Several of these coenzymes are derivatives of vitamins, and it is their role as precursors of coenzymes that accounts for the essentiality of several vitamins. Cofactors that are bound strongly to the enzyme and become an integral part of the enzyme structure are termed *prosthetic groups*. Other substances that are sometimes taken as dietary supplements can also act as coenzymes: these are not classified as vitamins because endogenous synthesis is considered sufficient to meet our needs (see Chapter 13).

Nature and functioning of ATP

Adenosine triphosphate consists of a purine base (adenine), a pentose sugar (ribose) and three phosphate groups. The hydrolysis of ATP to adenosine diphosphate (ADP), by removal of one of the phosphate groups, is a highly *exergonic reaction*; that is, a considerable amount of chemical energy is released during the reaction. This energy would be released as heat if the ATP hydrolysis were conducted in a test tube. Similarly, the hydrolysis of ADP to *adenosine monophosphate* (AMP) is also highly exergonic. Conversely, the conversions of AMP to ADP to ATP are highly *endergonic reactions*; that is, they absorb large amounts of energy. If these reactions were conducted in a test tube then one would expect to need to provide heat energy to make the thermodynamics of the reactions favourable.

$$ATP: adenine \text{---} ribose \text{---} P \text{---} P \text{---} P$$
$$ADP: adenine \text{---} ribose \text{---} P \text{---} P \text{---} P$$
$$AMP: adenine \text{---} ribose \text{---} P$$

$$P = phosphate\ group\ (PO_4)$$

Within the cell, highly exergonic reactions in the catabolism of foodstuffs are coupled to ATP synthesis. The combined reaction remains slightly exergonic, but much of the chemical energy of the exergonic, catabolic reaction is stored as ATP rather than being released into the cellular fluids as heat. For example, consider the hypothetical exergonic catabolic reaction:

$$A \longrightarrow B + large\ output\ of\ heat\ energy$$

In the cell:

$$A \longrightarrow B + a\ smaller\ output\ of\ heat\ energy$$
$$ADP \qquad ATP$$

Other reactions within the cell are endergonic (energy-consuming). One would expect that, if these reactions were being carried out in a test tube, it would be necessary to provide heat to make them thermodynamically favourable and allow them to occur. Within the cell, however, such an endergonic reaction can be coupled to ATP hydrolysis to make the combined reaction exergonic and thus thermodynamically favourable at body temperature. For example, consider the hypothetical endergonic reaction:

$$X + heat\ energy \longrightarrow Y$$

In the cell:

$$X \longrightarrow Y + small\ net\ output\ of\ heat\ energy$$
$$ATP \qquad ADP$$

Substrate-level phosphorylation

In catabolic pathways, some highly exergonic steps are directly linked to ATP formation (substrate-level phosphorylation), as illustrated by the theoretical A → B reaction above. For example, in the glycolysis pathway one reaction involves the conversion of diphosphoglyceric acid to mono-phosphoglyceric acid, and this reaction is directly coupled to ATP synthesis:

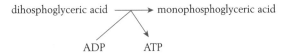

$$dihosphoglyceric\ acid \longrightarrow monophosphoglyceric\ acid$$
$$ADP \qquad ATP$$

Oxidative phosphorylation

Much of the energy release in the catabolic pathways of metabolism occurs as a result of oxidation. Many oxidative steps involve the removal of hydrogen atoms from substrate molecules and their acceptance by hydrogen acceptor molecules, such as nicotinamide adenine dinucleotide (NAD). For example, consider the hypothetical oxidative reaction:

$$XH_2 + NAD \longrightarrow X + NADH_2$$

In this reaction, XH_2 has been oxidized to X and NAD has been reduced to $NADH_2$. As a real example, in the citric acid cycle discussed below, malic acid is oxidized to oxaloacetic acid by the removal of hydrogen, and this reaction is coupled to the reduction of NAD by hydrogen addition:

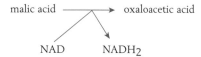

NAD is derived from the vitamin niacin. Niacin is essential because it is a precursor of NAD and the phosphorylated derivative NADP. Re-oxidation of these reduced hydrogen acceptors in the mitochondria of cells results in the production of large quantities of ATP (three molecules of ATP per molecule of $NADH_2$ re-oxidized):

$$NADH_2 + O_2 \longrightarrow NAD + H_2O$$
$$3\ ADP \qquad 3\ ATP$$

This mitochondrial process is called *oxidative phosphorylation*. In this process, there are a series of oxidation–reduction reactions, which culminate in the reduction of molecular oxygen to water. Reduced NAD ($NADH_2$) reduces the next compound on the electron transport chain and is itself re-oxidized; this reduced compound then reduces the next compound, and so on to molecular oxygen. This sequence is called the *electron transport chain* because reduction can be defined either as the addition of electrons or the addition of hydrogen.

During this sequence of oxidation–reduction reactions, there is considerable release of chemical energy. Some of this energy is released as heat, which helps to keep the body warm, but some of it is used to force hydrogen ions or protons (H^+) through the inner mitochondrial membrane. As the inner mitochondrial membrane is generally impermeable to protons, this creates a considerable proton gradient across this membrane. There are pores in the inner mitochondrial membrane where protons can pass back into the mitochondrion, and this controlled flow of protons provides the energy that drives ATP synthesis in the mitochondrion. This is the *chemiosmotic theory of oxidative phosphorylation*, which explains how the oxidation of reduced cofactors such as $NADH_2$ is linked to ATP synthesis.

If the inner mitochondrial membrane becomes more permeable to protons, this will compromise or 'uncouple' this link between oxidation and ATP synthesis. *Uncouplers* make the inner mitochondrial membrane more permeable to protons and so they cause oxidation to accelerate, but the energy is released as heat rather than being used to drive ATP synthesis. In a tissue known as *brown fat*, there is an uncoupling protein (UCP1) which, when activated by sympathetic nerve stimulation, allows protons to leak through the inner mitochondrial membrane and this generates heat. This tissue is capable of producing large amounts of heat to warm the body, and brown fat is prominent in small mammals, hibernating animals and human babies. There are other uncoupler proteins in other tissues (UCP2 and UCP3); their significance is discussed in Chapter 8. Some drugs and poisons (e.g. dinitrophenol) also uncouple oxidative phosphorylation. These substances increase body heat production and can cause rapid weight loss, but those currently available are too toxic to be used therapeutically for this purpose.

Oxidative phosphorylation normally yields the vast bulk of the energy released in catabolic metabolism. Cells that do not have mitochondria (e.g. red blood cells) or that have insufficient oxygen supply (e.g. a muscle working beyond the capacity of the blood system to supply oxygen) have to rely on the anaerobic metabolism of glucose to supply their energy needs. One molecule of glucose when metabolized anaerobically to lactic acid gives a net yield of only two molecules of ATP, whereas when metabolized aerobically to carbon dioxide and water it yields 38 ATP molecules.

METABOLISM OF GLUCOSE AND THE MONOSACCHARIDES

Dietary carbohydrates are digested to their component monosaccharides before being absorbed. Digestion of starch yields glucose and digestion of disaccharides yields glucose plus other monosaccharides, fructose from sucrose (cane or beet sugar) and galactose from lactose (milk sugar).

Glycolysis

Glycolysis is the initial pathway involved in the metabolism of carbohydrates and is summarized in

Figure 6.1. The first three steps in this pathway involve activation of the glucose molecule by the addition of phosphate groups and a molecular rearrangement (*isomerization*) of glucose phosphate to fructose phosphate. There is consumption of two ATP molecules during these activating steps. The fructose diphosphate thus produced is much more reactive (unstable) than glucose and the six carbon (6C) molecule can be split by an enzyme into two, three carbon (3C) molecules. The other major dietary monosaccharides, fructose and galactose, also feed into the early stages of this glycolysis pathway, as does glucose phosphate derived from the breakdown of body glycogen stores.

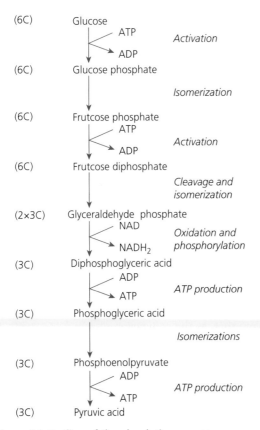

Figure 6.1 Outline of the glycolytic sequence.

During the steps that convert glyceraldehyde phosphate into pyruvic acid, there is production of two molecules of reduced NAD and four molecules of ATP from each starting molecule of glucose. Taking into account the two molecules of ATP used to generate fructose diphosphate, this gives a net yield of

2 ATP at the substrate level for each molecule of glucose. Under aerobic conditions, the reduced NAD will be re-oxidized in the mitochondria using molecular oxygen and will yield a further six molecules of ATP in oxidative phosphorylation. Under anaerobic conditions then this reduced NAD must be re-oxidized by some other means, otherwise the very small quantities of oxidized NAD within the cell would be quickly exhausted and the whole process halted. In mammalian cells this NAD is regenerated under anaerobic conditions by the reduction of pyruvic acid to lactic acid:

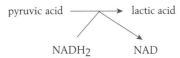

Lactic acid is the end-product of anaerobic metabolism in mammalian cells and anaerobic energy production is possible only from carbohydrate substrate. Red blood cells do not have mitochondria, so they metabolize glucose only as far as pyruvic acid and lactic acid. During heavy exercise, the oxygen supply to a muscle limits aerobic metabolism, so the muscles will generate some ATP anaerobically and produce lactic acid as a by-product. Accumulation of lactic acid is one factor responsible for the fatigue of exercising muscles. Note also that in thiamin deficiency (beriberi) there is effectively a partial block in the metabolism of carbohydrate beyond pyruvic acid because the conversion of pyruvic acid to acetyl coenzyme A requires a coenzyme, thiamin pyrophosphate, which is derived from thiamin. Lactic acid and pyruvic acid therefore also accumulate in victims of beriberi because of this metabolic block.

The lactic acid produced by anaerobic metabolism is used for the re-synthesis of glucose in the liver (the *Cori cycle*). This re-synthesis of glucose is effectively a reversal of glycolysis, so it is possible to synthesize glucose from any intermediate of the glycolysis pathway although the process does consume ATP.

Aerobic metabolism of pyruvic acid

Under aerobic conditions, pyruvic acid will normally be converted to acetyl coenzyme A (effectively activated acetate):

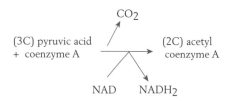

Coenzyme A is a large moiety that is derived from the B vitamin, pantothenic acid. Addition of the coenzyme A moiety increases the reactivity of acetate. It is released in the next reaction and recycled. This step cannot be reversed in mammalian cells, so glucose cannot be synthesized from acetyl coenzyme A.

The acetyl coenzyme A (2C) then enters a sequence known as the *Krebs cycle* or the *citric acid cycle* (Figure 6.2). It combines with oxaloacetic acid (4C) to give citric acid (6C). This citric acid then goes through a sequence of eight reactions, which ultimately result, once again, in the production of oxaloacetic acid, i.e. a cyclic process. During two of the reactions, a molecule of carbon dioxide is produced and in four of them a molecule of reduced coenzyme (e.g. $NADH_2$) is produced; in only one reaction is there direct substrate level ATP production. Each starting molecule of glucose yields two molecules of acetyl coenzyme A, so each molecule of glucose metabolized under aerobic conditions results in two 'turns' of the citric acid cycle.

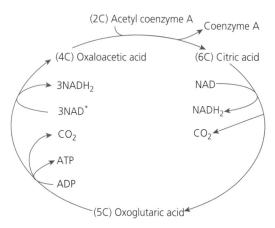

Figure 6.2 Outline of the Krebs cycle.

After undergoing the reactions of glycolysis and the citric acid cycle, all the six carbon atoms of the original glucose molecule will thus have been evolved as carbon dioxide. When the reduced coenzyme (e.g. $NADH_2$) is re-oxidized in the mitochondria this will result in the production of water. Thus overall, the glucose has been metabolized to carbon dioxide and water.

METABOLISM OF FATTY ACIDS AND GLYCEROL

Dietary fat, or the fat stored in adipose tissue, is largely triacylglycerol (*triglyceride*). It yields, for metabolism, one molecule of glycerol and three fatty acid molecules. The 3-carbon (3C) glycerol is converted to glyceraldehyde phosphate and enters glycolysis; it can thus be used directly as a source of energy or it can be used to generate glucose (by reversal of glycolysis). Fatty acids are metabolized to multiple units of acetyl coenzyme A, in a pathway known as the *β-oxidation pathway*. A 16-carbon fatty acid (e.g. palmitic acid) would thus yield eight 2C units of acetyl coenzyme A (summarized in Figure 6.3).

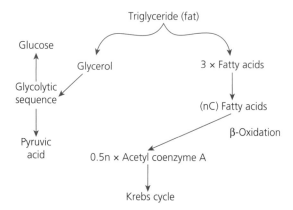

Figure 6.3 Outline of food metabolism.

Note that, as the conversion of acetyl coenzyme A back to pyruvic acid is not possible in mammalian cells, fatty acids cannot be used to generate glucose.

Brain cells do not have the enzymes necessary for β-oxidation, so they cannot directly use fatty acids as an energy source. When carbohydrate is available (e.g. when carbohydrates are eaten regularly) brain cells use glucose as their substrate but they are not, as was previously thought, totally dependent on carbohydrate as a substrate. During fasting, they can utilize certain ketones or *ketone bodies* that are made from acetyl coenzyme A. This means that during starvation the brain can indirectly utilize fatty acids that have been converted to these ketones in the liver (discussed more fully under metabolic adaptation to starvation in Chapter 7).

Fatty acids are synthesized by a process that is essentially a reversal of β-oxidation. For example, to synthesize 16C palmitic acid, eight units of 2C acetate (as acetyl coenzyme A) are progressively assembled. Thus fatty acids can be synthesized from carbohydrates via acetyl coenzyme A. Breakdown of fatty acids to acetyl coenzyme A is an oxidative process (hence β-oxidation), so the synthesis of fatty acids from acetyl coenzyme A is a reductive process. The reduced form of the phosphorylated derivative of NAD, $NADPH_2$, is used as the source of reducing power in this pathway: $NADPH_2$ is generated in the *pentose phosphate pathway* (see below).

METABOLISM OF AMINO ACIDS

Surplus amino acids from protein can be used as an energy source. The nitrogen-containing amino group is removed to leave a moiety, the keto acid, which can be converted to pyruvic acid, acetyl coenzyme A or one of the intermediates of the citric acid cycle. The amino group can be converted to the waste product urea, or it can be transferred to another keto acid and thus produce another amino acid – a process called *transamination*.

It is possible to make glucose from protein. If the amino acid (e.g. alanine) yields pyruvic acid, then glucose synthesis merely involves the effective reversal of glycolysis. If the amino acid (e.g. glutamic acid) yields a citric acid cycle intermediate, then this intermediate will be converted to oxaloacetic acid, which can then be converted to the phospho-enol pyruvate of glycolysis:

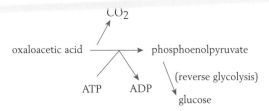

Note that acetyl coenzyme A (and thus fatty acids) cannot be used to synthesize glucose via this route because the two atoms of the acetate that enter the citric acid cycle have been lost as carbon dioxide by the time oxaloacetic acid has been

regenerated. Utilization of existing citric acid cycle intermediates to synthesize glucose is theoretically possible, but they would be so rapidly depleted that their contribution to glucose supply would be insignificant. The metabolic routes for the metabolism of the different foodstuffs are summarized in Figure 6.4.

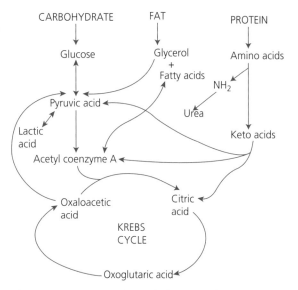

Figure 6.4 Summary of metabolic routes for foodstuffs.

During starvation or carbohydrate deprivation, the only routes available for the maintenance of carbohydrate supplies are by manufacture from amino acids or the glycerol component of fat. This process of generation of glucose from amino acids (*gluconeogenesis*) occurs in the liver, but it is inefficient and energy expensive and will, of course, lead to depletion of the protein in muscle and vital organs. Note, however, that the need for gluconeogenesis is limited during starvation or carbohydrate deprivation by the use of ketone bodies as an alternative to carbohydrate substrate (see Chapter 7).

THE PENTOSE PHOSPHATE PATHWAY

This pathway generates reducing power in the form of $NADPH_2$ (necessary, for example, in fatty acids biosynthesis) and also generates the pentose sugar, ribose phosphate, that is essential for nucleotide (e.g. ATP) biosynthesis and nucleic acid (RNA and DNA) synthesis. The first part of this pathway involves the conversion of glucose phosphate to ribose phosphate:

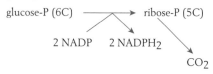

If the demand for $NADPH_2$ and ribose phosphate is balanced, these two will represent end-products of the pathway. If, however, the demand for $NADPH_2$, say for active lipid synthesis, exceeds the demand for ribose phosphate, the excess ribose is converted by a complex series of reactions to 3-carbon glyceraldehyde phosphate and 6-carbon fructose phosphate. The overall reaction is:

$$3 \times \text{ribose-P} (3 \times 5C) \longrightarrow \begin{array}{l} \text{glyceraldehyde-P} \\ + 2 \times \text{fructose-P} (2 \times 6C) \end{array}$$

The enzymes used in this series of reactions are called *transketolase* and *transaldolase*. The former requires thiamin pyrophosphate, derived from vitamin B_1, thiamin, as a coenzyme. The glyceraldehyde phosphate and fructose phosphate produced by these reactions can both enter glycolysis either to be metabolized to pyruvic acid or used to regenerate glucose phosphate.

If the demand for ribose phosphate exceeds that for $NADPH_2$, the reverse of the transketolase/transaldolase reaction can generate ribose phosphate from glyceraldehyde phosphate and fructose phosphate.

Wernicke–Korsakoff syndrome is a neuropsychiatric disorder caused by lack of dietary thiamin (see Chapter 14 for details). In industrialized countries it is usually associated with thiamin deficiency brought on by alcoholism. The symptoms of this syndrome are probably due to inadequate $NADPH_2$ synthesis leading to impaired synthesis of myelin, the fatty sheath that surrounds many neurones.

OVERVIEW OF MACRONUTRIENT HANDLING IN THE GUT

This chapter has been concerned with the final metabolic fate of the monomeric components of fats, carbohydrates and proteins; that is, how monosaccharides, amino acids and fatty acids are metabolized within the cell. However, most of the energy in food is present as complex macromolecules which must first be broken down into these monomers before they can be absorbed and utilized within cells. The processes of digestion of these macromolecules are discussed briefly in Chapters 10–12 dealing with carbohydrates, fats and proteins, but digestion and absorption of all three are overviewed briefly here.

Carbohydrates

Most of the available carbohydrate in food is consumed as either starches or the disaccharides sucrose (beet or cane sugar, glucose–fructose) and lactose (milk sugar, glucose–galactose) with usually just small amounts of free glucose and fructose. (Figure 10.1 in Chapter 10 gives a brief classification of the carbohydrates, and Figure 10.2 shows the structure of some carbohydrates and illustrates the nature of α1–4 and α1–6 links between glucose residues in starch.) Saliva in the mouth contains the enzyme α-amylase which breaks down α1–4 links between glucose residues in starch. Under most circumstances the contribution of salivary α-amylase to overall starch digestion will be relatively small because food usually only spends a short time in the mouth and the enzyme is denatured by the acid environment of the stomach. However, food entering the stomach will buffer the stomach acid and raise stomach pH for a while, and enzymes within a bolus of food may be protected from the effects of stomach acid.

Pancreatic juice secreted into the duodenum also contains an α-amylase. The end-products of starch digestion by α-amylase are mainly maltose (glucose–glucose), maltotriose (three glucose residues joined by α1–4 links), and so-called α-limit dextrin which is a small oligosaccharide produced from amylopectin with an α1–6 link that cannot be broken down by α-amylase.

On the mucosal surface of the small intestine are a series of enzymes which complete the digestion of carbohydrates into their component monosaccharides.

- Maltase breaks α1–4 links between maltose, maltotriose or slightly larger oligosaccharides with glucose residues joined solely by α1–4 links into glucose.

- Lactase digests any lactose present to glucose and galactose.
- Sucrase breaks sucrose into glucose and fructose.
- Isomaltase breaks the α1–6 links in the α-limit dextrin enabling it to be broken down into glucose. (Sucrase and isomaltase can also break α1–4 links between glucose residues.)

Glucose and galactose are absorbed actively across the intestinal brush border. They bind to a transporter protein called SGLT1 which also binds to sodium ions on the mucosal surface of the gut cell. Inside the cell the concentration of sodium is kept low by an active sodium–potassium pump and this low sodium concentration causes release of both sodium and glucose (or galactose) from the transporter protein. The high sodium gradient requires energy to maintain it and this accelerates glucose/galactose transport and makes it 'active' transport. High sodium concentration increases glucose or galactose binding to SGLT1, but low sodium concentration inhibits glucose or galactose binding. Fructose binds to a GLUT-5 transporter protein at the brush border, but this does not bind sodium and so fructose absorption is said to be sodium independent and not active; it is absorbed more slowly than the other monosaccharides. Fructose concentration within the mucosal cell is kept very low and so fructose absorption is essentially complete even though it is not active and fructose can only pass down a concentration gradient (i.e. it is absorbed by facilitated diffusion).

Protein

Amino acids are ingested as proteins which contain 20 different amino acids linked together in sometimes very long chains joined together by peptide bonds. Figure 11.1 in Chapter 11 illustrates the way in which amino acids are joined to make proteins and shows that at one end of every protein there is a free amino group (the N-terminal) and at the other end a free carboxyl group (the C-terminal). The different types of amino acid are described in the text.

In the acidic environment of the stomach, the enzyme pepsin starts to cleave the peptide bonds between amino acids in proteins. It is a type of proteolytic enzyme called an *endopeptidase* because it breaks peptide bonds within the protein

molecule. *Exopeptidases* break off the terminal amino acids from a peptide. Complete digestion of protein still occurs in conditions where there is an absence of pepsin and so it is not necessary for protein digestion. In the duodenum, proteolytic enzymes from the pancreas convert 70 per cent of dietary protein into oligopeptides of up to six amino acids, and the remaining 30 per cent is broken down to free amino acids. These pancreatic proteases are:

- *trypsin* – which breaks the links within proteins at lysine or arginine residues
- *chymotrypsin* – which breaks links at aromatic or neutral amino acids
- *elastase* – which breaks bonds at aliphatic amino acids
- *carboxypeptidases* – which break off certain C-terminal amino acids from proteins and peptides.

On the surface of the brush border there are a series of 20 further peptidases which complete the breakdown of dietary protein into free amino acids plus dipeptides and tripeptides. There are several amino acid transporter proteins and some that transport the small peptides; these have different amino acid specificities and some are sodium dependent. Any di- and tripeptides absorbed are digested by peptidases within the cytoplasm of the mucosal cells.

Fat

The digestion and absorption of fat are discussed extensively in Chapter 12 and so will only be outlined here. Most dietary fat is in the form of *triacylglycerol* made up of a glycerol 'backbone' to which are attached three fatty acid residues (see Figure 12.1 in Chapter 12). Fat is insoluble in water, and so, to allow water-soluble digestive enzymes to act upon it, it must first be emulsified (dispersed as small particles within the fluid gut contents). Churning of fats in the stomach with phospholipids and the effect of bile within the duodenum emulsify the dietary fat so that the pancreatic enzyme lipase can act on it to convert dietary triacylglycerol into *monoacylglycerol* plus two free fatty acids. Some shorter chain fatty acids pass directly into the mucosal cell, but most of the products of fat digestion form microscopically small particles with bile salts and phospholipids called *micelles*. An emulsion formed when fats are emulsified is cloudy because the particles are large enough to scatter light but micelles are so small that they appear clear as if a true solution had been formed.

Fat digestion products (and fat-soluble vitamins) within the micelles are in equilibrium with tiny amounts of these products that are in true solution within the intestinal contents. These small amounts in true solution diffuse across into the mucosal cells and are immediately replaced by amounts from within the micelles. Once inside the mucosal cell the monoacylglycerol and fatty acids are re-esterified into triacylglycerol, so the concentration gradient across the mucosal cell membrane is maintained and more fat digestion products can diffuse across; in this way fat absorption from the intestine is normally almost 100 per cent. The triacylglycerol produced within the mucosal cells is coated with protein to form particles called *chylomicrons*, which then enter into the lymphatic vessels that supply the intestine and these drain into the venous system. In the tissues, lipase in the capillaries breaks down triacylglycerol within chylomicrons to fatty acids and monoacylglycerol and fatty acids which diffuse into the tissues and may once again be re-esterified into triacylglycerol for storage or transport.

PART TWO

ENERGY, ENERGY BALANCE AND OBESITY

7   Introduction to energy aspects of nutrition   167
8   Energy balance and its regulation   187
9   Obesity   202

INTRODUCTION TO ENERGY ASPECTS OF NUTRITION

Sources of energy	167	Energy density	174
Units of energy	167	Nutrient density	176
How energy requirements are estimated	168	Sources of dietary energy by food groups	177
Variation in energy requirements:		Starvation	178
general trends	170	Eating disorders	182
Energy content of foods	171	Cancer cachexia	185
Sources of dietary energy by nutrient	172		

SOURCES OF ENERGY

Although the range of nutrients required by living organisms varies enormously, all organisms require an external supply of energy. Plants 'trap' energy from sunlight and use it to make sugars in the process of photosynthesis. Photosynthesis is the ultimate source of all the energy in living systems and fossil fuels. In human diets, the food macronutrients – fat, carbohydrate and protein (plus alcohol) – are the sources of energy.

UNITS OF ENERGY

The Standard International (SI) unit of energy is the *joule*, which is defined as the energy expended when a mass of 1 kilogram (kg) is moved through a distance of 1 metre (m) by a force of 1 newton (N). For nutritionists, the kilojoule (kJ, a thousand joules) and the megajoule (MJ, a million joules) are more practical units. Traditionally, nutritionists have used a unit of heat, the *kilocalorie* (kcal), as their unit of energy. Although a kilocalorie is strictly a thousand calories, most people, when dealing with nutrition, tend to use the terms 'calorie' and 'kilocalorie' as if synonymous. A kilocalorie is defined as the heat required to raise the temperature of 1 litre (L) of water by 1°C.

In practice, the kilocalorie is still widely used both by nutritionists and by non-scientists. The kilocalorie is a convenient unit because people with a limited knowledge of physics can understand its definition, and nutritionists may use heat output as their method of measuring both the energy yields of foods and the energy expenditure of animals and people.

To interconvert kilocalories and kilojoules:

$$1 \text{ kcal} = 4.2 \text{ kJ}.$$

Key points

- A joule is the energy expended when a mass of 1 kg is moved through a distance of 1 m by a force of 1 N.
- One kilojoule (kJ) is 1000 joules.
- One megajoule (MJ) is 1 000 000 joules (1000 kJ).
- One kilocalorie is 1000 calories, but in nutrition the term 'calorie' usually means kilocalorie.
- 1 kilocalorie (kcal) = 4.2 kJ.

HOW ENERGY REQUIREMENTS ARE ESTIMATED

Table 7.1 shows some selected UK *estimated average requirements* (EARs) for energy. Remember that these UK dietary standards for energy represent the best estimates of average requirements, whereas the most commonly used reference values for most nutrients – the reference nutrient intake (RNI) or recommended dietary allowance (RDA) – are the estimated needs of those with the highest requirements (see Chapter 3 for discussion and rationale).

Table 7.1 Selected current UK estimated average requirements (EARs) for energy (corresponding US recommended daily allowances (RDA) from the 1989 edition of dietary reference values are given for comparative purposes)*

Age (years)	UK EAR		American RDA[1]	
	kcal	MJ	kcal	MJ
1–3 boys	1230	5.15	1300	5.44
1–3 girls	1165	4.86	1300	5.44
7–10 boys	1970	8.24	2000	8.37
7–10 girls	1740	7.28	2000	8.37
15–18 men	2755	11.51	3000	12.56
15–18 women	2110	8.83	2200	9.21
19–50 men	2550	10.60	2900	12.14
19–50 women	1940	8.10	2200	9.21
75+ men	2100	8.77	2300	9.63
75+ women	1810	7.61	1900	7.96

*Data sources: COMA (1991) and NRC (1989a).
[1]Note that since 2002 (IOM, 2002) the American standards for energy have allowed an estimated energy requirement for an individual adult to be determined that takes account of their exact age, height category, weight category and activity level; this is discussed in the text.

The *basal metabolic rate* (BMR) is the minimum rate of energy expenditure in a conscious person or animal. It is determined by measuring the metabolic rate (see Chapter 3) of a subject who has been resting for some time in a warm room and after an overnight fast. BMR represents the energy required to keep the body's internal organs and systems functioning, including for breathing, circulation of blood and brain functioning. In a sedentary person, BMR accounts for more than two-thirds of total energy expenditure, and only in those who are extremely active will it make up less than half of total energy expenditure. If BMR is measured in large samples of individuals, then, within specified age and sex bands, there is a linear relationship between BMR and body weight. This means that one can derive regression equations that allow the average BMR of a group of people within an age band to be predicted from the average weight of the group. For example, in women aged 18–29 years the following regression equation allows prediction of average BMR from average weight:

$$BMR \ (kcal/day) = 14.8 \times weight \ (kg) + 487.$$

So, if the average weight of women in this age band is 60 kg, then:

$$Average \ BMR = (14.8 \times 60) + 487$$
$$= 1375 \ kcal/day.$$

To estimate the average daily energy requirement of this group, one must multiply the BMR by a factor that reflects the level of physical activity of the group; this is called the *physical activity level* (PAL). If this population is assumed to be sedentary in both their occupation and in their leisure time, a PAL value of 1.4 would be appropriate. So the average energy expenditure of the group (and thus their average requirement) would be estimated at:

$$BMR \times PAL = 1375 \times 1.4$$
$$= 1925 \ kcal/day.$$

This is essentially how the UK panel setting the dietary standards (COMA 1991) arrived at the figure of 1940 kcal/day (8.1 MJ/day) for women aged 19–50 in Table 7.1 (the slight difference in numbers occurs because of interpolation over the larger age band).

In principle, this is the method COMA used to set the EARs for energy for all adults and older children. They used regression equations like the one above to predict BMR from the average weight of Britons in each age group. For most groups they multiplied the BMR by a PAL of 1.4 to reflect the generally sedentary nature of the British population. In adults aged over 60 years, they used a PAL of 1.5. This higher PAL for elderly people seems surprising given the clear evidence that activity decreases in the elderly (the reasons for this anomaly are outlined in the next section). For younger children, estimates of energy requirements are largely based on measurements of average energy intakes.

Also shown simply for comparison in Table 7.1 are the 1989 RDAs for energy in the USA (see later for discussion of current US energy standards for individuals). The American panel that set the 1989 energy RDAs (NRC, 1989a) used very similar regression equations to predict the average BMR (or the resting energy expenditure, REE) of Americans in the various age bands and multiplied by an activity (PAL) factor. The large differences between the UK and US values in the table are mainly due to differences in the activity factor used by the two panels. Americans also tend to be a little heavier than Britons. The US panel used PAL multiples of between 1.55 and 1.7 in older children and adults up to 50 years, compared to the UK panel's 1.4. Like the British panel, NRC used a PAL multiple of 1.5 for older people.

It must be borne in mind when using figures such as those in Table 7.1 that these are estimates of average requirements. They are *not* intended to be used as an accurate statement of the requirements of individuals. Many factors will affect the energy expenditure – and thus the energy requirement – of an individual, such as those listed below:

- size – in general, the bigger the body the greater the energy expenditure
- body composition – lean tissue is metabolically more active and uses more energy than adipose tissue
- activity level
- environmental conditions such as the ambient temperature
- physiological factors such as hormone levels
- rate of growth in children
- individual genetic variability.

It is possible to roughly estimate the energy requirements of an individual. One could use the regression equation appropriate for the person's age to estimate his or her BMR from the person's weight (a list of regression equations can be found in COMA, 1991). Alternatively one can assume that, in adults aged under 50 years, the BMR is 0.9 kcal per hour for a woman (1.0 for a man). Such approximations assume average proportions of fat and lean in the body and so they become increasingly unreliable as one moves towards extremes of fatness or leanness. Using this rule of thumb, the estimated BMR of a 65 kg man would be:

$$65 \times 1.0 \times 24 = 1560 \,\text{kcal/day}.$$

This estimated BMR must then be multiplied by an appropriate PAL. Table 7.2 was offered by COMA as a guide to deciding on the appropriate PAL multiple. It uses three categories each for both occupational and non-occupational activity levels. Only those who are extremely active (e.g. athletes in training) or extremely inactive (e.g. elderly housebound people) will fall outside this range.

Table 7.2 Guide to predicting the physical activity level (PAL) multiple of an individual or group*

Non-occupational activity	Occupational activity					
	Light		Moderate		Moderate/heavy	
	M	F	M	F	M	F
Non-active	1.4	1.4	1.6	1.5	1.7	1.5
Moderately active	1.5	1.5	1.7	1.6	1.8	1.6
Very active	1.6	1.6	1.8	1.7	1.9	1.7

*After COMA (1991).
M, male; F, female.
It takes about half an hour's brisk walking to raise the PAL by 0.1 on that day.

The current US dietary reference intakes for energy make it possible to derive a more specific estimated energy requirement (EER) which reflects the height, weight, exact age and activity category of the individual. There is a standard table which gives the EER for a 30-year-old man and woman and there are 24 numerical values listed for each sex. There are three different heights and two different body weights for each height (corresponding to a BMI of either 18.5 or 25). For each of the six height and weight categories given for each sex there are four different activity levels to choose from (sedentary, low active, active and very active). Of course these 48 numerical values are only for men and women aged exactly 30 years – for each year less than 30 one must add on 10 kcal/day for men and 7 kcal/day for women, and for each year above 30 one must subtract these same amounts. This table can be found in Shils *et al.* (2006) or IOM (2002).

Key points

- The average BMR of a group can be estimated from their average body weight using regression equations derived from measurement of BMR and body weight in a large sample of people.
- This BMR can be used to estimate average energy requirements by multiplying it by a factor that reflects the activity level of the group – the physical activity level (PAL).
- This PAL can vary from under 1.3 in elderly housebound people to over 2 in athletes during training.
- In the UK, the dietary standard for energy is the estimated average requirement (EAR). Until 2002 in the USA it was the recommended dietary allowance (RDA).
- Both the EAR and the RDA are estimates of average requirements. Any individual's requirements will depend on many factors such as size, body composition, activity level, physiological state and environmental conditions.
- Current US energy standards allow an EER for an individual to be calculated which takes into account their exact age, height category, weight category, and activity level category.

VARIATION IN AVERAGE ENERGY REQUIREMENTS: GENERAL TRENDS

Table 7.1 suggests quite large differences between the estimated average energy requirements of Britons and Americans which largely reflect the different assumptions about activity levels and average body weights made by the panels who set these values. Other trends that are apparent on close inspection of the table are summarized here.

First, the energy requirements of males are generally higher than those of females. This is largely because the average male is bigger than the average female. In older children and adults, females also have a higher proportion of adipose tissue which is metabolically less active than lean tissue.

Second, the energy requirement per unit of body weight of growing children is higher than that of adults; so a 2-year-old may be only around a fifth of the weight of an adult but requires more than half of the adult energy intake. In the case of older teenagers, even the absolute energy requirement is higher than in adults. These relatively high energy requirements of children partly reflect the requirements for growth; but also, particularly in small children, it is partly a manifestation of the general inverse relationship between the relative metabolic rate and body size (see Chapter 3). Younger children also tend to be more active than adults.

The values given in Table 7.1 imply that there is a considerable reduction in energy needs in the elderly. This suggests that older people will need less energy and eat less food than younger adults. As requirements for most other nutrients are not thought to decline with age, this increases the vulnerability of elderly people to nutrient inadequacies (see Chapter 16 for further discussion). The amount of metabolically active lean tissue declines in old age and the proportion of body fat increases. There is also no doubt that activity levels show an accelerating decline in middle age and old age. This decline in activity is reflected in the use of a reduced PAL multiple for elderly people in the US values. However, the British panel took the surprising decision to use a PAL multiple of 1.5 for older adults compared to only 1.4 in younger adults. This decision was made because the panel was keen to discourage overconsumption of energy in younger people because of the prevalence of obesity. For elderly people, their priorities were (a) to maintain sufficient energy intake to allow adequate intake of other nutrients, and (b) to prevent elderly people becoming underweight. The values in Table 7.1 almost certainly understate the real decline in energy intake that occurs in the very elderly. The real PAL of elderly housebound people may be 1.3 or even less.

Key points

- Children have higher relative metabolic rates than adults and thus require more energy per kilogram of body weight.
- Men have higher average energy requirements than women because they are bigger and have a higher lean-to-fat ratio.
- Basal metabolic rate declines in the elderly owing to reduced lean body mass. This compounds with declining activity levels to substantially reduce the average energy requirements in the very elderly.

ENERGY CONTENT OF FOODS

The oxidation of foodstuffs in metabolism is often likened to the oxidative processes of combustion or burning. This would suggest that the heat energy released during the burning of a food should be an indicator of its metabolic energy yield. In a bomb calorimeter, a small sample of food is placed in a sealed chamber, which is pressurized with oxygen to ensure complete oxidation (burning). The food is then ignited electrically, and the heat energy that is released during combustion of the food sample is measured. In practice, the heat energy released during combustion will significantly overestimate the energy that is metabolically available from most foods. The predictive value of the energy of combustion is worsened if the food is high in indigestible material or high in protein.

Some components of a food may burn and release heat energy but not be digested and absorbed, so this fraction of the energy of combustion will be lost in the faeces (e.g. some components of dietary fibre and indigestible proteins like those in hair).

In the bomb calorimeter there is complete oxidation of protein to water, carbon dioxide and oxides of nitrogen, whereas in metabolic oxidation most of the nitrogen is excreted in the urine as urea.

Urea will burn and release energy and so this means that some energy released from protein when it is burnt is lost in the urine when it is metabolized. The metabolic energy yield from protein is only about 70 per cent of the heat energy released during combustion; the other 30 per cent is lost in the urine. To determine the *metabolizable energy* using a bomb calorimeter, the heat energy released during combustion has to be corrected for this energy lost in the faeces and urine.

The usual way of determining the energy value of foods is to measure the available carbohydrate, fat, protein and alcohol content of the food and then to use standard conversion values for the metabolizable energy of each of these nutrients (Box 7.1).

Box 7.1

Metabolizable energy yields

- 1 gram of carbohydrate yields 16 kJ = 3.75 kcal.
- 1 gram of protein yields 17 kJ = 4 kcal.
- 1 gram of fat yields 37 kJ = 9 kcal.
- 1 gram of alcohol yields 29 kJ = 7 kcal.

Generally, these approximations hold irrespective of the type of fat, carbohydrate or protein; the carbohydrate figure is applied to both starches and sugars. Small variations in these conversion factors are of little significance given the many other sources of error in estimating dietary energy intake. Dietary fibre has traditionally been assumed to contribute nothing to metabolizable energy, but it may yield small amounts via its fermentation by intestinal bacteria to volatile fatty acids which can be absorbed and metabolized.

Key points

- Foods yield less energy when metabolized than when burnt because of losses in faeces (undigested material) and in urine (mainly urea).
- The energy yields of the macronutrients are shown in Box 7.1.
- The metabolizable energy of foods is determined by measuring the content of fat, carbohydrate and protein and using the energy equivalents of these nutrients.

SOURCES OF DIETARY ENERGY BY NUTRIENT

Dietary recommendations and survey reports often quote carbohydrate, fat, protein and even alcohol intakes as a percentage of total energy. This method of presentation allows meaningful comparison of the diet composition of people with widely differing energy intakes. It can be seen as a way of comparing the 'concentration' of fat, carbohydrate or protein in different foods and diets. Quoting absolute values for intakes of these major nutrients (e.g. grams per day) may be of limited usefulness and may even on occasion be misleading. For example, someone eating 4.2 MJ (1000 kcal) per day and 30 g of fat will get the same proportion of their dietary energy from fat (27 per cent) as someone consuming 8.4 MJ (2000 kcal) and 60 g of fat.

As another example of the usefulness of this tool, absolute per-capita intakes of fat (g/day) in the UK dropped sharply between 1975 and 1995. However, this reduction was almost entirely due to a reduction in total food intake, and during this period the proportion of energy from fat remained almost constant.

To calculate macronutrient intakes as a percentage of total energy, the energy equivalents of fat, carbohydrate and protein given in the previous section are used in the following formula:

(nutrient consumed (g) × energy equivalent as in Box 7.1) × 100 *divided by* total energy intake.

For example, to calculate the proportion of energy from fat in an 11 000 kJ diet containing 100 g of fat:

$(100 \times 37) \times 100 / 11\,000 = 33.6\%$ of energy as fat.

Table 7.3 shows estimates of the contribution of the various energy-yielding nutrients to the total energy supplies of adults in the UK. This was measured directly using 7-day weighed inventories (Gregory *et al.*, 1990; Hoare *et al.*, 2004) or 4-day food diaries (Bates *et al.*, 2011).

The energy contribution of the major macronutrients is often expressed as a percentage of food energy (i.e. excluding alcohol), and selected values from Table 7.3 are shown in this way in Table 7.4.

A substantial amount of alcohol in a diet 'dilutes' the percentage contribution of the other food macronutrients to total energy intake. This means that, in high alcohol consumers, the proportion of total energy derived from fats and sugars will be reduced and may make the diet appear to be more in line with current DRVs for these. Thus the average contribution of fat to total energy is 3 per cent lower than its contribution to food energy for men in 2009; this difference would be much greater if the difference were compared in those men with high alcohol intakes. Another effect of excluding alcohol is to move the values for men and women closer together because men have higher average alcohol intakes than women.

Table 7.3 Changes in the sources of energy in the diets of British adults expressed as percentages of total energy*

Nutrient	Men			Women		
	1987	2001	2009	1987	2001	2009
Fat (%)	37.6	33.5	32.8	39.4	33.5	33.0
Protein (%)	14.1	15.4	16.4	15.2	15.9	16.6
Carbohydrate (%)	41.6	44.7	43.0	43.1	46.7	45.5
Sugars (%)	17.6		18.5	19.2		19.9
Non-milk extrinsic sugars (%)	16.2	12.8	11.7	16.2	14.6	11.5
Starches (%)	24.0		24.5	23.9		25.6
Starches + intrinsic and milk sugars (%)	25.4	34.9	33.8	26.9	37.0	34.1
Alcohol (%)	6.9	6.5	7.8	2.3	3.9	4.9
Total (kcal/day)	2450	2321	2255	1680	1640	1645
(MJ/day)	10.26	9.72	9.32	7.03	6.87	6.92

*Data sources: Gregory *et al.* (1990), Hoare *et al.* (2004) and Bates *et al.* (2011).

Table 7.4 Some of the figures in Table 7.3 expressed as a percentage of food energy (i.e. excluding alcohol)*

Nutrient	Men			Women		
	1987	2001	2009	1987	2001	2009
Fat (%)	40.4	35.8	35.5	40.3	34.9	34.7
Protein (%)	15.2	16.5	17.8	15.6	16.6	17.5
Carbohydrate (%)	44.7	47.7	46.8	44.2	48.5	47.8

*Data sources: for 1987 (Gregory *et al.*, 1990), 2001 (Hoare *et al.*, 2004) and 2009 (Bates *et al.*, 2011).

It is clear from Tables 7.3 and 7.4 that fat and carbohydrate together provide the bulk of the food energy in the UK – over 80 per cent of the total. This will also be true of most European and US diets, and indeed it will be true for all but the most unusual or extreme diets – such as 'high-protein' reducing diets where almost the only foods eaten are lean meat, white fish, eggs and skimmed milk. As the bulk of any diet's energy usually comes from fat and carbohydrate, this means that as the proportion of one goes up so the proportion of the other tends to go down. An inverse relationship between the proportion of dietary energy derived from fat and carbohydrate is almost inevitable and could be termed a *carbohydrate–fat seesaw*. This means that, in most Western diets, there also tends to be an inverse relationship between dietary fat content and the major classes of carbohydrate – sugars, starches and non-starch polysaccharide (NSP)/dietary fibre. The consequences of the *sugar–fat seesaw* are discussed in Chapter 5.

Tables 7.3 and 7.4 show that there were significant changes in the adult British diet between 1986 and 2009. Fat dropped as a percentage of food and total energy by over 5 per cent and is now close to the dietary reference value (DRV) of 35 per cent of food energy. As would be expected, because of the carbohydrate–fat seesaw there was an increase in the proportion of energy derived from carbohydrates, although it is still a little way below the DRV of 50 per cent of food energy. The protein contribution to energy intake has increased over this period by more than 2 per cent, owing partly to increased use of low-fat milk and low-fat milk products. The proportion of energy derived from non-milk extrinsic sugars (largely added sugars) fell quite sharply despite an overall increase in carbohydrates, although the average of 12.5 per

cent of food energy is still above the DRV of 11 per cent. Total recorded energy intakes dropped by 200 kcal (0.54 MJ) per day in men, and this is consistent with the long-term decline in average energy intake since the late 1950s indicated by household budget surveys; energy intakes of women declined only very slightly.

Table 7.3 shows an increase in the percentage of total energy derived from alcohol over this period, especially in women. Bates *et al.* (2011) reported that, in 2009, alcohol contributed 8 per cent of energy for men and 5 per cent for women. For those who consumed alcohol (86 per cent of men and 48 per cent of women) alcohol provided 10 per cent of total energy. This indicates that increased numbers of men and women are exceeding the published safe levels for alcohol intake (see Chapter 5).

Table 7.5 shows the percentage of energy derived from the major macronutrients in the UK as

Table 7.5 Percentage of energy obtained from fat, carbohydrate and protein in all food and drink purchases in the UK*

	Energy
Fat	36.4%
Protein	13.7%
Carbohydrate	46.5%
Sugars	22.3%
Non-milk extrinsic sugars	14.9%
Starches	24.1%
Alcohol	3.4%
Total energy per capita	
kcal	2239
MJ	9.4

*Data source: *Family Food 2004–5* (DEFRA, 2006).

estimated using the household budget method (DEFRA, 2006).

Key points

- The macronutrient content of diets and foods is often expressed as the percentage of the total energy derived from that nutrient. This is a measure of the 'concentration' of these nutrients in a diet.

- These nutrients can also be expressed as the percentage of food energy (i.e. excluding alcohol).

- High alcohol content of diets 'dilutes' the contribution of other macronutrients and thus, for example, lowers the apparent fat and sugar contribution.

- In most diets, fat and carbohydrate together provide most of the food energy (over 80 per cent in the UK).

- As the proportion of energy derived from fat in a diet goes up, so the proportion from carbohydrate tends to go down, and vice versa – the so-called carbohydrate–fat seesaw.

- In most Western diets there also tends to be a sugar–fat seesaw.

- Between 1986 and 2009, the contribution of carbohydrates to food energy of British adult diets rose from 44.5 to 47.8 per cent. Protein rose from 15.4 to 17.6 per cent, and fat fell from 40.4 to 35.1 per cent.

- The energy contributions of different macronutrients in 2009 were much closer to the DRV than those of 1987. Current values for carbohydrate were still below the DRV and those for non-milk extrinsic sugars still above the DRV.

- There have been marked increases in the proportion of total energy derived from alcohol, which in 2009 contributed almost 10 per cent of total energy in those who consumed it (86 per cent of men and 48 per cent of women). These alcohol figures suggest that many more people are now exceeding the published safe limits for alcohol consumption.

ENERGY DENSITY

The energy density of a food or diet is the metabolizable energy yield per unit weight of food (e.g. kcal or kJ per 100 g of food). If a food is of high energy density then a little of it provides a lot of energy, whereas one can eat a lot of a food with low energy density and yet obtain little energy. This is illustrated in Table 7.6 where the weights of various foods required to provide 4.2 MJ (1000 kcal) are shown. The range of energy densities is very large. For example, just over a tenth of a kilo of vegetable oil will provide 4.2 MJ but one needs over 9 kg of boiled swede or 7 kg of lettuce. A number of the general trends illustrated by Table 7.6 are summarized below.

- As fat yields more than twice as much energy as either carbohydrate or protein, so fat content must be a major factor increasing the energy density of foods or diets. High-fat foods are inevitably of high energy density (e.g. nuts, seeds and oils) whereas low-fat foods are generally of low or moderate energy density.

- Most fruits and vegetables are almost fat-free and are high in water and fibre. They thus have very low energy densities (e.g. grapes and lettuce). Drying fruits (e.g. raisins) or adding sugar to them (e.g. strawberries canned in syrup) increases their energy density. Cooking or preparing vegetables with fat or oil greatly increases their energy yield (e.g. French fried potatoes, hummus, and fried tofu).

- When boiled, starchy cereals and roots are low in fat and absorb substantial amounts of water. This means that, despite their importance as major sources of energy in many diets, their energy density is rather modest (e.g. boiled potatoes, boiled rice and corn grits).

- Very lean meat and white fish are low in fat and so their energy density is moderate or low (e.g. roast chicken meat), especially if boiled (e.g. lean boiled ham, poached cod). The meat in our ancestors' diets (and even a few populations today) would have come from wild animal carcasses and this is usually low in fat.

- Many of the modern processed foods in Table 7.6 have a relatively high energy density. Many modern methods of preparing and processing foods tend to remove water and fibre, but they add fat and/or sugar (e.g. fish fingers, chicken nuggets, fruit/meat pies, cornflakes, cookies and cakes).

The modern diets of affluent populations are of much higher energy density than those of our hunter-gatherer ancestors or in subsistence

Table 7.6 Weights of selected foods that would need to be eaten to obtain 4.2 MJ (1000 kcal)*

Food	Weight (g)
Fruits	
Orange	5950
Banana	2280
Grapes	1667
Raisins	368
Strawberries	3704
Strawberries (canned in syrup)	1538
Fruit pie (individual purchased)	271
Vegetables	
Lettuce	7143
Tomato	5882
Green beans	4000
Broccoli	4167
Boiled swede	9091
Red kidney beans (boiled)	971
Soya beans (boiled)	709
Tofu (fried)	383
Chick peas (boiled)	836
Hummus	535
Starchy staples and products	
Boiled potatoes	1389
French fries	357
Potato crisps (chips)	183
Boiled yam	752
Boiled sweet potato	1190
Boiled rice	725
Spaghetti (boiled)	962
Wheat bread	464
Corn grits (made with water)	1666
Porridge made with water	2041
Porridge made with whole milk	862
Tortilla/chapatti (no added fat)	478
Cornflakes	278
Weetabix	279
Chocolate biscuits (cookies)	191
Fruit cake	282
Doughnuts (ring)	252
Pizza (cheese and tomato)	400

Food	Weight (g)
Dairy foods	
Whole milk	1515
Skimmed milk	3030
Double cream	223
Cheddar cheese	243
Butter	136
Meat, fish and products	
Boiled egg	680
Fried egg	560
Lean boiled ham	758
Roast chicken meat	606
Southern fried chicken	350
Chicken nuggets	338
Grilled rump steak with fat	459
Grilled rump steak trimmed	595
Cheeseburger	380
Salami	204
Sausage rolls	210
Grilled pork sausage	314
Poached cod	1064
Cod fried in batter	503
Steamed salmon	508
Boiled prawns	935
Fish fingers (fried)	429
Fried scampi (breaded)	316
Nuts, seeds and oils	
Peanuts (raw)	177
Walnuts	145
Sunflower seeds	167
Margarine	136
Low-fat spread	256
Vegetable oils	112
Miscellaneous	
Sugar	254
Chocolate	189
Quiche	318

*Adapted from Webb (2003).

agricultural communities today. The cross-population changes in diet that are associated with increasing affluence also increase the energy density of the diet, by the partial replacement of vegetables and starchy, fibre-rich foods with foods rich in fats and sugars but low in fibre. These compositional changes produce diets that, as well as being more energy-dense, are also more palatable. This combination of high palatability and high energy density may increase the likelihood of energy intake exceeding requirements and encourage weight gain. If gut-fill cues (e.g. stomach distension) play any role at all in the regulation of energy intake, then one would expect high energy density of the diet to reduce the effectiveness of food intake-regulating mechanisms. This may be particularly so if there is also low energy expenditure through inactivity. It is widely believed that a reduction in the energy density of adult diets in affluent, industrialized countries will help people to control their energy intake better and so lessen the risks of excessive weight gain.

Diets high in fat, and therefore of high energy density, have often been used to induce obesity in rodents. According to Miller (1979), high energy density, rather than fat content *per se*, is the primary obesifying influence. Varying the energy density and the proportion of fat independently (by using an inert bulking agent) produced a strong correlation between the fatness of the animals and dietary energy density but not between body fatness and dietary fat content.

At the other end of the spectrum, it is now widely believed that the low energy density of some children's diets, especially weaning diets, may be a major precipitating factor for malnutrition. Weaning diets, particularly in some developing countries, may have energy densities that are so low that, even under optimal conditions, children may have difficulty in consuming sufficient volume of food to satisfy their energy needs. Children fed these low-energy diets may be in energy deficit (i.e. starved) despite apparently being fed enough to satisfy their demands. These low-energy diets are based on starchy staples, are often practically fat-free, and have large amounts of water added to produce a consistency considered suitable for babies and young children. Children fed such low-energy-density diets

may need to consume anything up to eight times the weight of food that children on a typical Western weaning diet would need to obtain the same amount of energy.

Key points

- Energy density is the number of kJ (or kcal) per unit weight in a food or diet.
- Fat is a concentrated source of energy, so high-fat foods are energy-dense and adding fat to foods (e.g. by frying) raises their energy density.
- Foods with high water content (e.g. fruits and vegetables) have very low energy density.
- Starchy foods have only modest energy density despite being the major energy source in most pre-industrial human diets.
- Modern diets of affluent populations tend to be much higher in energy density than those eaten by hunter gatherers or subsistence farmers.
- High-energy-density diets probably predispose to obesity.
- Weaning diets that have very low energy density may precipitate malnutrition because children are unable to eat enough of the diluted food to satisfy their energy needs.

NUTRIENT DENSITY

Nutrient density is the amount of nutrient per unit of energy in the food or diet (e.g. μg nutrient per kcal or kJ). In the diets of the affluent, nutrient density is often almost a mirror image of energy density; adding ingredients to foods or diets, which contain much energy but few nutrients (e.g. fats, sugar and alcohol) raises the energy density but reduces the overall nutrient density. Diets and foods high in nutrient density help to ensure nutritional adequacy, but those low in nutrient density increase the possibility that their energy requirements may be met and appetite satisfied without also fulfilling their needs for essential nutrients. People consuming relatively small amounts of energy (e.g. those on reducing diets or elderly, immobile people) or those requiring higher amounts of some nutrients (e.g. pregnant women) may need to take particular care to ensure that their diet is nutrient-dense.

It is possible to predict the likely adequacy of a combination of foods for any particular nutrient by multiplying the nutrient density of the mixture by the estimated average requirement (or RDA) for energy:

nutrient density × energy EAR (or RDA) = amount of nutrient consumed by subjects meeting their energy needs.

If this figure exceeds the RNI (RDA) for that nutrient then that diet is probably adequate for that nutrient.

Similar calculations are also often made for individual foods in order to illustrate their value as a source of particular nutrients; some examples are shown in Table 7.7. Clearly, oily French fries from a burger bar are a poor source of vitamin C. Even fresh home-made chips (fries) are much worse than boiled new potatoes. Oranges, peppers and grilled tomatoes are clearly good sources of the vitamin. Addition of sugar (canned oranges) or fat (fried tomatoes or potatoes) reduces the nutrient density because it adds energy but no more vitamin C. Avocados have relatively modest amounts of vitamin C and the nutrient density is further depressed because they are relatively high in fat and energy.

Table 7.7 Amount of energy from various foods that would need to be consumed in order to obtain the UK adult reference nutrient intake (RNI) for vitamin C (40 mg)*

Food	Amount of energy	
	kcal	kJ
New potatoes (boiled)	175	735
French fries (burger bar)	2764	11 611
French fries (home-made)	840	3528
Avocado pear	1266	5317
Banana	345	1499
Orange	27	113
Mandarin oranges (canned in syrup)	139	584
Green pepper (capsicum)	5	21
Tomatoes (grilled)	45	189
Tomatoes (fried in oil)	228	958

*Compare with the UK estimated energy requirement (EAR) for an adult male of 10.6 MJ (2550 kcal) per day.

Key points

- Nutrient density is the amount of nutrient per kJ or kcal in a food or diet.
- Adding sugar, alcohol or fat to foods lowers nutrient density because it adds energy but little or no nutrient.
- A nutrient-dense diet helps to ensure nutritional adequacy whereas low nutrient density increases the chances that appetite can be satisfied without fulfilling all nutrient requirements.
- People with low energy intakes especially need to ensure that their diet is nutrient-dense. This includes elderly housebound people and those on reducing diets.

SOURCES OF DIETARY ENERGY BY FOOD GROUPS

NDNS surveys and household budget surveys can also be used to estimate the contribution that the major food groups make to the energy intake. Table 7.8 gives a summary of the food sources of dietary energy using these different approaches.

Considering the very different methodologies of the surveys used to devise Table 7.8, the results of the weighed inventory of Hoare et al. (2004) and the household budget survey of DEFRA (2006) are reassuringly similar. Comparison of the results obtained by Gregory et al. (1990) and Hoare et al. (2004) also suggests that these proportions remained fairly stable over the period 1987 to 2001. The recent NDNS results of Bates et al. (2011) are also shown and these were based on a sample of 500 adults and used a 4-day food diary; some of the slight differences between these results and those of the earlier NDNS surveys could be due to differing methodology and differences in the sample size.

Some particular factors that would cause differences between the weighed-inventory/food-diary approach and the household budget survey are:

- in a weighed inventory or food diary, cooking fats and oils will be incorporated into other foods, whereas in an expenditure survey they are measured as purchased and incorporated into the fats and sugars group
- the NDNS survey results in Table 7.8 are only for adults under 65 years but the expenditure survey includes all age groups.

Table 7.8 Percentage contributions of the major food groups to total energy intakes in the UK*

Food group	Hoare et al. (2004) (Gregory et al., 1990)	DEFRA (2006)	Bates et al. (2011)
Cereals and cereal products	31 (30)	32	28
Milk and milk products (including cheese)	10 (11)	12	9
Meat, fish, eggs and products	21 (20)	17	23
Fats and sugars (including soft and alcoholic drinks and confectionery)	21 (21)	21	20
Fruits and vegetables (about half of this energy comes from potatoes and potato products)	16 (14)	13	15

*As measured by weighed inventory (Hoare *et al.*, 2004; and in parenthesis from Gregory *et al.*, 1990), and by family expenditure survey (DEFRA, 2006). Figures from Bates *et al.* (2011) were from a 4-day food diary.

Comparison of Table 7.8 with the 'ideal diets' suggested by the UK *food guide plate* or the US *food guide pyramid* (see Chapter 6) shows that the fats and sugars would seem much too prominent; these provide few nutrients but lots of energy largely as fat and sugar. Cereals plus potatoes are the largest contributors of energy (almost 40 per cent), but a deeper analysis would indicate that highly refined products and those with considerable added fat and/or sugar are much more prominent than would be considered ideal. Fruits and vegetables (excluding potatoes) provide only around 6–7 per cent of total energy. This is lower than ideal, but a very low energy yield from these foods is almost inevitable given the very low energy density of most of them.

Key points

- According to household budget data (DEFRA, 2006):
  - almost 40 per cent of the energy in the UK diet comes from cereals and potatoes
  - 12 per cent from milk and milk products
  - 17 per cent from the meat group
  - 21 per cent from fats and sugars (including drinks and confectionery)
  - 6–7 per cent from the fruit and vegetable food group (excluding potatoes).
- These figures are quite similar to those obtained by weighed inventory or food diary using representative samples of British adults.
- Ideally, more of the energy should come from unrefined cereals and potatoes, fruits and vegetables, slightly less from the milk and meat groups and much less from the fats and sugars group.

STARVATION

Immediate causes of starvation

For most of the world's population, starvation results from local food shortages or from lack of money to buy food. Some children may also be unwittingly starved because they are fed foods of such low energy density that they are unable to consume sufficient volume of the dilute food to meet their energy needs. Inadequate food intake usually results in hunger and, if food is available, in eating. In some circumstances hunger may not occur or be suppressed, and in some circumstances nourishment will not reach the tissues despite hunger and eating. In affluent countries, because of the ready availability of high-energy-density food, such causes of inadequate intake may result from various causes.

- Illness, injury or therapy may result in loss of appetite.
- Infirmity may reduce the ability to eat or to obtain and prepare food.
- Illness and injury result in hypermetabolism which increases nutritional needs.
- Some illnesses lead to loss of nutrients (e.g. the glucose and ketones lost in the urine of diabetics – see Chapter 17).
- Psychological state or psychological illness may result in inadequate food intake despite its ready availability (e.g. in anorexia nervosa).
- Some diseases may result in poor digestion and absorption of nutrients (e.g. in coeliac disease and cystic fibrosis – see Chapter 17).

Physiological responses and adaptations

The most obvious physiological response to starvation is *wasting*. If energy intake is not sufficient to cover expenditure then the deficit must be made up by burning the body's energy reserves. All tissues, with the exception of the brain, will waste during starvation; the most obvious wasting will be in body fat and muscle, but other vital organs will also waste. After prolonged starvation, the heart may be only half its original weight and this wasting of heart muscle can lead to death from circulatory failure. The intestines of starving people will atrophy. They become thin and have greatly reduced digestive and absorptive capacity. This may cause problems in re-feeding people after prolonged starvation.

A healthy and well-nourished non-obese man should be able to lose more than 25 per cent of his initial body weight before his life is threatened. During such a 25 per cent weight loss, the man would lose around 70 per cent of his stored fat and around 25 per cent of his body protein. Total carbohydrate content of the body is small (say 500 g) even in well-fed people, so the small loss of carbohydrate during this prolonged period of weight loss would make an insignificant contribution to total losses of body energy. The energy yield of this 25 per cent loss of body weight represents around 6–7 weeks' energy expenditure in a totally starved and sedentary man. This means that well-nourished adults can survive several weeks of total starvation provided they maintain hydration. This was strikingly illustrated by the IRA hunger strikers in the Maze prison in Northern Ireland during the 1980s: it took up to 10 weeks of total starvation for these healthy young men to reach the point of death (obese people may survive much longer).

This capacity of people to survive long periods of food shortage, or even complete starvation, clearly represents a very considerable aid to the survival of the species. If there is a temporary food shortage, there is a good chance that many people will survive until food supplies are restored. Children are more vulnerable to starvation than adults; survival times of completely starved babies or children may be measured in days rather than weeks depending on age.

Many cells can utilize either glucose or fatty acids as an energy source. As body stores of carbohydrate are minimal, during a fast such cells will increasingly switch to using fatty acids as an energy source. The cells of some tissues, including the brain and red blood cells, cannot use fatty acids directly as an alternative energy source and most tissues have a limited capacity to use fatty acids. Glucose can be manufactured in the liver from the glycerol component of stored fat and from amino acids protein breakdown (see *gluconeogenesis* in Chapter 6), but glucose cannot be synthesized from fatty acids. This process of gluconeogenesis is energy expensive (i.e. wasteful) and supplies of amino acids are limited because they are being taken from protein in muscles and essential organs. A maximum of around 5 kg of protein is available for gluconeogenesis in an adult man.

It was once thought that the brain relied exclusively on glucose as its substrate for energy production. As there are negligible carbohydrate stores, this would mean that the brain would have to rely entirely on glucose produced from gluconeogenesis during prolonged fasting. The brain normally uses the equivalent of around 100 g of glucose per day and, unless some adaptation occurred, use of protein in gluconeogenesis would lead to rapid depletion of body protein reserves and the size of these protein reserves would limit the duration of survival during fasting. Starving people would be likely to die from depletion of body protein reserves long before body fat stores were exhausted. If one monitors nitrogen excretion (i.e. protein breakdown) during fasting, one finds that it declines as the fast is extended and after a week or so is down to about 30 per cent of the initial rate. An important adaptation to starvation has occurred that preserves lean tissue during prolonged fasting. During the course of fasting, the blood levels of substances called *ketone bodies* rise as they are produced from fatty acids in the liver. After a few days of fasting, these ketone bodies become the most abundant metabolic fuel in the blood. It is now clear that they act as alternative substrates for the brain and other tissues during prolonged fasting. These ketones are synthesized in the liver from the acetyl CoA produced during the β-oxidation of fatty acids; this is illustrated in Figure 7.1 and discussed in Chapter 6 (p.160).

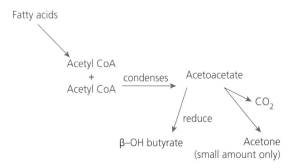

Figure 7.1 The origins of ketone bodies.

After prolonged fasting, as much as three-quarters of muscle energy production and more than half of the brain's energy supply will be from β-OH butyrate and acetoacetate (acetone is produced in small amounts as a by-product of the process but is not metabolized). The brain is thus indirectly using fatty acids as an energy source. During a prolonged fast, the brain's requirement for glucose will fall from 100 g/day to 40 g/day and most of this will come from the glycerol component of stored fat. This use of ketones as a substrate thus represents a substantial brake on the depletion of lean tissue during starvation.

For many years, these ketones were thought of solely as abnormal metabolic products produced during uncontrolled diabetes. In severe diabetes they are produced to excess and their concentration builds up to the point where they become highly toxic. They are toxic principally because they are acidic and produce a metabolic acidosis. Acetone is responsible for the 'pear drops' smell on the breath of persons in diabetic (hyperglycaemic) coma. Persons on severe reducing diets or diets in which carbohydrate intake is severely restricted will experience mild ketosis.

A third important adaptation to starvation is a reduced rate of energy expenditure. This slows the rate at which reserves are depleted and extends the survival time. Below are listed some of the very obvious reasons why energy expenditure decreases during fasting (or severe dieting).

- With little or no eating, there is less food to digest, absorb and assimilate. These processes each have an energy cost and eating raises resting metabolic rate.
- Most starving people curtail their physical activity. (Many anorexics are an exception to this

generalization – they exercise to lose yet more weight.)

- As the body wastes, it gets smaller and so the energy costs of maintenance decrease.
- The energy costs of any activity are also reduced if the body is smaller.
- There is an increase in metabolic efficiency perhaps related to changes in body temperature regulation.

This means that, during starvation, the rate of energy expenditure decreases and the rate at which energy stores are used up also decreases. During deliberate weight loss, the amount of energy needed to maintain body weight also declines. Many dieters find that a diet initially succeeds in achieving weight loss but then their weight sticks and they need to reduce their intake still further to get continued weight loss. Prentice *et al.* (1991) estimated that the crude reduction in energy expenditure during dieting might exceed 25 per cent but when corrected for changes in lean body mass it varies between 5 per cent and 15 per cent depending on the severity of the intake restriction.

Some adverse consequences of starvation

Some of the consequences of starvation are summarized in Box 7.2. Those suffering from anorexia nervosa (see later in the chapter) vividly illustrate these consequences in developed countries.

Box 7.2

Some consequences of starvation (after Webb, 2003)

- Wasting of lean tissue and vital organs
- Shrinkage of heart muscle, irregular heart rhythm and risk of heart failure
- Reduced digestive and absorption capability in the gut often leading to diarrhoea
- Reduced growth and development in children and young people, perhaps intellectual as well as physical development
- Depressed immune function and increased susceptibility to infections
- Delayed puberty, lack of menstruation, infertility and loss of sex drive   →

- Reduced bone density (osteoporosis) and increased risk of fractures, especially stress fractures in anorexic athletes
- Slow healing of wounds
- Reduced strength and physical work capacity and impaired performance in dancers and athletes
- Hypothermia
- Insomnia, changes in personality and brain function

Endocrine function becomes deranged during starvation. Pituitary gonadotrophin secretion is greatly depressed in starvation and this manifests itself outwardly in a cessation of menstruation in starving women. Puberty is delayed by malnutrition. In industrialized countries, the age of onset of menstruation has decreased very markedly over the last century as children have become better nourished and grow faster. Women need a minimum threshold amount of fat to maintain their fertility and proper menstrual cycling. Underweight women may have difficulty in conceiving a child and they are more likely to have an underweight baby. The reduced secretion of sex hormones also leads to loss of bone mass. This makes fractures more likely and may, for example, predispose women who have suffered from anorexia nervosa to osteoporosis fractures later in life.

Malnutrition predisposes to *infection*, and infection in turn increases the severity of malnutrition or may precipitate malnutrition in areas where there is no overt food shortage. Thereby a cycle of infection and malnutrition is set up. Sick children (or adults) may have reduced appetite and increased requirement for nutrients. They may also be starved or fed a very restricted diet in the belief that this is the correct way to treat sick children. Malnutrition has very profound, specific and deleterious effects on the functioning of the immune system – these are discussed at some length in Chapter 17. Cohort studies in malnourished children in which nutritional status has been related to subsequent death rate showed that the risk of dying increases exponentially as one moves from the better nourished to the mildly, moderately and severely malnourished (Waterlow, 1979).

There may also be very pronounced psychological effects and personality changes produced by starvation. During the 1940s in Minnesota, a group of young male volunteers were subjected to a period of partial starvation that resulted in a 25 per cent body weight loss (Keys *et al.*, 1950). The feeding behaviour of these men changed markedly during their period of deprivation including a dramatic decline in their speed of eating. They became preoccupied with food, it dominated their conversations, thoughts and reading. They became introverted and selfish and made irrational purchases of unwanted items. Personality tests conducted during the period of starvation showed a considerable movement towards the neurotic end of the scale as starvation occurred. Towards the end of the period of weight loss, the results from personality tests with these starved men became comparable with those of people with frank psychiatric disease.

Key points

- Worldwide, starvation is usually the result of famine or poverty but it can also be a consequence of illness or infirmity.
- During starvation the body uses stored fat and tissue protein to make up its energy deficit.
- Healthy non-obese adults can survive 10 weeks or more of total starvation and for much longer on restricted rations, provided hydration is maintained.
- During starvation, ketone bodies (β-OH butyrate and acetoacetate) produced from fatty acids become the major body substrates.
- Ketone use reduces the need to produce glucose and spares body protein.
- More than half of even the brain's energy needs are met by ketones during prolonged starvation.
- Starvation leads to a large fall in energy expenditure (less digestion and assimilation, reduced activity, reduced tissue mass and some apparent increase in metabolic efficiency).
- Adverse consequences of starvation include tissue wasting, reduced growth and healing, depressed immune function, reduced physical performance, endocrine disturbances and reproductive impairment, and psychological disturbances.

EATING DISORDERS

The term 'eating disorder' is used to describe the diseases anorexia nervosa (AN) and bulimia nervosa (BN). The term also encompasses many other people who have some symptoms of these conditions but who do not meet the formal diagnostic criteria for either condition; these are termed EDNOS (eating disorder not otherwise specified).

Characteristics and consequences

Anorexic people have very low energy intakes and are severely underweight; occasionally they may starve themselves to death. *Anorexia nervosa* is characterized by an obsessive desire to be thin and an intense fear of being fat even though the victim may be severely emaciated. The disease has significant mortality, estimated at between 1 and 13 per cent. Perhaps half of patients show little improvement or make only a partial recovery. They continue to eat very restricted diets, to maintain a very low body weight, and fail to start menstruating. Perhaps as many as a fifth of patients continue to suffer severe and unremitting symptoms of the condition. The consequences of this self-starvation are essentially the same as for starvation generally (summarized earlier in Box 7.2). Some symptoms are particularly associated with anorexics, such as excessive growth of dry brittle facial and body hair ('lanugo hair'), constipation and peripheral oedema. Those who take purgatives or resort to induced vomiting are also likely to suffer from adverse consequences of these behaviours, including:

- electrolyte imbalances, which may lead to muscle weakness, fatigue and increased susceptibility to cardiac arrhythmias
- irritation of the throat and damage to the teeth caused by the corrosive effects of vomitus.

The diagnostic characteristics of anorexia nervosa are:

- low body weight – at least 15 per cent below expected minimum for age and height
- intense fear of gaining weight or becoming fat even though underweight
- distorted body image – self-perception as fat even though alarmingly emaciated to the impartial observer

- lack of menstrual periods in females for three consecutive months.

Many anorexics also frequently exhibit one or more of the following behaviours:

- frequent use of purgatives, induced vomiting or emetics
- high levels of physical activity, in contrast to most other victims of starvation.

Victims of the disease may also go to great lengths to hide their restricted food intake and their physical emaciation from relatives and friends. They may wear loose clothing, avoid social eating situations, eat very slowly, choose only foods very low in calories, conceal food that they have pretended to eat and then dispose of it, or induce vomiting after they have eaten. It is, of course, important to rule out other physical and psychological causes of under-nutrition and weight loss before concluding that an underweight person is suffering from anorexia nervosa.

Bulimia nervosa is characterized by recurrent bouts of binge-eating. Periods of restricted eating are interspersed with sometimes huge binges where massive quantities and bizarre mixtures of foods may be consumed in very short periods of time. This voracious eating may continue until abdominal pain, sleep or interruption trigger its end. Often the binge is followed by self-induced vomiting or purging. The morbid fear of fatness and distortion of body image seen in anorexia are also seen in this condition. A diagnosis of bulimia would be made if the following features are present in a person who is not very underweight:

- recurrent bouts of binge-eating in which large amounts of food are consumed and in which the person loses control of her or his eating
- recurrent bouts of inappropriate compensatory behaviour to prevent weight gain after binges (e.g. induced vomiting, purging, excessive exercise or fasting)
- bouts of bingeing and compensation occurring at an average rate of twice a week for 3 months
- the person's self-image being unrelated to the true body shape and weight.

This condition can also have serious repercussions on the health of individuals with the condition, including:

- damage to the throat, teeth, oesophagus (gullet) and stomach caused by overloading or the induced vomiting, with consequent risk of infection
- possible harmful side-effects of laxatives or emetics used.

Mortality associated with this condition is less than that of anorexia nervosa; it is estimated at between 0 and 3 per cent. If binge-eating occurs in someone who is seriously underweight, they are classified as having a form of anorexia nervosa.

Incidence

Some surveys among college students and among more random samples of women in the UK and USA have suggested disturbingly high proportions of subjects exhibiting bulimic behaviour (as many as 20 per cent of sampled women in some surveys). Gilbert (1986) concluded that 'at any one time up to 2 per cent of women up to the age of forty may be experiencing problems with controlling their eating'.

Anorexia nervosa is the best known of the eating disorders. The condition was first described more than a century ago but there is general agreement that the disease has become more prevalent in recent decades. It affects fewer than 0.5 per cent of women. Anorexia nervosa affects mainly females who typically are:

- white
- aged 15–19 years (about 40 per cent of cases are within this age range although it can occur at any time between 12 and 44 years)
- from middle- and upper-class families, well educated and with a good knowledge of nutrition.

Cases do occur in men (less than a tenth of the frequency in women), and among other social and racial groups. As it becomes more common, so anorexia is radiating out from its traditional risk group and is being reported increasingly in Asian and African-Caribbean women and in women of other social classes.

Bulimia nervosa occurs in people whose weight is within the normal range. Since they are guilty and secretive about their behaviour, this makes it difficult to diagnose and difficult to make estimates of its incidence; hence the wide variability in the estimated frequency of eating disorders noted earlier. Perhaps the best estimates of frequency are about 1 per cent of adolescent girls and young women and about a tenth of this frequency among the corresponding male population.

Estimates of the frequency of EDNOS are higher than for anorexia nervosa or bulimia nervosa at 2–3 per cent, with a much lower female-to-male ratio and tending to onset later in life – often between 30 and 50 years.

Causes of eating disorders

There seems to be a general acceptance that these eating disorders have become more prevalent in recent decades, although part of this apparent increase may be due to better detection and increased awareness of the conditions. There are genetic influences on the susceptibility to an eating disorder. Close relatives of those with an eating disorder have a much higher prevalence of an eating disorder than controls. Monozygotic twins have higher concordance than dizygotic twins, and twin studies suggest that heritability accounts for >50 per cent of the risk of developing an eating disorder.

It is widely believed that they are triggered in genetically susceptible people by dieting and social pressures on young people to be thin, pressures that may be particularly acutely felt by young women. The majority of adolescent girls have tried dieting, and preoccupation with body weight and dieting has been reported in children as young as 10 years old. Many bulimic patients have a history of cycles of weight loss and regain – so-called 'yo-yo dieting'. The average woman (and man) in most industrialized countries is getting fatter as judged by surveys of weight and height, whereas images of the ideal woman are apparently getting thinner. Many of the models used in classical painting of the female form would be overweight by present standards, and studies of American winners of beauty contests and models for men's magazines indicated that the 'ideal' body shape got thinner during the 1960s and 1970s. Almost all of the models used by fashion photographers are lean and many appear to be emaciated. Young women aspire to a body shape that is unhealthy and unattainable except by the most extreme restrictive diets. These disorders do seem to occur more often in girls and women for whom thinness is a career requirement (e.g. models, ballet dancers and airline stewardesses). In some male athletes and ballet dancers, eating disorders are almost as common as in women despite their general rarity in men.

Over the years, many suggestions have been made as to the individual causes of anorexia nervosa and related eating disorders. Social conditions may favour increasing prevalence of the disease, but what individual factors make some women develop the disease? It is likely that the cause of these diseases is multifactorial and that there is no one simple cause that applies to all sufferers.

The effects of starvation on the men in Minnesota in Keys' experiment were discussed earlier and may be of some relevance in understanding the development of anorexic behaviour. The slowness of eating seen in these starving men is typical of anorexics. The men's unsociability, their obsessive interest in food and their curtailment of other activities are all recognized as traditional symptoms of anorexia nervosa. These men also developed personality profiles that were characteristic of people with frank psychiatric disease as they starved. During the period of re-feeding and rehabilitation of these men, many of them showed a marked tendency to binge-eat, behaviour in many ways similar to that found in bulimia. Some months after the re-feeding period, a high proportion of the men had put themselves on a reducing diet; men who had previously had a normal interest in food became preoccupied with dieting after this bout of starvation.

These observations on starving individuals have encouraged the suggestion that anorexia and bulimia may be triggered by social and cultural conditions that require young women, in particular, to be thin. The dieting itself may, in genetically susceptible individuals, cause some of the grossly aberrant and apparently irrational behaviour characteristic of anorexia and bulimia. Weight loss and leanness are generally admired and praised in our culture, so the initial positive reactions to the results of anorexic behaviour may serve as powerful reinforcement or reward and thus encourage learning of anorexic behaviour. In someone whose self-esteem is low and who feels that, because of the family environment, she or he lacks control, this (initially praised) ability to totally control some aspect of her or his life may also act as positive

reinforcement and encourage continuation and intensification of the anorexic behaviour.

Coughlin and Guarda (2006) suggest that parents' comments about weight are the most consistent factor associated with children's concerns and behaviour regarding their weight and shape. They suggest that each of the following factors relating to family life is associated with increased risk of a child developing an eating disorder:

- the child frequently eats alone
- perception of poor family communication and caring
- low parental expectations
- parents who are not married.

Trials of the use of family therapy in the treatment of anorexia have provided only limited support for it being an effective approach to therapy (Fisher *et al.*, 2010).

There are numerous other theories about the origins of anorexia nervosa. Some have suggested that there is some defect in the hypothalamic mechanisms regulating intake, but this idea is largely discounted these days and the frequent occurrence of binge-eating suggests suppression of appetite rather than lack of appetite.

Some adherents to Freudian psychological theories have suggested that the subconscious goal of these women and girls is to avoid adult responsibility and sexuality by starving themselves. The cessation of menstruation, inhibition of sexual development and lack of adult female form found in anorexics are seen as the aims and rewards of anorexic behaviour. This theory has attracted much attention over the years and is probably the one theory about anorexia that non-specialists will have heard of. It would be fair to say that this theory has gone out of fashion as has, to some extent, the Freudian view of psychology.

Some have suggested that anorexia is a symptom of a frank affective psychiatric disorder like clinical depression. This is supported, to some extent, by claims of successful treatment of anorexics with antidepressant drugs; although a systematic review by Claudino *et al.* (2006) found that there was at this time no clear published evidence that antidepressants were an effective treatment. One major problem of trying to investigate the psychological and physiological characteristics that bring about the disease is that, by the time the disease is recognized, it will be impossible to decide which abnormalities are due to starvation and which are causes of the self-starvation.

A more detailed discussion of either the causes or treatment of eating disorders is beyond the scope of this book. The aim of this brief discussion has been to increase the awareness of non-specialists and to help them to recognize potential sufferers. The disease requires specialist management; the non-specialist's role can only be to be able to recognize likely sufferers, appreciate that this is a 'real' and potentially life-threatening illness, and direct them towards specialist help.

The discussion may also give those in contact with anorexics some insight into the psychological consequences of anorexia/starvation and thus help them to deal more sympathetically with difficult and incomprehensible behaviour.

A detailed and well-referenced account of eating disorders may be found in Gilbert (1986), and a shorter more recent summary may be found in Coughlin and Guarda (2006).

Key points

- The term 'eating disorder' encompasses the two well-defined conditions anorexia nervosa and bulimia nervosa but could also include many other people with some features of these diseases but who fail to meet the formal diagnostic criteria – referred to as EDNOS (eating disorder not otherwise specified).

- People with anorexia nervosa starve themselves, sometimes to the point of death, because of an obsessive preoccupation with their weight and a pathological fear of fatness even when they are grossly emaciated.

- People with bulimia nervosa are not seriously underweight but engage in recurrent bouts of bingeing followed by inappropriate compensatory behaviour to prevent weight gain.

- The consequences of anorexia nervosa are similar to those of starvation. In addition, people with eating disorders may suffer adverse consequences associated with induced vomiting, use of purgatives or emetics, and overloading of the stomach during binges. →

Key points *continued*

- Eating disorders are predominantly found in adolescent girls and young women. Estimates of frequency vary widely, but in young women estimates of 0.5 per cent for anorexia and 1 per cent for bulimia may be reasonable. The frequency in men is less than a tenth of that in women. The frequency of EDNOS is higher and it tends to onset later in life.

- There are many theories about the causes. There is a widespread belief that they may be triggered in genetically susceptible people by dieting and preoccupation with being slim. Family relationships are seen as important predisposing factors.

- Eating disorders are more common in women (and sometimes men) for whom thinness is a career requirement.

CANCER CACHEXIA

Severe emaciation and malnutrition are frequently associated with terminal malignant diseases, and starvation may, in many cases, be the immediate cause of death. It is seen in about half of all terminally ill cancer patients, especially those with lung, pancreatic and stomach cancers. This is termed *cancer cachexia*. There may be a readily identifiable cause for the loss of weight, including:

- malignancy affecting the alimentary tract
- eating made difficult or painful
- appetite depressed in a patient who is in great pain or extremely distressed
- anti-cancer therapy that induces nausea and anorexia.

There are nonetheless occasions when a patient with a malignant disease may lose weight initially for no clearly apparent reason. Sometimes weight loss may be the symptom that triggers the investigation leading to the diagnosis of malignancy. Hypermetabolism (increased energy expenditure) seems to be partly responsible for such weight loss and this may be a reflection of the metabolic activity associated with rapidly dividing malignant cells. There is additionally thought to be an anorexic effect of tumour growth. The metabolic disturbance or metabolic by-products of tumour growth have a depressing effect on appetite. In simple starvation, around three-quarters of weight loss is via adipose tissue, whereas in cancer cachexia a much higher proportion of the weight loss is via lean tissue. This accelerated loss of lean tissue hastens death in the cachectic patient. Increasing food intake does not always reverse the cachectic process, and some studies have found that even intravenous feeding fails to stabilize weight in the long term. In the short term, intravenous feeding does seem to increase body fat but does not reverse the loss of muscle and lean tissue.

Cytokines are proteins that are secreted as part of the immune response, and several cytokines are known to be produced as a response to tumour growth; an example is tumour necrosis factor (TNF). These cytokines may be partly responsible for the anorexia and metabolic changes seen in malignant disease. All the cytokines produced in cancer cause anorexia and weight loss. Once cancer is suspected or confirmed, the psychological reactions to the disease, the effects of any treatment, the pain and discomfort caused by disease or treatment, as well as the direct pathological effects of the disease will all interact to reduce appetite and hasten weight loss. A short referenced review of cancer cachexia may be found in Tisdale (1997).

There have been suggestions that n-3 fatty acids – particularly eicosapentaenoic acid (EPA) from fish oil – may be beneficial in the management of this cachexia. The underlying basis for this proposition is that EPA inhibits fat and muscle degradation by cytokines, specifically by decreasing the production by the tumour of a factor that stimulates protein breakdown, proteolysis-inducing factor (PIF). Dewey *et al.* (2007) conducted a meta-analysis of five clinical trials of EPA in the management of cancer cachexia published up to 2005. They found that there were insufficient data to establish whether EPA was more effective than a placebo in improving the symptoms of cancer cachexia when used alone or in combination with protein energy supplements or an appetite-stimulating drug.

Key points

- Large weight losses due to both reduced appetite and hypermetabolism are a usual feature of malignant disease. This is cancer cachexia.

- In cancer cachexia there is greater loss of lean tissue than in simple starvation.

- Many factors contribute to the weight loss in cancer. In particular, cytokines such as tumour necrosis factor produced as part of the immune response depress appetite and play a part in this response to malignancy.

- Neither raised food intake nor intravenous feeding seems able to correct the excess loss of lean tissue seen in cancer, even if body weight is increased or maintained.

8

ENERGY BALANCE AND ITS REGULATION

The concept of energy balance	187	Is energy expenditure regulated?	189
Physiological regulation of energy		External influences on food intake	192
balance	188	Control of energy intake	192
The 'set point' theory	189	The leptin story	198

THE CONCEPT OF ENERGY BALANCE

When we digest and metabolize food, the oxidation of fats, carbohydrates, protein and alcohol releases chemical energy that can be used for body functions. The first law of thermodynamics states that energy can neither be created nor destroyed but only changed from one form to another. This means that all of the energy released during the oxidation of the macronutrients in food (the *metabolizable energy*) must be accounted for. It must be used to keep the body's internal systems functioning (this is ultimately lost from the body as heat energy), to do external work (e.g. move something), or be stored within the body (e.g. as fat in adipose tissue).

If an adult's energy intake (the metabolizable energy in food) exactly equals his or her energy expenditure (as internal and external work), the person is in *energy balance* and his or her total body energy content (and therefore fat stores) will remain constant (Figure 8.1).

The 'energy in' is the sum of the metabolizable energy yields of all the food and drink consumed, so it will normally be influenced only by the nature and amount of food and drink consumed. The 'energy out' can be directly measured by determining heat output in a whole-body calorimeter or, as is more usual, by predicting the heat output from measurements of oxygen consumption and carbon dioxide evolution (see Chapter 3). This output figure will be influenced

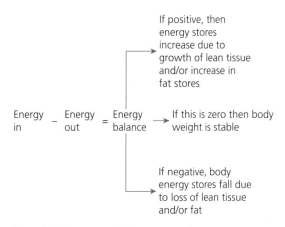

Figure 8.1 The energy balance equation.

by a number of factors (listed below) that raise heat output above the resting level (i.e. factors that have a thermogenic (heat-producing) effect.

- *The thermogenic effect of exercise.* Metabolic rate rises as exercise load is increased. The sweating and rise in skin temperature induced by exertion are obvious outward signs of this thermogenesis. Some of this extra energy output may also be used to do external work.
- *Thermoregulatory thermogenesis.* There is an increase in metabolic rate, and therefore heat output, associated with shivering or non-shivering mechanisms used for heat generation in a cold

environment. Energy expenditure also increases in a very hot environment.

- *Drug-induced thermogenesis.* This is the increase in heat output brought about by certain drugs (e.g. caffeine) that have a stimulating effect on metabolic rate.
- *The thermic effect of feeding or postprandial thermogenesis.* This is the increase in metabolic rate and heat output that follows feeding and is the energy expended in digesting, absorbing and assimilating the food (e.g. in the synthesis of fat and glycogen).
- *Adaptive thermogenesis.* This is an increase in metabolic rate as a consequence of overfeeding that is claimed to help in the maintenance of energy balance.

For a healthy adult whose weight is stable, over a period of time the energy intake and output must be matched. There is a zero balance; that is, the energy content of the body remains constant. There is very wide variation in the energy intakes that different individuals require to maintain balance (see Chapter 7).

If energy intake exceeds output then that individual is said to be in *positive energy balance*. Under these circumstances, body energy content must be increasing because 'energy cannot be destroyed'. The surplus energy is converted from chemical energy of food to chemical energy of body tissues. An increase in body energy content leads to either an increase in lean body mass (growth) or an increase in body fat deposition, or both. Children, pregnant women, and those regaining weight after a period of illness or starvation would all properly be expected to show a positive balance. For most of the rest of the population, sustained positive balance means increasing fat stores which will ultimately lead to obesity.

If energy output exceeds intake then that individual is said to be in *negative energy balance*. Since 'energy cannot be created', the shortfall must be made up from body energy stores. Individuals in negative energy balance must be losing body energy and this will almost certainly be reflected in weight loss. It is possible that body energy content can fall without weight loss if fat loss is compensated for by increases in lean tissue and/or water content; for example, in starvation there may be excess accumulation of tissue fluid (oedema). Loss of body energy may be due to

loss of lean tissue (protein) or loss of fat or, as is most likely, both. People who are starving or successfully dieting will be in negative energy balance, as will:

- many sick or seriously injured people
- those losing large amounts of nutrients (e.g. uncontrolled diabetics)
- those whose expenditure is particularly high (e.g. people with a hyperactive thyroid gland or those undertaking intense physical activity for prolonged periods).

Key points

- Energy can neither be created nor destroyed, only changed from one form to another.
- Energy intake is the metabolizable energy content of food and drink.
- Energy expenditure comprises basal metabolic rate (BMR) plus extra energy expended as a result of exercise, thermoregulation, drug action, feeding, etc.
- If energy intake exactly equals expenditure then a person is in energy balance and his or her weight should remain stable.
- If energy intake exceeds expenditure (positive energy balance) then there must be either growth of lean tissue or extra fat accumulation. Growing children, pregnant women and those recuperating after illness or starvation would all be expected to show a positive energy balance.
- If expenditure exceeds intake (negative energy balance) then there must be a corresponding decrease in body energy stores. Negative energy balance occurs in starvation, serious illness, and in those undertaking intense physical activity. Reducing diets are intended to achieve a negative energy balance.

PHYSIOLOGICAL REGULATION OF ENERGY BALANCE

Many adults maintain their body weight within a very narrow range over periods of years or even decades. Consider a normal 65 kg man who consistently takes in 420 kJ (100 kcal) per day more than he uses. This small surplus represents only 3–4 per cent of his estimated requirement and would be equivalent in food terms to not much more than the generous layer of butter or margarine on a slice of bread. If one assumes that 1 kg of adipose tissue yields about 30 MJ (7000 kcal), then if this surplus were maintained for a year it would be energetically equivalent to 5 kg of adipose tissue and in 10 years to 50 kg of adipose tissue! Now consider the 'opposite' scenario. If this man had the same constant daily *deficit* then he would lose adipose tissue at this rate and his fat stores would be totally exhausted in 1–2 years.

Such calculations imply that, unless there is extraordinarily precise long-term matching of energy intake to expenditure, over a period of decades massive changes in fat stores will occur. Of course, in reality these changes would tend to be self-limiting. In the man taking in the small daily surplus, his energy requirements would tend to rise in response to the constant surplus intake, for several reasons.

- Even adipose tissue uses some energy, so as he gets bigger it 'costs' more energy to maintain his bigger body. In other words, his basal metabolic rate increases with his size.
- The energy 'costs' of all activities increase as he gets bigger.
- He uses up some energy in converting surplus food energy into stored fat, especially if the surplus is in the form of carbohydrate or protein.

These changes would tend to bring him back into balance after a modest weight gain, unless he increased intake or curtailed his activity to maintain the imbalance. We saw in Chapter 7 a corresponding list of changes that occur when there is an energy deficit – changes that tend to reduce energy requirements and weight loss.

Key points

- Long-term weight stability requires very accurate matching of energy intake and expenditure. Even tiny sustained imbalances can lead to significant changes in body fat stores over years or decades.
- Weight losses or gains do *tend* to be self-limiting because over-consumption increases expenditure and under-consumption decreases expenditure. This implies that there is some 'automatic' regulation of energy balance.

THE 'SET POINT' THEORY

According to the 'set point' theory, body-weight control mechanisms operate to maintain a fixed level of body fat stores. If healthy volunteers are weighed accurately every day for a period of months, their day-to-day weights do tend to fluctuate and seem to oscillate around an individual's 'set point'. This is analogous to the oscillations in temperature that occur in a room where the temperature is controlled by a thermostat:

- weight decreases during periods of food restriction or illness
- during times of feasting, weight tends to increase
- when normal conditions are restored, the subject's weight tends to return to the 'set point'.

Similar observations have been made in animals. Even rats that have been made obese by damage to the brain centres that control energy balance seem to control their body weight to a set point, albeit a higher set point than in normal animals. Unfortunately, over the course of adulthood the set point of many people seems to drift upwards, so that the majority of middle-aged Europeans and Americans become overweight or obese (see Chapter 9).

Key points

- Physiological control mechanisms may operate to maintain a constant level of body fat stores – the 'set point' theory.
- Body weight appears to oscillate around this set point, although in the longer term there is often an upward drift in body fat stores.

IS ENERGY EXPENDITURE REGULATED?

Regulation of energy balance could be achieved by regulation of energy intake or expenditure or by a combination of the two. The sensations of hunger and satiation are universally experienced manifestations of some energy intake regulating mechanism. Traditionally, therefore, studies on the regulation of energy balance have focused on the mechanisms regulating food intake and these are discussed at length later in this chapter.

The regulation of energy expenditure as a mechanism for controlling the energy balance has been a more controversial topic. We have already seen that overfeeding increases energy expenditure and that energy restriction reduces expenditure, and these changes tend to restore balance. An apparent increase in 'metabolic efficiency' occurs during fasting and food restriction; the BMR drops by up to 15 per cent even when one allows for any decrease in lean body mass (Prentice *et al.*, 1991). The point of controversy is whether any mechanism exists whose primary purpose is to compensate for overeating by 'burning off' surplus calories.

In 1902, the German scientist Neumann coined the term *Luxoskonsumption* to describe an adaptive increase in energy expenditure in response to overfeeding. The term *adaptive thermogenesis* is often used today. Essentially, it is envisaged that some energy-wasting metabolic process is activated when people overeat and that this 'burns off' the surplus calories in order to restore energy balance or to reduce the imbalance.

Rats can be persuaded to overeat and become obese by the provision of a variety of varied, palatable and energy-dense human foods ('cafeteria feeding'). This mode of feeding in caged animals is designed to mimic the affluent human lifestyle. Rothwell and Stock (1979) reported that some rats fed in this way stored much less of the surplus food energy than they predicted and appeared to burn off some of this extra energy. Sims *et al.* (1973) did similar experiments with young men who were persuaded to consume an extra 3000 kcal (13 MJ) per day for a period of 8 months. At the end of this period, only about 15 per cent of the surplus energy that had been eaten could be accounted for in the increased fat stores. This implied that some adaptive thermogenesis had occurred.

Many subsequent shorter and less extreme overeating experiments have failed to find evidence of significant adaptive thermogenesis in human subjects. If there is any significant capacity for adaptive thermogenesis, then one would expect that under conditions of abundant food supply people might eat more than their bare minimum requirements and burn off some energy. The apparent increase in metabolic efficiency seen during fasting might represent a switching off of this adaptive thermogenesis and there might be limited further capacity to increase thermogenesis under conditions of experimental overfeeding.

Rothwell and Stock proposed that *brown adipose tissue* (BAT) or *brown fat* is the site of adaptive thermogenesis. Brown fat is the major site of cold-induced heat production (non-shivering thermogenesis) in small mammals and is particularly prominent in hibernators where it is important in generating heat during arousal from hibernation. The sympathetic stimulation of brown adipose tissue results in an uncoupling of oxidative phosphorylation; that is, oxidation accelerates but does not result in ATP production. The chemical energy produced during oxidation is released as heat and this warms the body during cold exposure. This mechanism is well established for thermoregulatory thermogenesis in small mammals (and human babies), and Rothwell and Stock suggested that this also occurs during overfeeding. The heat generated during overfeeding is then dissipated from the relatively large surface of the small animal. This theory was given added credence by evidence of abnormal thermoregulation in several animal models with inherited obesity. The most widely used of these models, the *ob/ob* mouse, is homozygous for a mutation at a gene locus referred to as *obese*, or *ob*. These mice have low body temperature, reduced heat production and die during cold exposure. They were said to have a 'thermogenic defect' which made them prone to a metabolic obesity as they would have little capacity for adaptive thermogenesis. A similar thermogenic defect might also predispose people to obesity.

It would be unwise to be too ready to extrapolate these findings in laboratory rodents to people. Adult human beings have very limited capacity for non-shivering thermogenesis, and brown adipose tissue has traditionally been regarded as vestigial in adult humans. People keep warm largely by heat conservation supplemented by shivering rather than by non-shivering thermogenesis. A large animal with a relatively small surface-area to volume ratio is less able to dissipate large amounts of surplus heat generation; this might also make adaptive thermogenesis a less advantageous strategy for maintenance of energy balance in people. Accurate long-term measurements of metabolic rate in obese people provide no evidence for any thermogenic defect in obesity, and indeed basal metabolic rates and total energy expenditure of obese people are increased because of their higher body mass

(Prentice *et al.*, 1989). Drugs that are highly specific activators of the β-3 adrenoreceptor on brown fat (β-3 *agonists*) cause big increases in metabolic rate in rodents but have very little effect in humans.

Even in the ob/ob mouse the abnormal thermoregulation probably represents an adaptation rather than a defect (Webb, 1992b). If the genetic defect of these mice makes them unable to detect their large fat stores, they would respond as if being continually starved (see discussion of leptin later in the chapter). One of the strategies that mice employ to conserve energy during fasting is to reduce their heat output and lower their body temperature. Fasting mice can enter a state of torpor where they allow their body temperature to fall by as much as 15°C for several hours at a time (Webb *et al.*, 1982). The low body temperature of ob/ob mice could represent a permanent semi-torpid state, as an adaptation to perceived starvation, and their poor cold tolerance might represent a form of disuse atrophy of their brown fat. Torpor is not a usual human response to starvation. Children have now been identified who have an analogous gene defect to that of the *ob/ob* mouse but these very obese children have normal body temperature and thermoregulation (Montague *et al.* 1997). See Webb (1990, 1992b or 2009) for critical discussion of the applicability of these studies on small animal models of obesity to people.

The publication of this brown fat theory by Rothwell and Stock in 1979 generated a flurry of interest and excitement in the early 1980s. It raised the prospect that adaptive thermogenesis could represent a major component of human energy expenditure and that differences in thermogenic capacity might explain the apparent variation in the susceptibility of people to obesity. It also raised the prospect of thermogenic drugs that would specifically stimulate adaptive thermogenesis. These might offer an attractive alternative to appetite suppressants for the pharmacological treatment of obesity. β-3 adrenoreceptor agonists that specifically stimulate brown fat thermogenesis have shown promising results in rats but not in humans. This is probably because of the low capacity for brown fat thermogenesis in people. It would be fair to say that the initial enthusiasm for this theory has cooled considerably over the last 30 years. There is little evidence that adaptive thermogenesis makes a major contribution to human energy balance control.

Later work further undermined the theory that adaptive thermogenesis is a major factor in controlling body weight. Enerback *et al.* (1997) produced transgenic mice that lacked the key protein required for the uncoupling of oxidation and phosphorylation in brown fat (UCP1). This protein is the key initiator of heat generation in brown fat. These mice are cold sensitive but they are not obese and their ability to regulate their body weight is normal. This work seemed to be a decisive blow against the brown fat theory of obesity. There are, however, now known to be other uncoupling proteins called UCP2 and UCP3. UCP2 is expressed not only in both white fat and brown fat but also in other tissues (Fleury *et al.* 1997); UCP3 is found mainly in skeletal muscle (Hirsch, 1997). The role of these other uncoupling proteins (UCP2 and UCP3) in the control of human metabolic rate is as yet unclear, but Schrauwen *et al.* (1999) suggested that they may be important. Uncoupled oxidative phosphorylation (proton leakage) may account for up to 20 per cent of the resting metabolic rate in people.

Nevertheless the idea of a thermogenic defect being a major cause of human or even mouse obesity is now largely discounted.

Key points

- Food intake is undoubtedly regulated, but can surplus energy be burnt off as an adaptive response to overfeeding (adaptive thermogenesis), and can this limit weight gain?
- Rothwell and Stock (1979) proposed that overfeeding increases sympathetic stimulation to brown fat which uncouples oxidative phosphorylation in this tissue and so increases heat generation. This mechanism is well established as a means of heat generation in small mammals and human babies during cold exposure (non-shivering thermogenesis).
- They also proposed that genetically obese mice (*ob/ob*) and humans might get fat because of some thermogenic defect that impaired their capacity for adaptive thermogenesis.

→

- Adaptive thermogenesis is not now thought to be a major component of human energy expenditure. There is no evidence of any thermogenic defect in most obese people, and indeed the basal metabolic rate and total energy expenditure of obese people tend to be higher than those of lean people.
- Transgenic mice that lack a key protein required for brown fat thermogenesis (UCP1) are hypothermic but not obese. Even the well-documented hypothermia of some obese mice probably represents an energy-conserving response in animals whose brains falsely perceive that their fat stores are depleted.
- The uncoupler proteins UCP2 and UCP3 are expressed in tissues outside brown fat.
- It is possible that regulated uncoupling of oxidative phosphorylation may play some role in controlling human metabolic rate. Up to 20 per cent of resting metabolic rate may be due to uncoupled oxidative phosphorylation (proton leakage).
- The proposal that a thermogenic defect is a major cause of human obesity is now discounted by most nutritionists and physiologists.

EXTERNAL INFLUENCES ON FOOD INTAKE

The remainder of this chapter considers the physiological regulation of energy intake. However, it is not only 'internal' physiological factors that influence when, what, where and how much we eat. Eating is also a conscious voluntary act that is affected by a host of 'external' influences.

- *The palatability of food and the pleasure derived from eating.* We do not have to be hungry to eat. Indeed, we may be persuaded to eat some delicious item even when feeling distinctly full.
- *Habit.* An example is always eating a particular snack when reading, driving or watching a favourite TV programme.
- *Psychological state.* We sometimes eat to relieve psychological states other than hunger (e.g. anxiety, boredom or unhappiness).

- *Eating for social rather than physiological reasons.* We might participate in a social 'feast', or eat to please someone who has offered us food.

It is perhaps only in newborn babies that eating is regulated largely by internal physiological hunger-control mechanisms uncluttered by these external influences. We may, on occasion, ignore or override our physiological mechanisms that control food intake, and this may be one reason why we are so prone to obesity.

Key points

- Even though physiological control mechanisms affect feeding, eating is a voluntary activity that is also influenced by a host of social, cultural and psychological factors.
- The external influences on feeding may reduce the effectiveness of physiological control mechanisms.

CONTROL OF ENERGY INTAKE

Early work with experimental animals

Over the last hundred years or so there have been several reports in the medical literature of patients becoming very obese after damage to their *hypothalamus* caused by trauma or tumour. This pointed to a role for the hypothalamus in weight control, and it is now well established that the hypothalamus is involved in other physiological regulatory systems such as:

- body temperature control
- control of water balance
- control of the female reproductive cycle.

Around 1940, the development of the stereotaxic apparatus allowed experimenters to make discrete and accurately located lesions deep within the brains of experimental animals. Over the next couple of decades this lesioning technique showed that damage to certain areas of the hypothalamus could profoundly affect a rat's eating and drinking behaviour. Damage to the ventromedial region of the hypothalamus in many mammalian species, ranging from mice to monkeys, produces a period of massive overeating and weight gain, which leads to severe and permanent obesity. The weight of rats with such lesions stabilizes at a much higher level than that of unoperated rats and their food intake returns to a level which maintains this 'new set point'. If these rats are slimmed down they will go through a second bout of overeating and they appear to defend their new set point. It was also found that lesions in the lateral part of the hypothalamus completely abolished eating and drinking behaviour in rats and they died unless tube-fed.

As a result of such observations, a simple theory of food intake regulation was proposed, the *dual-centre hypothesis* (Figure 8.2). A spontaneously active feeding centre that initiates food seeking and eating behaviour was envisaged as being located in the lateral hypothalamus. Its destruction by a lateral hypothalamic lesion results in a cessation of eating behaviour. This feeding centre was said to be periodically inhibited by a satiety centre located in the ventromedial region of the hypothalamus. This satiety centre would become active in response to certain satiety signals, which strengthen after feeding; it would then inhibit the feeding centre and produce satiation. As time after feeding elapses so one would envisage these satiety signals dying away, the satiety centre would become quiescent, allowing the feeding centre to become active again and producing hunger. Destruction of this satiety centre would reduce satiation and result in excessive food consumption and obesity. The hypothalamus is thus envisaged as acting like a meter or 'appestat' that adjusts the feeding drive in response to a variety of physiological signals that reflect the short- and long-term energy status of the body. Energy intake is thus matched to output and energy balance is maintained.

The dual-centre hypothesis: a more recent perspective

The dual-centre hypothesis has had enormous influence on thinking about control of energy balance and body weight. It was prominent in many textbooks published in the 1960s and 1970s and it may still be found in some modern texts. It is now regarded as a rather simplistic model of a complex process. Since these early studies, much detailed work has been done in trying to identify hypothalamic and extra-hypothalamic brain areas

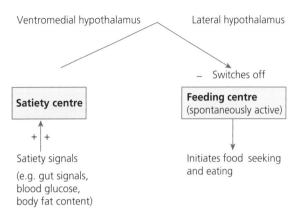

Figure 8.2 The dual-centre hypothesis.

that are involved in the control of feeding and body weight. Detailed discussion of the anatomical locations and interconnections of neural centres controlling energy balance is beyond the scope of this book, but several hypothalamic and other brain areas are known to play a role. I will generally use the term *appestat* (cf. thermostat) as a term to collectively describe the centres in the hypothalamus that control energy balance. References to the early experimental work on the hypothalamic mechanisms regulating food intake have been excluded. Interested readers will find detailed and well-referenced accounts of this work in editions of many texts published during the 1960s and 1970s or by reference to Mayer (1956, 1968), Kennedy (1966) or Brobeck (1974), three of the most prolific and influential researchers in this field.

Despite nowadays being regarded as simplistic, the dual-centre hypothesis does have the three basic elements that any system for controlling food intake must have (Figure 8.3).

- It has a series of physiological inputs to the appestat that provide information about the feeding status and the level of body energy stores – so-called *satiety signals*.
- There are areas within the brain that integrate information about feeding status and level of body energy stores – the *appestat*.
- It includes a hunger drive that can be modified by the appestat in response to the information received from the satiety inputs (also mechanisms for controlling energy expenditure).

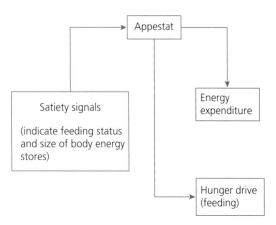

Figure 8.3 The three major elements of the physiological control of energy balance.

The arcuate nucleus of the hypothalamus seems to play a key role in receiving and responding to both short- and long-term signals that reflect the body's feeding and nutritional status and thus control body weight. Circulating factors can interact directly with neurones of the arcuate nucleus because it is incompletely separated from the general circulation by the blood–brain barrier. Within the arcuate nucleus are sub-populations of neurones involved in food intake regulation, some that are appetite inhibiting and some that are appetite stimulating. These neurones release peptides such as neuropeptide Y (NPY) and Agouti-related peptide (AgRP) which bind to receptors within the central nervous system to produce appetite stimulation, while α-melanocyte- stimulating hormone (α-MSH) causes an anorectic response (Murphy and Bloom, 2004).

Cannabis use is known to stimulate appetite, a phenomenon commonly referred to as 'the munchies'. The cannabinoids present in cannabis bind to a cannabinoid receptor (CB1) in the brain and this mimics the effects of endocannabinoids produced naturally in the brain and other tissues. These endocannabinoids are like prostaglandin derivatives of the fatty acid arachidonic acid. The first of these endocannabinoids was characterized in 1992 and was named *anandamide*. The endocannabinoid system plays a role in the normal regulation of food intake and may be responsible for producing pleasurable sensations associated with eating. It has been shown in rats that just the taste of fat (without eating it) can induce large increases in

endocannabinoid production in the small intestine, and this could have a positive feedback effect, increasing fat consumption (DiPatrizio *et al.*, 2011). Antagonists of endocannabinoids that bind to the CB1 receptor are being investigated as potential anti-obesity drugs (see rimonabant in Chapter 9).

Various satiety signals have been proposed and investigated over the years. These fall into the three major categories below.

- *Signals emanating from the alimentary tract and transmitted via sensory nerves or hormones released from the gut.* These would provide information about the amount and the nature of food in the gut.
- *Blood substrate levels.* After eating, the blood concentrations of substrates including glucose and amino acids rise as they are absorbed from the gut. These concentrations fall in the post-absorptive state. If we eat three meals per day and they each take around 4 hours to digest and absorb, then for most of our waking hours we are absorbing food. The notion that blood glucose concentration or the rate of glucose utilization is a major satiety signal has historically been very popular – the *glucostat theory*.
- *Signals that emanate from adipose tissue.* These are hypothesized to indicate the level of body fat stores – the *lipostat theory*.

Gut-fill cues

We experience the feeling of stomach fullness that occurs after a meal and the feelings of stomach emptiness and hunger contractions that occur during fasting. Feeding normally finishes before there have been detectable changes in blood substrate levels (or changes in blood leptin levels – see later in this chapter). These observations suggest that signals from the alimentary tract play some part in signalling satiation and have some role in short-term appetite regulation. This could be mediated either through sensory nerves in the gut directly affecting the appestat, or perhaps through the effect of hormones released from the gut by the presence of food.

One can greatly alter the energy density of the diets of laboratory rats by the use of an inert bulking agent (e.g. methylcellulose) or by the addition of energy-rich fat. Rats fed diluted diets are able to maintain their body weight and compensate for the dilution by increasing the volume of food they eat. However, long-term feeding with diets of high energy density causes obesity in rats, which suggests that over-concentration of the diet may reduce the effectiveness of feeding control mechanisms. It is widely believed that reducing the energy density of human diets will help to prevent excessive weight, which implies widespread acceptance of the belief that dietary bulk has some modulating effect on appetite. One could, for example, envisage alimentary signals playing an important role in signalling satiety at the end of a meal but, when food is very dilute, being overridden or dampened by other physiological signals indicating the need for more energy intake. The mechanisms regulating energy balance are generally more effective in preventing under- rather than over-consumption (see Chapter 9).

The hormone *cholecystokinin* (CCK) is released from the intestine when food is present. It induces satiety and reduces feeding, and pre-prandial administration of substances that block the CCK receptor lead to increases in meal size in animals and people. It was the first gut hormone identified as playing a role in the control of appetite. It is said to act by activating sensory branches of the vagus nerve in the gut and these relay the information to the appestat. Prolonged administration of CCK to animals leads to rapid diminution in its anorectic effect, and animals that have been bred with no CCK receptors have normal food intake and body weight. Animals adapt to oversupply of CCK and also adapt to an absence of the CCK response.

A more recently discovered hormone, *ghrelin*, is the only known peripherally produced hormone that has an appetite-stimulating effect. It is a small peptide (28 amino acids) produced mainly in the stomach. Plasma ghrelin levels are inversely correlated with body weight, and they rise during fasting and weight loss and fall rapidly after a meal. It has been suggested that ghrelin may play a role in meal initiation. Peripherally administered ghrelin binds to appetite-stimulating cells in the arcuate nucleus of the hypothalamus and this leads to increased production and release of appetite-stimulating peptides within the hypothalamus. Chronic administration of ghrelin leads to overeating and weight gain in rats, while anti-ghrelin antibodies lead to a reduction in the amount of food consumed after fasting.

Pancreatic peptide (PP) and polypeptide YY (PYY) are two appetite-suppressing hormones produced in the gut that are both structurally related to the appetite-inhibiting brain peptide neuropeptide Y (NPY). PP is produced in the pancreas and when administered peripherally to rats it reduces food intake and slows stomach emptying; it also suppresses food intake in humans. Increases in blood levels of PP lead to increases in hypothalamic levels of NPY. PYY is produced by endocrine cells within the gut and levels in the blood rise after eating. When PYY is administered to rats or people in amounts that mimic the normal levels found post-prandially in the blood, this leads to activation of appetite-suppressing neurones in the arcuate nucleus and markedly reduces food intake.

Glucagon-like peptide 1 (GLP-1) and oxyntomodulin (Oxm) are peptides that are produced in the small intestine and colon and released into the blood after eating. They both have appetite-suppressing effects. GLP-1 receptors are found in the arcuate nucleus and in other parts of the brain and their administration to rats or people inhibits food intake. Oxm has similar anorectic effects and it may act via GLP-1 receptors.

Murphy and Bloom (2004) and Druce *et al.* (2004) have written concise referenced reviews of the role of the gut in regulating appetite and both reviews can be accessed freely online.

The glucostat theory

In this theory it is envisaged that there are glucose receptors or sensors in the appestat and perhaps elsewhere that respond to blood glucose concentration (Mayer, 1956). These glucose receptors induce satiety when blood glucose concentration is high and hunger when it is low. The occurrence of both high blood glucose and hunger in uncontrolled diabetes was explained by the suggestion that the glucoreceptor cells needed insulin for glucose entry in the same way as, say, resting muscle cells do. In the absence of insulin (i.e. in diabetes), despite a high blood glucose concentration, the glucoreceptor cells are deprived of glucose – resulting in hunger. As the brain was regarded at this time as being exclusively dependent on a supply of glucose in the blood, hypothalamic glucoreceptors sensitive to fluctuations in blood glucose concentration seemed a logical homeostatic device.

This theory was given an important boost in the 1950s by work that showed that a glucose derivative, *gold thioglucose*, produced both obesity and lesions in the ventromedial region of the hypothalamus of mice. No other gold thio compounds produced this effect; the glucose moiety appeared to be essential. This supported the proposal that there are glucoreceptors in this region that bind the gold thioglucose and this leads to accumulation of neurotoxic concentrations of gold in their vicinity (reviewed by Debons *et al.*, 1977). Later versions of this theory suggested that a high rate of glucose metabolism might produce satiation rather than high blood concentration *per se*. Satiation correlates very well with the difference between arterial and venous blood glucose concentration, which is a measure of the rate of glucose utilization.

When the rate of glucose metabolism is high then fat use is low. In healthy people, this high-glucose/low-fat usage occurs after eating carbohydrate and produces satiation. When glucose metabolism is low then that of fat is high, and this results in hunger. High-fat/low-glucose utilization occurs:

- during fasting
- in the absence of insulin (uncontrolled diabetes)
- if meals with little or no carbohydrate are eaten.

Insulin, when released after a meal, causes glucose to be taken up and metabolized by the cells and this leads to satiation. Use of fat in metabolism is associated with hunger. Carbohydrate intake increases use of carbohydrate and reduces use of fat, but fat intake has little effect on either fat or carbohydrate metabolism (Schutz *et al.*, 1989). As fat is absorbed, much of it is shunted directly into our fat stores. This may help explain why high-fat diets may be less satiating than high-carbohydrate diets and why high-fat diets seem to predispose to weight gain and obesity (see Chapter 9).

The evidence that some glucostat mechanism plays an important role in the short-term control of appetite is very persuasive (reviewed by Penicaud *et al.*, 2002).

The lipostat or adipostat theory

It is difficult to see how short-term satiety signals like gut-fill, blood glucose concentration or even the rate of glucose utilization could produce long-term weight stability (i.e. over a period of months, years or decades). They are more likely to fulfil functions such as:

- limiting the size of meals to prevent overload of the gut and the body's metabolic processes for assimilating nutrients
- ensuring a regular flow of energy and nutrients to maintain optimal metabolic functioning even when body fat stores are substantial, and so reducing the need for regular and prolonged activation of starvation mechanisms. (Note that the need to avoid excessive fat stores may have played a relatively minor role in shaping our physiology – see Chapter 9.)

This lipostat or adipostat theory was used to explain how body energy stores (i.e. fat) could be regulated in the long term by regulation of apparently short-term phenomena like hunger and satiety. It was first proposed by Gordon Kennedy in the 1950s (see Kennedy, 1966). It is envisaged that some appetite-regulating chemical (a satiety factor or satiety hormone) is released from adipose tissue so that its concentration in blood indicates, to the appestat, the total amount of stored fat. This would allow total amount of body fat to have a modulating effect on appetite and would offer a relatively simple mechanism for long-term control of energy balance. This lipostat theory would fit well with the notion of a set point for body weight discussed earlier in the chapter.

Some very persuasive but indirect evidence for the existence of such a satiety hormone (now called *leptin*) came from the work of Coleman (1978) using two types of genetically obese mice.

Obese (ob/ob) and *diabetes (db/db)* are two forms of genetic obesity in mice. Both *ob/ob* and *db/db* mice inherit a very severe obesity associated with diabetes. On a similar genetic background the two syndromes are practically identical and yet are caused by mutations at different gene loci. Coleman proposed that in the *ob/ob* mouse the genetic defect is in the leptin (satiety hormone) gene, leaving them unable to produce this satiety hormone (leptin) and making their appestat unable to detect any fat stores. As a consequence of this they overeat and get very fat. He suggested that, in the *db/db* mouse, the abnormal protein is one that allows the appestat to respond to leptin (the leptin receptor). *db/db* would thus produce lots of leptin because they have lots of fat in their adipose tissue. However, without any leptin receptor their appestat cannot detect the leptin and so once again they cannot sense any fat stores and so they overeat. At this time, leptin had not been discovered and was a purely hypothetical hormone. These suggestions were the result of an ingenious series of parabiosis experiments (pairs of animals are surgically linked together so that hormones and other substances can pass between their blood systems). The results obtained from four of these parabiotic pairings are explained in Table 8.1.

Key points

- The hypothalamus plays a major role in the control of feeding. Experimental lesions in the hypothalamus profoundly affect feeding behaviour.
- The hypothalamic 'appestat' receives input of satiety signals that indicate the feeding state and level of body fat stores.
- The hypothalamus alters the feeding drive and rate of energy expenditure in response to these satiety inputs.

→

Key points

- Satiety signals relay information to the appestat about the amount and nature of food in the gut, the level or rate of usage of blood substrates, and the amount of fat stored in adipose tissue.
- Sensory nerves in the gut and hormones released from the gut indicate the nature and amount of gut contents.
- In the *glucostat* theory it is envisaged that information from glucose sensors in the hypothalamus and elsewhere have a major role in the short-term control of feeding.
- In the *lipostat* theory, Kennedy proposed that some satiety factor (leptin) is released from adipose tissue in proportion to the amount of stored fat. This would enable the appestat to regulate feeding and energy expenditure to maintain a constant level of these stores.
- Indirect evidence has suggested that obese mice with mutations at the *obese* locus (*ob/ob*) do not produce this satiety factor whereas mice with mutations at the *diabetes* locus (*db/db*) do not respond to it.

Table 8.1 Results of parabiotic pairings of lean and obese rodents

Pairing	A normal animal paired with one that has had its ventromedial hypothalamus (part of the appestat) destroyed	A normal mouse and an *ob/ob* mouse	A normal mouse and a *db/db* mouse	An *ob/ob* mouse and a *db/db* mouse
Result	The animal with the damaged hypothalamus overeats and gains weight as expected. The normal animal eats less and loses weight	The *ob/ob* mouse eats less and loses weight	The normal mouse stops eating and starves	The *ob/ob* mouse eats less and loses weight
Explanation	The animal with its hypothalamus damaged gets fat because the area where the leptin acts in the brain has been destroyed and so it cannot respond to leptin. As this lesioned animal gets fatter, its adipose tissue produces large amounts of leptin. This extra leptin enters the blood of the normal animal and this animal's appestat responds by reducing food intake	The *ob/ob* mouse cannot produce its own leptin, but it can respond to leptin produced by its lean partner, so it eats less and loses weight	The *db/db* mouse cannot respond to leptin and so gets fat and produces excess leptin. This leptin enters the blood of the normal mouse and acts on this animal's appestat to suppress food intake	The *ob/ob* mouse is responding to the excess leptin produced by its *db/db* partner

THE LEPTIN STORY

In 1994, Zhang and co-workers published a paper that radically changed scientific thinking about the physiological mechanisms that control energy balance. Zhang *et al.* (1994) identified the *obese* (*ob*) gene and the protein that is produced by it in healthy lean mice. The *obese* gene produces a secretory protein of 167 amino acids that seemed to be produced exclusively in adipose tissue and has been named *leptin*. (Note that later studies have shown that it is also produced in the placenta and stomach.) It seems to have all the characteristics of the hypothetical satiety factor from adipose tissue that was proposed in the lipostat theory of weight control. In normal mice, leptin production falls during starvation and it increases in environmentally induced obesity. Leptin production seems to be proportional to the mass of adipose tissue. In genetically obese (*ob/ob*) mice, a mutation in the *ob* gene results in the production of a shorter, inactive protein that is not secreted. This leaves the appestat of *ob/ob* mice with no input from adipose tissue. The appestat perceives this as absence of fat stores and so initiates appropriate starvation responses.

Leptin administration to *ob/ob* mice causes weight loss and normalization of body composition, and it corrects all the other metabolic and hormonal abnormalities of these mice. Leptin also causes reduced food intake, increased energy expenditure and loss of body weight when it is administered to normal mice. Leptin administration has no effect in the *db/db* mouse, an observation that is entirely consistent with the earlier suggestion of Coleman (1978) that the genetic defect in these mice was in a gene that codes for the satiety factor (i.e. leptin) receptor. In 1995, Tartaglia and co-workers were able to identify and characterize the leptin receptor. They confirmed that the mutation in *db/db* mice leads to abnormalities in the leptin receptor. The leptin receptor can be detected in all the areas of the hypothalamus known to be involved in control of energy balance and in the vascular region where leptin is conducted across the blood–brain barrier (the choroid plexus).

Leptin seems to play a central role in the long-term regulation of energy balance (Figure 8.4). During starvation and weight loss, leptin production from adipose tissue decreases. This decrease in leptin is detected by the hypothalamic appestat which then triggers the normal responses to starvation that are seen at their most extreme in the *ob/ob* mouse, such as:

- increased food intake if food is available
- reduced activity and resting energy expenditure, including reduced body temperature and the permanent semi-torpid state of *ob/ob* mice
- reduced production of hormones in the pituitary gland (gonadotrophins) that leads to delayed puberty and infertility
- other changes in the secretion of hormones from the pituitary, which in turn regulate most of the other endocrine glands. (The output of pituitary hormones is controlled by the hypothalamus.)

During weight gain, as the fat content of adipose tissue increases, so increasing leptin production should act via the hypothalamus to reduce food intake and increase energy expenditure. However, it does seem that, while the absence of leptin in the circulation caused by depletion of adipose tissue or genetic defect has profound effects on appetite, fat storage and fertility, the effects of elevated leptin levels are much less dramatic. This may be just another manifestation of the general observation that the body's weight control mechanism seem to be much more geared to preventing underweight and maintaining adequate fat stores (the evolutionary priority) than preventing excessive weight gain (see Chapter 9 for further discussion). Nevertheless obesity would theoretically occur under either of the following circumstances:

- complete failure of leptin production (as in *ob/ob* mice) or inadequate leptin production – a failure to produce sufficient leptin to reflect the level of fat stores to the hypothalamus
- a complete lack of response to leptin (as in *db/db* mice) or a reduced response to leptin.

The observation that leptin levels are high in most induced animal obesities suggests that reduced leptin sensitivity is the likely scenario in most obesity. Increasing the fatness of animals by feeding them a high-fat diet does indeed lead to a decrease in their sensitivity to leptin. There is thus a complete spectrum of leptin sensitivity in mice, from the high

a) Too little fat

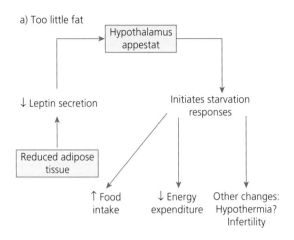

b) Too much fat

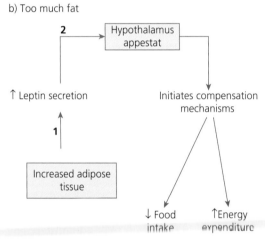

1 If production of leptin is absent (*ob/ob* mice) or insufficient then obesity will result.

2 If leptin sensing is absent (*db/db* mice) or reduced (mice fed high-fat diets) then obesity results.

Figure 8.4 Role of leptin in responses of mice to excess or inadequate fat stores.

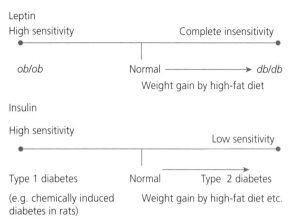

Figure 8.5 Variations in leptin and insulin sensitivity.

disease (type 1) that starts in childhood and requires regular insulin injections for survival. In type 2 diabetes, an affluent Western lifestyle (inactivity, high-fat diet and excessive weight gain) triggers a progressive decrease in the sensitivity to insulin, probably as a response to high insulin secretion. In genetically susceptible people, this eventually leads to symptoms of diabetes. Zhang and Scarpace (2006) review results from several studies which suggest that, as with the insulin/type 2 diabetes analogy, high circulating leptin levels lead directly to reduced leptin sensitivity by reducing the number of leptin receptors in the hypothalamus and reducing the signalling efficiency of these receptors. They argue that the increased leptin production associated with increased adipose tissue mass directly contributes to leptin resistance and thus promotes further weight gain, leading to a vicious cycle of:

weight gain → elevated blood leptin → leptin resistance → weight gain → obesity.

Leptin appears to play a key role in long-term energy balance control even though other factors such as blood glucose and gut-fill cues seem to control meal spacing and the short-term control of hunger and satiety. Leptin levels do not rise noticeably after a meal and it is not thought to immediately induce satiety during feeding and signal the end of a meal. However, the observation that some leptin is produced in the stomachs of rats and that it is released during feeding may indicate some role for leptin in short-term hunger and satiety control. Administration of the hormone cholecystokinin

sensitivity of *ob/ob* mice through to the complete insensitivity of *db/db* mice (Figure 8.5). Normal mice lie between these two extremes, but inducing obesity by dietary means reduces leptin sensitivity.

There is a clear precedent for diet and lifestyle causing increased production and declining sensitivity to a hormone. The most common and mildest form of diabetes begins in middle or old age and does not normally require insulin injections (type 2 diabetes). There is no primary failure of the pancreas to produce insulin as there is in the severe form of the

(CCK) also causes release of leptin from the stomach (Bado *et al.*, 1998). CCK is released from the gut during feeding and, along with several other gut hormones, is known to induce satiety or – in the case of ghrelin – increase appetite (see under gut-fill cues earlier in this chapter).

So far, this discussion has been largely confined to studies in experimental animals. What is the relevance of this work to people and – more especially – what future role can leptin play in human obesity therapy?

In their original leptin paper, Zhang *et al.* (1994) identified a human version of leptin produced in human adipose tissue. Measurements of serum leptin concentrations in people with varying levels of fatness suggest that leptin concentration rises in proportion to the adipose tissue mass. This means that, in general, leptin levels are higher in obese people than in lean people. For example, in a large sample of Polynesian men and women, Zimmet *et al.* (1996) found a very high correlation ($r = 0.8$) between serum leptin concentration and body mass index (BMI, i.e. body fat content).

In 1997, the first two cases of people with obesity caused by mutations in their leptin genes were identified; they were two British cousins of Pakistani origin (Montague *et al.*, 1997). These are the apparent human equivalents of *ob/ob* mice. These two children were extremely obese: at 8 years the girl weighed 86 kg and at 2 years the boy weighed 29 kg. There are technical reasons why one would expect that this mutation (analogous to the *ob* mutation seen in *ob/ob* mice) would be expected to be extremely rare in humans (Sorensen *et al.*, 1996). It is thus no coincidence that these children were from a close-knit immigrant community with a history of consanguineous marriage which increases the chances of people being homozygous for any rare harmful recessive trait and thus having a genetic disease. According to Friedman and Halaas (1998), only about 5–10 per cent of obese humans may

have relatively low leptin levels. One group who are particularly prone to obesity, the Pima Indians, tend to have low leptin levels which may explain their extreme propensity to obesity. The first identified cases of people obese because they have a mutation in their leptin receptor gene, the human equivalent of *db/db* mice, were found in three members of a French immigrant family (Clement *et al.*, 1998).

When humans with leptin or leptin receptor mutations reach the normal age for puberty, they show similar reproductive abnormalities to *ob/ob* and *db/db* mice; they do not go through normal pubertal changes and the females do not menstruate. Studies such as these provide confirmation that leptin plays a similar role in the regulation of energy balance in mice and humans (see Figure 8.4). However, as noted earlier, both types of obese people, unlike their mouse equivalents, have apparently normal thermoregulation and there is no suggestion that their obesity is caused by any thermogenic defect.

When the discovery of leptin was first announced, an American pharmaceutical company paid millions of dollars for the patent on the leptin gene. Leptin seemed to offer the prospect of a major advance in the treatment of obesity, even though most obesity seems to be associated with leptin resistance rather than reduced leptin production. Leptin is a protein that needs to be administered by injection, a major drawback to its potential therapeutic usage. Early trials of leptin injections in obese people suggest that, even though it does produce a small average weight loss over a month of use, the individual response is variable and in general its efficacy as an anti-obesity 'drug' is very limited. As with *ob/ob* mice, leptin has proved to be effective in human patients who have a congenital leptin deficiency (Murphy and Bloom, 2004).

For a fully referenced review of the first few years of leptin developments, see Friedman and Halaas (1998).

Key points

- In 1994, the protein produced from the *obese* gene in healthy mice and people was identified and characterized.

- The *obese* gene product is a secreted protein called leptin that is mainly produced in adipose tissue.

- Leptin seems to be the hypothetical satiety factor from adipose tissue that was predicted in the lipostat theory of weight control.

- In general, leptin concentration in blood is proportional to the amount of stored fat.

- Obesity could result from inadequate leptin production or inadequate response to leptin, as this would cause the appestat to 'underestimate' the fat content of adipose tissue.

- In general, low blood leptin caused by congenital deficiency or adipose tissue depletion seems to have more profound effects than high blood leptin levels.

- The leptin system, like other regulatory mechanisms, seems more effective at maintaining adequate fat stores than preventing excessive accumulation of fat and obesity.

- Obese mice with mutations at the *obese* locus (*ob/ob*) do not produce functional leptin, and mice with mutations at the *diabetes* locus (*db/db*) do not respond to leptin because they have a defective receptor protein.

- A few very obese children have been identified with mutations at the leptin gene locus (analogous to *ob/ob* mice) and at the leptin receptor locus (analogous to *db/db* mice).

- Only a small proportion of obese people have low leptin levels. Most have high leptin levels that reflect their large amounts of stored fat.

- Most human obesity is probably due to an environmentally induced reduction in sensitivity or response to leptin. By analogy, most human diabetes is due to reduced insulin sensitivity.

- In experimental animals, leptin sensitivity declines if they are made obese by environmental means (e.g. feeding a high-fat diet).

- High leptin secretion caused by excessive weight gain causes leptin insensitivity which predisposes to further weight gain.

- Leptin is effective in treating *ob/ob* mice and in treating humans with congenital leptin deficiency, but it has low efficacy with other obese people.

OBESITY

Defining obesity 202
Prevalence of obesity 203
Consequences of obesity 211
The metabolic syndrome or 'syndrome X' 219
Causes of obesity 219
Prevention and treatment of obesity in populations 229
Obesity treatment in individuals 232
'Aggressive' treatments for obesity 237

DEFINING OBESITY

Obesity strictly refers to an excess accumulation of body fat, but body fat content is difficult to measure quickly and accurately in people. For this reason, the *body mass index* (BMI) is now very widely used to determine whether or not someone is excessively fat. (See Chapter 3 for a critical discussion of the use of BMI.). The BMI classification system in Table 9.1 is now used internationally and the World Health Organization (WHO) defines clinical obesity as a BMI of over 30.

This classification is a simple one because it uses:

- a small number of ranges
- mainly whole rounded numbers
- the same cut-off points for men and women.

This simplicity must have a cost in terms of accuracy and sensitivity, and so these ranges should be used as a general guide rather than absolute cut-off points. A small difference in BMI is still small even if one value is above and one below a boundary. Note that 20–25 was for some time used as the 'normal range', and some older data sources referenced in this book use that for 'normality'. However, at the upper end, the cut-off points for the definitions of overweight and obese have remained constant.

In this book, *overweight* always refers to a BMI in excess of 25 and *obese* to a BMI of over 30, unless otherwise specified.

Table 9.1 Internationally recognized classification of people according to their body mass index (BMI)

BMI range (kg/m²)	Classification
Under 18.5	Underweight
18.5–25	Ideal range
25–30	Overweight
Over 30	Obese
Over 40	Morbidly obese

BMI = weight (kg) divided by height squared (m²).

Waist circumference and *waist-to-hip ratio* (WHR) are two measures of fat distribution around the body. High levels of abdominal fat are thought to have more serious health consequences than fat stored subcutaneously (e.g. around the hips). High waist circumference and high WHR are considered to be risk factors for type 2 diabetes and cardiovascular disease.

'High waist circumference' and 'high WHR' are defined by the following criteria:

- men – waist circumference >102 cm, WHR >0.95
- women – waist circumference >88 cm, WHR >0.85.

Key points

- Body mass index is the standard way of classifying people according to fatness.

PREVALENCE OF OBESITY

There is little doubt that overweight and obesity are more common in the UK and the USA than in previous generations and that the prevalence is still rising. There have been particularly rapid increases in prevalence since the start of the 1980s. Almost two-thirds of English adults are currently overweight or obese (BMI >25) and almost a quarter are clinically obese (BMI >30). Figure 9.1 shows the proportion of English adults in various BMI categories. Most of the data for English adults quoted in this chapter are from *Health Survey for England* (see, for example, www.ic.nhs.uk/webfiles/publications/003_Health_Lifestyles/opad11/Statistics_on_Obesity_Physical_Activity_and_Diet_England_2011_revised_Aug11.pdf). In the USA the situation is even worse, with around 68 per cent adults having BMIs that are above 25 and 34 per cent classified as obese.

Even the high frequency of obesity indicated in Figure 9.1 somewhat understates the problem in middle-aged people. Figure 9.2 shows how the proportion of people who are overweight or obese changes with age in English adults. This proportion rises steeply throughout early adulthood and middle age, and only in the over-75s do the proportions start to fall back slightly. Well over 70 per cent of adults aged between 45 and 64 years are either overweight or obese. Essentially similar age-related changes in prevalence are seen in the USA, and Figure 9.3 shows the prevalence of obesity in various age groups of men and women in 2000. Obesity peaks in US adults in the 60- to 69-year age group where 40 per cent of adults are classified as obese. Note also the

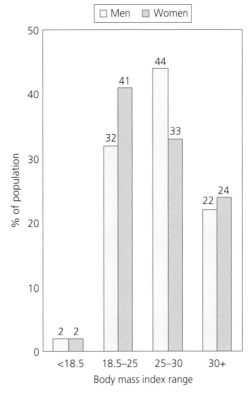

Figure 9.1 Distribution of English adults according to body mass index (BMI) category.

substantial fall in obesity prevalence in old age, especially in the over-80s; many people tend to lose weight at the end of their lives, or perhaps the increased mortality of the obese is selectively removing them from the population. (However, Chapter 16 presents evidence to suggest that, in older age groups, excess weight seems to be associated with reduced mortality – an apparent protective effect of extra fat stores in old age.)

Figure 9.4 shows changes in the estimated prevalence of obesity in England; obesity prevalence has trebled since 1980. In 1992, the British government set a target of reducing clinical obesity prevalence in England to no more than 6 per cent of men and 8 per cent of women by the year 2005 (DH, 1992). Even at the time they were set, these seemed to be very ambitious targets and they now seem to have been totally unrealistic, yet these targets represent the estimated prevalence of obesity in 1980. This target date of 2005 is now long gone and yet obesity prevalence is around three times the target values and still shows no sign of falling.

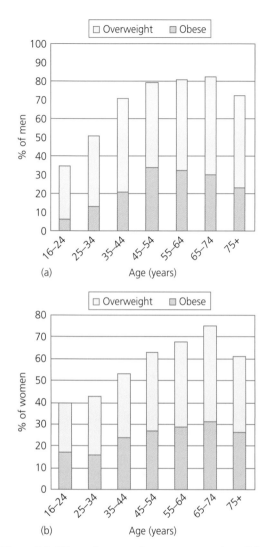

(a)   Age (years)

(b)   Age (years)

Figure 9.2 Effect of age on the percentage of English (a) men and (b) women who are overweight or obese.

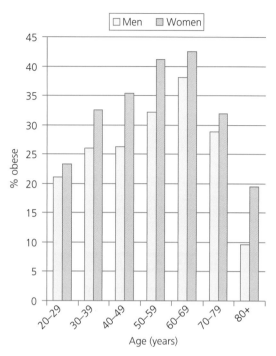

Age (years)

Figure 9.3 Prevalence of obesity in American men in a range of age groups.

Flegal *et al.* (2006) and Ogden *et al.* (2010) have reported similar rapid increases in obesity prevalence in the USA. Between 1960 and 1980 the prevalence of adult obesity in the USA rose slowly from 13.5 to 15 per cent of adults aged 20–74 years. However, between 1980 and the end of the millennium the US rate of adult obesity doubled to 31 per cent and is now around 34 per cent (Figure 9.5). The stated aim of the US government in 1992 (DHHS, 1992) was that, by the year 2000, no more than 20 per cent of Americans should have BMIs that exceed 27.8 for men and 27.3 for women (these cut-off points were widely used in the USA at this time). The number

of people exceeding these thresholds in 2000 was at least twice this 20 per cent target. A more recent US target is to reduce adult obesity prevalence (BMI >30) to 15 per cent.

Table 9.2 shows the percentage of English adults who have high waist circumferences and high WHR. Over 30 per cent of men have a waist measurement in excess of 102 cm and almost 45 per cent of women a measurement of over 88 cm. As with BMI, the prevalence of high waist measurement and high WHR increases greatly with age in both sexes up to 75 years of age, but declines in the over-75s. Table 9.2 shows that there were modest increases in overall prevalence of high waist circumference in men and women between 2003 and 2009 but closer examination of the data shows that there were substantial increases in prevalence in the older age groups, especially in women.

A worldwide perspective

The prevalence of obesity is rising not just in the UK and USA but throughout the industrialized world. According to WHO (2006), more than a billion

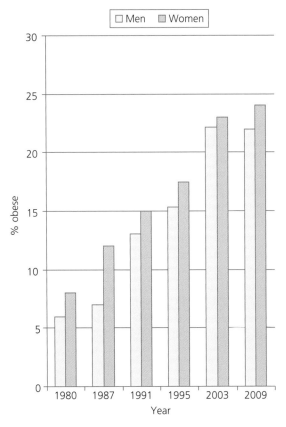

Figure 9.4 Changes in the prevalence of obesity in English adults.

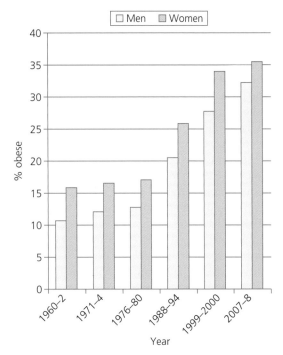

Figure 9.5 Changes in the prevalence of adult obesity in the USA.

Table 9.2 Percentages of English men and women above the threshold values indicative of raised waist-to-hip ratio and raised waist circumference, by age*

Age (years)	Waist-to-hip ratio (WHR)[1]		Waist circumference[1]	
	Men	Women	Men	Women
16–24	4	11	9 (8)	21 (18)
25–34	14	18	20 (19)	30 (26)
35–44	32	26	30 (27)	37 (39)
45–54	41	28	38 (41)	42 (51)
55–64	54	42	41 (48)	51 (58)
65–74	57	45	49 (54)	61 (68)
75+	51	54	31 (40)	41 (56)
All ages	33	30	31 (32)	41 (44)

*Most data are from Sproston and Primatesta (2004), but the figures in parentheses are the latest available waist circumference values from the *Health Survey for England*.
[1] WHR is 0.95 for men, 0.85 for women; raised waist circumference is 102 cm for men, 88 cm for women.

adults around the world were overweight, with at least 300 million of them clinically obese (BMI >30), and these figures will undoubtedly have increased substantially since 2006. The WHO data suggest that obesity rates have trebled since 1980 in eastern Europe, the Middle East, the Pacific Islands,

Australasia and China. The epidemic of obesity is not just confined to industrialized countries but is also affecting many developing countries; indeed, the rate of increase in some developing countries is even higher than in the industrialized world. In some developing countries there is obesity in parts of the country (often urban areas) or in affluent sectors of the population while in other areas or in the poorer sectors of society there may be widespread under-nutrition.

Figure 9.6 shows WHO estimates of prevalence of obesity and overweight in 10 selected European countries and 10 from outside Europe.

Figure 9.6a shows that, in the each country in the European sample, 40 per cent or more of adults are classified as overweight. The prevalence of obesity in these same European countries is shown in Figure 9.6c, and the rate of obesity varies from around 10 per cent or less in France, the Netherlands and Sweden to around 20 per cent or even more in Greece, the UK, Germany and Finland. The data for

the Russian Federation show a very large sex difference, with fewer than 10 per cent of Russian men classified as obese but approaching 25 per cent of Russian women. Data from individual countries suggest that rates of overweight and obesity are rising in almost all European countries.

Figures 9.6b and 9.6d show rates of overweight and obesity in the 10 selected non-European countries. The variation in prevalence is much greater than with the European countries because this sample includes countries at varying stages of industrial development. In the most industrialized countries including Australia, Israel and the USA rates are similar to those seen in Europe, but rates are much lower in China, Nigeria, Tanzania and India. The data for Samoa (WSM) in 9.6b and 9.6d are particularly striking: almost 80 per cent of Samoan adults are overweight and over 45 per cent are obese (about 54 per cent of Samoan women are obese). Hodge *et al.* (1994) reported that, in urban areas of what was then Western Samoa, 60 per cent

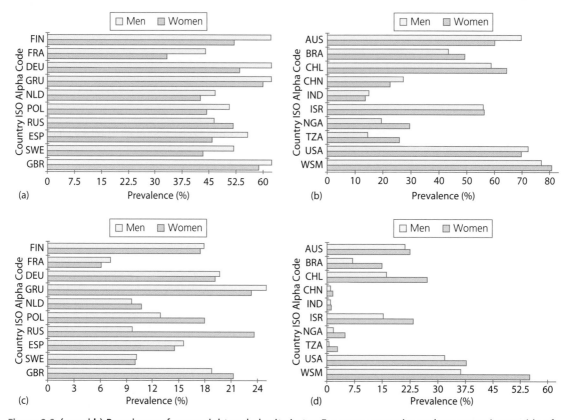

Figure 9.6 (**a and b**) Prevalence of overweight and obesity in ten European countries and ten countries outside of Europe. (**c and d**) Overweight defined as BMI > 25 and obesity as BMI > 30.

of men and 75 per cent of women were obese, and fewer than 10 per cent were not overweight. Hodge's team also reported large increases in obesity rates in all regions of Western Samoa over the period 1978–91, but increases in the rural areas were particularly dramatic; for example, in men in the rural Tuasivi region, obesity rates quadrupled in 13 years. In 1978 there was a large urban–rural difference in obesity rates in Western Samoa. Obesity rates were much higher in the urban areas where many people were employed in sedentary jobs and had ready access to imported Western foods, but less prevalent in the rural areas where the diet and lifestyle were more traditional. With increasing development and industrialization, the rural populations are rapidly becoming as obese as their urban neighbours (see sample figures in Table 9.3).

The four graphs that make up Figure 9.6 have been produced using a WHO website: http://infobase.who.int. This site gives access to a regularly updated database containing statistical information on rates of non-communicable diseases (including diabetes and stroke) in most countries of the world, and about risk factors for non-communicable diseases (including BMI, blood pressure, blood cholesterol concentration, alcohol and tobacco use and physical activity).

Effects of ethnicity and social status on obesity prevalence

The normal ranges and cut-off levels for BMI, WHR and waist circumference have largely come out of work with Europeans, so their suitability for use

Table 9.3 Changes in the prevalence of obesity (percentage with BMI >30) in selected areas of (Western) Samoa*

Region	1978	1991
Apia (urban)		
Men	38.7	58.5
Women	61.2	77.7
Tuasivi (rural)		
Men	9.9	39.3
Women	26.6	57.2

*Data are from Hodge et al. (1994).

with other ethnic groups has not been fully evaluated. It has been suggested, for example, that the threshold value for overweight in South Asians should be $23\,kg/m^2$ because the health risks associated with being overweight are greater in this group. A 4 cm reduction in the threshold for healthy waist circumference has also been suggested for South Asian and Chinese men. However, as no generally agreed alternative ethnic specific ranges and cut-off points have been agreed, those listed at the start of the chapter are still used for all ethnic groups in this chapter.

Within the UK and USA, there are marked differences in the prevalence of obesity between socioeconomic and ethnic groups. In the USA, obesity (and type 2 diabetes) is much more prevalent among certain Native American tribes like the Pima of Arizona than it is in the white population. Table 9.4 shows the prevalence of overweight/obesity (BMI >25) and obesity (BMI >30) in the three major ethnic groupings in the USA. At the beginning of this millennium, substantial ethnic differences were apparent in women with considerably greater rates of overweight and obesity in Mexican-American and black women than in white women; more recent data confirm this pattern. In American men, rates of obesity in 2000 were similar in the three ethnic groups, although Mexican-American men were much more likely to be overweight. The more recent data suggest that obesity prevalence has risen in men in all three ethnic groups but has risen faster in the black and Mexican-Americans so that obesity prevalence is now significantly greater in men from these two ethnic groups than in the white population in men as well as in women.

Table 9.5 shows the percentage of women of various ethnic groupings in England who have a BMI of over 25 or over 30. Obesity in women is more prevalent in black Africans, black Caribbeans and Pakistanis than it is in the general population, but much lower in Chinese women. In men, the prevalence is lower in black Africans, Indians and Pakistanis and much lower in Chinese and Bangladeshi men.

It has been generally accepted that South Asians are more prone to abdominal obesity than some other ethnic groups and have a higher WHR or waist circumference at any given BMI than Europeans.

Table 9.4 Ethnic differences in prevalence of overweight and obesity in the USA*

	BMI 25+ (%)	BMI 30+ (%)
Men		
White	67.4	27.3 (31.9)
Black	60.7	28.1 (37.3)
Mexican-American	74.7	28.9 (35.9)
Women		
White	57.3	30.1 (33.0)
Black	77.3	49.7 (49.6)
Mexican-American	71.9	39.7 (45.1)

*Most data are from Flegal *et al.* (2002), but figures in parentheses are the latest 2007–8 obesity rates from Ogden *et al.* (2010). BMI, body mass index.

Table 9.5 Prevalence of obesity and overweight among adults of ethnic groupings in England

Ethnic group	BMI 25+ (%)		BMI 30+ (%)	
	Men	Women	Men	Women
Black Caribbean	67	65	25	32
Black African	62	70	17	38
Indian	53	55	14	20
Pakistani	55	62	15	28
Bangladeshi	44	51	6	17
Chinese	37	25	6	8
Irish	67	58	25	21
General	67	57	23	23

BMI, body mass index.

Table 9.6 shows the percentage of men and women in different ethnic groups in England who have waist circumferences or WHR that exceed the healthy threshold values. Some values for South Asians in this table are indeed significantly above those for the general population – WHR for Pakistani and Bangladeshi women and waist circumference for Pakistani women. However, some other values are well below those for the general population – waist circumference for Indian and Bangladeshi men. The WHR values for Asian men are at or above those of the general population despite the lower levels of obesity in these groups shown in Table 9.5; that is, they are consistent with the suggestion that WHR is higher in South Asian men at any given BMI.

Table 9.6 Percentage of English adults from selected ethnic groups who have a high weight-to-hip ratio or high waist circumference

Ethnic group	Waist-to-hip ratio (WHR)[1]		Waist circumference[1]	
	Men	Women	Men	Women
Black Caribbean	25	37	22	47
Indian	38	30	20	38
Pakistani	36	39	30	48
Bangladeshi	32	50	12	43
All	33	30	31	41

[1] WHR is > 0.95 for men, > 0.85 for women; raised waist circumference is > 102 cm for men, > 88 cm for women.

In the industrialized countries, obesity is more prevalent in the lower socioeconomic groups and among the less well educated. Table 9.7 shows obesity rates in different socioeconomic groupings using a descriptive classification. The table shows a pronounced trend for increased prevalence of obesity in English women as one looks down the socioeconomic scale. This class-related pattern of obesity is less clear in English men, although rates in the two highest social categories are significantly lower than those in the lower three.

Table 9.8 shows data from the *Health Survey for England* in which rates of overweight, obesity and high waist circumference are shown in English men and women grouped according to quintile of household income. In women, the prevalence of both obesity and high waist circumference tends to

Table 9.7 Percentages of English adults who are obese (BMI 30+) in different socioeconomic groupings*

Grouping[1]	Men	Women
Managerial/professional	20.9	18.7
Intermediate	19.7	18.7
Small employers and own account workers	26.7	20.5
Lower supervisory and technical	24.9	28.8
Semi-routine and routine	21.6	29.1

*Data are from Sproston and Primatesta (2004).
[1] This socioeconomic classification is based on the current or former occupation of the household reference person (HRP).

Table 9.8 Percentages of English adults by quintile of household income who are overweight (BMI 25–30) or obese (BMI 30+) or have a high waist circumference

Income quintile	Overweight		Obese		Waist circumference[1]	
	Men	Women	Men	Women	Men	Women
Highest	48	31	20	17	28	36
2nd	44	33	21	21	32	45
3rd	48	31	21	27	32	42
4th	37	33	28	27	37	49
Lowest	36	33	22	33	32	51

[1] A high waist circumference is defined as at least 102 cm for men and 88 cm for women.

rise with declining household income – similar to the pattern seen in the earlier data shown in Table 9.7. In men, there is no clear trend across the income groups; perhaps this is because some men in the lower social grouping are still employed in manual jobs which may lower obesity rates in these groups.

There is a strong inverse correlation between level of educational attainment and obesity; those with higher levels of education are less likely to become obese than those with more limited education. Molarius *et al.* (2000) related BMI to educational attainment in 26 populations around the world using WHO data. They found that lower educational attainment was associated with higher BMI in almost all the 26 female populations and in about half of the male populations. They also found that these differences between BMI in groups with different levels of educational attainment had widened over a 10-year period. Sobal and Stunkard (1989) reviewed the influence of socioeconomic status on obesity around the world. They concluded that, in industrialized countries, obesity tends to be more prevalent among the lower socioeconomic groups, whereas in poorer countries it is more common in the upper social groups because only the relatively affluent have the opportunity to get fat. This is most obviously seen in countries where obesity and under-nutrition co-exist in different sections of the population; one of the major factors leading to obesity in such countries is a relatively affluent urban lifestyle.

Overweight and obesity in children

One problem with estimating the prevalence of overweight and obesity in children has been the lack of agreed international standards of classification. In Chapter 3, a set of international standards devised by Cole *et al.* (2000) is discussed. This estimated the BMI of girls and boys at various ages that are equivalent to the cut-off values for overweight (BMI $>25 \text{ kg/m}^2$) and obesity ($>30 \text{ kg/m}^2$). Sample numerical values are given in Chapter 3 and these standards are shown in graphical format in Figure 9.7.

Until quite recently, obesity in children, although rising, was still relatively uncommon. However, a WHO fact sheet (WHO, 2006) indicated that childhood obesity is now epidemic in some parts of the world and rising in other areas. The International Obesity Task Force (Lobstein *et al.*, 2004) estimated that about 10 per cent of school-aged children were overweight (155 million) and 30–40 million of these could be classified as obese; that is, 2–3 per cent of all the world's children aged 5–17 years. In addition, around 22 million children aged under 5 years are estimated to be overweight.

Using the international classification of Cole *et al.* (2000), 22 per cent of boys and 27.5 per cent of girls in the UK aged 2–15 years were estimated to be overweight in 2002, and this included 5.5 per cent of boys and 7.2 per cent of girls classified as obese. These percentages translate into around 2.4 million British children being overweight and 700 000 of these being obese. The trends for overweight and obesity in UK children between 1974 and 2002 are very like those already described for adults, with levels of overweight rising from around 7 per cent of children being overweight and only around 1 per cent being obese in the mid-1970s to an estimated 27 and 7 per cent, respectively, in 2002. Rates of increase have been particularly high in children in the 7–11 years age band: Figure 9.8 shows changes

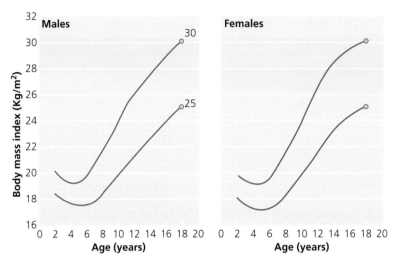

Figure 9.7 Body mass indices in children at different ages, corresponding to adult values of BMI of 25 and 30. Redrawn from Cole *et al.* (2000) by kind permission of BMJ Publishing Group.

in the prevalence of overweight and obesity in this age group over this 25-year period.

Data from the 2009 *Health Survey for England* are not directly comparable to those in Figure 9.8 because the results are reported in different age bandings and a UK-based classification

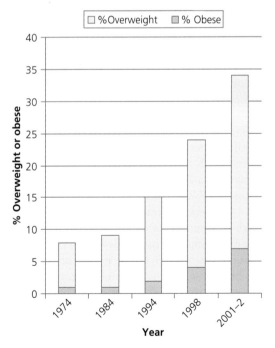

Figure 9.8 Changes in the prevalence of overweight and obesity in English children aged 7–11 years.

system is used to define overweight and obesity; this gives numerical values that may be substantially different but shows similar trends. This survey found that, between 1995 and 2009, average BMI increased by 0.6 kg/m² for boys and 0.4 kg/m² for girls aged 2–15 years. Over this same period, the prevalence of obesity increased in boys (from 11 to 16 per cent) and girls (from 12 to 15 per cent) and the prevalence of overweight also increased in both boys (from 24 to 31 per cent) and girls (from 26 to 28 per cent). There is some indication from these data that rates of overweight and obesity in both sexes appeared to peak in 2004–5 and fell slightly in the 4 years to 2009.

Similar trends to those in the UK have been documented in US children. The number of overweight children (6–11 years) has more than doubled since 1980 and the number of overweight adolescents (12–17 years) has trebled over the same period. Rates of increase have been particularly high in black and Mexican-American children. Numerical values for US children along with graphical analysis may be found in Ogden *et al.* (2002); they are summarized on the website of the National Center for Health Statistics. (Numerical values have not been given here because they have been calculated using American standards, not those of Cole's team.)

Key points

- Obesity rates are rising rapidly in most industrialized countries and in many developing countries.
- In England in 2009, 23 per cent of adults were obese and a further 44 per cent of men and 33 per cent of women were overweight.
- More than two-thirds of US adults have a BMI of over 25 and 34 per cent are classified as obese.
- In 1980 it was estimated that only 6 per cent of English men and 8 per cent of women were obese.
- The proportion of people who are overweight or obese rises steeply throughout early adulthood and middle age. Well over 70 per cent of English people aged 45–64 years have a BMI above 25.
- In the USA, obesity peaks in the 60- to 69-year age group where 40 per cent are obese.
- Over 30 per cent of English men and 45 per cent of women have a high waist measurement (>102 cm or >88 cm respectively).
- Prevalence of high waist circumference and high waist-to-hip ratio increases with age in a similar pattern to overweight and obesity.
- Prevalence of raised waist circumference increased modestly between 2003 and 2009, but there were substantial increases in prevalence in older age groups of both sexes.
- In the USA, obesity is much more prevalent among certain tribes of Native Americans. It is also more prevalent in Mexican-Americans and black Americans than it is in white Americans.
- In 2000, rates of obesity in US men were similar in the three ethnic groupings. In the last decade, rates have increased faster in Mexican and black American men.
- In women in England, obesity is more prevalent in black Africans, black Caribbeans and Pakistanis but much less prevalent in Chinese women than in the general population.
- In men in England, obesity is less prevalent in black Africans, Indians and Pakistanis and much lower in Chinese and Bangladeshi men.
- Data for waist circumference and WHR in different ethnic groups are consistent with the suggestion that South Asians have a higher WHR for any given BMI than the white population.

→

Key points *continued*

- There is some debate about whether the thresholds used for BMI, WHR and waist circumference are appropriate for all ethnic groups. In particular, a lower BMI threshold for obesity has been suggested for South Asians and a lower waist threshold for Asian men.
- In industrialized countries, obesity is more prevalent in the lower socioeconomic groups and less well-educated sectors of the population. In England, this trend is particularly pronounced in women.
- Internationally there is a marked tendency for BMI to be higher in those with the lowest educational attainment.
- In some developing countries, obesity may be more prevalent in the upper socioeconomic grouping because it is only these groups that have the opportunity to get fat by overeating and being sedentary.
- Overweight and obesity in children are also rising rapidly, with perhaps 10 per cent of the world's school-aged children overweight and 2–3 per cent obese. A quarter of UK children aged 2–15 years are overweight and 7 per cent of them are obese, using international standards.
- Prevalences of overweight and obesity in UK and US children have increased several-fold since the mid-1970s. There is some very preliminary indication that obesity rates in UK children may have peaked in 2004–5.

CONSEQUENCES OF OBESITY

The relationship between BMI and life expectancy

Studies conducted by life insurance companies since early in the twentieth century have found that being overweight or obese is associated with excess mortality and that mortality rises steeply when BMI is over 30; mortality ratio is doubled at a BMI of around 35. In a study of 200 morbidly obese American men, death rates were 12 times higher than normal in those aged 25–34 and still three times higher than normal in the 45–54 age group when the total number of deaths is much higher (Drenick *et al.*, 1980).

According to life insurance studies, the health effects of obesity seem to be greater in men than in women. Such studies usually show some increase in mortality in those who are underweight as well as in those who are overweight; that is, there is a so-called *J-curve* when mortality is plotted against BMI. This idea of a J-curve is now generally accepted (e.g. Hill *et al.*, 2006). The higher death rate at low BMI has usually been explained by suggesting that being underweight is often an indicator of poor health, or the result of smoking or of alcohol or drug abuse. Smoking, for example, is known to depress body weight and is also a cause of much ill-health and many premature deaths. Figure 9.9 uses data from the Nurses' Health Study discussed in Chapter 3 and shows a typical J-curve of mortality against BMI. However, the figure also shows the results from this study when the following 'corrections' were made:

- those who died within the first 4 years were excluded (i.e. already in poor health when the study started?)
- when only those whose weight was stable at the start of the study were included (recent

unintentional weight loss may be an indicator of existing ill-health)
- when only women who had never smoked were included (smoking damages health and lowers body weight).

The J-curve disappears when these women are excluded. The increase in death rate with increasing BMI is also more pronounced. These data suggest that raised mortality among smokers and women whose weight is depressed by poor health tends to obscure the strength and steepness of the association between BMI and mortality.

The mortality risk associated with being overweight or obese seems to be greater in young people. Andres *et al.* (1985) used life insurance data to calculate the BMI associated with the lowest risk of dying during the follow-up period in various age bands. This analysis is summarized in Figure 9.10. It seems to indicate that the 'ideal BMI' (the one associated with lowest mortality risk) appears to rise progressively with age. Although the data used to construct Figure 9.10 are now more than 25 years old, more recent evidence is presented in Chapter 16 which indicate an apparent protective effect of overweight in the elderly and very elderly.

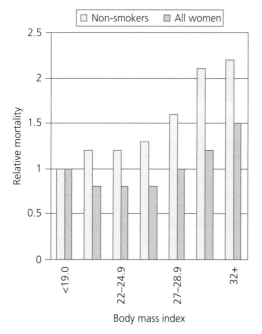

Figure 9.9 The J-curve of BMI and mortality, and the effects of smoking – see text for details. Data from Manson *et al.* (1995).

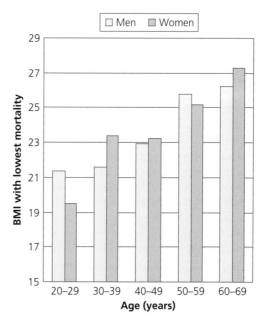

Figure 9.10 Effects of age on the apparent 'ideal' BMI. Data from Andres *et al.* (1985).

Box 9.1 shows a list of conditions that are associated with high BMI and which are probably caused or worsened by obesity. Increased numbers of premature deaths from some of these conditions are largely responsible for the increased mortality and reduced life expectancy of obese people. Death rates from stroke, coronary heart disease, type 2 diabetes, diseases of the liver and digestive system and certain cancers in women are particularly high in the obese. The WHO has suggested that approximately 58 per cent of diabetes, 21 per cent of ischemic heart disease and 8–42 per cent of cancers in the world are attributable to a BMI in excess of 21 kg/m².

Box 9.1

Some conditions thought to be caused by obesity or worsened by it

Heart and circulatory system

- Coronary heart disease
- Stroke
- Hypertension
- Angina pectoris
- Sudden death due to ventricular arrhythmia (abnormal heart rhythm)
- Congestive heart failure
- Varicose veins, haemorrhoids, swollen ankles, and venous thrombosis

Joints

- Osteoarthritis – knees

Endocrine/metabolic

- Type 2 diabetes (maturity-onset diabetes)
- Gout
- Gallstones

Cancer

- In women – increased risk of cancer of the ovary, cervix (neck of womb), breast and endometrium (lining of womb)
- In men – increased risk of prostate cancer and cancers of the colon and rectum

Other

- Increased risk of pregnancy complications
- Reduced fertility
- Menstrual irregularities
- Increased risk during anaesthesia and surgery
- Reduced mobility and agility, and increased risk of accidents

➜

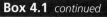

Box 4.1 *continued*

- Adverse psychological, social and economic consequences (see later in the chapter)

Risk factors

- Raised blood lipids, including blood cholesterol
- Raised blood uric acid levels
- Elevation of blood pressure
- Insulin resistance
- Increased plasma fibrinogen concentration

Obesity and the quality of life

Some of the conditions listed in Box 9.1 may cause ill-health and disability even if they are unlikely to be a primary cause of death (e.g. gout and arthritis). Type 2 diabetes increases the risk of cardiovascular disease and strokes and also leads to a number of problems that are disabling even though not necessarily acutely fatal (e.g. blindness, peripheral neuropathy, gangrene and progressive renal failure – see Chapter 17).

One Finnish study (Rissanen *et al.*, 1990) found that overweight people were much more likely to claim a disability pension than people with a normal weight. The authors concluded that being overweight is a major cause of disability in Finland. This effect of overweight on disability seemed to start at relatively low BMIs where the effect on mortality is usually small or non-existent (>25 for women and >27 for men). The effect of overweight on disability also seemed to be more pronounced in women than in men. Being overweight or obese not only shortens life but also reduces the proportion of life that is spent free of major illness and disability. More recently, Walter *et al.* (2009) found no association between BMI and mortality in a large sample of older Europeans. They did, however, find that increased BMI was associated with a higher risk of becoming and remaining disabled, so more of the life expectancy in obese people comprised years of living with a disability. In the USA, it has been reported that obese workers take increased amounts of sick leave and have higher numbers of disability claims. The direct medical costs of obesity in the USA were estimated to represent more than 7 per cent of the total healthcare budget in 1995, and that the costs of higher rates of sick leave and disability claims cost US businesses more than $3 billion at 1996 prices (about $4.5 billion at 2011 prices).

Also listed in Box 9.1 are several risk factors for heart disease that are elevated in the obese. Risk factors are parameters that predict the risk of developing or dying of particular diseases and in many cases are assumed to contribute to the cause of the disease. It is increases in these risk factors that probably cause much of the excess mortality of obese people. In a large survey of English adults, Bennett et al. (1995) found the following examples of associations between BMI and cardiovascular risk factors.

- Overweight and obese people have high blood pressure. In this survey, people with a BMI over 30 had double the risk of hypertension compared with people with a BMI in the 20–25 range. Blood pressure rose with increasing BMI in all age and sex groups. Sproston and Primatesta (2004) have confirmed a progressive increase in systolic blood pressure in both men and women in England as one goes up the standard BMI categories shown in Table 9.1.
- Overweight and obese people have reduced insulin sensitivity and high average blood glucose concentrations (early indications of the onset of type 2 diabetes). Glycosylated haemoglobin concentration in blood tends to rise with average blood glucose concentration and so it is used as a marker for high blood glucose concentration. In this survey, obese people had the highest levels of glycosylated haemoglobin and those with a BMI of less than 20 had the lowest levels.
- People who are overweight or obese tend to have the highest blood cholesterol levels. In this survey there was a clear tendency for blood cholesterol to rise with increasing BMI.
- Obese people in this survey tended to have increased plasma uric acid levels
- Plasma fibrinogen concentration is used as an indicator of the blood's tendency to clot and form thromboses. Plasma fibrinogen concentration rose with increasing BMI in this survey.

In general, these risk factors tend to rise during weight gain and they tend to fall during weight reduction. This indicates that weight gain per se, or the behaviours that lead to weight gain, are the direct cause of these elevated risk factor levels. Type 2 diabetes seems to be triggered by a decline in target tissue sensitivity to insulin (insulin resistance) rather than a primary failure of insulin secretion. In experimental studies, deliberate overfeeding and weight gain reduce insulin sensitivity in animals and people; insulin sensitivity increases during weight loss (e.g. Sims et al., 1973). Weight loss is known to lessen the symptoms of type 2 diabetes. According to Chan et al. (1994), for men in their forties, being moderately obese (BMI >31) increases the risk of developing type 2 diabetes by tenfold, and in those with a BMI over 35 the risk is 77 times higher. More recently it has been reported that obese English women were 13 times more likely than lean women to develop type 2 diabetes and obese men five times more likely to develop the disease (Information Centre, 2006). Type 2 diabetes has been regarded as a disease that is almost exclusively confined to older adults, but the disease has increasingly been found in young people and in children who are obese (Alberti et al., 2004).

Weight loss is also an accepted part of the treatment for hypertension and gout. Gout is the painful joint condition caused by crystals of uric acid forming in the joints when blood uric acid levels are elevated.

In addition to higher morbidity and mortality, there are major social and economic disadvantages to being obese. In some cultures, obesity may be admired as a symbol of wealth and success and fatness regarded as physically attractive. In most Western countries, however, the obese have long been poorly regarded and discriminated against. In his book on obesity, Mayer (1968) devotes a whole chapter to largely literary examples of hostility towards the obese, and Gilbert (1986) also includes a short, referenced review of negative attitudes towards the obese.

Several studies have been conducted in which children have been asked to rate the likeability of other children from pictures and to assign various character traits to them. They consistently rate the obese children in these pictures as less likeable than the lean and, in some studies, even less likeable than children with physical deformities such as missing limbs or facial disfigurement. They attribute unpleasant characteristics to the obese children in the pictures – comments like they are 'lazy', 'dirty', 'stupid', 'ugly' and that they are 'cheats' and 'liars'.

Basically similar attitudes are also widespread among adults of all social classes. Even among those professionally involved in the treatment of obesity, the obese may be seen as self-indulgent people who lack willpower and overeat to compensate for their emotional problems – these early studies are reviewed and referenced in Wadden and Stunkard (1985).

Obese people are subject to practical discrimination as well; they are less likely to be accepted for university education and for employment. Gortmaker *et al.* (1993) did a 7-year follow-up of 10 000 young people in Boston who were aged 16–24 years at the start of the study. They found that, particularly among women, there were substantial social and economic disadvantages to being obese. After 7 years, those women who were obese at the start of the study:

- had completed fewer years at school
- had lower household incomes and were more likely to be below the poverty line
- were less likely to be married (another study has reported that lower class women are much less likely to marry men of higher social class than lean lower class women).

Similar trends were seen in the men but the magnitude of the disadvantages attributed to being obese were substantially smaller. The investigators concluded that prejudice and discrimination were the main causes of these socioeconomic disadvantages of being obese. They were not due to differences in the socioeconomic status of the obese subjects at the start of the study, nor to differences in levels of ability as measured by initial performance of the young people on intelligence and aptitude tests. This conclusion was also supported by their finding that there was no evidence of similar reduced socioeconomic prospects for those subjects who at the start of the study were suffering from a chronic physical condition such as asthma, diabetes or a musculoskeletal problem. Such conditions could well have reduced physical performance, but being obese was more of a socioeconomic handicap over this 7-year period than suffering from one of these chronic conditions. It was noted earlier in this chapter that, in industrialized countries, obesity, especially among women, is more common in those with the lowest socioeconomic status and the least well-educated groups (see Tables 9.7 and 9.8). This is usually presented as low educational attainment and low social status being risk factors for obesity, but these observations also suggest that perhaps obesity may restrict educational opportunities and lower social status.

These negative attitudes to the obese may well be rooted in the historically assumed association between overweight, excessive food intake and inactivity; that is, obesity is widely assumed to be due to greed and laziness. The obese are seen as responsible for their own condition owing to the presence of these two undesirable personality traits.

Is all body fat equally bad?

Studies in the early 1980s indicated that the *waist-to-hip ratio* (WHR) was an important determinant of the health risks associated with obesity. This measure is the circumference of the body at the waist divided by that around the hips and it is used as a simple indicator of body fat distribution; waist circumference is also used as an even simpler indication of abdominal obesity. The health risks seem to be greater if the obesity is associated with a high WHR or large waist circumference – *abdominal obesity*. People with this type are sometimes called 'apple-shaped' and this is the typically male (ovoid) pattern of fat distribution. There is much less risk if the obesity is associated with a low WHR; this is termed 'pear-shaped' or gynoid and is the typically female pattern (early work reviewed by Seidell, 1992).

Figure 9.11, and data presented earlier in the chapter, indicate that – as with BMI – the numbers of people with a raised WHR and waist circumference rises with age in both sexes. They are also higher in women from lower socioeconomic groups, and seem to be a particular problem for some people of South Asian origin. Inactivity, smoking and high alcohol consumption also seem to be associated with high WHR and waist circumference. Sex hormones also affect fat distribution, and hormone replacement therapy (HRT) in post-menopausal women seems to reduce central fat deposition (Samaras and Campbell, 1997). Table 9.9 shows how the prevalence of high WHR and waist circumference increases progressively and sharply with decreasing activity level; WHR in the least active tertiles is almost double that in the most active (note that Figure 9.14 later in the chapter shows that BMI and prevalence of obesity also rise with decreasing activity level).

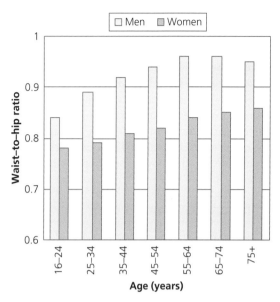

Figure 9.11 Rise in average waist-to-hip ratio (WHR) with age. Data from Sproston and Primatesta (2004).

Table 9.9 Percentages of English adults who have a raised waist-to-hip ratio (WHR) or raised waist circumference classified according to reported activity level

Activity level	Raised WHR		Raised waist circumference	
	Men	Women	Men	Women
High	24.3	22.1	23.4	30.4
Medium	29.4	26.1	28.9	36.2
Low	47.4	39.3	42.4	52.5

This research on waist-to-hip ratio and related measures suggests that fat deposited in the abdominal cavity may be largely responsible for the detrimental health consequences of being overweight or obese. Table 9.10 shows the guidelines for the UK's National Institute for Health and Clinical Excellence (NICE) about how having a raised waist circumference affects the health risks associated with different BMI categories. At BMI of up to 35, having a raised waist circumference increases the health risks associated with any particular BMI even for people within the normal range. Once BMI exceeds 35, all waist categories are classified as very high risk – although it is still probable that having a higher waist measurement compounds the risk.

Large amounts of abdominal fat seem to predispose people to diabetes and heart disease. The increase in heart disease may be largely a consequence of the predisposition to diabetes. South Asians seem to be particularly prone to diabetes and heart disease and have higher WHRs than Caucasians at any given BMI (see Chapter 18). The fat cells in the abdominal cavity have different metabolic characteristics and hormone receptor profiles from those of fat cells taken from subcutaneous sites. The abdominal fat cells of obese women have fewer insulin receptors and the receptors have lower affinity for insulin compared to fat cells taken from a subcutaneous site in the same women. Thus high levels of abdominal obesity predispose individuals to type 2 diabetes and the other adverse health consequences of abdominal obesity are probably secondary to this increased risk of diabetes (Bolinder *et al.*, 1983; Zierath *et al.*, 1998).

Table 9.10 Health risks associated with a raised BMI and high waist circumference

BMI	Waist circumference		
	Low	High	Very high
(Men)	(<94 cm)	(94–102 cm)	(>102 cm)
(Women)	(<80 cm)	(80–88 cm)	(>88 cm)
18.5–25	No ↑ risk	No ↑ risk	↑ risk
25–30	No ↑ risk	↑ risk	High risk
30–35	↑ risk	High risk	Very high risk
35–40	Very high risk	Very high risk	Very high risk
40+	Very high risk	Very high risk	Very high risk

Weight cycling

In line with the high prevalence of obesity, there is also a high prevalence of weight dissatisfaction and dieting, particularly among women. At any one time, perhaps a third of American women are dieting and studies in England and Ireland have found that most adolescent girls have tried to lose weight (Ryan *et al.*, 1998). Many dieters fail to lose significant amounts of weight, whereas many others do achieve substantial short-term weight losses only to regain this weight once their diet is relaxed. This cycle of weight loss and regain has been termed *weight cycling* or *yo-yo dieting*.

It is a common perception that people find it increasingly difficult to lose weight after previous cycles of weight loss and regain. One obvious explanation for this observation is simply that it becomes increasingly difficult for people to summon up the effort and willpower to stick to a weight reduction programme after being dispirited by previous experiences of rapid weight regain. It has also been suggested that cycles of weight loss and regain might lower metabolic rate and so predispose people to weight gain because of the replacement of lean tissue by fat during these cycles of loss and regain. Studies that have attempted to test this hypothesis with animals or people have generally not found evidence to support it (e.g. Jebb *et al.*, 1991).

Weight fluctuation is also associated with increased mortality risk, leading to speculation that yo-yo dieting might have detrimental health effects *per se*. One large American study did indeed find that men who had experienced weight loss or weight fluctuation had an elevated mortality risk. However, when smokers and those with existing ill-health were excluded from the analysis, this association between weight fluctuation and elevated mortality risk disappeared. This led the authors to conclude that any association between weight fluctuation and elevated mortality is due to the effects of pre-existing illness and smoking and that weight cycling is not, in itself, directly harmful to health (Iribarren *et al.*, 1995). A major report in the USA (National Task Force, 1994) concluded that possible concerns about any hazards associated with weight cycling should not deter obese people from trying to lose weight. Note, however, that many patients with eating disorders do have a history of yo-yo dieting.

Does high BMI directly cause an increase in mortality?

The earlier observation that risk factors (e.g. blood pressure and insulin resistance) tend to rise and fall with induced changes in body weight provides persuasive support for the belief that the association between BMI and mortality is a cause-and-effect relationship. There are two probable scenarios:

- *either* the presence of excessive amounts of body fat directly hastens death via development of the diseases in Box 9.1
- *or* the behaviours that cause people to gain weight also increase the risk of ill-health.

Such a subtle distinction might seem to be pedantic because in either case changes in behaviour that prevent or reduce obesity should lead to corresponding improvements in health and longevity. Some work at the University of Texas by a group led by Dr Steven Blair (e.g. Lee *et al.*, 1998) suggests that this may be a significant distinction. They related measured fitness to all-cause mortality in a large sample of men divided into strata on the basis of their BMIs. They found, as one might expect, that in each BMI stratum, mortality was inversely related to fitness (i.e. the fit were less likely to die). More surprisingly, they also found that men in the high and moderate fitness categories had similar death rates irrespective of BMI category (even those in the BMI 30+ category) and that men in the unfit category had high death rates again irrespective of their BMI category. This suggests that men with high BMIs have high mortality because they are much more likely to be inactive and unfit, so the inactivity and lack of fitness are the common cause of both their high BMI and high mortality risk. More encouragingly, this would also suggest that increasing activity and improving fitness could substantially reduce the adverse health consequences of overweight and obesity even if it does not lead to substantial weight loss.

This lends support to the suggestion in an editorial in the influential *New England Journal of Medicine* (Byers, 1995) that the emphasis of research and health education should be shifted away from body weight *per se* and focus more on the behaviours that lead to excessive weight gain. Rather than focusing on body weight reduction, we should concentrate more on encouraging healthier food choices and increased physical activity and on reducing the behavioural and cultural barriers that prevent people from adopting this lifestyle pattern.

In a recent review, McCauley and Blair (2011) reiterated the conclusion that physical fitness offsets the excess mortality associated with obesity. They go on to suggest that low cardiorespiratory fitness and inactivity are a greater risk to health than obesity *per se*, and so more emphasis should be given to increasing fitness and physical activity as a strategy for reducing mortality risk in the general population of overweight and obese adults. They also suggest that being what they termed *pre-obese* (BMI 25–30 kg/m^2) is associated with reduced mortality risk.

This is an important point for those working in health education and health promotion to take on board. Huge numbers of people go on diets and spend lots of money on a variety of books and products in order to try, usually unsuccessfully, to achieve an 'ideal' body shape. The severe social and psychological consequences of being obese mean that very few people are content to be obese and many people are desperate to become or remain lean and are willing to adopt desperate measures to achieve this. Despite this, obesity rates continue to increase. The work of Harris (1983) exemplifies this almost universal wish to be lean. She asked Australian psychology students how they would feel about being obese themselves. All of the students gave negative responses to this question and 60 per cent chose the highest level of negative response offered. Studies with teenage girls in the UK and Ireland have found a high level of dissatisfaction with their body weight. For example, Ryan *et al.* (1998) found that 60 per cent of a sample of 15-year-old Dublin schoolgirls wanted to be slimmer and 68 per cent had tried to lose weight. Most worryingly, many normal-weight and even underweight girls also expressed this wish to be thinner. Many of these girls reported using a variety of unhealthy practices to try to lose weight, including purging, smoking, periodic fasting and avoidance of staple foods.

Health promotion campaigns that focus on body fat *per se* are, at best, probably pointless because most people already desperately want to become or remain lean. At worst, they may increase the prejudice and discrimination against obese people and push some impressionable young people into trying to lose weight when it is inappropriate and using methods that are harmful.

Key points

- An elevated BMI is associated with reduced life expectancy, increased risk of illness and disability, and increased levels of cardiovascular risk factors.

- Increased prevalence of childhood obesity means that type 2 diabetes, once a disease confined to older adults, is now being increasingly recorded in children and adolescents.

- The health consequences of obesity are greater in the young and probably greater in men.

- Low BMI is also associated with reduced life expectancy, but this is probably because of an excess of smokers and those with existing ill-health in this category.

- Obesity has adverse social and economic consequences for the individual; obese people, especially women, are the subject of widespread prejudice and discrimination.

- Obesity that is associated with a high waist-to-hip ratio or a high waist circumference is more harmful than if the waist-to-hip ratio is low. Excess fat stored in the abdominal cavity is largely responsible for the adverse health consequences of obesity.

- Abdominal fat cells from obese subjects have fewer insulin receptors and these receptors have lower affinity for insulin than those taken from subcutaneous sites.

- Increased predisposition to type 2 diabetes caused by high levels of abdominal fat is probably responsible for the adverse health consequences of abdominal obesity.

- There is no convincing evidence that cycles of weight loss and regain (yo-yo dieting) are directly harmful to health or have physiological consequences that predispose to obesity. Excess mortality associated with yo-yo dieting may be largely due to the weight instability of many smokers and those with existing ill-health.

→

- Cardiovascular risk factor levels (e.g. insulin resistance and blood pressure) tend to rise and fall with weight gain and loss. This suggests that the relationships are probably causal; that is, either weight gain *per se* or the behaviours that cause weight gain are responsible for the elevated risk factor levels.

- The inactivity and low physical fitness of many obese people may be largely responsible for both their obesity and their reduced health prospects.

- Health promotion should concentrate on encouraging and enabling people to increase their activity and fitness and to eat a healthy low-fat diet.

- Most people already desperately want to become or remain lean, so health promotion campaigns that focus on body weight *per se* may achieve little. They may simply:
  - increase prejudice and discrimination against the obese
  - increase the dissatisfaction and unhappiness of overweight and obese people
  - encourage some young people to aim for an inappropriately low body weight and adopt harmful strategies to achieve it.

THE METABOLIC SYNDROME OR 'SYNDROME X'

Type 2 diabetes accounts for 85 per cent of all diabetics in the UK and is by far the most common endocrine disorder. This type of diabetes is now known to be caused by insulin resistance rather than a primary failure of insulin supply. In type 2 diabetes, lifestyle factors including inactivity, high food intake, obesity (particularly abdominal obesity) and a high-fat diet lead to insulin resistance. Those people who develop type 2 diabetes are unable to produce sufficient insulin to compensate for the decline in sensitivity and so there is a progressive shortfall in insulin supply leading to gradually increasing symptoms of diabetes. Many people with insulin resistance are able to compensate by raising their insulin production and thus are able to avoid the immediate symptoms of diabetes such as severe hyperglycaemia, glucose in the urine, high urine flow and excessive thirst and drinking. These non-diabetic but insulin-resistant individuals are,

however, subject to other metabolic consequences of insulin resistance, including:

- hyperinsulinaemia
- moderate glucose intolerance
- hypertension
- raised plasma triacylglycerol levels
- lowered plasma high-density lipoproteins (HDL) levels.

This cocktail of metabolic consequences of insulin resistance is termed the *metabolic syndrome*, or sometimes 'syndrome X'. While people with this syndrome do not have the acute symptoms of diabetes, their condition does nevertheless predispose them to cardiovascular disease in just the same way as does having overt type 2 diabetes. Many people with syndrome X will go on to develop overt type 2 diabetes. Any individual who meets three of the following criteria would be classified as having syndrome X:

- high waist circumference
- moderate fasting hyperglycaemia
- elevated blood pressure
- elevated blood triacylglycerol
- low plasma HDL.

Numerical thresholds for these criteria have been suggested by an American expert panel (APC III, 2002).

- Insulin resistance in the absence of overt type 2 diabetes still leads to hypertension, high blood triacylglycerol, reduced plasma HDL and some degree of hyperglycaemia.

- These metabolic consequences of insulin resistance are called the metabolic syndrome or syndrome X.

- Some people with syndrome X will develop diabetes and all of them will be predisposed to cardiovascular disease by their metabolic abnormalities.

CAUSES OF OBESITY

Evolutionary selection pressures?

During the course of human evolution, intermittent food shortages and an active lifestyle would have been the norm. The assured availability of a varied, highly palatable and energy-dense diet coupled with a negligible requirement for physical work would not have been a general experience. The reality would often have been a general state of food shortage or insecurity interspersed with occasional gluts of food. Those best equipped to cope with limited rations and to survive prolonged bouts of severe food shortage would be the most likely to survive, reproduce and pass on their genes. Some deposition of extra fat reserves during periods of abundance to act as a buffer during the almost inevitable periods of food shortage would have been a considerable aid to survival. Permanent and severe obesity is unlikely under these circumstances because, as explained in Chapter 8, energy expenditure tends to rise under conditions of energy surplus and this tends to restore energy balance. The monotony, low palatability and low energy density of primitive diets would have tended to limit excess consumption. Overweight and obese people may also have been at a disadvantage in the competition for food. Only where people have an unlimited supply of palatable, varied and energy-dense food, and where they can curtail their activity as they gain weight, would obesity be likely to be prevalent, progressive and often severe. The struggle to ensure energy adequacy and security would have been major selection pressures shaping our mechanisms of energy balance control. The need to prevent excess fat accumulation would have been a more minor influence.

Given these selection pressures, one would expect our regulatory mechanisms to be more efficient at preventing energy deficit rather than preventing energy surplus. Those best equipped to cope with periods of famine and shortage would be more likely to survive and reproduce, while those best equipped for conditions of continual plenty and inactivity would tend to be selected out during times of famine. It is therefore not too surprising that, under conditions of affluence and plenty, many people store more body fat than is desirable for their long-term health prospects. Some populations seem to be even more prone to obesity than Europeans and their descendants, examples being the Polynesian people of Samoa and some Native American tribes like the Pima Indians of Southern Arizona where the majority of the adult populations are clinically

obese. Often populations that have only recently adopted Western dietary and lifestyle habits and are historically accustomed to a harsher energy supply environment seem to be particularly prone to obesity and diabetes. They may have evolved a 'thrifty' genotype that makes them better able to survive such conditions. There is also some evidence that a period of food shortage in early life (or other adverse circumstances like cold exposure) may programme people to become obese in later life if environmental conditions allow it (Phillips, 1998).

Nature or nurture?

Both genetic and environmental influences must be involved in the genesis of obesity; only the relative contributions of nature and nurture are disputed. As explained in Chapter 8, certain rare genetic defects can cause profound obesity in animals and people. It is also possible to selectively breed animals for leanness or fatness. Dietary and environmental changes can also markedly affect the degree of fatness of laboratory or farm animals; for example, offering rats a varied, palatable and energy-rich diet when confined in cages ('cafeteria feeding') causes them to get fat. The situation of the cafeteria-fed rat seems to mimic the situation of many affluent humans.

There is a strong correlation between the fatness levels of parents and their children and between the fatness levels of siblings, but it is difficult to dissect out how much of this is due to common environmental factors and how much to shared genes. Several lines of enquiry point towards a considerable genetic component in this tendency of obesity to run in families.

- There is a much higher correlation between the fatness of monozygotic (identical) twins than between dizygotic (non-identical) twins. When they share the same environment, the fatness levels of the monozygotic twins are closer because they have the same genotype.
- When monozygotic twins are adopted and reared apart, their fatness levels are still very similar. Despite their differing environments, their identical genes mean that they show similar levels of fatness.
- Large studies of adopted children in Denmark suggest that correlations between the BMI of

adopted children and their natural first-degree relatives (parents and siblings) are similar to those in natural families. This suggests that family resemblances in adiposity are mostly due to genetic factors.

Of course, the environmental and dietary variation between Danish families may be relatively small and this will tend to exaggerate the prominence of genetic factors in determining obesity levels. See Sorensen (1992) for a referenced review of these genetic aspects of obesity.

While the papers upon which the above bullet-point statements are based are now rather old, Hill *et al.* (2006) have quoted a series of more recent papers that essentially repeat and confirm the findings. Hill's team also conclude that perhaps 40 per cent of the variation in BMI is explained by genetic factors.

Clearly, certain environmental conditions are necessary for the expression of any genetic tendency to obesity, but equally some individuals and some populations (e.g. the Samoans and Pima Indians mentioned earlier) do seem to be more susceptible than others.

The widespread use of animal models with some inherited or induced lesion that produces extreme obesity may have encouraged the view that 'obese' and 'lean' are two distinct categories. In reality, there will be a continuum of genetic susceptibility to obesity in people, ranging from very resistant to very susceptible. As the conditions in affluent countries have increasingly favoured the development of obesity, so more and more people's 'threshold of susceptibility' has been reached and so the number of overweight and obese people has risen. The recent large rises in the prevalence of obesity in many populations cannot be due to genetic change, they must be caused by lifestyle changes. The increase in obesity as one looks down the socioeconomic classes is also unlikely to be due primarily to genetics, particularly as it is much less obvious in men than women. The relatively low rates of obesity in some affluent European countries suggest that very high rates of obesity and rapid increases in its prevalence are not an inevitable consequence of affluence. The fact that obesity rates in England in 1980 were less than a third of current levels confirms that this change

must be the result of dietary and/or lifestyle changes. If English people reversed some of the lifestyle and dietary changes of the last few decades then one could expect corresponding falls in the levels of obesity.

Studies of the Pima Indians provide striking evidence of the need for environmental triggers to produce widespread obesity even in a population considered genetically susceptible to obesity. Several centuries ago, one group of Pima Indians settled in southern Arizona and another group settled in the mountains of Mexico. These two groups remain genetically very similar. Present-day Mexican Pimas do not suffer from widespread obesity; they are subsistence farmers who spend many hours each week in hard physical labour and still eat a fairly traditional low-fat high-carbohydrate diet. In contrast, the Arizona Pimas have ceased to be subsistence farmers; they are now a sedentary population, eating a typical high-fat American diet, so they have one of the highest rates of obesity in the world (Gibbs, 1996).

A weakening link between hunger and eating?

The internal/external hypothesis and behaviour therapy

Hunger is the drive or need to eat food that is initiated by the appestat in response to internal physiological signals such as the absence of food in the gut, low blood glucose concentration or depleted fat stores. As noted in Chapter 8, many 'external' factors in addition to physiological need determine when, where, what and how much we eat. Appetite, the desire to eat palatable food, may persist even after hunger has been quenched. Social convention, emotional state or just the hedonistic pleasure of eating may cause us to eat in the absence of hunger. Hunger will usually drive us to eat but absence of hunger will not necessarily prevent us from eating. By analogy, we do not have to be thirsty to make a cup of tea or to accept the offer of a social drink. Thirst will cause us to drink but we may drink for pleasure or to be sociable when we are not thirsty. We can easily excrete excess fluid but we are less well equipped to burn off surplus calories – notwithstanding the discussion of adaptive thermogenesis in Chapter 8.

Do modern diets and lifestyles weaken the link between hunger and eating and make us more prone to excessive consumption and weight gain?

Consider the following. For the majority of people in affluent populations:

- food is more consistently abundant than it has ever been
- less effort is required to prepare food and there is more encouragement to consume it (e.g. by advertising) than ever before
- food is more varied, palatable and energy-dense than it has ever been
- the requirement for food has never been lower because of our inactive lifestyles and the high energy density of our diets.

Schachter (1968) proposed that lean people regulate their food intake primarily in response to their internal physiological hunger mechanisms whereas obese people are much more responsive to external, non-physiological influences on their feeding behaviour. Schachter and Rodin (1974) identified certain behavioural characteristics of obese rats and then, in an ingenious series of experiments, demonstrated very similar behavioural characteristics in obese people. Some examples are given below.

- Obese rats and people consumed more food than leans when it was readily available but less than leans when they were required to work for the food. Obese rats generally ate more than leans, but if they were required to run through a maze to obtain food then the leans ate more than the obese. In another experiment, lean and fat people were offered nuts to eat in a disguised situation. If these nuts were opened and easy to eat, the obese subjects ate many more than the leans, but when the subjects had to crack them open for themselves the obese ate far fewer nuts than the leans.
- Obese rats and people consumed more than leans when the food was palatable but less when it was made unpalatable (e.g. by the addition of bitter-tasting quinine). They were more finicky.
- The feeding behaviour of obese rats and people was more affected by their anxiety state than was that of the leans.

Schacter and Rodin concluded that the feeding behaviour of obese rats and obese people was motivated primarily by appetite (the learned, hedonistic desire to eat food) rather than by hunger (the physiological need to eat food). The leans appeared to be driven to eat by hunger but the obese were persuaded to eat by ease of access, high palatability and for emotional comfort.

This theory has lost favour in recent years for the reason that external orientation of food regulation is not confined to the obese. Nevertheless, this theory has had a great practical influence on the treatment of obesity. Much of the behavioural treatment of obesity is based on this concept of external orientation of food intake regulation in obese people.

Behaviour is envisaged as being initiated by certain cues or antecedents. Then, if the behaviour results in pleasure, this acts as a reward or reinforcement and that behaviour is learned. If the behaviour has unpleasant consequences then this acts as negative reinforcement and discourages repetition of the behaviour (Figure 9.12). Thus obese people are triggered into inappropriate eating behaviour by certain circumstances or cues and their inappropriate behaviour is rewarded, and thus learned, because of the pleasure or relief of anxiety that results from the inappropriate eating behaviour. *Behaviour therapy* seeks to identify the cues or antecedents to inappropriate behaviour (e.g. eating high-energy foods). It then involves devising ways of avoiding these cues and ways of reinforcing or rewarding appropriate behaviours (e.g. taking exercise or achieving weight loss targets) so that they are 'learned'.

To identify the antecedents or cues that trigger inappropriate eating behaviour, patients are often asked to keep a diary of when and what they eat, and in what circumstances they eat it. They are then encouraged to modify their habits and environment to reduce these cues using techniques such as those below.

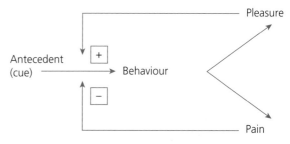

Figure 9.12 Pain or pleasure elicited by an action encourages learning and repetition of that action.

- They may be encouraged to avoid the temptation to buy high-energy foods on impulse, by shopping strictly from a list.
- They may reduce casual, impulse consumption of high-energy snacks by making them less accessible – for example, keeping them on a high shelf or in a locked cabinet so that this snacking has to be a premeditated act.
- They may reduce the temptation to pick at food they are preparing by encouraging other family members to prepare their own snacks.
- They can reduce the temptation to eat leftovers by throwing them away immediately.

They may be encouraged to modify the *process* of eating by:

- always using utensils and never eating with fingers
- slowing down the eating process by chewing food thoroughly, using a smaller spoon, pausing between mouthfuls or introducing a short gap in the meal
- never eating alone but always with other family members
- leaving some food on their plate at the end of a meal.

They are also encouraged to increase the cues to appropriate behaviour by, for example:

- keeping walking shoes and equipment for active pursuits in easily accessible and visible locations
- keeping low-energy snacks ready prepared and in a prominent place in the refrigerator.

Most therapists avoid the use of active 'punishment' in their schemes. Clients are encouraged to eat with others and ask them to praise and encourage appropriate behaviour but to pointedly ignore inappropriate behaviour and simply withhold praise. Scolding is seen as attention-giving and thus a form of reward, whereas withholding of attention is seen as punishment.

In the past, some behaviour therapists have used punishment as an active part of their programme – so-called *aversion therapy*. Patients were shown images of problem foods followed by painful electric shocks or some other unpleasant image in the hope that they would learn to associate these foods with unpleasant sensations and so avoid them.

A thorough and referenced review of the behavioural methods employed to treat obesity may be found in Gilbert (1986).

Food variety and sensory-specific satiety

Rolls *et al.* (1982) reviewed a series of experiments which seemed to suggest that increasing food variety may encourage increased consumption. Volunteers were asked to rate the pleasantness of foods after eating particular foods. Previous consumption of a food reduced its pleasantness rating and the desire to consume more of it, but had little effect on that of other foods; they termed this phenomenon *sensory-specific satiety*. When people ate sausages then their rating for sausages was reduced but the pleasantness rating for other foods (e.g. fruit or cookies) was largely unaffected by eating sausages. Subjects offered successive plates of sandwiches ate more if the sandwiches contained different fillings than if they were all the same. More surprisingly, subjects offered successive plates of pasta ate more if the pasta shape was varied than if the shape was the same. Variation in taste or appearance increased the amount eaten. So, if a diet is monotonous then we are less likely to overeat than if it is varied. This is not too surprising a conclusion – most of us can usually be persuaded to accept a little dessert even when satiated by earlier courses of the meal. Even laboratory rats eat much more when they are offered a variety of foods ('cafeteria feeding').

Sensory-specific satiety should increase the range of foods that people eat and limit the consumption of any single food. It should therefore decrease the likelihood of nutritional inadequacies because they are unlikely if the diet is varied. It would also reduce the likelihood that any of the toxins found in small amounts in many foods would be consumed in sufficient quantities to be hazardous. In an affluent population, nutrient deficiencies are unlikely; food is always plentiful and its variety appears almost limitless. Under such conditions, sensory-specific satiety probably encourages overeating and excessive weight gain.

Since these early studies, the concept of sensory-specific satiety has become widely accepted. A decline in sensory-specific satiety with age may explain why elderly people consume a more monotonous diet and may play a role in the decline in appetite frequently reported in older people (Rolls, 1993). Other studies have shown formally that increased variety leads to increase in food and energy intake and may lead to positive energy balance in the short to medium term. (Sensory influences on food intakes are reviewed by Sorensen *et al.* (2003).) For example, McCrory *et al.* (1999) found that, with each of 10 food groups, energy intake was positively associated with variety. They suggested that increased variety within certain food groups was positively associated with body fatness (e.g. sweets, snacks, condiments, entrees and carbohydrates) and that increased variety from vegetables was negatively associated with body fatness.

Key points

- Evolutionary pressures may have caused the mechanisms that regulate energy balance to be relatively ineffective at preventing excess energy storage.
- Some populations (e.g. the Pima Indians and Samoans) are extremely prone to obesity. A harsh environment in the past may have caused them to evolve with a 'thrifty' genotype.
- Studies with twins and adopted children suggest that much of the family resemblance in fatness levels is due to genetic factors.
- Clearly both environmental and genetic influences determine an individual's or a population's fatness.
- Certain environmental conditions are necessary before any inherited predisposition to obesity is expressed.
- Recent changes in obesity prevalence must be due to lifestyle changes.
- Even in those groups with an extreme propensity to obesity (like the Pima Indians) it only becomes prevalent when environmental conditions are conducive to obesity.
- Hunger will drive us to eat during fasting or fat depletion but absence of hunger will not always prevent us from eating.

→

Key points *continued*

- 'External' influences like pleasure of eating, habit, social pressures or anxiety may cause us to eat in the absence of hunger.
- The feeding of obese people was said to be more influenced by external factors than that of lean people, who were thought to be more responsive to their internal regulatory mechanisms.
- Behavioural therapy is based on the notion of external orientation of feeding control in obese people. Obese people are encouraged to identify and avoid the external cues that trigger inappropriate eating and to facilitate and reward appropriate behaviour (e.g. taking exercise).
- The availability of a wide variety of food encourages higher consumption. As one food is eaten, so satiation for that food develops but the desire to eat other foods is much less affected. This has been called sensory-specific satiety.
- Increased variety within some food groups encourages over-consumption of food energy and leads to weight gain.

Is fat more fattening than carbohydrate?

This topic was reviewed by Livingstone (1996) and some of the earlier uncited references are listed here. For many years it was very widely held that carbohydrates, and especially sugar, were the most fattening components of the diet. This notion was reinforced by a string of popular diet books that promoted a variety of low-carbohydrate diets as the best for weight loss. These popular diet books included one written by an eminent British professor of nutrition (John Yudkin: *This Slimming Business*).

Yudkin made the point that severe restriction of dietary carbohydrate would not only affect the carbohydrate foods that provided a high proportion of the dietary energy but would also indirectly reduce the fat that is normally consumed with these foods. He expected that, on his diet, fat consumption would either drop or stay the same. Thus the carbohydrate in bread, sugary foods and drinks, breakfast cereals, rice, pasta, potatoes, cakes, biscuits, etc. is deliberately restricted, but so indirectly is, for example, butter/margarine that is spread on bread, fat used to fry potatoes, rice or other carbohydrate foods, the fat in battered or breadcrumbed fish or meat, and the fat in pies, pastries, biscuits and cakes. Some low-carbohydrate diets may also put milk (especially low-fat milk!) on the prohibited or restricted list because of its lactose content. Under these circumstances it is difficult to make up the lost carbohydrate calories by replacing them with fat because concentrated fat is nauseating. The net result would often be a reduction in total energy intake, and this accounts for the frequent short-term successes of fashionable low-carbohydrate diets like the Atkins diet.

Current wisdom and advice are the opposite to these earlier views. Fat is now regarded as more fattening than carbohydrate and the current consensus among nutritionists is that diets that are rich in starch, fibre, fruits and vegetables but low in fat are most likely to prevent excessive weight gain and achieve long-term weight control.

There are, of course, other important reasons for moderating fat intake – as discussed in Chapter 12. In cross-sectional studies of populations, dietary and anthropometric data are collected from large samples of people. It is often found in such studies that there is a positive correlation between the proportion of energy derived from fat and the BMI; put bluntly, those who get the highest proportion of their energy from fat are the most likely to 'be fat'. Given the carbohydrate–fat and sugar–fat seesaws discussed in Chapter 7, it almost inevitably follows that, as the proportion of energy from carbohydrate or even sugar increases, so BMI tends to fall; those who get more of their energy from carbohydrate or sugar tend to be leaner. In one study of more than 11 500 Scots, Bolton-Smith and Woodward (1994) found that the prevalence of overweight and obesity decreased with an increase in the proportion of energy derived from carbohydrate or from sugar, but it increased with increases in the proportion of energy that came from fat. In the 20 per cent of the men in this Scottish population who had the highest fat-to-sugar ratios, rates of obesity were 3.5 times higher than in the 20 per cent with the lowest ratios (double in women). Other examples of these

cross-sectional studies are discussed briefly in Prentice (2001).

There is evidence that very low-fat diets (say under 20 per cent of energy from fat) are associated with weight loss even when total energy intake is not restricted. High-fat diets, in contrast, lead to over-consumption of energy (positive energy balance) in animal studies and others using free-living human subjects. Stubbs et al. (1995) monitored body fat balance in men over a 7-day period when they were fed a diet where fat provided 20, 40 or 60 per cent of the energy. When fed the 60 per cent fat diet there was an average body fat gain of around 400 g during the week; when fed the 40 per cent fat diet there was no significant change in body fat; but when fed the 20 per cent fat diet the men lost an average of around 150 g of fat. Note that these diets were designed to make the changes covert so that they should not be obvious to the subjects. Prentice (2001) suggests that if such studies are repeated using a diluent to equalize the energy density of the high-fat diets then they no longer cause weight gain; that is, the effect of the variation in fat could be due largely to the effect that it has on the energy density of the diet.

Lissner et al. (2000) discuss data obtained from a prospective study of middle-aged and elderly Swedish women which indicates that increases in dietary fat content predict the long-term development of central obesity as measured by waist-to-hip ratio. They conclude that their data 'may reflect a causal role for total fat intake in the development of central adiposity'. Astrup et al. (2000) did a meta-analysis of studies that had used ad-libitum (i.e. not calorie-restricted) low-fat diets in intervention trials. Their analysis indicated that low-fat diets prevented weight gain in individuals with normal weight but led to modest weight loss in overweight and obese subjects. The magnitude of weight loss in these studies was greatest in those who were most overweight at the start of the trial. So, effective population-based messages aimed at reducing the proportion of dietary calories derived from fat may achieve some weight loss, but the greatest benefit is likely to be in preventing excess weight gain in the first place. In a later review, Astrup (2005) suggests that meta-analyses indicate that specifically fat-reduced diets result in 3–4 kg greater weight loss than normal-fat diets.

There may well be an interaction between activity and dietary fat content in their effects on energy balance control. In one study, the proportion of energy from fat was varied between 20, 40 and 60 per cent in active and sedentary men. The active men were in negative energy balance on the 20 per cent diet and still in slight negative balance at 40 per cent, but had a small positive balance when fat was raised to 60 per cent of energy. The inactive men, however, only achieved balance on the 20 per cent fat diet and were in substantial positive balance on the other two diets.

These observations suggest that, in sedentary populations, diets with fat contents typically found in Western industrialized societies are likely to promote positive energy balance and weight gain. As we become more sedentary so our high-fat diets will make us increasingly *susceptible* to obesity.

This interaction between high-fat high-energy-density diets and activity is also briefly reviewed in Prentice (2001).

Theoretical reasons why one might expect fat to be more fattening than carbohydrate

- *Fat is energy-dense.* It yields more than twice as much energy as the same weight of carbohydrate or protein. This means that high-fat diets are inevitably energy-dense. This may be the predominant reason why high-fat diets encourage over-consumption in free-living situations. (There is a discussion of energy density in Chapter 7.)
- *Fat increases the palatability of food.* This will tend to encourage over-consumption, especially if it replaces bland starch. Overweight and obese people seem to have an increased preference for high-fat foods.
- *Conversion of excess dietary fat to body fat is a very efficient process.* Only about 4 per cent of the energy is wasted in the conversion process. In contrast, the conversion of dietary carbohydrate to fat leads to the loss of about 25 per cent of the energy, and the conversion of dietary protein into fat is even more wasteful. In practice, on normal high-fat Western diets, there is very little conversion of dietary carbohydrate to fat, and

most carbohydrate is either used directly as an energy source or converted to glycogen.

- *Calorie for calorie, fat seems to be less satiating than carbohydrate.* Numerous experiments have been performed in which subjects are given iso-energetic pre-loads of varying composition and the effect on their subsequent hunger ratings and the amount consumed at a subsequent meal is compared. These studies consistently suggest that fat is slightly less satiating than carbohydrate (usually sugar), and that this difference is more pronounced in obese than in lean subjects.
- *Consumption of carbohydrate leads to an accelerated use of glucose in metabolism and a reduction in fat oxidation.* These are conditions that are associated with satiation. Consumption of fat has little effect on the metabolism of fat or carbohydrate.

Key points

- Obesity was at one time widely blamed on high-carbohydrate (and especially high-sugar) diets.
- Low-carbohydrate diets have been widely recommended for weight reduction. They often achieve short-term success because they reduce total energy intake and tend also to reduce total fat consumption.
- In cross-population studies, people who get the highest proportion of their energy from fat tend to have the highest BMIs. Those who obtain the highest proportion from carbohydrate or even sugar tend to have the lowest BMIs.
- An increase in dietary fat content may be a causal factor in the development of central obesity.
- Very low-fat diets are associated with weight loss even when total intake is not restricted. In contrast, high-fat diets encourage weight gain.
- Active people may be able to tolerate medium- and high-fat diets without weight gain, but in inactive people they lead to weight gain.
- High fat intake encourages weight gain because fat is energy-dense, palatable, less satiating than carbohydrate, and more efficiently converted to stored fat.

Inactivity as a cause of obesity

Less requirement for physical activity is strongly implicated as an important cause of the rapid increases in the number of overweight and obese people in Europe, the USA and elsewhere (Prentice and Jebb, 1995). Car ownership and automation in the home, garden and workplace have substantially reduced our mandatory energy expenditure – the amount we must use to accomplish the tasks of everyday life. Few people in the USA and western Europe now have jobs that are physically demanding. Some have increased their leisure-time activities to compensate – recreational walking, jogging, exercise classes, participation in sports and active games. However, for most people any increase in recreational activity does not compensate for the decline in mandatory activity.

There is persuasive evidence that per-capita energy intakes have dropped substantially in Britain in recent decades. According to Durnin (1992), average energy intakes of teenagers were up to a third higher in the 1930s than they were in the 1990s. According to the old National Food Survey, per-capita household food consumption in the UK dropped by more than a quarter between 1950 and 1992, and a similar trend is seen using wider measures of energy consumption (Figure 9.13). The 2004–5 Expenditure and Food Survey reports that average energy intake was 1.8 per cent lower than in the previous year and the long-term trend of a gradual fall in energy intake was continuing.

Unlike those expenditure surveys, the National Diet and Nutrition Surveys (NDNS) attempt to measure what people actually eat. NDNS data go back 25 years. They indicate that, between 1986–7 and 2009, average daily energy intake for men fell from 10.26 MJ (2450 kcal) to 9.48 MJ (2255 kcal); in women there was little change, from 7.0 MJ (1680 kcal) to 6.92 MJ (1645 kcal).

This fall in daily energy intake has corresponded with the very large increases in the number of people who are overweight and obese detailed earlier in the chapter; that is, we are eating less but getting fatter. The only explanation for these opposing trends seems to be that activity levels have declined sharply. The fall in intake has lagged behind the fall in expenditure.

Prentice and Jebb (1995) have reported that increases in obesity prevalence in the UK since 1950

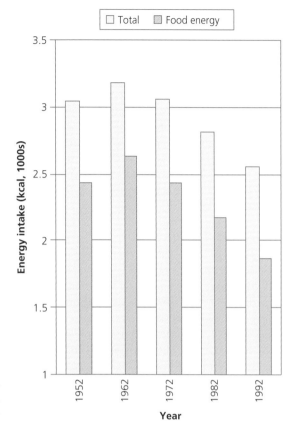

Figure 9.13 The apparent decline in average energy intake in the UK. Principal data source: COMA (1984).

have tended to mirror increases in car ownership and the number of hours that Britons spend in watching television.

Large cross-sectional surveys in both the USA and the UK have found that those who report being the least active are the most likely to be overweight or obese. Bennett *et al.* (1995) recorded BMI and assessed activity by questionnaire in a large representative sample of English adults. In both men and women, obesity was more than twice as common in the lowest activity band compared to the highest.

Information on physical activity was collected by questionnaire in the 2003 *Health Survey for England* (Sproston and Primatesta, 2004) and this found that only 37 per cent of men and 24 per cent of women were meeting the current recommended target of at least 30 minutes of activity of at least moderate intensity on at least five occasions per week. In men the proportion who met this recommended level declined sharply with age, while in women it remained fairly stable until around 55 years of age and then declined. This survey, as in previous years, found a strong inverse relationship between reported physical activity and BMI. Participants were classified as high, medium or low activity and the proportion of those with high activity declined as BMI rose whereas the proportion of those classified as low activity rose with increasing BMI category. Figure 9.14 shows the odds ratio (relative risk) of having a BMI of over 25 or over 30 kg/m^2 in the three activity categories: the chances of having a BMI of >25 declines highly significantly with increasing activity, and this trend is even more pronounced for a BMI >30.

In women there is a very pronounced class variation in obesity prevalence. Prentice and Jebb (1995) showed that hours of TV viewing, number of people reporting being inactive and obesity rates all rise as one looks down the social classes. Gregory *et al.* (1990) reported that BMI increased with declining social class but that recorded energy intake was also lower in the lower social classes. Women in the lower classes were fatter but reported eating less, again an indication of reduced activity in the most overweight categories.

One note of caution must be sounded about all of these studies. Both food consumption and activity level are self-reported in most studies, and there is

persuasive evidence that food intake tends to be under-recorded and activity level over-estimated in such studies. This tendency to be over-optimistic about activity levels and energy intakes is probably more pronounced in the obese.

Television viewing is now the most popular recreational activity in most industrialized countries. The average Briton spends twice as much time watching television as in 1960, and the average American child watches 28 hours of television each week. Many people spend more time watching television each week than they do at work or at school. Dietz and Gortmaker (1985) analysed data on TV viewing in American children when they were aged 6–11 years and again when they were aged 12–17 years. When they divided the children up according to the number of hours of TV watched, they found that at both times the prevalence of obesity rose with increased TV viewing hours. This trend was most marked in adolescence, and at this stage there was a 2 per cent rise in obesity prevalence for every extra hour of TV viewing. They also found that the number of hours of TV watching in the 6- to 11-year-olds was significantly correlated with the prevalence of obesity 6 years later. Those 6- to 11-year-olds who watched the most TV were the most likely to be obese when they reached adolescence – a strong indication that the relationship is cause and effect.

That study by Dietz and Gortmaker is now more than 25 years old, but numerous studies since 1985 have generally confirmed their findings. In the USA, Jago *et al.* (2005) conducted a longitudinal study of girls and found that those who watched more than the recommended 2 hours per day when younger were 13.2 times more likely to be overweight at the age of 11 years than those who watched less than 2 hours per day. In the UK, Viner and Cole (2005) found that a higher number of hours of weekend TV viewing at the age of 5 years predicted a higher BMI at 30 years of age. Each additional hour of TV viewing at age 5 increased the risk of being obese at 30 years by 7 per cent. In New Zealand, Hancox *et al.* (2004) did a 26-year follow-up of 1000 children and found that higher average TV viewing between the ages of 5 and 15 years was associated with a higher BMI at 26 years and was associated with other adverse health indicators.

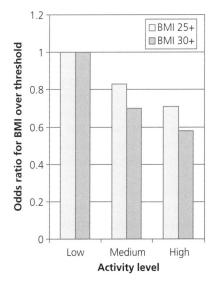

Figure 9.14 Risk of being overweight or obese according to activity level.

Of course, even strong and consistent associations between obesity and inactivity in a variety of studies

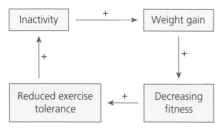

Figure 9.15 The inactivity–obesity cycle.

do not prove that inactivity *causes* obesity. Apart from the difficulty of measuring activity levels, it is also likely that excess weight gain reduces fitness and exercise tolerance and this discourages activity – an effect-and-cause relationship. There is almost certainly a large element of truth in both of these suggestions, so a dangerous obesity/inactivity cycle is created (Figure 9.15).

Key points

- Reduced requirement for activity to travel and to accomplish household and occupational tasks has led to a general decline in energy expenditure.
- Average energy intake in the UK has fallen substantially over recent decades and yet levels of fatness have also increased markedly. Energy intake has fallen more slowly than energy expenditure, leading to increased levels of fat stores in the population.
- Indirect measures of population inactivity in the UK, such as the amount of television viewing and car ownership, have mirrored increases in obesity rates.
- There is persuasive evidence in children that the amount of television viewing is positively linked to the risk of obesity.
- Inactivity is a major factor in recent increases in the prevalence of overweight and obesity. Inactivity encourages weight gain and weight gain probably discourages activity, leading to a cycle of inactivity and weight gain.

PREVENTION AND TREATMENT OF OBESITY IN POPULATIONS

Adopting a lower risk lifestyle

For effective, long-term weight control one needs to identify dietary and lifestyle patterns that are associated with low risk of obesity without the need for continual restraint on food consumption and calorie counting. From the earlier discussion of the *causes* of obesity, there appear to be two changes that would lessen an individual's risk of becoming overweight:

- an increase in activity and fitness level (or perhaps just a reduction in inactivity)
- a reduction in the proportion of dietary energy that is derived from fat.

If these principles were generally adopted we could expect a levelling off and eventually a fall in the population prevalence of overweight and obesity. Both changes would also be likely to have substantial health benefits. High-fat diets are implicated in the genesis of cardiovascular disease, cancer and perhaps diabetes. The many health benefits of regular exercise are detailed in Chapter 18.

The most obvious way of increasing activity and fitness is by participation in games, sports or formal exercise sessions and, of course, these need to be encouraged and facilitated. However, the major reason why affluent populations are now so inactive is because mandatory activity has been almost eliminated from everyday life for many people. To bring about a substantial increase in the weekly energy expenditure of most people, we also need to find ways of incorporating more activity into everyday living. Examples are suggested below.

- Make more journeys on foot or bicycle rather than by car. In the UK, journeys of less than a mile account for a third of all car journeys and these have been growing rapidly as a proportion of the total. More of these short journeys need to be made on foot or bicycle.
- Make more use of stairs rather than always taking lifts (elevators) or escalators.
- Become less reliant on labour-saving gadgets and do some tasks by hand.
- Engage in more leisure-time pursuits that, although not formally exercise, do have a physical activity element – gardening, home improvements or maintenance, playing with children, walking a dog, etc.
- Limit the time spent in passive pursuits such as watching television or playing computer games.

Studies with obese children have found that simply reducing access to these sedentary activities was more effective in long-term weight control than programmes involving strenuous exercise sessions. Evidence was given earlier that children who watch the most TV have the highest risk of becoming obese in adolescence or even in adulthood.

Health promotion campaigns that are aiming to improve population weight control need to concentrate on the following.

- Make it clear that the priorities for improving weight control are increased activity and a reduction in dietary fat.
- Educate people about the ways in which they can achieve these objectives. Impart information on the sources of fat in the diet and dietary choices that would reduce fat consumption. Suggest how more activity can be incorporated into everyday living, and encourage participation in formal or informal exercise sessions.
- Identify and then look for ways to minimize the barriers that make it difficult for people to be active and consume less fat.

It must be said that personal choice is a major reason why people are inactive and eat high-fat diets. High fat and sugar content makes food more palatable. Many affluent people have no necessity to be active, and indeed their sedentary occupations may force them to be inactive during long working and commuting hours. To fill their leisure time they have access to pleasurable and almost addictive pursuits that are also totally inactive. It is therefore not surprising that many people choose to be very inactive. Health promoters can only try to encourage people to go against their natural inclinations and adopt healthier lifestyle patterns. However, there may also be circumstances that encourage unhealthy lifestyles, or barriers that prevent people adopting healthier lifestyles.

Some barriers to being more active

- There might be a lack of access to sports facilities, or to safe, attractive open spaces (e.g. no local facilities, inconvenient opening hours, high cost of entry or membership fees, lack of money to buy sports clothing or equipment).

- There may be a real or perceived danger when walking or cycling (e.g. vulnerability to injury by motor vehicles, fear of mugging or molestation, noise and pollution caused by motor vehicles).
- Town planning decisions can assume that the car is the only mode of transport and make no provision for pedestrians or cyclists.
- Long hours may be spent in the workplace, in sedentary jobs in an environment that discourages physical activity and with no opportunity to do anything active.

Some barriers to reducing fat consumption

- Low-fat diets tend to be less palatable than high-fat diets.
- Low-fat foods might not be available. In fact, the availability of low- or reduced-fat foods has increased in line with consumer demand for these products. Low-fat spreads, reduced-fat cheese, low-fat milk and yoghurts, reduced-fat crisps (chips) and savoury snacks, extra-lean meat, reduced-fat French fries, low-fat cakes and biscuits (cookies) and reduced-fat ready meals are all readily available now. Note that some of the products listed still contain substantial amounts of fat and/or sugar even though their fat content is lower than the standard product (e.g. reduced-fat crisps and savoury snacks, reduced-fat cheddar cheese). Until recently the food provided in restaurants and some fast-food outlets usually had much more limited low-fat options, but this is starting to change and even many of the large fast-food chains have introduced 'healthier options'. But these may still not be ideal choices (e.g. salads with lots of high-fat dressing).
- There can be an increased cost associated with a diet that is lower in fat and yet still palatable. Starchy foods are cheaper but rather bland. Many low- or reduced-fat products carry a price premium over the standard product and almost all do if one expresses cost as calories (or joules) per penny. Fruits and vegetables, lean meat and white fish are all relatively expensive using this criterion. These extra costs may be significant for those on low incomes.
- There may simply be lack of knowledge about the sources of dietary fat.

Suggesting measures to reduce these barriers takes us firmly into the political arena. An increased risk of obesity is just one of many health consequences of poverty and poor educational attainment. If we are to substantially increase activity levels in the population as a whole then the safety and comfort of pedestrians and cyclists need to be given a higher priority by politicians, town planners, property developers and law enforcement agencies. This may have to include active measures to discourage car usage, especially for short urban journeys.

Targeting anti-obesity measures or campaigns

Is it possible to identify an age group where intervention to prevent or reduce obesity is likely to be most effective? Intuitively, childhood would seem to be a crucial time because this is when good dietary and lifestyle patterns can be set for the rest of life and this would seem like a better option than trying to change bad habits later in life. Most obese adults were not obese as children, but the majority of obese children do become obese adults and it may well be bad habits learned earlier in life that are responsible for much adult-onset obesity. The observation noted earlier that the number of hours spent viewing television in early childhood predicts higher BMI in adulthood supports this intuitive belief. Some possible measures that could be directed towards children are listed below.

- Give proper weighting to food and nutrition, including food preparation skills, in the school curriculum. If people are advised to reduce their fat consumption they must have a clear idea of where their dietary fat comes from and what practical measures would reduce fat consumption. They should have the skills and confidence to prepare appealing low-fat dishes.
- Recognize the importance of physical education to the long-term well-being of children. It should not be sacrificed to make room for more academic work in the school timetable.
- Physical education sessions should seek to involve all children, not just the talented minority. There should also be more emphasis on those activities that are more likely to be continued into adulthood. We would think

poorly of a school that concentrated all of its academic efforts onto the brightest pupils and on subjects that were unlikely to be used in later life. It may require considerable innovation and ingenuity to engage some of the less athletically minded pupils with physical education programmes that they will enjoy and willingly participate in.
- Try to limit the time spent in watching TV and playing computer games. Ideally this should be by persuasion rather than coercion, for example by offering children more attention and more opportunities to spend some of their leisure time in enjoyable alternative activities.
- Every effort should be made to facilitate activity in children, for example by ensuring that they can walk or cycle to school safely. One can try to change the subjective norm by making activity more fashionable, such as by emphasizing the environmental benefits of walking to school.

At one time, the *fat-cell theory* (Hirsch and Han, 1969) gave a formal theoretical basis for this belief that childhood was the best time to act. Hirsch and Han suggested that early overfeeding permanently increased the number of fat cells and thus predisposed children to obesity in later life. This theory was based on some dubious extrapolation of experiments with rats to people. Hirsch and Han reported that adipose tissue in rats, in the first few weeks of life, grew by both cell division (increasing the number of fat cells) and by increases in fat cell size. According to this theory, at about 6 weeks old the number of fat cells in the rat was fixed and any increases in adipose tissue in adult rats could occur only by increases in the size of existing fat cells. Overfeeding before 6 weeks of age permanently increased rats' numbers of fat cells and so might have permanently increased their susceptibility to obesity.

Pond (1987) provided very persuasive arguments for not applying these ideas to people. Pond found that fat cell numbers could be increased throughout life in primates and that the capacity of primate fat cells to increase by expansion alone was rather limited compared to the rat. She suggested that the key premise of this fat-cell theory was false. It has also been suggested that a period of deprivation in early life may programme people to become obese in later life if conditions allow it.

OBESITY TREATMENT IN INDIVIDUALS

Realistic rates of weight loss

To lose substantial weight, energy expenditure must exceed energy intake for a considerable time. A moderately low-fat diet and a reasonably active lifestyle may be effective in preventing excessive weight gain. However, to lose a substantial amount of excess fat that has accumulated over time will probably require a prolonged period of deliberate and uncomfortable food restriction (dieting). Most treatments for obesity represent different strategies for making this dieting easier, more effective and more acceptable. This applies even to most anti-obesity drugs and surgical treatments.

If one assumes that 1 kg of adipose tissue yields about 29 MJ (7000 kcal), even a daily deficit of 4.2 MJ (1000 kcal) will result in the loss of only 1 kg of adipose tissue per week. This is probably the most that can be hoped for with conventional dieting, and for small women or inactive people as little as half of this might be a more realistic target.

During the first week of a diet or in severe dieting, weight loss may be much faster than this because of loss of glycogen reserves and protein (lean tissue). Each kilogram of body glycogen or protein is associated with three or more kilograms of water, so to lose 1 kg via these routes requires an energy deficit of only about 4.2 MJ (1000 kcal). However, body glycogen reserves are very limited and loss of lean tissue is not the aim of dieting. Any weight lost via these routes can be rapidly regained once the diet is relaxed. It also takes significantly more than 29 MJ (7000 kcal) to synthesize 1 kg of adipose tissue; and so – on a more positive note – an occasional lapse in an otherwise successful diet (say two chocolate bars at 1 MJ (250 kcal) each) is not going to undo weeks of hard-won losses.

The aim of dieting is to lose fat but to minimize losses of muscle and other metabolically active lean tissue. It is inevitable and proper that some of the weight lost during slimming is lean tissue because obese people have more lean tissue as well as more fat, and even adipose tissue has a cellular, protein component. A ratio of about three-quarters fat to one-quarter lean may be a reasonable rule of thumb for planned weight loss. Extreme dieting and very rapid weight loss increase the proportion of lean that is lost, whereas exercise seems to protect against lean tissue loss during dieting (reviewed by Prentice *et al.*, 1991).

As noted in Chapter 7, starvation reduces resting metabolic rate (RMR) and this conservation of energy during starvation is an aid to survival during food shortages. It will also tend to thwart the efforts of the dieter. This decline in RMR remains even after correcting for changes in lean body mass and is rapid. It can be detected within 24 hours of the start of dieting, and a rise in RMR occurs within 24 hours of a return to normal eating. The magnitude of this protective response to dieting is not so large as to present an insurmountable barrier to successful weight loss. According to Prentice's team, even in severe dieting (say under 3 MJ or 700 kcal per day) the decline in RMR per unit of lean body mass rarely exceeds 15 per cent, and in more moderate dieting (over 5 MJ or 1200 kcal per day) it is only about 5 per cent.

The reducing diet

The diet should aim to produce a daily energy deficit of 2–4 MJ (500–1000 kcal). It should achieve this by selectively restricting fat, added sugars and alcohol. Such measures will drastically reduce the energy density of the diet but will actually increase the nutrient density, which makes nutrient deficiencies unlikely despite the reduced energy intake.

As noted in Chapter 7, most fruits and vegetables have extremely low energy yields and so can be eaten in large quantities without adding much energy to the diet. Starchy foods like potatoes and cereals are relatively low in energy density, and whole-grain cereals have the added advantage of high amounts of dietary fibre/non-starch polysaccharide, which may increase their satiation value (see Chapter 10). Low-fat milk, very lean meat, white fish, pulses or the vegetarian options in the meat group will also be essential components of a healthy reducing diet. Foods from the fats and sugars group of the food plate (or pyramid) – high-fat meats and dairy products, fried foods and other foods with added fats and sugars – are the prime candidates for reduction in a healthy reducing diet.

Note that evidence discussed earlier in the chapter suggested that low-fat diets with no more than 20 per cent of the dietary energy as fat lead to weight loss even without caloric restriction. Evidence is discussed in Chapter 10 which indicates that low *glycaemic index* produced more weight loss in controlled trials than other types of diets (e.g. a systematic review by Thomas *et al.*, 2007). Glycaemic index is a ranking of foods according to their effect on blood glucose levels. Foods with a

low glycaemic index – for example, dried peas and beans, pasta and porridge/oatmeal – produce a slow sustained release of glucose into the blood and less insulin is released than with food with a high glycaemic index, such as white bread, corn flakes and most cakes (see Chapter 10 for further discussion).

Alternative diets

There are numerous alternative diets presented in popular books which often employ strategies and recommendations that seem totally at odds with the low-fat, low-sugar, low-energy-density but high-nutrient-density diet recommended in this book and by the bulk of orthodox nutritionists and dieticians. Many of the books offer some new gimmick that will allow the reader to achieve large and rapid weight loss with relatively little inconvenience. These books often contain impressive case histories of people who have lost considerable weight using the author's plan, or an account of how the author stumbled upon this new diet and how it transformed their life. If all of these diets are so successful then why, despite the publication of dozens of new 'spectacularly successful' diet books each year, do rates of obesity and overweight spiral ever upwards?

In practice these diet books usually employ one or more strategies that will tend to reduce energy intake if the reader sticks to the rules. Consider, for example, the fashionable low-carbohydrate diets which forbid consumption of foods that normally provide the bulk of our daily energy intake. Cereal products, potato products, milk and milk products, sugar, sweets, soft drinks, many sauces, coated meat and fish products, pies, etc. are all excluded from the acceptable foods, and yet these normally account for well over 70 per cent of our energy intake. Exclusion of these foods will also limit the consumption of fats that are normally eaten with carbohydrates, like spreading and cooking fats. It is not surprising that total energy intake tends to fall if people stick to this very restrictive and monotonous diet, which may become nauseating after a short while. Where people lose weight on low-carbohydrate diets this is principally associated with reduced calorie intake and increased diet duration but not with reduced carbohydrate intake *per se*

(Bravata *et al.*, 2003). Some other strategies employed in these books are considered below.

Making the diet monotonous and reducing its palatability Obese people may be particularly sensitive to reductions in palatability. Remember that rats given access to a variety of palatable and energy-dense foods tend, like people, to gain weight. Some 'popular' diets seem to be aiming to almost reverse this process and persuade people to eat the human equivalent of the rat's pellet diet.

Giving unlimited access to low-energy foods Examples are certain fruits and vegetables. Conventional diets also do this.

Making eating hard work or expensive For example, certain so-called 'food combining diets' forbid the mixing together within a meal of foods that are high in protein and those that are high in carbohydrate, as well as other restrictions. This theory is based on a book written in the early twentieth century which falsely suggested that the gut is incapable of digesting carbohydrates and proteins at the same time because different conditions are required for their digestion. This diet excludes many of the culturally normal meals such as:

- cereal with milk
- cheese, meat, egg or fish sandwiches
- pasta with meat, fish or cheese sauce
- potatoes or rice with meat, fish, eggs or cheese
- pizza
- hamburger.

The role of exercise

The evidence that inactivity is strongly implicated as a cause of obesity seems very persuasive. This would also mean that regular exercise should be of major importance in preventing excessive weight gain. However, evidence that exercise has a major impact on rates of *weight loss* during dieting is less persuasive.

Most studies that have looked at the contribution of exercise to weight loss programmes have concluded that the exercise contributed only modestly to weight loss. However, there is evidence that an exercise component increases the chances of long-term success; that is, it helps to prevent rapid regaining of lost weight. Wadden *et al.* (2006) came to a similar conclusion – that exercise in the absence of dieting produces very little weight loss in the short or medium term and that the benefits of exercise are to prevent weight gain, maintain weight losses and to improve health rather than induce weight loss.

Shaw *et al.* (2006) conducted a meta-analysis of 43 weight-reduction controlled trials that involved increased physical activity as one of the treatments. When exercise was compared to no treatment then it resulted in small weight losses, but when combined with a reducing diet it resulted in greater weight loss than the diet alone. Increasing the intensity of the exercise increased the amount of weight lost. In these trials, exercise also resulted in significant beneficial changes in several risk factors for cardiovascular disease: reduced blood pressure, reduced blood triacylglycerol concentrations and reduced fasting blood glucose. Higher intensity exercise resulted in bigger changes in these risk factors.

Thus exercise alone produces small weight losses and reduces risk factors for several cardiovascular diseases and when used in conjunction with a reducing diet it increases the effectiveness of the diet.

It takes a long time to *walk* off 2–4 MJ (500–1000 kcal) – say 2–6+ hours depending on speed and the person's size. Very few people have this much time to devote to formal exercise. Many very overweight people will have a low exercise tolerance and so the amount of energy that can be consumed in a formal exercise session will be small. These observations highlight the need to incorporate more activity into everyday living as well as in formal exercise sessions. Earlier in the chapter it was suggested that inactivity and weight gain become part of a vicious cycle (see Figure 9.15). Increased activity should break this cycle and create a virtuous cycle: exercise improves tolerance and so enables more exercise to be taken, as depicted in Figure 9.16.

The energy expenditure and energy requirements of an individual are determined by his or her *basal metabolic rate* (BMR) and *physical activity level* (PAL), discussed fully in Chapter 7. PAL is the factor that BMR is multiplied by to allow for the increase in energy expenditure caused by all activities:

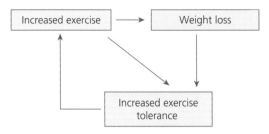

Figure 9.16 The hoped for virtuous cycle of increased activity and weight loss.

$$energy\ expenditure = BMR \times PAL.$$

Table 9.11 shows how the energy a woman needs to achieve balance and to produce a 2.1–4.2 MJ (500–1000 kcal) deficit increases with her PAL multiple.

A sedentary, largely housebound woman with a PAL multiple of 1.3 can eat less than 3.4 MJ (800 kcal) per day if she is aiming for a 4.2 MJ (1000 kcal) daily energy deficit. As the PAL multiple rises so the amount that can be eaten and still achieve this deficit rises; so a woman with a PAL multiple of 1.7 could eat over 5.5 MJ (1300 kcal) and still achieve this deficit. A higher PAL multiple increases the amount that can be eaten while

maintaining an energy deficit, and this also reduces the likelihood that dieting will lead to inadequate intakes of other nutrients. About 30 minutes' walking per day increases the PAL multiple by 0.1.

These calculations suggest that achieving and maintaining long-term energy deficits of the required magnitude may be much easier in people who are active and may be impracticable in people who are very inactive. It should also be borne in mind that exercise may protect against lean tissue loss during diet and so increase the quality of weight loss.

Are the obese less 'vigilant'?

In 1992, Garrow suggested that one major reason why some people remain relatively lean while others get very fat is that the lean are more vigilant. Lean people monitor their body weight more closely and take steps to correct any weight gain (i.e. eating less and exercising more) before it has become a major problem. Garrow argued that the obese are less vigilant and do not initiate corrective steps until the condition has progressed to the point where the person cannot cope with the magnitude of weight loss required to target a normal body weight.

Table 9.11 Energy needs of a 65 kg woman at various physical activity levels (PALs) to achieve energy balance or a 500 kcal (2.1 MJ) or 1000 kcal (4.2–MJ) deficit*

Status	PAL multiple[1]					
	1.0	1.3	1.5	1.7	2.0	2.2
kcal	1375	1788	2063	2338	2750	3025
MJ	5.78	7.51	8.66	9.82	11.55	12.71
500 kcal (2.1 MJ) deficit						
kcal	875	1288	1563	1838	2250	2525
MJ	3.68	5.41	6.56	7.72	9.45	10.61
1000 kcal (4.2 MJ) deficit						
kcal	375	788	1063	1338	1750	2025
MJ	1.58	3.31	4.46	5.62	7.35	8.51

*Modified from Webb (1998).

[1] 1.3 represents an extremely inactive person, e.g. a largely housebound elderly person.

1.5 represents someone (e.g. a teacher) who walks around quite a bit while working.

1.7 represents a person who walks around quite a bit at work and also takes part in some regular leisure-time physical activity (e.g. jogs several times a week).

2.0 represents someone whose job involves a lot of heavy manual work and probably also takes part in regular vigorous leisure-time pursuits.

2.2+ represents a serious athlete during training.

Note that a brisk 30- to 40-minute walk would increase the PAL by around 0.1 on that day.

This reasoning has been used to partly explain the social class and educational influences on obesity prevalence. Are those in the lowest socioeconomic or educational groups less vigilant in monitoring their body weight, and is this why they are more prone to becoming obese? This class/educational difference in body weight vigilance would be consistent with the general trend for the upper social groups and better educated to be more health-aware. They are, for example, more likely to choose foods with 'healthy images' and more likely to take dietary supplements. Similar lack of vigilance, it has been argued, allows regain of weight after successful slimming: the weight creeps back on unnoticed by the person until it is not readily correctable. Once the weight loss or re-loss required is high then the person feels unable to control the situation, becomes disheartened, and no longer makes any sustained effort to control his or her weight.

Garrow (1992) also reported the use of an adjustable weight cord to increase the vigilance of his patients. The patient is able to adjust the length of this cord only by an amount that allows for normal day-to-day fluctuations in waist size. Any increase in waist size above the adjustable range makes the cord uncomfortable and immediately signals the need for corrective measures. Garrow has used such a cord to reduce the risk of weight regain during and after slimming. The cord is shortened by the physician as slimming proceeds. It could also be used as a preventative measure. A cherished or expensive item of clothing that becomes uncomfortably tight may serve as a similar early warning signal for many of us who struggle to keep our weight within certain tolerance limits.

Key points

- Substantial weight loss will require a sustained period of dieting and negative energy balance.
- A daily deficit of 4.2 MJ (1000 kcal) is equivalent to a weekly loss of about 1 kg of adipose tissue, which is around the realistic maximum for conventional dieting.

→

Key points *continued*

- It is inevitable that both fat and lean are lost during slimming. A ratio of three-quarters fat to one-quarter lean is a realistic guideline figure.
- Extreme energy restriction increases the proportion of lean that is lost, while exercise reduces lean tissue losses.
- Resting metabolic rate (RMR) falls during dieting and rises when the diet is relaxed. In severe dieting, the RMR per unit of lean body mass may fall by up to 15 per cent but only by about 5 per cent in moderate dieting.
- The reducing diet should selectively restrict fat, added sugars and alcohol, which will reduce the energy density of the diet but increase its nutrient density.
- Exercise alone has only a modest direct effect on rates of weight loss, but it increases the effectiveness of reducing diets and also leads to beneficial changes in cardiovascular risk factors.
- Weight loss programmes that include an exercise element seem to have better long-term success rates.
- It takes a long time to expend 2–4 MJ (500–1000 kcal) in a formal exercise session. This highlights the need to incorporate more activity into everyday life.
- Many overweight and obese people will have limited exercise tolerance, but increased activity should increase tolerance and create a virtuous cycle as depicted in Figure 9.16.
- An active lifestyle increases the amount of food that can be consumed while still achieving the target energy deficit. It may be impracticable for inactive people to aim for an energy deficit of 4.2 MJ (1000 kcal) with a conventional diet.
- A moderate diet increases the quality of weight gain (more of it is fat) and causes a smaller decrease in RMR.
- Obese people may be less vigilant in monitoring their body weight. Lean people are able to initiate corrective measures early while the obese may not start them until the magnitude of weight loss required is large and very difficult to achieve.

'AGGRESSIVE' TREATMENTS FOR OBESITY

Drug therapy

There are a number of potential pharmacological treatments of obesity and these are briefly outlined here. Some have resulted in licensed drugs while others are approaches that may have longer term potential.

Appetite suppressants

Appetite suppressants aim to affect neurotransmission in the brain centres that regulate feeding. When noradrenalin (norepinephrine) is injected into the brains of experimental animals it reduces hunger and food intake and also stimulates the sympathetic nervous system. Amphetamine has a noradrenalin-like effect and was the first appetite suppressant to be widely used. Amphetamine itself also increases the activity of the nerve transmitter dopamine, and this produces a potentially addictive euphoric effect. Modified amphetamines maintain the noradrenalin-like effect but the addictive dopamine-like effect is minimized. They have been widely used in the USA because until 1996 they were the only appetite suppressants approved by the FDA. In controlled trials they produce only modest extra weight loss as compared to placebos, and then only in the first few weeks of treatment.

Until 1997, *fenfluramine* and *dexfenfluramine* were the most widely used anti-obesity drugs in the UK and Europe. They act to increase the activity of the nerve transmitter serotonin or 5HT (5-hydroxytryptamine) in the brain. They block the reuptake of serotonin which is the normal mechanism for inactivation of this transmitter after its release. When serotonin (5HT) is injected into the brains of animals it also decreases feeding. These drugs mimic the actions of serotonin but do not have the addictive dopamine-like effects of the amphetamines. They act not by reducing the desire to eat but by causing the patient to feel full or satiated earlier. Fenfluramine was in use for about 30 years and tens of millions of Europeans took these drugs over that period (more than 60 000 Britons in 1996 alone). In 1996 they were finally approved by the FDA for use in the USA. Long-term studies of over a year have reported significantly greater weight loss in people treated with drug and diet as compared

to diet and placebo. Rare but potentially fatal side-effects of these drugs have been known for some time (pulmonary hypertension) and there have been suggestions from animal experiments that they may damage serotonin-producing brain cells. However, in 1997 new evidence was produced in the USA suggesting that they might cause damage to heart valves. This led to both drugs being withdrawn from the market in both Europe and the USA.

Sibutramine is a licensed drug available in both the UK and USA. It has combined noradrenalin and serotonin effects. Large controlled trials of sibutramine in association with a reducing diet show that it does increase weight losses compared to diet alone and substantially increases the proportion of obese patients who maintain most of their weight loss after 2 years (James *et al.*, 2000). The sibutramine group also showed significant improvements in blood concentrations of high-density and very-low-density lipoproteins (HDLs, VLDLs) and some other risk factors, but also showed some increases in blood pressure and heart rate; and some patients from the sibutramine group were withdrawn because of increases in their blood pressure. High blood pressure would thus be a contraindication for sibutramine use; it should be regularly monitored in patients receiving this drug. It is also not suitable for patients taking the most popular form of antidepressant, selective serotonin-reuptake inhibitors (SSRIs).

It is interesting to look at the detailed numbers in the trial of James *et al.* (2000). Initially 605 obese patients were selected from several centres and given individual weight loss programmes based on a 600 kcal/day energy deficit. After 6 months, 467 patients (over three-quarters of the total) had lost more than 5 per cent of their initial weight. These were then used in the second stage, with 352 receiving sibutramine with their diet and 115 the placebo. After a further 18 months, 204 patients remained on sibutramine treatment and 57 in the placebo group. In the sibutramine group, 89 patients retained 80 per cent or more of their initial weight loss, but only nine of the placebo group. This dramatically demonstrates the earlier observation that even those obese patients who lose weight initially rarely retain their initial weight losses – perhaps only 8 per cent of the original placebo group – despite an individualized programme and regular monitoring. The figures for the sibutramine group were substantially higher, with at least 19 per cent maintaining most of their initial weight loss.

Nevertheless, even with an individually tailored weight reduction programme and labour-intensive monitoring and follow-up, the vast majority of patients did not maintain their initial weight loss. Although pharmacotherapy helped, it did not change this qualitative summary. It still requires great motivation and willpower for obese individuals to lose substantial amounts of weight and maintain that weight loss even in the medium term.

Rimonabant is a new type of anti-obesity agent that was licensed for a short period for use in the UK. This compound blocks the endocannabinoid receptors in the brain where active ingredients of cannabis (*cannabinoids*) bind and where endogenously produced cannabinoids also bind (see Chapter 8). Endogenous cannabinoids and those taken in the form of cannabis are known to increase appetite (when associated with cannabis use this is sometimes referred to as 'the munchies'). This drug was licensed in 2006 in the UK after successful clinical trials in the USA and in Europe, and was for a time licensed for use in over 50 countries. Curioni and André (2006) did a meta-analysis of four controlled trials of rimonabant for weight loss. They found that a daily dose of 20 mg for a year resulted in around 5 kg greater weight loss than with a placebo. Rimonabant also led to improvements in several cardiovascular risk factors. A daily dose of 5 mg produced only a quarter of the weight loss and did not lead to significant beneficial changes in cardiovascular risk factors. At the higher dose, the meta-analysis found that a significant number of adverse effects were reported, which were mainly psychiatric and gastro-intestinal problems. Rimonabant was withdrawn from sale by its manufacturers in 2008 and its approval as a medicine was formally withdrawn in 2009 because it was felt that the beneficial effects did not outweigh its adverse effects, particularly its adverse psychiatric effects.

Drugs that block digestion

Orlistat is a drug that blocks pancreatic lipase, resulting in up to 30 per cent of dietary fat not being digested but passing through the gut into the faeces.

This drug has been approved for use in the UK, USA and several other countries. This compound irreversibly and selectively inhibits gut lipase by modifying a serine residue at the active site of lipase. At therapeutic doses it blocks absorption of about a third of the fat in a meal. Patients taking this drug need to eat a low-fat diet; otherwise, if they eat a lot of fat it produces adverse symptoms owing to the high fat entry into the large bowel, such as oily stools, anal leakage, urgency of defecation and increased intestinal gas production. These adverse symptoms may, in fact, encourage patients to stick to a low-fat diet, which may additionally help them to lose weight. The increased faecal loss of fat may decrease absorption of fat-soluble vitamins, so supplements are advised. Long-term trials do suggest that orlistat in combination with a low-fat diet leads to modest but significant and clinically useful extra loss of weight compared to diet alone (Wadden *et al.*, 2006).

Padwal *et al.* (2003) did meta-analyses of controlled trials that had used orlistat, sibutramine or rimonabant for weight reduction. They concluded that all three drugs were moderately effective in reducing weight when used for a year or more. However, trials of all three drugs had high dropout rates of 30–40 per cent. Orlistat produced less weight loss than the other two drugs, at around 3 kg more than the placebo after a year, and it also reduced diabetes incidence, improved glycaemic control and reduced LDL cholesterol and blood pressure. The most common side-effects were, as might be expected, gastro-intestinal.

Olestra is a synthetic fat that is not digested in the gut and so it passes out with the faeces. It has the palatability benefits of fat but yields no calories. Its use is permitted in the USA in savoury snacks such as potato crisps (chips) but not in the EU. Compounds like olestra are being promoted as potentially able to replace up to 30 g of fat per day in the diet. In the short term, they can cause problems because of the entry of indigestible fatty material into the large bowel, including diarrhoea, bowel urgency, anal 'leakage', abdominal cramps, and greasy staining of toilets and underwear. They also reduce the absorption of fat-soluble substances including vitamins and cholesterol. In the USA, foods containing olestra have to be fortified with fat-soluble vitamins to compensate. Olestra is currently restricted to use in savoury snacks in the USA on the grounds that these foods are not usually eaten with meals and so the olestra will not interfere with the absorption of vitamins in normal meals. In a 9-month trial with a relatively small number of obese men, Lovejoy *et al.* (2003) used a diet in which olestra was substituted for a third of the dietary fat. Men on the olestra diet lost more weight than men on either control or fat-reduced diets, and there were significant improvements in cardiovascular risk factors.

Drugs based on gut hormones

In Chapter 8, several gut hormones were noted as having appetite-suppressing effects, so drugs that mimic the actions of these hormones might have potential as anti-obesity agents. *Cholecystokinin* (CCK) is a gut hormone released during feeding that causes satiety, and it is also a transmitter in the brain where it seems to depress feeding. Despite early promise, CCK has limited potential as an obesity agent because animals rapidly adapt to excess CCK and become tolerant to it; and even when animals are produced who lack CCK receptors they are still able to regulate their body weight normally (Murphy and Bloom, 2004).

Some preliminary experiments suggest that another gut hormone, oxyntomodulin (discussed in Chapter 7), may have potential as an anti-obesity agent, although the research is still in its early stages. In small-scale trials it caused decreased body weight in obese people by both reducing energy intake and increasing activity-related energy expenditure (Wynne *et al.*, 2006).

Suzuki *et al.* (2011) have recently reviewed the role of gut hormones in appetite regulation. They suggest that changes in gut hormone levels may contribute to the long-term successes of some surgical treatments for obesity. Following gastric banding there is a decrease in the level of *ghrelin* (an appetite-stimulating hormone) and increases in some gut hormones that have anorectic effects (discussed in Chapter 8). Suzuki's team suggests that mimicking the changes in gut hormone levels produced by obesity surgery could also produce weight reduction. They conclude that these gut hormones offer a promising treatment for obesity; this conclusion has been made in several other reviews by Professor Bloom and his associates over the last couple of decades.

Drugs that increase energy expenditure

In the early 1980s, drugs that increase energy expenditure – or 'thermogenic agents' – were considered to have major potential for the treatment of human obesity. At this time the 'brown fat theory' was at its height; that is, the belief that adaptive thermogenesis in brown fat could have a major effect on human energy expenditure and protect against obesity when people overeat. Drugs that stimulate the rat β_3-adrenergic receptor and lead to uncoupling of oxidative phosphorylation in rat brown fat have been developed but these have limited effects in people. It would be fair to say that few nutritionists now believe that brown fat thermogenesis plays a major role in any human adaptive thermogenic response to overfeeding, and so the theoretical basis for this approach to obesity treatment has weakened substantially.

Leptin and leptin analogues

Early trials of recombinant *leptin* in obese people have been disappointing. It was associated with only modest weight loss so that, according to Wadden *et al.* (2006), the manufacturer is unlikely to seek FDA approval for its use in the USA. Leptin is a protein and so it needs to be administered frequently by injection. In the longer term, perhaps orally active agents may be found that mimic or potentiate the actions of leptin. The fact that most human obesity seems to be associated with leptin resistance weakens the theoretical basis for this approach.

Surgical treatment for obesity

Surgery is a treatment of last resort for severe and intractable obesity. All surgical procedures carry some risks and these are much higher in obese people. Surgical treatment does seem to offer some help in losing weight to severely obese people, and it may even be the most effective treatment for this extreme group judged purely on the basis of weight lost.

A number of surgical treatments have been used in the treatment of obesity; they are summarized below.

- *Gastric stapling or gastric banding.* These procedures involve reducing the capacity of the stomach by surgically stapling off a large part of it or by use of an adjustable silicone band. This small pouch may have a capacity of just 30 mL, which means that the patient can eat only small meals; if they eat too much then this may cause them to vomit. This is the most common surgical approach in Europe and it has a low mortality rate (<0.1 per cent).

- *Gastric bypass.* This is the most common procedure used in the USA with around 125 000 operations in 2004. A small pouch is created at the base of the oesophagus and this is then linked directly to a part of the jejunum, thus bypassing the stomach and the duodenum. The mortality rate from this procedure in the month after surgery is 0.5–1 per cent, and many patients experience a number of side-effects in the months after surgery, including vomiting, nausea, bloating and extreme diarrhoea. Patients may need iron and vitamin B_{12} supplements.

Weight losses of up to 30 per cent have been reported for both of these procedures, with associated improvements in other risk factors (Wadden *et al.* 2006). In a systematic review of surgical treatments for obesity, Colquitt *et al.* (2009) found that surgery did produce more weight loss than other treatments in obese and very obese people. Some procedures (e.g. gastric bypass) seemed to be more effective than others, although such comparisons were based on limited numbers of trials. There were insufficient data for them to compare the safety of different procedures.

- *Jaw wiring.* This involves wiring the jaws together so that the intake of solid food is restricted whereas the intake of liquids is relatively unhindered. This procedure is often effective in producing short-term weight loss while the jaws are actually wired, but patients usually regain the weight once the wires are removed. It may be useful for achieving short-term weight loss prior to surgery.
- *Fat removal.* This can be achieved by cutting or by liposuction (literally sucking out areas of adipose tissue). This unpleasant procedure may be judged by some people to be worthwhile for its short-term, localized, cosmetic effects.
- *Intestinal bypass.* This procedure involves surgically bypassing a large section of the small intestine and shunting food past most of it. This hinders digestion and absorption. Patients often suffer from chronic diarrhoea and nutrient deficiencies and may also suffer from liver and kidney damage. This risky procedure has now been largely superseded by gastric banding or gastric bypass.

Very low-energy diets (VLEDs)

These are commercial products that are formulated to contain all of the essential vitamins and minerals but provide only 1.6–3.2 MJ (400–800 kcal) per day. The product is consumed as a flavoured drink and is used to replace normal food. It is very difficult, using normal food, to provide all of the essential nutrients with such a low energy intake. Sometimes a cheaper 'milk diet' is used as an alternative to these commercial products; that is, skimmed or semi-skimmed milk plus a multivitamin and mineral supplement. The attraction for dieters is that they are absolved of all responsibility for food choice: the regimen is very clearly prescribed, significant mistakes are not possible, and weight loss must occur if one sticks to the regimen. For people who comply, the diet must produce substantial and rapid weight loss. Some of the disadvantages of VLEDs are listed below.

- The patient gets no experience of eating a real diet that is capable of maintaining the weight losses induced by this 'controlled starvation'. It has even been argued that this could be viewed as an advantage of these products because it minimizes contact with food and breaks bad eating habits. However, patients are likely to regain any weight as soon as control of their eating is returned to them; in practice, maintenance of weight loss after use of a VLED is poor (Wadden *et al.*, 2006).
- The rapid weight loss leads to high loss of lean tissue. It is difficult to measure this change in body composition accurately, and some advocates of these products claim that this problem has been exaggerated.
- The energy deficit is so severe that ketosis occurs.
- Might this 'controlled starvation' risk precipitating an eating disorder?
- They are potentially dangerous, especially if used for prolonged periods without proper supervision.

Despite these issues, some physicians and nutritionists do consider that these products may have a role in the *supervised* treatment of people with moderate or severe obesity (BMI well in excess of 30) which poses a larger threat to their health.

In a similar vein, there are many 'meal replacement' products on the market that are designed to replace one or more meals each day with a drink or snack. These products have a clearly defined energy yield and so are supposed to make it easy for dieters to control their energy intake. Often these products are nutrient-enriched, but in some cases they have similar energy yields to much cheaper conventional equivalents.

Notes on use of the more aggressive treatments

All drugs have potential side-effects, all surgical procedures entail some risk, and prolonged use of VLEDs may have adverse consequences. They are all relatively extreme measures that are inappropriate for people who are only moderately overweight, and even more inappropriate for people of healthy weight who wish to be thinner to enhance their self-esteem and perception of their appearance. The commercial motivation may persuade some unscrupulous 'counsellors' and even physicians to recommend them to people who are not even overweight. In people who are obese, the health and other consequences of the obesity may justify their use if there is some reasonable prospect that they are likely to be effective. This must be a matter for individual clinical judgement.

As a general guide, surgical treatment should normally be reserved for patients with a BMI in excess of 40, although the presence of other risk factors like high blood pressure and glucose intolerance may lower this threshold to patients with a BMI of over 35. Pharmacotherapy would normally be considered for those who are clinically obese (BMI >30), but once again the presence of other risk factors might lower this threshold, so patients in the upper end of the overweight range might be considered suitable for drug therapy.

Wadden *et al.* (2006) suggest the following guidelines for selection of obesity therapy:

- BMI 25–27: treat with diet and exercise if other risk factors are present
- BMI 27–30: use diet and exercise therapy but consider pharmacotherapy if other risk factors are present
- BMI 30–35: use diet and exercise therapy together with anti-obesity drugs
- BMI 35–40: as for 30–35, but consider surgery if other risk factors are present
- BMI >40: consider all available options including surgery.

These more extreme treatments are not alternatives to diet and exercise. In most cases their aim is to make it easier for patients to comply with their weight loss programmes. Appetite suppressants may reduce hunger during dieting, psychotherapy may help people to control their hunger, and dietary changes may maximize the satiating value of each food calorie. Despite this, dieting will inevitably involve a considerable period of discomfort and the dieter will have to exercise a considerable degree of sustained willpower to achieve substantial weight loss. A VLED will not produce weight loss if it is supplemented by other eating, an appetite suppressant will only produce weight loss if food intake is actually reduced. Some patients who have had their stomach capacity reduced by 90 per cent by surgical stapling still manage to consume enough to prevent weight loss.

Key points

- Drugs can combat obesity by interfering with the digestion and absorption of food, by decreasing appetite, or by increasing energy expenditure.
- Amphetamines suppress appetite by increasing the activity of noradrenalin (norepinephrine) in the brain. Their effects on appetite diminish after a few weeks.

- The appetite suppressants fenfluramine and dexfenfluramine suppress appetite by increasing the activity of the transmitter serotonin in the brain. These were the most commonly used anti-obesity drugs in Europe and had been available for 30 years prior to their withdrawal from sale in 1997 after new doubts were raised about their safety.

→

- Sibutramine is a licensed appetite suppressant in both the UK and USA that increases the effects of both noradrenalin and serotonin in the brain.

- Rimonabant was licensed for use as an appetite suppressant in the UK between 2006 and 2009. It blocks receptors in the brain that are normally involved in the response to endogenous cannabinoids and those from the drug cannabis.

- Several gut hormones and their analogues bring about satiety and preliminary data suggest that oxyntomodulin may have potential in obesity treatment.

- Orlistat interferes with fat digestion by blocking pancreatic lipase and has been approved for use in the UK and the USA.

- Gastric reduction in Europe and gastric bypass in the USA are the most popular surgical treatments for obesity. Jaw wiring, intestinal bypass and lipid reduction are some of the other surgical treatments that have been used.

- Gastric reduction involves reducing the stomach capacity by stapling or banding off a large part of it and thus severely limiting meal size.

- Current surgical procedures are more effective than other treatment for obese and very obese patients, but there are insufficient data to fully assess and compare their safety.

- Very low-energy diets (VLEDs) are liquid formulae designed to provide all the essential nutrients but only a very low energy yield of 1.6–3.2 MJ (400–800 kcal) per day. They are used to replace all solid food or perhaps just some meals.

- The most severe measures inevitably carry some risks, which make them suitable only as treatments for people in whom the risks of their obesity are likely to outweigh any risks of therapy.

- These treatments are adjuncts to conventional dieting rather than substitutes for it. They make it easier for the patient to maintain an energy deficit and work only if it is maintained.

PART THREE

THE NUTRIENTS

---

10   Carbohydrates   245

11   Protein and amino acids   268

12   Fats   285

13   The micronutrients   324

14   The vitamins   357

15   The minerals   393

CARBOHYDRATES

10

Introduction	245	Starches	255
Nature and classification of carbohydrates	246	Non-starch polysaccharide	257
Dietary sources of carbohydrates	247	Resistant starch	260
Sugars	248	The glycaemic index	261
Artificial sweeteners	250	Dietary factors in the aetiology of bowel cancer	262
Diet and dental health	252	Dietary factors in heart disease	266

INTRODUCTION

Carbohydrates have traditionally supplied the largest part of the energy in most human diets. They still provide most of the energy intake for the majority of the world's population whose diets are based on cereals or starchy roots. Dietary carbohydrates are almost exclusively derived from the vegetable kingdom and the carbohydrate content of most foods of animal origin is dietetically insignificant. The only major exception is lactose or milk sugar, which provides about 40 per cent of the energy in human milk and 30 per cent of the energy in cow milk. It is usually only in populations consuming large amounts of meat, oily fish and dairy produce that fat challenges carbohydrates as the principal source of dietary energy. Some affluent vegetarian populations may derive a high proportion of their dietary energy from fat in the form of extracted vegetable oils and margarine.

In some developing countries, over 75 per cent of dietary energy is derived from carbohydrate which is predominantly starch. In the affluent countries of western Europe, Australasia and North America, carbohydrates may provide only about 45 per cent of total dietary energy, and close to half of this is in the form of simple sugars in some instances. These affluent populations are currently being advised to increase the proportion of their energy derived from carbohydrates to 50–60 per cent of the total, and yet – at the same time – substantially reduce their consumption of simple sugars, perhaps limiting 'extracted' sugars to no more than 10 per cent of the total energy intake.

Key points

- Historically, carbohydrates have provided most of the energy in human diets.
- Carbohydrates, principally starch, still provide as much as 75 per cent of the energy in many diets in developing countries.
- In many affluent countries, only about 45 per cent of dietary energy comes from carbohydrate, and close to half of this may be in the form of simple sugars.
- Almost all dietary carbohydrate is from plant foods. An exception is the lactose in milk.
- In populations consuming large amounts of animal foods and/or extracted vegetable oils, fat will challenge carbohydrate as the major energy source.
- Western consumers are advised to take 50–60 per cent of their energy as carbohydrate, but ideally with less than 10 per cent of their energy coming from added sugars.

NATURE AND CLASSIFICATION OF CARBOHYDRATES

Carbohydrates are monomers or polymers of simple sugar units or *saccharides*. Carbohydrates may be described according to the number of saccharide units they contain: the *mono*saccharides (one), the *di*saccharides (two), the *oligo*saccharides (a few), and the *poly*saccharides (many). Although a range of monosaccharides are present in human diets, three of them make up the bulk of the monosaccharide that is released for absorption and utilization during the digestion of most diets: *glucose*, *galactose* and *fructose*. These three monosaccharides each contain six carbon atoms and are therefore termed *hexoses*. The two five-carbon sugars (*pentoses*) are *ribose* and *deoxyribose*; these are released from the digestion of the nucleic acids DNA and RNA in food.

Carbohydrates must be broken down (digested) to their component monosaccharide units before they can be absorbed in the small intestine. Saliva and pancreatic juice contain an enzyme known as α-*amylase* that breaks up digestible polysaccharides (starches) into oligosaccharides and disaccharides. The enzymes *maltase* and *isomaltase* that are present on the absorptive surface of the small intestine complete starch digestion by cleaving the products of the partial digestion by α-amylase into glucose. The enzymes *lactase* and *sucrase*, which are present also on the absorptive surface of the small intestine, digest any of the lactose and sucrose present in the diet.

Dietary carbohydrates are usually classified into three major subdivisions: the *sugars*, the *starches* and the *non-starch polysaccharides* (NSPs) (Figure 10.1). Sugars and starches are readily digested and absorbed in the human small intestine, so they clearly serve as a source of dietary energy and are sometimes termed the 'available carbohydrates'; they all yield about 16 kJ (3.75 kcal) per gram. The non-starch polysaccharides are resistant to digestion by human gut enzymes and are thus referred to as the 'unavailable carbohydrates', although they may yield some energy if they are fermented by bacteria in the large intestine. This fermentation yields volatile fatty acids (e.g. propionate, butyrate and acetate) which can be absorbed and metabolized.

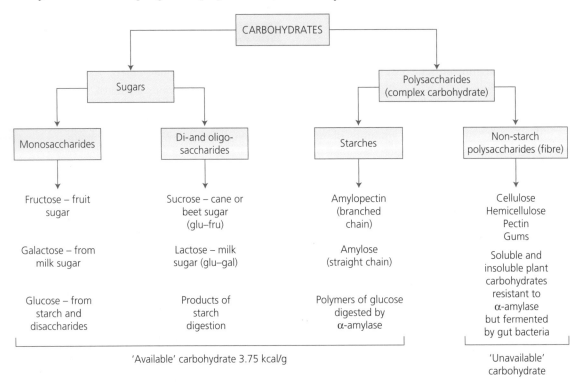

Figure 10.1 A summary of carbohydrate classification.

Key points

- Carbohydrates may be monosaccharides (1 sugar unit), disaccharides (2), oligosaccharides (a few) or polysaccharides (many).

- Only monosaccharides can be absorbed from the gut.

- α-Amylase in saliva and pancreatic juice breaks down starches to di- and oligosaccharides. Other enzymes on the surface of the small intestine complete the digestion of carbohydrates to monosaccharides.

- Sugars, starches and non-starch polysaccharides are the major subdivisions of the carbohydrates.

- Sugars and starches are digested and absorbed in the small intestine.

- Non-starch polysaccharides are indigestible and enter the colon undigested but may be fermented by bacteria in the colon.

DIETARY SOURCES OF CARBOHYDRATES

Carbohydrates provide about 48 per cent of the food energy (excluding alcohol) purchased in the UK, with 23 per cent coming from simple sugars (15.5 per cent from non-milk extrinsic sugars) and 25 per cent from starch (DEFRA, 2006). Likewise, 48 per cent of the food energy in food eaten also came from carbohydrate, with 12.8 per cent from non-milk extrinsic sugars. According to the National Food Survey, between 1952 and 1996 the carbohydrate content of household food (excluding alcohol, soft drinks and confectionery) fell from 324 to 228 g/day; that is, from 53 per cent of food energy in 1952 to 46 per cent in 1996. More recent values (estimated from DEFRA, 2006) expressed in the same way are approximately 230 g/day and 43 per cent.

About 75 per cent of the starch in British household food comes from cereals and cereal products and about 20 per cent from vegetables (mostly from potatoes). About 4 per cent of our starch comes from cereals added to meat and fish products (e.g. breadcrumb coatings). Just under half of the non-starch polysaccharide in British diets comes from fruits and vegetables, while most of the rest comes from cereal foods.

Table 10.1 shows the sources of total sugars in the British diet as estimated in the previous edition of this book, derived from MAFF (1997), and for comparison more recent estimates of the food sources of non-milk extrinsic sugars have been added. Clearly foods in the sugars and fats group of the *food guide plate* or pyramid (see p. 152–3) are the major sources of added sugars in the British and other Western diets. Most of the sugar in the milk group and in fruits and vegetables is sugar that is naturally present in the food.

Table 10.1 The estimated contribution of food groups to the total sugars and non-milk extrinsic sugars (NMES) in the average British diet.

Food	Total sugars	NMES
Milk & milk products inc. cheese	16%	5%
Sugar, preserves, confectionery, soft & alcoholic drinks	39%	64%
Vegetables	6%	1%
Fruit inc. fruit juices	14%	7%
All cereals	18%	17%
(Cakes, pastries & biscuits)	10%	10%

Key points

- Carbohydrates comprise about 48 per cent of food energy in the UK and about 50–55 per cent of this carbohydrate is starch.

- The carbohydrate content of British diets has fallen since the 1950s both in absolute terms and as a proportion of food energy.

- About 90 per cent of the starch in British diets comes from cereal foods and potatoes.

- The NSP in British diets is derived roughly equally from cereal foods and from fruits and vegetables.

- Almost two-thirds of the non-milk extrinsic sugars in British diets comes from sweetened drinks, sweets, preserves and sugar itself.

- Sweetened cereal products, including cakes and biscuits, are another major source of added sugars.

SUGARS

Sugars may be monosaccharides, disaccharides or oligosaccharides; they are characteristically soluble in water and have a sweet taste. The monosaccharides glucose and fructose are present in some fruits and vegetables and in honey. Fructose is three times as sweet as glucose and is largely responsible for the sweet taste of fruits and some vegetables.

Sucrose (relative sweetness 100) is used as the standard against which the sweetness of other sugars and artificial sweeteners is measured. The relative sweetnesses of the other major dietary sugars are: lactose 30, glucose 50 and fructose 170.

Lactose or milk sugar

Lactose is a disaccharide found exclusively in milk and is the least sweet of the major dietary sugars. It comprises one unit of glucose and one of galactose. Lactose is the only significant source of galactose in the diet. Galactose is essential in several synthetic pathways but can be readily synthesized from glucose and so it is not an essential nutrient.

On rare occasions, babies may inherit an enzyme deficiency that renders them unable to metabolize dietary galactose. If such babies are fed with breast milk or lactose-containing infant formula, galactose accumulates in their blood (*galactosaemia*). This results in a range of symptoms (e.g. vomiting, weight loss and jaundice) and, if untreated, may result in death or permanent disability (e.g. cataracts, retarded physical and mental development). Infants with this condition must be fed on a lactose-free formula and will need to continue to avoid milk and milk-containing foods after weaning.

Some babies are born deficient in the enzyme lactase that cleaves lactose into its component monosaccharides in the small intestine (*congenital lactase deficiency*). This deficiency results in a failure to digest and absorb dietary lactose. Such infants will fail to thrive. They will suffer from diarrhoea because of the osmotic effect of undigested lactose causing retention of water within the gut, and bloating because of fermentation of lactose by intestinal bacteria. These infants, too, need to be fed on a lactose-free formula.

In most human populations (and other mammals), lactase activity in the small intestine declines with age after about 4 years. This reduces the capacity of the gut to digest and absorb lactose in older children and adults (*primary lactase non-persistence*). This decline in lactase activity is genetically determined; it is not prevented by continued consumption of lactose and is exhibited to some degree by up to two-thirds of the world's population. Lactase activity does not usually decline with age in the white populations of North America and northern Europe. People who exhibit primary lactase non-persistence are termed 'lactose intolerant' and they experience symptoms of diarrhoea and bloating when challenged with a high dose of lactose. Lactose intolerance may also occur as a secondary consequence of intestinal infection, inflammatory gut diseases and parasitic infestations of the gut (*secondary lactase deficiency*).

The high prevalence of lactose intolerance has led to suggestions that milk and milk products are inappropriate for use in nutritional support programmes in many countries. In a detailed review, Rosado (1997) confirms that many adults and older children in developing countries are indeed intolerant to the 50 g of lactose (equivalent to 1.5 L of milk) used in standard lactose tolerance tests. However, he suggests that only about 30 per cent of these people are intolerant of the smaller amounts of lactose that are likely to be consumed, for example in a glass of milk. Even this 30 per cent, whom he terms 'lactose maldigesters', can tolerate smaller amounts of milk without symptoms and their colon metabolism will adapt to regular milk intake to eliminate symptoms. He suggested that the problem of primary lactase non-persistence does not warrant elimination or severe restriction of milk intake in developing countries.

Sucrose

Sucrose is a disaccharide composed of one unit of glucose and one unit of fructose. It is digested by the enzyme sucrase, which is located on the absorptive surface of the small intestine. Sucrose is found in several fruits and vegetables and is present in large quantities in sugar beet and sugar cane – from which it is extracted and purified on a vast industrial scale. Sucrose is readily available in highly purified or partly purified forms (e.g. white sugar, brown sugar, treacle or syrup). It is also very widely used by food processors to sweeten, preserve and texturize a variety of foods. The terms 'sucrose' and 'sugar' are often used as if they are synonymous.

High sucrose consumption has frequently been blamed for many of the illnesses that afflict affluent populations. The poor health image of sucrose was encapsulated in the phrase 'pure, white and deadly'. Its poor health image has led many food manufacturers to use other sugars, or sugar-containing extracts, in their products so that they can imply in advertising claims that their product is 'healthier' because it has reduced levels of sucrose. The term *extrinsic non-milk sugar* has been used to cover all of the dietary sugars (still principally sucrose) that are not present as natural components of the fruits, vegetables and milk in the diet. Conversely, sugars that are naturally present within the cell walls of plants are termed *intrinsic sugars* (note that the sugars in fruit juice are classified as part of the extrinsic non-milk sugars).

A simpler classification is to divide sugars into those naturally present in food and drinks (milk and fruit juices) and that added by manufacturers or consumers (added sugars).

Sucrose is a natural plant sugar. It happens to be present in large enough amounts in readily cultivatable plants to make it convenient for extraction in industrial quantities. It seems reasonable to suppose that, if sucrose is indeed innately harmful, as it is used in affluent countries, then other sugars used in the same ways and quantities are also likely to be harmful. Substitution of sucrose by other extracted sugars that have not yet acquired the poor health image of sucrose does not appear to offer a high probability of dietary 'improvement'. Extrinsic non-milk sugars comprise roughly 10–20 per cent of the total energy intake in most affluent populations.

Sucrose and other sugars have a very high, almost addictive, sensory appeal, and this might be expected to encourage over-consumption of food energy and thus predispose to obesity. Providing sugared drinking water to rats and mice has been used as an experimental means of inducing obesity. In these experiments with rodents, increasing sugar consumption depresses intake of solid food (and therefore also nutrient intake) but not by enough to fully compensate for the extra energy in the sugar (e.g. Kanarek and Hirsch, 1977). However, as noted in Chapter 9, most of the epidemiological evidence suggests that people who take in a high proportion of their energy as sugar are less likely to be obese than those who consume a lower sugar diet. The proportion of energy derived from fat and sugar tends to be inversely correlated in Western diets (the sugar–fat seesaw), and there are good reasons to expect fat to be more fattening than carbohydrates including sugar. There is thus no convincing evidence to link high sugar intake *per se* to increased risk of obesity.

There is little convincing evidence that, at levels typical of UK and US diets, added sugars are directly implicated in the aetiology of cardiovascular diseases, diabetes or hypertension. There is convincing evidence to link some dietary fats to these conditions, and the sugar–fat seesaw means that high sugar consumers will often consume less of these fats. At very high intakes, 30 per cent or more of total calories, they may elevate serum cholesterol levels and lead to insulin resistance which is important in the aetiology of the maturity-onset form of diabetes (COMA, 1991).

When extracted sugars are added to foods, they add energy but no nutrients. They reduce the nutrient density of the diet, and the phrase 'empty calories' has been coined. The significance of this reduction in nutrient density will depend on the general level of nutrient adequacy. In populations or individuals with high nutrient intakes it will be of less significance than in those whose nutrient intakes are more marginal. Some nutrient-rich foods may become palatable only if sugar is added (e.g. some sour fruits). In groups, such as the elderly, where high nutrient density is considered a nutritional priority, moderation of added sugar to no more than 10 per cent of total energy should help to raise nutrient density. However, when appetite is poor, any reduction in dietary palatability resulting from reduction in sugar intakes may simply depress both energy and nutrient intake.

Key points

- Sugars have a sweet taste and are soluble in water.
- The relative sweetnesses of sugars and artificial sweeteners are graded in relation to sucrose (relative sweetness 100). Fructose is the sweetest dietary sugar (170) and lactose the least sweet (30).
- Lactose is a disaccharide of glucose and galactose that is found exclusively in milk.
- Babies with congenital galactosaemia are unable to metabolize galactose. Babies with congenital lactase deficiency are unable to digest and absorb lactose. These infants need a lactose-free formula.
- In most non-European populations, lactose activity in the gut declines after early childhood, leading to lactose intolerance (primary lactase non-persistence). Most lactose-intolerant people can tolerate moderate amounts of milk, so lactose intolerance does not warrant the elimination of milk from diets in the developing countries.
- Lactose intolerance may also occur as a secondary consequence of gut disease.
- Sucrose is a disaccharide of glucose and fructose and is the major added sugar in the diet.
- The term 'non-milk extrinsic sugars' covers all sugars (largely sucrose) that are not present naturally in the fruits, vegetables and milk that we eat; it includes the sugar in fruit juice.
- Sugars contained within the cell walls of plants are termed intrinsic sugars.
- A simpler classification is between sugars added by manufacturers and consumers (added sugars) and those naturally present in food and drinks (milk and fruit juice).
- There is little evidence that high sugar intake is causally linked to diabetes, heart disease or obesity.
- The proportion of energy derived from fats and sugars tends to be inversely correlated – the sugar–fat seesaw.
- Low-fat diets, which because of the sugar–fat seesaw tend to be high in sugar, are associated with reduced risk of obesity.
- High sugar consumption does reduce the nutrient density of diets. This may be particularly important in groups, such as the very elderly, with marginal intakes of essential nutrients.

ARTIFICIAL SWEETENERS

Artificial sweeteners have been developed and manufactured to satisfy our craving for sweetness without the necessity to consume sugars. Saccharin, aspartame and acesulfame K are not sugars or carbohydrates and are essentially calorie-free. They are also intensely sweet; those three examples are typically 200–300 times as sweet as sucrose and so very small quantities are needed to replace the sweetness normally provided by sugar. Their use is particularly prominent in drinks. Low-calorie soft drinks, containing artificial sweeteners, account for more than 40 per cent of the soft drinks consumed by British adults, with women more likely than men to choose a low-calorie soft drink.

Saccharin was the first artificial sweetener and has been in use for over a century. Saccharin is absorbed and excreted unchanged in the urine. Very large intakes have been reported to increase the incidence of bladder tumours in rats; despite this, it is still a permitted sweetener in most countries, including the USA and UK, because at practical intake levels it is not thought to represent a significant hazard. Saccharin has a bitter after-taste. It is destroyed by heating, which means that it cannot be used as a substitute for sugar in cooking, limiting its usefulness to food manufacturers.

Aspartame is a more recent addition to the sweetener range. It is a dipeptide made up of the amino acids aspartic acid and phenylalanine. Despite being digested to its constituent amino acids and absorbed, it has a negligible calorific yield because so little is used. In the rare inherited condition phenylketonuria (PKU), there is an inability to metabolize dietary phenylalanine and so it can accumulate in the blood, causing severe brain damage and mental retardation in affected children (see Chapter 17). Obviously, PKU sufferers should avoid aspartame, but there have been some largely unsubstantiated suggestions that consuming large amounts of phenylalanine in the form of aspartame might cause brain damage also in non-PKU sufferers.

Sucralose is the most recent addition to the list of approved sweeteners; it was licensed for use in 1998 in the USA and in 2002 in the UK. Sucralose is made from cane sugar. Three of the hydroxyl groups of sucrose are replaced by chlorine atoms, and taste tests suggest that it is perceived to taste very much like sugar. The chemical modification of sucrose produces a compound that is 600 times as sweet as sucrose but is not metabolized to yield energy; most of it passes through the gut unchanged. A major advantage of sucralose is its stability; it is heat-resistant and so, unlike the other major sweeteners, can be used in cooked and baked goods. It is also retains its stability and sweetness at low pH.

Although these intense sweeteners mimic the sweetness of sugar they do not have the preservative or textural effects of sugar. This means that, even with sucralose, recipes need to be modified if the sugar is serving other functions besides just adding sweetness.

These artificial sweeteners would seem to offer great potential benefits especially to people who are trying to lose weight. If a glass of regular cola is replaced by a 'diet' version sweetened with one of these, this would reduce energy intake by 75 kcal (300 kJ). If a sweetener is used to replace two spoonfuls of sugar in a cup of tea or coffee then this avoids 40 kcal (150 kJ) each time. Consumption of these artificial sweeteners is equivalent to billions of sugar calories in Europe and North America each year, and this saved energy is equivalent to several kilos of theoretically prevented weight gain for these people. However, the massive growth in the use of these products has not been accompanied by corresponding reductions in sugar use, and it has coincided with a large rise in the prevalence of obesity.

These intense sweeteners do not provide energy, but neither do they have the satiating effect of sugar. This means that, unless users are consciously restricting their energy intake (i.e. dieting), they will tend to replace any lost sugar calories with more of their usual mixed food. The net effect is that there tends to be some replacement of carbohydrate calories (sugar) by fat calories and so the proportion of energy derived from fat tends to rise. Given the arguments about the greater fattening effects of fat compared to carbohydrate in Chapter 9, this would not be a desirable outcome for improving weight control. Data from the USA show that there has been no significant decline in sugar use to parallel the growth in sales of intense sweeteners, so are they really substituting for sugar or largely an addition to the usual diet? Of course these sweeteners may be helpful to those who are

consciously dieting but who do not want give up sweet drinks and other sweet products. They may also have benefits for dental health and nutrient density if they really reduce sugar consumption.

These effects of sugar substitutes on food choice and dietary composition were reviewed by Mela (1997). A more recent review by Yang (2010) came to the following conclusions.

- In epidemiological studies in children and adults there was generally a positive association between artificial sweetener use and weight gain.
- The consensus from intervention studies suggests that simple substitution of beverages sweetened with artificial sweeteners for those sweetened with sugar did not help to reduce weight.
- Some short-term experiments with rats and people suggest that a sweet taste may enhance appetite. Yang discusses possible neurological mechanisms for this effect in his review.

Mattes and Popkin (2009) also concluded that use of artificial sweeteners offers no benefit for weight control unless it is coupled with energy restriction.

Sugar replacers

In recent decades there has been a growth in the use of bulk sweeteners or sugar replacers that have a similar sweetness to sucrose on a weight-for-weight basis (typically 40–90 per cent of the sweetness of sucrose). These compounds are mostly sugar alcohols (e.g. xylitol, sorbitol and isomalt) that yield fewer calories than sugar because they are incompletely absorbed or metabolized; they typically yield 40–60 per cent of the energy of an equivalent weight of sucrose. They can be used in similar amounts to sugar in some food products. They add not just sweetness but also the textural and mouthfeel properties of sugar. They may be used in combination with intense artificial sweeteners to boost their sweetness. These sugar replacers do not promote dental caries and, because they are only slowly and partially absorbed, they do not cause the same large rises in blood glucose and insulin that sugar does – which may be particularly useful for diabetics. However, if they are eaten in large amounts then (because of their limited absorption) a large amount of carbohydrate may enter the large bowel. This can have an osmotic effect and increase bacterial fermentation, leading to diarrhoea and flatulence. Sugar replacers have been reviewed by McNutt (1998).

Key points

- Artificial sweeteners like saccharin, sucralose and aspartame are intensely sweet and so only need to be used in minute amounts. They are practically calorie-free.

- Saccharin and aspartame are destroyed during cooking. Sucralose is stable when heated and retains its sweetness at low pH.

- Aspartame is a source of phenylalanine and so must be avoided by those with phenylketonuria.

- These sweeteners do not have the preservative or textural effects of sugar. This limits their usefulness in cooking and food processing.

- Artificial sweeteners can cut total energy intake if they replace sugar in a calorie-controlled diet.

- Sweeteners do not have the satiating effect of sugar and so, in unregulated diets, any 'saved' sugar calories are likely to be replaced by calories from other foods.

- In epidemiological studies, high use of artificial sweeteners is positively associated with body mass index (BMI).

- Simple replacement of beverages sweetened with sugar by those with artificial sweeteners does not prevent weight gain or lead to weight loss unless accompanied by calorie restriction.

- If sweeteners really do replace sugar intake, they may have benefits for dental health and should improve the nutrient density of the diet.

- Sugar replacers are mostly sugar alcohols (e.g. sorbitol) that have similar sweetness to sugar but yield less energy because they are incompletely absorbed and metabolized. Sugar replacers provide similar textural effects to sugar in food processing. Sugar replacers do not promote dental caries.

- Sugar replacers may be useful for diabetics because their slower absorption means they cause smaller rises in blood sugar and insulin release than sugar.

- In large doses, sugar replacers spill into the large bowel and can cause flatulence and diarrhoea.

DIET AND DENTAL HEALTH

COMA (1989a) and Binns (1992) have published referenced reviews of the role of sugars in the aetiology of dental caries. Moynihan (1995) reviewed the relationship between all aspects of diet and dental health. Most of the older uncited references used in this section are listed in these reviews.

The notion that sugar is implicated in the aetiology of dental caries (tooth decay) stretches back to the Ancient Greeks. The evidence that sugars, and sucrose in particular, have some effect on the development of dental caries is overwhelming; only the relative importance of sugar as compared to other factors, like fluoride intake and individual susceptibility, is really disputed. There is a strong correlation across populations between average sugar consumption and the number of decayed, missing and filled (DMF) teeth in children. In populations with low sugar consumption (less than 10 per cent of energy intake), dental caries are uncommon. Observations with island populations and other isolated communities have shown a strong correlation between changes in the sugar supply and changes in the rates of tooth decay. In the UK during the Second World War, rates of tooth decay fell when sugar was rationed. In the past, low rates of tooth decay have been found in diabetic children living in institutions whose sugar intake would have been kept very low as part of their diabetic management. Studies of other groups of people with habitually low sugar intakes have also found low levels of dental caries (e.g. children living in children's homes, Seventh Day Adventists and children of dentists). Conversely, groups with high habitual sugar intakes have high rates of caries (e.g. sugar cane cutters and those working in factories producing confectionery).

In a study conducted over 60 years ago in Swedish mental hospitals, the Vipeholm study, groups of patients were exposed to not only differing levels of sugar intake but also differences in the form and frequency of that sugar intake. Not only was the amount of sugar important in determining rates of tooth decay, but form and frequency had an even greater impact:

- sugar taken between meals was found to be the most cariogenic
- frequent consumption of small amounts of sugar was more harmful than the same amount consumed in large infrequent doses

- the most cariogenic foods were those where the sugar was in a sticky form that adhered to the teeth (e.g. toffees).

Studies with animals have found that:

- the presence of sugar in the mouth is required for caries to occur
- all common dietary sugars are cariogenic to some extent
- increased frequency and duration of eating sugar-containing foods increase the risk of caries production.

The key event in the development of dental caries is the production of acid by the bacteria *Streptococcus mutans* in dental plaque. Plaque is a sticky mixture of food residue, bacteria and bacterial polysaccharides that adheres to teeth. The bacteria produce acid by fermenting carbohydrates, particularly sugars, in foods. When the mouth becomes acidic enough (i.e. pH drops below 5.2), this causes demineralization of the teeth. This can lead to holes in the hard outer enamel layer, exposing the softer dentine and enabling decay to proceed rapidly. This is not a one-way process. Between periods of demineralization there will be phases of remineralization or repair, and it is the balance between these two processes that will determine susceptibility to decay.

The key role of oral bacteria in the development of caries is highlighted by experiments with germ-free animals. Rats born by caesarean section into a sterile environment and maintained germ-free throughout their lives do not develop dental caries even when their diets are high in sucrose.

Tooth decay can therefore be considered a bacterial disease that is promoted by dietary sugar. Sugars are ideal substrates for the acid-producing bacteria of the plaque. When sugars are consumed as part of a meal then other constituents of the food can act as buffers that 'soak up' the acid and limit the effects on mouth pH of any acid produced. High saliva production also reduces acid attack by buffering and diluting the acid. The more frequently sugar-containing snacks or drinks are consumed, and the longer that sugar remains in the mouth, the longer is the period that the overall pH of the mouth is below the level at which demineralization occurs. In the UK, there is a target for reducing extrinsic

non-milk sugars to less than 11 per cent of total energy intake. Reducing between-meal sugar in drinks and sugary snacks is regarded as the priority in the prevention of dental caries. Prolonged sucking of sugary drinks through a teat by infants and young children is particularly damaging to teeth, so manufacturers of these drinks recommend that they be consumed from a cup. Some foods contain factors that protect against caries, particularly milk and cheese. Despite containing large amounts of lactose, milk is regarded as non-cariogenic. Chocolate may also contain factors that protect against caries, but this is counterbalanced by its high sugar content.

In a review of the role of sugars in caries induction from the sugar industry viewpoint, Binns (1992) emphasized the importance of other factors in determining caries frequency. Binns gave evidence of a substantial reduction in caries frequency in industrialized countries between 1967 and 1983 (Table 10.2). During the period covered, sugar consumption did not change substantially and Binns suggested that consumption of sugary snacks between meals might even have increased. Moynihan (1995) summarized UK data which suggested that, between 1983 and 1993, the number of 15-year-old children who were free of caries rose from 7 to 37 per cent and the average number of decayed, missing and filled teeth fell from 6 to 2.5. There have been similar improvements in the dental health of adults; between 1968 and 1988 the number of Britons aged 65–74 years who had no natural teeth dropped from three-quarters to under half.

Table 10.2 Changes in the average number of decayed, missing and filled (DMF) teeth in 12-year-old children over the period 1967 to 1983. Data source: Binns (1992).

Country	1967	1983
Australia	4.8	2.8
Denmark	6.3	4.7
Finland	7.2	4.1
Netherlands	7.5	3.9
New Zealand	9.0	3.3
Norway	10.1	4.4
Sweden	4.8	3.4
United Kingdom	4.7	3.0
United States	3.8	2.6

The decline in the prevalence of caries in children in the UK and other industrialized countries may be attributed in large part to the effect of increased *fluoride intake*. Some water supplies have been fluoridated, some parents give children fluoride supplements and, most significantly, almost all toothpaste is now fluoridated. The evidence that fluoride has a protective effect against the development of dental caries is very strong. There is an inverse epidemiological association between the fluoride content of drinking water and rates of DMF teeth in the children. These epidemiological comparisons suggest that an optimal level of fluoride in drinking water is about 1 part per million (1 mg/L). At this level there seems to be good protection against tooth decay without the risk of the mottling of teeth that is increasingly associated with levels much above this.

Intervention studies where the water supply has been fluoridated (see the example in Chapter 4) and studies using fluoridated milk and salt have also confirmed the protective effects of fluoride. In a systematic review, Marinho *et al.* (2003) found solid evidence that regular use of fluoridated toothpaste helps to prevent dental caries in children and adolescents.

The major effect of fluoride in preventing tooth decay is thought to be by its incorporation into the mineral matter of the tooth enamel; incorporation of fluoride into the calcium/phosphate compound hydroxyapatite to give fluorapatite renders the tooth enamel more resistant to demineralization. This means that fluoride is most effective in preventing dental caries when administered to young children (the under-5s) during tooth formation. Fluoride in relatively high doses also inhibits bacterial acid production and inhibits bacterial growth; it may concentrate in plaque to produce these effects at normal intake levels. Fluoride at low concentrations in the mouth decreases the process of demineralization and increases the remineralization (healing) of early carious lesions in the teeth. Several expert committees have made specific recommendations to ensure adequate intakes of fluoride, especially in young children, and these quantitative recommendations are summarized in Chapter 15.

Despite the very strong evidence for a beneficial effect of fluoride on dental health, there has been limited fluoridation of water supplies in the UK – in contrast to the USA where it is widespread. Only about 12 per cent of England has optimally fluoridated water even though water companies have had the power to add fluoride to drinking water at the request of the health authority since the passage of the Water (Fluoridation) Act in 1985. This is because of strong opposition from some pressure groups. Opposition to fluoridation has been partly on the grounds that addition of fluoride to the public water supply amounts to mass medication without individual consent. There have also been persistent concerns expressed about the long-term safety of this level of fluoride consumption; it is very difficult, for example, to prove beyond any doubt that there is no increased cancer risk associated with lifetime consumption. The consensus is that fluoride in drinking water at optimal levels for dental health is not associated with any increase in risk of cancer or other diseases. The difference between the therapeutic levels proposed and the dose associated with early signs of fluoride overload (mottling of the teeth) is also relatively small (2- to 3-fold). There may also be a relatively small number of people who are sensitive to fluoride. A map showing current levels of natural and artificial fluoride in drinking water in England and Wales can be found at http://dwi.defra.gov.uk/consumers/advice-leaflets/fluoridemap.pdf.

Dental caries is not the only cause of tooth loss. In adults, gum disease (periodontal disease) is the most frequent cause of tooth loss. *Gingivitis* is an inflammation of the gums caused by the presence of plaque. It can lead to receding of the gums which exposes the roots of the teeth to decay and eventually may lead to loosening and loss of teeth. As with caries, sugar is a major causative factor for gum disease, but attainable reductions in sugar consumption are unlikely to have much impact on this condition. Improved oral hygiene may be the most effective way of controlling this condition. Deficiencies of vitamins A, C, E and folic acid have detrimental effects on gum health but it is unclear whether increased intakes would improve general standards of oral health.

Key points

- Cross-cultural comparisons, time trends and observations on groups with high or low sugar intakes all suggest that high sugar intake promotes dental caries.

- Sugar is most damaging to teeth when it is taken frequently, between meals and in a form that adheres to the teeth.

- Bacteria in the mouth ferment carbohydrates in food, especially sugars, to produce acid. This acidity leads to demineralization of teeth, making them prone to decay. Germ-free experimental animals fed sugar do not get dental caries.

- When sugar is taken as part of a meal, other components of the meal may buffer any acid produced. Saliva also buffers and dilutes mouth acid.

- Some foods contain factors that protect against dental caries; they include milk, cheese and chocolate.

- A reduction in the consumption of added sugar with a particular emphasis on reducing sugary snacks and drinks between meals is recommended to improve dental health.

- Infants should not be allowed to suck sugary drinks slowly through a teat.

- Rates of dental caries in children have fallen in recent decades in many countries, owing largely to higher fluoride intakes particularly from fluoridated toothpaste.

- In areas with naturally high fluoride content in drinking water of 1 mg/L, rates of child dental disease are low and there are no indications of any adverse effects.

- Fluoride is incorporated into the tooth enamel in young children and makes teeth more resistant to acid demineralization. Fluoride in the mouth also decreases tooth demineralization and helps remineralization of carious lesions.

- Expert committees in both the USA and UK have recommended that adequate intakes of fluoride should be ensured, especially in infants and young children. Some areas have artificially fluoridated their water up to a level of 1 mg/L, but there has been considerable resistance to widespread fluoridation largely because of →

Key points *continued*

- unsubstantiated concerns about the long-term safety of this level of fluoride intake.

- In adults, gum disease is the most frequent cause of tooth loss. Gum disease is promoted by sugar, but improved dental hygiene may be the most effective way of reducing tooth loss by this route.

STARCHES

Plants use starches as a store of energy in their roots and seeds. Animals also manufacture and store a form of starch – *glycogen* – in muscle and liver, but the amounts present in most flesh foods are dietetically insignificant. The amount of energy that animals and people store as glycogen is very small. Total glycogen stores of people amount to only a few hours' energy expenditure. Glycogen is an inefficient bulk energy store because it yields only about 4 kcal (16 kJ) per gram and because it holds with it probably four times its own weight of water. (Fat yields 9 kcal per gram and does not hold water.) Glycogen serves as a store of carbohydrate that can maintain blood glucose concentration during normal intervals between meals.

Starches are polymers of glucose. The glucose may be arranged in predominantly straight chains (*amylose*) or, more frequently, in highly branched chains (*amylopectin*). The glucose residues in starches are joined together by linkages that can be broken (hydrolysed) by human digestive enzymes. These linkages are mainly α 1–4 linkages with some α 1–6 linkages that cause the branching of the glucose chain. Amylose has few α 1–6 linkages whereas amylopectin has many, and the latter's extensively branched structure has been likened to a bunch of grapes (Figure 10.2). The dimers and trimers of glucose that are produced as a result of digestion by α-amylase are then finally cleaved by enzymes on the mucosal surface of the small intestine to yield glucose. The enzyme *maltase* breaks α 1–4 linkages in these dimers and trimers, and the enzyme *isomaltase* breaks α 1–6 linkages.

Starches provide approximately the same energy yield as sugars (3.75 kcal/g or 16 kJ/g). They have low solubility in water and they do not have a sweet taste.

Glucose

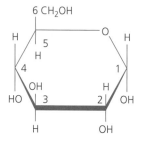

Maltose
Glucose joined by α 1–4 links

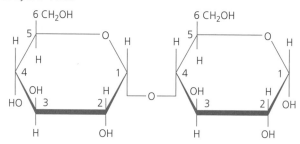

Amylose
Long chains of glucose residues joined by α 1–4 links

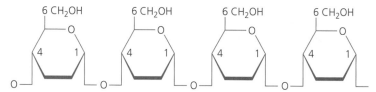

Amylopectin
An α branch point in amylopectin due to an α 1–6 link

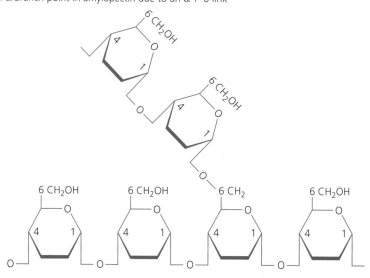

Figure 10.2 Some carbohydrate structures.

As starches are bland, starchy foods also tend to be bland. This is one reason why affluent populations take the opportunity to select foods with more sensory appeal and tend to reduce the proportion of their dietary energy that is supplied by starch and replace it with fats and sugars. If both sugar and fat intakes are to be reduced in line with the recommendations discussed in Chapter 5, this must inevitably involve a large increase in starch consumption – perhaps a doubling of current intakes. Something like 90 per cent of the starch in the British diet comes from cereals and potatoes, so any major increase in starch consumption must mean eating more potatoes, bread and other cereals.

Key points

- Animals store glycogen, a form of starch, in liver and muscles, but the starch content of meat is insignificant.
- Glycogen is an inefficient bulk energy store for animals because it has a lower energy yield than fat and holds large amounts of water.
- Starches are polymers of glucose.
- Amylose is starch in which the glucose residues are joined in long, straight chains by α 1-4 links.
- In amylopectin there is considerable branching of the glucose chain caused by the presence of α 1–6 links.
- The enzyme α-amylase in saliva and pancreatic juice cleaves starches to dimers and trimers of glucose by hydrolysing α 1-4 links.
- The enzymes maltase and isomaltase located on the surface of the small intestine complete the digestion of starch to glucose.
- Starches are insoluble in water and are bland, so affluent populations tend to replace much of the starch that predominates in peasant diets with fats and sugars.
- Reducing fat and sugar intakes to recommended levels will involve large increases in starch consumption, which means eating more potatoes, bread and other cereals.

NON-STARCH POLYSACCHARIDE

Non-starch polysaccharides (NSP) are structural components of plant cell walls (cellulose and hemicellulose) and viscous soluble substances found in cell sap (pectin and gums). They are resistant to digestion by human gut enzymes. Animal-derived foods can be regarded for dietetic purposes as containing no NSP. NSP contains numerous different sugar residues but it passes through the small intestine and into the large bowel undigested. The term 'non-starch polysaccharide' is used interchangeably with the term 'dietary fibre', although the latter term would also include *lignin* and *resistant starch* (see next section). Lignin is an insoluble, chemically complex material that is not carbohydrate; it is found in wood and is the woody component of cell walls. Dietary lignin comes from mature root vegetables, wheat bran and the seeds of fruits such as strawberries.

Americans and Britons are currently being advised to substantially increase their consumption of NSP or fibre; the recommendations suggest increases over current intakes of 50–100 per cent. NSP and starches are usually found within the same foods, particularly in cereals and starchy vegetables like potatoes. This means that increasing NSP and starch intakes are likely to go hand in hand. The milling of cereals so that all or part of the indigestible outer layers of the cereal grains (bran) is removed substantially reduces the NSP and micronutrient content of the end-product, but without removing significant amounts of starch. Whole-grain cereals therefore contain substantially more NSP than refined cereals; for example (per 100 g):

- wholemeal bread   5.8 g
- white bread – 1.5 g
- brown rice — 0.8 g
- white rice– 0.2 g.

Current average intakes of NSP in the UK are about 14 g/day with a wide individual variation, and this compares with the dietary reference value (DRV) of 18 g/day. About 72 per cent of men and 87 per cent of women appear to take in less than the 18 g/day target value.

Non-starch polysaccharide is frequently categorized into two major fractions:

- the soluble substances that form gums and gels when mixed with water (the gums and pectins plus some hemicellulose)
- the water-insoluble fraction (cellulose and some hemicellulose).

The NSP in the UK diet is made up of similar proportions of soluble and insoluble NSP. The insoluble forms predominate in the bran of wheat, rice and maize, but oats, rye and barley contain higher proportions of soluble NSP. The proportions of soluble and insoluble NSP in fruits and vegetables vary, but they generally contain a substantially higher proportion of soluble NSP than wheat fibre, the principal cereal NSP in the British diet. Table 10.3 shows the total NSP content of a number of common foods and the proportion of the NSP that is soluble.

Table 10.3 The soluble non-starch polysaccharide (NSP) content of some common foods. Data source: Halliday and Ashwell (1991).

Food	Total NSP	% soluble NSP
	g/100g	
Wholemeal bread	5.8	17
Brown rice	0.8	12
Oatmeal (raw)	7.0	60
'All-bran'	24.5	17
Cornflakes	0.9	44
Potatoes	1.2	58
Apples	1.6	38
Oranges	2.1	66
Bananas	1.1	64
Carrots	2.5	56
Peas	2.9	28
Sprouts	4.8	52
Cabbage	3.2	50
Baked beans	3.5	60
Roasted peanuts	6.2	31

Although NSP is resistant to digestion by human gut enzymes and passes through the small intestine largely intact, in the large intestine most of the components of NSP are fermented to variable extents by gut bacteria. The pectins are very readily fermentable, but cellulose remains largely unfermented in the human colon and in general soluble NSP is more fermented than insoluble NSP. NSP thus acts as a substrate for bacterial growth within the large intestine; the by-products of this fermentation are intestinal gases and short-chain fatty acids (acetate, butyrate and propionate). The short-chain fatty acids thus produced can be

absorbed from the gut and can serve as a human energy source. (Note that in ruminating animals like sheep and cattle, the short-chain fatty acids produced by the fermentation of starches and NSP by microbes in the rumen are the animal's principal energy source. Even in pigs, whose gastrointestinal physiology is much more like that of humans, such fermentation in the large intestine, and the resulting short-chain fatty acids, can make up a substantial proportion of the total dietary energy.)

Increasing levels of NSP in the diet can be convincingly shown to have a number of physiological effects in the short term.

1

Increased NSP content of food slows down the rate of glucose absorption from the gut and thus reduces the postprandial peak concentrations of glucose and insulin in blood. This effect is attributed to the soluble components of NSP and it is thought to be partly due to the mechanical effect of the viscous NSP components in reducing the contact of dissolved glucose with the absorptive surface of the intestinal epithelium. Soluble NSP may also slow down the mixing of gut contents with digestive enzymes and so slow the digestive process. Guar gum (a soluble NSP that forms a viscous solution when mixed with water) has been shown to reduce the outflow of dissolved glucose even in in-vitro experiments using a dialysis bag made from synthetic materials. The NSP can only produce this effect if taken with the glucose or digestible carbohydrate – it cannot work if taken a few hours before or after the ingested glucose. Increased intakes of dietary fibre have been shown to improve glucose tolerance; diabetics, in particular, may benefit from this improvement. Dietary guidelines for diabetics now include a recommendation to ensure good intakes of high-NSP foods.

2

Increased intake of NSP increases the volume of stools produced and reduces the transit time (i.e. the time it takes for an ingested marker to pass out in the faeces). The fermentable components of NSP lead to increased proliferation of intestinal bacteria and thus increase the bacterial mass in the stools. The short-chain fatty acids produced during fermentation also tend to acidify the colonic contents and act as substrates for the intestinal cells, and this may increase gut motility. The unfermented components of NSP hold water, so they also increase the stool bulk and make the stools softer and easier to pass. The increased bulk and softness of stools, together with more direct effects on gut motility, produced by the products of fermentation, combine to accelerate the passage of faeces through the colon.

These effects of fibre/NSP on the gut are often presented as being only relatively recently recognized but they do in fact have a very long history. The following statements are quoted from a booklet published by the Kellogg Company in 1934:

> It is imperative that proper bulk be included in the foods that are served. Otherwise, the system fails to eliminate regularly. Common constipation, with its attendant evils, sets in. ... This bulk is the cellulose or fibre content in certain natural foods. ... Within the body, it [bran] absorbs moisture and forms a soft mass which gently helps to clear the intestines of wastes.

Even back in the 1880s, Dr Thomas Allinson was championing the cause of wholemeal bread. He suggested many benefits of wholemeal over white bread (i.e. of bran) that are widely accepted today, including prevention of constipation and the prevention of minor bowel disorders such as haemorrhoids ('piles').

3

Non-starch polysaccharide and some of the substances associated with it (e.g. phytate) tend to bind or chelate minerals and probably also vitamins, and thus may hinder their absorption. In compensation, foods rich in NSP tend also to have higher levels of micronutrients than refined foods. If the NSP is fermented in the colon then this releases bound minerals. At intakes of NSP consumed by most Britons or Americans this is unlikely to pose a significant threat to micronutrient supply.

4

In recent years there has been considerable interest in the possible effects that increased intakes of soluble NSP may have in reducing the serum cholesterol concentration. A number of controlled studies have indicated that consumption of

relatively large quantities of oats, which are rich in soluble NSP, can have a significant cholesterol-lowering effect in subjects with either elevated or normal cholesterol levels. One explanation for this effect is that the soluble NSP binds or chelates both dietary cholesterol and bile acids (produced from cholesterol), and this reduces their absorption or re-absorption in the small intestine and thus increases the rate of faecal cholesterol loss. Most of the considerable quantity of bile acids and cholesterol secreted in the bile each day are reabsorbed and recycled (see enterohepatic recycling of bile acids in Chapter 12). High NSP intake may reduce this recycling.

5

High-fibre diets tend to be high in starch and low in fat, so the energy density of such diets tends to be low. There is a widespread belief that such dietary bulking may contribute to maintaining energy balance and thus to reducing overweight and obesity. Blundell and Burley (1987) reviewed evidence that NSP may also have a satiating effect and thus may be a useful aid to regulating energy balance in those prone to overweight and obesity (another effect of bran proposed by Allinson in the 1880s). Some possible reasons why high NSP foods could be more satiating are listed below.

- They reduce eating speed because they require increased chewing (this also stimulates saliva production and may be beneficial to dental health).
- Soluble NSP slows gastric emptying and may contribute to feelings of fullness.
- NSP slows down the absorption of glucose and other nutrients and reduces the insulin response to absorbed nutrients. A large insulin response to absorbed nutrients may cause blood glucose concentration to fall below resting levels (the rebound effect), triggering feelings of hunger.

Key points

- Non-starch polysaccharides are carbohydrates such as cellulose, hemicellulose, pectin and some gums that are all resistant to digestion by α-amylase.
- NSP passes into the large bowel undigested.

Key points *continued*

- The term dietary fibre would include not only NSP but also lignin, a complex, woody material that is not carbohydrate, as well as starch that resists digestion by α-amylase.
- UK and US consumers are curently recommended to increase their fibre/NSP intakes by 50–100 per cent.
- Most of the NSP in cereal grains is in the bran layer, and so milling cereals to remove the bran removes much of their NSP.
- Whole-grain cereals contain much more fibre/ NSP than refined cereals.
- Some components of NSP are soluble and form gels when mixed with water, whereas other components are insoluble.
- Insoluble NSP predominates in wheat, rice and maize bran. Other cereals (e.g. oats) and most fruits and vegetables contain higher proportions of soluble NSP.
- In the bowel, most components of NSP are fermented to varying extents by bacteria to yield short-chain fatty acids. These acids can be absorbed and may yield significant amounts of metabolizable energy.
- Soluble NSP slows glucose absorption and reduces the postprandial peaks of glucose and insulin.
- NSP increases the volume of stools and reduces transit time because it increases the bacterial mass and water content.
- NSP may bind vitamins and minerals and hinder their absorption. However, many high-NSP foods are relatively rich in micronutrients and any bound nutrients will be released if the NSP is fermented.
- Soluble fibre has a lowering effect on plasma cholesterol because it hinders the recycling of bile acids and so increases faecal losses of cholesterol.
- High-fibre foods may help in the regulation of energy intake because:
  - they reduce eating speed
  - NSP slows gastric emptying
  - NSP slows glucose absorption and may help to prevent rebound hypoglycaemia caused by a large insulin response to a rapid absorption of glucose.

RESISTANT STARCH

Many starchy foods such as bread, cornflakes and boiled potatoes contain starch that is resistant to digestion by α-amylase *in vitro*. If resistance to α-amylase digestion is used in the chemical determination of NSP in food, this resistant starch would be classified as part of the NSP. Studies on patients with ileostomies (i.e. whose small intestine has been surgically modified so that they drain externally into a bag rather than into the large intestine) show that this resistant starch also resists digestion by gut enzymes *in vivo*. Like NSP, resistant starch enters the large intestine undigested. Resistant starch acts as a substrate for bacteria in the large bowel and this affects bowel function. Resistant starch could therefore be regarded as part of the 'dietary fibre' with health benefits similar to those of NSP.

Starch that is within starch granules is in a partial crystalline form that is insoluble and relatively resistant to α-amylase digestion. During cooking (heating with moisture) this crystalline starch is disrupted (gelatinized), rendering it much more digestible. During cooling the starch starts to re-crystallize (retrogradation) which reduces its digestibility. There are essentially three reasons why starch may be resistant to digestion in the gut.

- It may inaccessible to digestive enzymes because it is enclosed within unbroken cell walls or in partly milled grains or seeds.
- Some forms of raw crystalline starch (e.g. in raw potatoes and green bananas) are resistant to α-amylase digestion.
- Retrograded starch in food that has been cooked and cooled is indigestible.

This resistant starch is usually only a small component of total starch in any food. However, it may make a considerable contribution to the apparent NSP content of some foods. For example, resistant starch would represent about 30 per cent of the apparent NSP in white bread, 33 per cent in boiled potatoes and 80 per cent in boiled white rice. The amount of resistant starch in any given food may vary quite a lot depending on slight differences in preparation. In freshly cooked potatoes, about 3–5 per cent of the starch is not digested in the small intestine but this rises to 12 per cent when potatoes are cooked and cooled before being eaten. In greenish under-ripe bananas, as much as 70 per cent of the starch reaches the large intestine. It has been estimated that average intake of resistant starch in Europe is about 4 g/day. It would be possible to alter the resistant starch content of processed food by manipulating the choice of raw materials and the processing conditions.

Resistant starch is just one of a number of factors that complicate the measurement of dietary fibre intakes of a population. Englyst and Kingman (1993) give values for the estimates of fibre intake in several foods, which vary by as much 100 per cent depending on the analytical methods used to estimate it. This clearly represents a major hindrance to epidemiological investigations of the effects of NSP/fibre on health. For example, several oriental populations with rice-based diets have lower fibre intakes than the British because of the very low NSP content of white rice. These oriental diets are, however, often high in starch and inclusion of resistant starch with NSP would significantly change the fibre position of these diets. The Englyst method specifically measures the NSP content of food. Starch is completely removed by enzyme hydrolysis and then the amount of sugars released by acid hydrolysis of the food is determined and used as the measure of NSP content. Resistant starch has been reviewed by Asp *et al.* (1996).

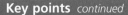

Key points

- Some starch resists digestion by α-amylase and enters the large bowel undigested – the resistant starch.
- Resistant starch is fermented in the large bowel and behaves like a fermentable component of NSP.
- Some starch resists digestion because it is inaccessible to gut enzymes (e.g. it is within cell walls).
- Raw crystalline starch is resistant to α-amylase (e.g. the starch in raw potatoes).
- When crystalline starch is cooked it gelatinizes and becomes digestible. During cooling some of it re-crystallizes (retrogradation) and becomes indigestible again.
- The way in which foods are processed can have a big influence on the resistant starch content.

→

Key points *continued*

For example, cooling boiled rice and potatoes greatly increases their resistant starch content.

- White rice has very little NSP but does contain significant amounts of resistant starch. This could make a significant difference to the functional NSP content of the diets of several Oriental populations that are based on white rice.

THE GLYCAEMIC INDEX

Ingested carbohydrate foods differ markedly in the way they affect blood glucose. If pure glucose is ingested, it is absorbed rapidly and causes a rapid large rise in blood glucose which in turn stimulates a large release of the hormone insulin to bring the blood glucose down again. Other foods like oat-based breakfast cereals are absorbed more slowly, produce a smaller rise in blood glucose concentration and a smaller insulin response.

Jenkins and Wolever (1981) coined the term *glycaemic index* (GI) to describe, in a quantitative way, the rise in blood glucose that different carbohydrate foods produce. Time-course curves of blood glucose concentration are plotted in the two hours after consumption of matched amounts of carbohydrate (usually 50 g) contained within different foods. The area under the curve for each food is then expressed as a percentage of that induced by the same amount of pure glucose. (Note that 50 g of carbohydrate contained in white bread is sometimes used as the standard.) Foods can be classified as having a high, medium or lower glycaemic index:

- high GI (≥70 per cent of the area under the glucose curve) – includes foods such as white bread and most white rice, most potatoes, corn flakes, most cakes, pancakes and crackers made from white flour
- medium GI (56–69) – includes wholemeal bread, baked potatoes, Basmati rice and sweet corn
- lower GI (<55) – includes dried beans and peas, most pasta, all bran, porridge (oatmeal), muesli and German black bread (pumpernickel).

The GI of a meal can be estimated by taking the average for the foods it contains weighted according to their contribution to the total carbohydrate content of the meal.

The following factors are some that will affect the GI of an isolated food:

- the speed of digestion (and ingestion) of the carbohydrate – the slower the digestion, the lower the GI
- the amount and type of dietary fibre – dietary fibre, especially soluble fibre, delays gastric emptying and slows absorption and so lowers the glycaemic response to a food or meal
- the presence of monosaccharides like fructose which are slowly absorbed from the gut and thus lower GI
- the ripeness of a fruit.

The form in which the food is consumed affects its digestion and absorption, and therefore its GI. For example, bread can be digested more rapidly than pasta and so has a higher GI.

Since the presence of other foods in a meal will modify the glycaemic response to a certain food, the glycaemic response *to a meal* may be difficult to predict from the GIs of foods measured individually. It is generally accepted that foods with low glycaemic index would be beneficial for glycaemic control in diabetes management. Manipulation of GI has in the past been regarded as too complex to be usefully incorporated into formal individual dietary advice for diabetics. However, a series of popular books (e.g. Leeds and Brand-Miller, 2005) has sought to increase popular awareness and to encourage the use of this concept in food selection for better weight control, diabetic management and general healthy eating. It is, for example, suggested that low-GI foods/meals will have a more sustained satiating effect that high-GI foods and thus aid in control of appetite – and thus in obesity management.

There is a growing body of research data to support some of the claimed benefits of a low-GI diet. Livesey *et al.* (2008) concluded from a meta-analysis of 45 published studies that low-GI diets reduced fasting blood glucose and longer term measures of blood glucose control such as glycated haemoglobin (see the section dealing with diabetes in Chapter 17). These would be beneficial outcomes for type 2 diabetics and for overweight and obese people. Thomas *et al.* (2007) in a meta-analysis of six published trials found that overweight and obese

people given a low-GI diet lost more weight and had bigger improvements in their blood lipoprotein profiles than those prescribed conventional reducing diets. In experiments with rats and mice, Pawlak *et al.* (2004) found that those fed high-GI diets had more body fat and less lean tissue than those fed a low-GI diet.

An extensive database of the GIs of a variety of foods together with other information and views about GI can be found on the website of the Glycemic Index Foundation, which is based in the Human Nutrition Unit at the University of Sydney (www.glycemicindex.com).

DIETARY FACTORS IN THE AETIOLOGY OF BOWEL CANCER

Background

The recent preoccupation with the protective effects of dietary fibre against bowel problems – constipation, diverticular disease, appendicitis, haemorrhoids and perhaps cancer of the colon and rectum – can be traced back to the work of Burkitt, Trowell, Painter and others in the 1960s and 1970s. These workers noted the rarity of bowel diseases in rural African populations consuming high-fibre diets and their much greater frequency in populations consuming the 'Western' low-fibre diet. Burkitt (1971) suggested that dietary fibre might protect against bowel cancer by diluting potential carcinogens in faeces and speeding their elimination so that the intestine is exposed to them for less time.

Bingham (1996) has reviewed the role of NSP and other dietary factors in the aetiology of bowel cancer, and Halliday and Ashwell (1991) have written a general review of non-starch polysaccharide. Evidence from many studies published before 1996 showed fairly consistently that a diet that was low in meat and fat but high in vegetables and fibre was associated with a reduced risk of *colorectal cancer*. Several possible explanations for these observations were put forward, as below.

- High dietary NSP/fibre intake directly protects against bowel cancer.
- High animal fat intake promotes bowel cancer.
- High intake of meat protein increases the risk of bowel cancer.

- NSP/fibre protects against the cancer-promoting effects of high dietary fat or meat protein.
- High fruit and vegetable intake protects against bowel cancer, perhaps because of their high content of anti-oxidants.

These proposals are not mutually exclusive and it is quite possible that more than one is correct. The inverse relationship between dietary fibre intake and fat/meat intake makes distinguishing between a direct promoting effect of fat or meat protein and a protective effect of dietary fibre difficult.

Mechanisms by which dietary factors might affect bowel cancer risk

Human faeces contain substances that induce mutation in bacteria (mutagens) and these are also found to be carcinogenic:

- bile acid breakdown products
- nitrosamines from cured meats and beer
- heterocyclic amines present in cooked meat and fish.

High-fat and/or high-meat diets may thus increase the mutagen content of faeces. A high-fat diet increases the production of bile acids and these may be converted to mutagens within the gut. High consumption of meat protein increases levels of heterocyclic amines, nitrosamines and other nitrogenous carcinogens.

Several proposed effects of high intakes of dietary fibre could help protect against bowel cancer.

- By increasing the volume and water content of stools, it would dilute any carcinogens in stools.
- Decreasing transit time reduces the time that the gut cells are exposed to faecal carcinogens.
- Butyrate and other short-chain fatty acids produced during fibre fermentation can act as substrates for the epithelial cells of the gut, and butyrate inhibits the proliferation of mutated cells into cancerous tumours.
- The acidic bowel environment produced by fibre fermentation may inhibit the conversion of bile acids to their mutagenic derivatives.
- Bran has been found to protect the bowels of experimental animals when they are exposed to chemical carcinogens. In human studies, bran fibre has been reported to reduce the mutagenicity of faeces (Bingham, 1990, 1996).

Descriptive epidemiology

In the UK, bowel or colorectal cancer is the second most common site for cancer in both men (after lung cancer) and women (after breast cancer). There were 40 000 new cases of bowel cancer (65 cases per 100 000 people) recorded in the UK, representing 13 per cent of all new cancers. Age-standardized rates for bowel cancer are even higher in the USA than the UK. There are very large international variations in the incidence of bowel cancer, with generally higher rates in the USA, Australasia and northern Europe but lower rates in, for example, India, China and rural Africa. Bingham (1996) suggests that age-standardized rates of bowel cancer may vary between countries by as much as 15-fold.

Figure 10.3 shows more recent comparative data for colorectal cancer incidence in parts of the world. The rate shown for Australia/New Zealand is close to 15 times that shown for Middle Africa. An extensive body of statistical data relating to bowel and other cancers can be found on the website of Cancer Research UK (http://info.cancerresearchuk.org/cancerstats).

The large international variations in bowel cancer could be the result of genetic differences between populations, or they could be due to dietary and other environmental differences. Migration studies, together with time trends for populations such as the Japanese, clearly indicate the predominance of environmental factors in the aetiology of bowel cancer – which also implies that bowel cancer is a potentially preventable disease. Rates of bowel cancer have increased among migrants and their descendants who have moved from areas with lower incidence to areas with higher incidence; an example is Japanese migrants to Hawaii in the late nineteenth and early twentieth centuries. Over the last 50 years there have been marked changes in the diets of people living in Japan and this has been accompanied by major increases in the incidence of colon cancer. In 1960, age-standardized rates of bowel cancer in Japan were about a third of those in the UK, but now they are similar.

Naturally high-fibre diets tend to be low in fat and low-fibre diets tend to be high in fat. This means that much of the evidence linking low-fibre diets to

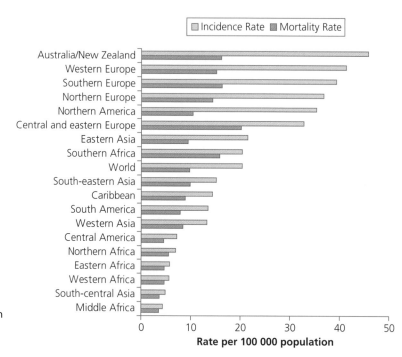

□ Incidence Rate ■ Mortality Rate

Figure 10.3 International variation in the rates of colorectal cancer (Source: Cancer Research UK).

increased risk of bowel cancer could equally well be used to implicate high-fat diets. This is another example of the recurring problem of confounding variables that plagues the epidemiologist. Cross-cultural comparisons indicate that populations with diets high in meat and fat but low in NSP, starch and vegetables are at high risk of bowel cancer. There is thus a general trend for populations with high-fibre intakes to have low rates of bowel cancer but the negative relationship between fibre intake and incidence of bowel cancer is very sharply reduced when this relationship is corrected for differences in fat and meat consumption. Vegetarian groups, like Seventh Day Adventists in the USA, have lower rates of bowel cancer than other Americans and they also have higher intakes of dietary NSP. Once again, low meat and fat intakes or even high intakes of anti-oxidant vitamins in fruits and vegetables make it impossible to finally attribute these low cancer rates to a direct protective effect of dietary NSP.

According to Bingham (1996), the cross-cultural data suggest that high meat and fat intakes are prerequisites for a population to have high incidence of bowel cancer, but that in such populations high intakes of NSP seem to exert a protective effect. High starch and vegetable intakes may also be protective; high vegetable intake would mean a high

intake of the anti-oxidant vitamins (e.g. β-carotene, vitamin E and vitamin C) and high starch intake probably also means high intake of resistant starch.

As already noted, there has been a 3-fold rise in incidence of bowel cancer in Japan since 1960. During this period there has been no significant change in overall NSP intakes but major increases in consumption of meat, dairy produce and wheat and a large decrease in rice consumption. Even though fibre intakes have not changed over this period, there has been a very substantial decline in the proportion of calories derived from starch, and most of the functional dietary fibre in white rice is resistant starch. Measures of the fibre intake that have taken no account of residual starch may thus be misleading. The reduction in the amount of carbohydrate in the Japanese diet over this period has been offset by increased fat consumption; consumption of animal fat has more than doubled over this period.

Case–control and cohort studies

According to Bingham (1990), a large majority of case–control studies indicate that cases of bowel cancer were more common in people who ate less vegetable fibre than controls. According to Willett *et al.* (1990), most case–control studies also indicate a significant positive association between total fat intake and bowel cancer. Bingham (1996) concluded that these studies have indicated similar trends to those found in cross-cultural studies; that is, individuals with high intake of fat and meat but low intake of fibre and vegetables are at increased risk of bowel cancer.

The limitations of case–control studies are noted in Chapter 4. As Bingham (1996) points out, diseases of the large bowel produce pain and altered bowel function, so one of the effects of bowel disease may be to make patients change their diet to try to avoid the symptoms. The low-fibre intakes of the cases in these case–control studies might be a consequence of the disease rather than an indication of its cause. Note that many studies do attempt to address this problem by asking cases about their past diets, but other studies suggest that recall of past diet is strongly influenced by current diet.

Willett *et al.* (1990) found no significant association between total fibre intake and risk of developing colon cancer in a cohort of 90 000 American nurses over a 6-year follow-up. They did find significant positive associations between total fat intake and colon cancer risk, and an even stronger association with animal fat intake (illustrated in Figure 4.3 in Chapter 4); 'red meat' (beef, pork and lamb) consumption was also positively associated with bowel cancer risk. There was the expected negative association between fibre intake and animal fat intake in their population. Their results provided little support for a causal link between low fibre intakes and bowel cancer but did provide evidence that high animal fat intake is linked to increased risk of colon cancer. Despite the very large sample size, the analysis is based on only 150 total bowel cancer cases, and only 103 cases if those developing in the first 2 years of follow-up were excluded.

In an overall assessment of all the cohort studies published up to 1996, Bingham (1996) concluded that there is only weak evidence for a slightly increased risk for high meat and fat consumers and for a slightly decreased risk in those with high vegetable and NSP intakes. All of the cohort studies published prior to 1996 had major drawbacks, including:

- poor dietary assessment methodology
- sample populations that had too narrow a range of dietary habits.

Since that time several large, well-designed cohort studies using sample populations with diverse dietary habits have been published. The European Prospective Investigation of Cancer and Nutrition (EPIC) used a cohort of over half a million individuals from 10 European countries (details may be found at http://epic.iarc.fr/). Bingham *et al.* (2003) published data from this study which found that there was a 40 per cent lower risk of bowel cancer in those with the highest quintile of fibre intake compared to those in the lowest quintile. In a later review, Bingham (2006) responded to criticisms that the earlier report did not take adequate account of confounding factors and suggested that correcting for confounding variables confirmed the inverse relationship between fibre intake and bowel cancer risk. She reports that incidence of bowel cancer decreased by about 9 per cent for each quintile increase in dietary fibre intake. Park *et al.* (2005) conducted a large pooled analysis of cohort studies with a total of 8081 cases of colorectal cancer; they found that there was a significant inverse association between dietary fibre intake and colorectal cancer incidence. However, when they corrected for confounding variables this association was reduced and was no longer statistically significant.

A fibre-rich diet is consistently associated with reduced risk of colorectal cancer but there is still doubt about whether this is a direct effect of the dietary fibre.

The EPIC study also found a strong positive association between the amount of red and processed meats consumed and colorectal cancer but a reduced risk associated with a higher intake of fish (Norat, 2005). This positive association between meat consumption and colorectal cancer has been a consistent finding of pooled analyses of other prospective cohort studies (e.g. Larsson and Wolk, 2006).

In a reasoned and referenced assessment of the current evidence relating other dietary factors to colorectal cancer, Cancer Research UK (2012) came to the following conclusions.

- There may be a modest protective effect of fruits and vegetables, although this could be due to confounding factors.
- There is no direct association independent of meat intake between high fat intake and bowel

cancer risk. There is some evidence that dairy fat is protective.

- A high-folate diet may be protective (see Chapter 14 for further discussion).
- Several studies suggest a significant reduction in bowel cancer risk in people with good biochemical status for vitamin D.
- Obesity and overweight are associated with increased risk of colon cancer especially in men.
- High alcohol consumption increases colorectal cancer risk.

In their conclusions on the relationship between dietary factors and colorectal cancer they reiterate the earlier recommendations of COMA (1998):

> There is moderately consistent evidence that diets with less meat and more vegetables and fibre are associated with reduced risk of colorectal cancer.

They go on to suggest that increasing intake of fish and milk is also probably associated with reduced risk.

There is thus fairly consistent agreement about the type of diet that leads to reduced colorectal cancer risk but still considerable uncertainty about the role of individual dietary constituents in this reduced risk. A diet that is naturally rich in fibre will probably protect against bowel cancer, but it is by no means clear that this is a direct effect of the dietary fibre.

DIETARY FACTORS IN HEART DISEASE

In general, populations with high rates of coronary heart disease (CHD) also tend to have high incidences of bowel cancer. This means that much of the evidence that implicates fibre or any other dietary factor in the aetiology of bowel cancer – as analysed in the previous section – could also be used to implicate it in the aetiology of heart disease. This link between bowel cancer and CHD is not inevitable: there are populations, including British Asians, that have high rates of CHD and low rates of bowel cancer. Recent increases mean that the modern Japanese population now has a relatively high rate of bowel cancer but still has a relatively low rate of CHD.

Some of the possible mechanisms by which NSP/fibre might have a specific influence on CHD risk are listed below.

- As noted earlier, soluble fibre may help to lower the plasma cholesterol concentration.

- A high intake of soluble fibre improves glucose tolerance, reduces insulin secretion and decreases the glycaemic index of a meal (diabetes is a strong risk factor for heart disease).
- High-fibre diets may reduce CHD by reducing the risk of obesity. It reduces the energy density of the diet and increases satiety by decreasing the glycaemic index of the diet.

Evidence supporting a direct link between fibre intake and CHD is limited or weak. There is a much stronger case for suggesting that dietary changes that would increase fibre intake would lead to reduced CHD risk. Consumption of more foods naturally rich in fibre and complex carbohydrates is more likely to reduce CHD (or bowel cancer) risk than using foods in which the fibre content has been 'amplified' by food manufacturers.

Key points

- High-fibre diets have long been thought to protect against bowel cancer as well as alleviate other bowel problems, including constipation, diverticular disease and haemorrhoids.
- Diets low in meat but high in vegetables and fibre are consistently associated with a lowered risk of colorectal cancer. This could be because:
  - fibre is directly protective
  - animal fat and/or meat protein is a causative influence
  - fibre protects against the effects of meat fat/protein
  - fruits and vegetables are protective because of their anti-oxidant content
  - a combination of these.
- Fibre intake tends to be inversely related to fat and meat protein intake when individual or population diets are compared.
- It is difficult to differentiate the contributions of high meat, high fat, low fibre/NSP and low vegetable intakes to the aetiology of bowel cancer.
- Human faeces contains carcinogenic substances including bile acid derivatives, nitrosamines from cured meats and beer and heterocyclic amines from cooked meat and fish.
- High meat and fat consumption increases the carcinogenicity of faeces.

→

Key points *continued*

- Fat increases bile acid production.
- NSP could protect against bowel cancer by causing dilution and more rapid elimination of faecal carcinogens.
- Increased production of butyrate from fibre fermentation may inhibit the proliferation of mutated cells and reduce the conversion of bile acids to potential carcinogens.
- Bowel is the second most common site for cancer in the UK for men and women.
- Internationally, rates of bowel cancer vary 15-fold. There are high rates in the USA, Australasia and northern Europe but low rates in India, China and rural Africa.
- Migration studies and recent changes in bowel cancer frequency in Japan show that environmental factors are largely responsible for the variations in bowel cancer incidence.
- Vegetarian groups and populations with diets low in meat and fat but high in fibre and vegetables have low rates of bowel cancer.
- Bingham (1996) suggested that high meat and fat intakes are prerequisites for high population rates of bowel cancer and that NSP is protective in these circumstances.
- Most case–control studies indicate higher fat and/or lower NSP intakes in bowel cancer cases, but this could reflect the effect of disease rather than indicate its cause.
- Cohort studies published prior to 1996 provide weak evidence for a slightly increased bowel cancer risk in high fat and meat consumers and a slightly decreased risk in those with high vegetable and NSP intakes. Most studies published before1996 used subjects with a narrow range of dietary habits and/or used inadequate means for assessing dietary intake.
- Data from a very large European cohort study (EPIC) suggest that, for each quintile of rise in dietary fibre intake, the incidence of bowel cancer drops by about 9 per cent; that is, more than 40 per cent lower in the highest compared to the lowest fibre quintile.
- In the EPIC study, the relationship between colon cancer risk and dietary fibre intake was not diminished by correction for several confounding variables.

→

Key points *continued*

- Large pooled analyses of other cohort studies have also reported a significant inverse association between fibre intake and risk of colorectal cancer, but this became not significant when corrected for confounding variables.
- EPIC data also show an increase in bowel cancer risk associated with increasing red meat consumption but a reduced risk associated with high fish intake.
- A summary of other dietary influences on bowel cancer risk concluded that:
  - there may be a protective effect of fruits and vegetables
  - there is no association between fat consumption and bowel cancer risk independent of meat intake
  - dairy fat may have a protective effect
  - a folate-rich diet may be protective
  - good vitamin D status may be protective
  - obesity and overweight are associated with increased risk especially in men
  - high alcohol intake increases risk
  - diets with less meat, more vegetables, fibre, fish and milk are associated with reduced bowel cancer risk
  - diets that are naturally high in fibre probably protect against bowel cancer but it is not clear whether this is a direct effect of the fibre.
- High rates of bowel cancer and high rates of CHD tend to go together, although there are exceptions (e.g. British Asians and the present-day Japanese population). This means that some of the evidence linking high-fibre diets with reduced bowel cancer risk could also be used to suggest they lower CHD risk.
- NSP might reduce CHD risk by:
  - reducing the re-absorption of bile acids and lowering plasma cholesterol
  - improving glucose tolerance
  - indirectly by helping to prevent excessive weight gain
  - decreasing the glycaemic index of the diet.
- Choosing a diet that is naturally high in fibre is more likely to reduce the risk of CHD (or bowel cancer) than artificially enhancing the fibre content of existing diets.

11

PROTEIN AND AMINO ACIDS

Introduction	268	Protein quality	274
Chemistry and digestion	268	The significance of protein in human nutrition	278
Intakes, dietary standards and food sources	270	Concluding remarks	284
Nitrogen balance	271		

INTRODUCTION

Experiments stretching back over the last two centuries have demonstrated the principle that all animals require an exogenous supply of protein. In humans, and in other non-ruminating mammals, this protein must be present in the food they eat. (Some ruminants can survive without dietary protein if their diet contains alternative sources of nitrogen. This is because bacteria in the rumen can make protein from non-protein nitrogen sources such as urea, and the animals can digest and absorb this bacterial protein.)

In the early 1800s, François Magendie fed dogs with single foods that were regarded as highly nutritious but lacked any nitrogen (e.g. sugar, olive oil or butter). These unfortunate dogs survived much longer than if they had been completely starved, but they lost weight, their muscles wasted dramatically and they all died within 40 days. Several modern writers, including myself, had assumed that Magendie completed the cycle of evidence by showing that the dogs recovered when nitrogen-containing foods were added back to their diets. In his excellent book on the history of protein nutrition, Carpenter (1994) points out that Magendie did not actually do these positive controls. Despite this he is still usually credited with the discovery that nitrogen-containing foods are essential in the diet. In later years it became clear that Magendie's initial conclusions were correct: adequate amounts of nitrogen-containing foods were essential to allow growth and even survival in experimental animals. Such experiments demonstrated the need for nitrogen-containing foods (i.e. protein) even before the chemical nature of dietary protein was known.

Further details of amino acid synthesis, catabolism and conversion to other nitrogen-containing compounds can be found in Matthews (2006), which also gives more details on protein turnover and amino acid kinetics and the methods used to study these phenomena.

> **Key points**
>
> - Protein is an essential nutrient for all animals.
> - Even before protein was chemically characterized it was clear that animals need foods that contain nitrogen.

CHEMISTRY AND DIGESTION

Protein is the only major nitrogen-containing component of the diet. It is composed of long chains of 20 different amino acids that are linked together by peptide bonds. Figure 11.1 illustrates the chemical nature of amino acids and proteins. The amino acid side-chain (the R-group in the figure) is the group that varies between amino acids, and some examples of the R-groups in particular amino acids are shown.

Generalized chemical formula of amino acids

$$NH_2 \!-\!\! \underset{\underset{H}{|}}{\overset{\overset{R}{|}}{C}} \!\!-\! COOH$$

amino group   carboxyl (acid) group

Examples of amino acid side-chains

R = H   amino acid = glycine
R = CH_3 amino acid = alanine
R = CH_2SH amino acid = cysteine
R = $(CH_2)_4NH_2$ amino acid = lysine
R = CH_2OH amino acid = serine

Two amino acids linked by a peptide bond

$$NH_2 \!-\!\! \underset{\underset{H}{|}}{\overset{\overset{R}{|}}{C}} \!\!-\! \overset{\overset{O}{\|}}{C} \!-\! \underset{\underset{H}{|}}{\overset{\overset{H}{|}}{N}} \!-\! \overset{\overset{R}{|}}{C} \!-\! COOH$$

Diagrammatic representation of a protein

$$NH_2 \!-\!\! \overset{\overset{R}{|}}{AA} \!\!-\! (\overset{\overset{R}{|}}{AA})_n \!\!-\! \overset{\overset{R}{|}}{AA} \!\!-\! COOH$$

N-terminal   C-terminal

Figure 11.1 The chemical nature of proteins and amino acids.

Amino acids are usually classified into groups according to the nature of the side-chain or R-group. These side-chains vary in size, shape, charge, hydrogen bonding capacity, affinity for water and reactivity, and these properties determine the three-dimensional structure of any given protein. The groupings can be described as follows.

- *Glycine* has just a hydrogen atom (H) as its side-chain and is the only amino acid without two optical isomers.
- *Alanine*, *valine*, *leucine* and *isoleucine* have aliphatic (hydrocarbon) side-chains.
- *Serine* and *threonine* have hydroxyl aliphatic side-chains and contain an OH group.
- *Proline* is an aliphatic amino acid but it has a ring structure because the amino group binds to the terminal methyl group of the side-chain (it is a secondary amine).
- *Phenylalanine*, *tyrosine* and *tryptophan* have aromatic side-chains and an aromatic or benzene ring.
- *Lysine*, *arginine* and *histidine* have basic side-chains owing to the presence of an amino group in the side-chain and these are positively charged at neutral pH.

- *Glutamic and aspartic acids* have carboxyl groups in the side-chain and these are negatively charged at neutral pH.
- *Cysteine* and *methionine* have sulphur-containing side-chains.
- *Glutamine* and *asparagine* have amide groups ($CONH_2$) in their side-chains.

Note that some amino acids may be modified after they have been incorporated into a protein. For example, proline in collagen is hydroxylated to hydroxyproline (this reaction requires vitamin C), and the glutamate in prothrombin and other clotting factor proteins is carboxylated (this reaction requires vitamin K).

The way in which amino acids are linked together by peptide bonds is illustrated in Figure 11.1. The nitrogen atom in the amino group of one amino acid is linked to the carbon atom of the carboxyl group in the adjacent amino acid. A protein may comprise hundreds of amino acids linked together in this way; each protein will have a free amino group at one end (the *N-terminal*) and a free carboxyl group at the opposite end (the *C-terminal*).

Dietary proteins are digested to their constituent amino acids prior to absorption in the small intestine. About a quarter of dietary protein is absorbed as dipeptides and tripeptides. This absorption of small peptide fragments is important in a rare genetic condition (*Hartnup disease*) in which there is an inability to absorb phenylalanine but it can be absorbed when administered as a dipeptide. Small amounts of some intact proteins can also be absorbed, including some bacterial toxins and IgG antibodies from milk in many newborn mammals. *Peptidase enzymes* in gastric and pancreatic juice break (hydrolyse) the peptide bonds between specific amino acids in dietary proteins, yielding small peptides, dipeptides and free amino acids. Other peptidase enzymes located on the mucosal surface of the small intestine continue the digestion of these small protein fragments. Some peptidases are classified as *endopeptidases* because they hydrolyse the bonds between certain amino acids within the protein or peptide molecule. The major endopeptidases in the gut are:

- *pepsin* in gastric juice
- *trypsin* in pancreatic juice

- *chymotrypsin* in pancreatic juice
- *collagenase* (which breaks down collagen) and *elastase*, also in pancreatic juice.

The peptidases below break off one of the amino acids at the end of the peptide chain and these are termed *exopeptidases*:

- *carboxypeptidases* in pancreatic juice break off the C-terminal amino acid
- *aminopeptidases* located on the surface of the small intestine break off the N-terminal amino acid.

Also located on the surface of the small intestine are *dipeptidases* and *tripeptidases*, which break down dipeptides and tripeptides. Dipeptidases and tripeptidases within the cells complete the digestion of any dipeptides and tripeptides that are absorbed intact into the intestinal cells.

Key points

- Protein is made up of 20 different amino acids joined together in long chains by peptide bonds.
- There are 20 amino acids used in protein synthesis and these can be classified according to the nature of their side-chains.
- The amino acid side-chains differ in size, charge, ability to form hydrogen bonds, reactivity and affinity for water. This largely determines the three-dimensional shape of a protein.
- Protein is largely digested to its constituent amino acids in the gut by peptidase enzymes, although some peptide fragments and even some intact protein is absorbed.
- Endopeptidases – including pepsin, trypsin and chymotrypsin – in gastric and pancreatic juice break proteins into peptide fragments by breaking peptide bonds within the protein chain.
- Carboxypeptidases (cleave the C-terminal amino acid), aminopeptidases (cleave the N-terminal amino acid) and a range of dipeptidases and tripeptidases complete the digestion of dietary protein.

INTAKES, DIETARY STANDARDS AND FOOD SOURCES

Table 11.1 shows the *reference nutrient intake* (RNI) for protein of selected population groups,

expressed both as an absolute value and as a percentage of dietary energy; some sample US recommended daily amounts (RDAs) are included for comparison.

Table 11.1 Reference nutrients intakes (RNIs) for protein expressed in absolute terms and as a percentage of average energy requirements*

Age (years)	RNI (g/day)	Percent of energy
1–3	14.5	4.7
7–10	28.3	5.7
Male		
11–14	42.1	7.7
19–50	55.5	8.7
65–74	53.3	9.2
Female		
11–14	41.2	8.9
19–50	45.0	9.3
Pregnancy	+6[1]	9.5–10.5[2]
Lactation	+11[1]	8.9–9.4[2]
Some sample American RDA (g/day) for comparison**		
1–3	14.3	
9–13	34.2	
Male		
14–18	51.9	
18+	56	
Female		
14–18	45.9	
18+	46.4	

*Data source: COMA (1991). ** Data source: IOM (2002).
[1] Additional to that of non-pregnant or lactating women.
[2] Varies as the energy EAR varies during pregnancy and lactation.

The UK values for all adults are based on a notional daily 0.75 g per kilogram of body weight. Values for children are set at a higher value per kilogram of body weight to reflect the extra protein requirements for growth, with the maximum value being 1.65 g/kg daily for 4- to 6-month-old children. The protein requirements of children are discussed more fully later in the chapter, and values for pregnancy and lactation are discussed in Chapter 16.

According to Bates *et al.* (2011), average adult intakes of protein in the UK are over 150 per cent of the RNI and contribute about 17.5 per cent of the food energy. Intakes of protein were lower in the younger age groups, but average intakes did not drop below 130 per cent of the RNI in any age group. Fewer than 2.5 per cent of adults (and children) had a protein intake that was below the estimated average requirement (EAR) of 45 g/day for men and 33 g/day for women. If one assumes a lower RNI (LRNI) that is set two standard deviations below the EAR, then no healthy individuals would be likely to fall below this level. Intakes of essential amino acids (see later in the chapter) are not considered as a specific issue because COMA (1991) concluded that any group in the UK who are consuming food that supplies sufficient energy and sufficient protein would be very unlikely to receive insufficient amounts of the essential amino acids; and similar conclusions have been made in the USA. Almost no individuals would be consuming more than twice their RNI, which is the guideline upper limit suggested in both the UK and USA.

These estimates of protein requirements are for healthy people and it is well known that both infection and trauma lead to a hypermetabolic state in which there is an increase in metabolic rate and protein breakdown. This 'metabolic response to injury' is discussed in Chapter 17.

The main food sources of protein for UK adults are summarized below:

- cereals and cereal products – 23 per cent
- milk and milk products – 16 per cent
- meat and meat products – 37 per cent
- fish and fish dishes – 7 per cent
- eggs and egg dishes – 3 per cent
- vegetables, including potatoes – 9 per cent.

The categories have been chosen partly to reflect the effect of different types of vegetarian diets. Bear in mind that, although a vegan would exclude foods that normally provide two-thirds of the daily protein, they would consume much larger amounts of other foods with relatively high protein contents, including pulses, soya milk, nuts, cereals and possibly vegetarian meat substitutes.

Key points

- The protein RNI for adults in the UK is set at a notional 0.75 g/kg per day.
- The RNI for children ranges up to 1.65 g/kg to reflect the extra requirements for growth.
- Average adult protein intakes are 1.5 times the RNI. Almost no healthy person in the UK is at risk of primary protein deficiency.
- Anyone consuming sufficient energy and sufficient protein will almost certainly get enough of all the essential amino acids.
- Foods from the meat and milk groups provide about 63 per cent of average adult protein intakes, but vegans and other vegetarians will inevitably consume larger amounts of other protein-containing vegetable foods.

NITROGEN BALANCE

Estimation of protein content

Early in the nineteenth century the German chemist Liebig noted that proteins from different sources all contained approximately 16 per cent by weight of nitrogen. This observation remains the basis of estimating the protein content of foods. The nitrogen content is determined by a relatively simple chemical analysis.

Using the Kjeldahl method, first the food is boiled with concentrated sulphuric acid and a catalyst, which converts the nitrogen into ammonium sulphate. Alkali is then added to the digest and liberated ammonia is distilled into acid and the amount of ammonia liberated is determined by titration. The result is then multiplied by 6.25 (i.e. 100/16) to give an estimate of the protein content:

$$\text{weight of protein} = \text{weight of nitrogen} \times 6.25.$$

The 6.25 factor is an approximation and more precise values may be used for some foods. Some foods may contain non-protein nitrogen, but in most this is largely amino acid and so would not produce any dietetic error. The Kjeldahl method can also be used to estimate the nitrogen content of urine; if this is multiplied by 6.25 it indicates how much protein has been broken down to produce this amount of nitrogen. Sweat and faeces can also be analysed for nitrogen to give a complete picture of protein losses by catabolism or direct protein loss in faeces.

Key points

- All proteins contain about 16 per cent nitrogen by weight.
- Protein content of food can be estimated from its nitrogen content and the rate of protein catabolism can be estimated from the nitrogen loss in urine.
- Nitrogen can be estimated using the Kjeldahl method.

The concept of nitrogen balance

Intakes and losses of nitrogen are used as the measure of protein intake and protein breakdown, respectively, and the difference between intake and total losses is the nitrogen balance:

nitrogen balance = nitrogen input − nitrogen losses.

The nitrogen input is from food protein. Nitrogen losses arise from the breakdown of dietary and body protein. Most nitrogen is lost in the urine but small amounts are lost in faeces and via the skin. If the nitrogen balance is zero then this means that intake completely offsets losses and that the body protein content (lean mass) remains constant.

A negative nitrogen balance

A negative balance indicates that body protein is being depleted because more nitrogen is being lost than is taken in the diet. Injury, illness, starvation (including dieting) or inadequate protein intake *per se* may lead to negative nitrogen balance. The minimum amount of protein, in an otherwise complete diet, that enables an adult to achieve balance indicates the minimum requirement for protein. A deficit in energy supplies would be expected to lead to negative nitrogen balance for the following two reasons.

- A diet that has insufficient energy will also tend to have a low protein content.
- During energy deficit, the protein that is present will tend to be used as a source of energy rather than being used for protein synthesis.

Requirements for balance

The protein requirement of an adult is the minimum intake that results in nitrogen balance. When adults are put onto a protein-free but otherwise complete diet, their rate of nitrogen loss drops sharply during the first 3 days as they adapt to this situation and stabilizes after about 8 days. Even after adaptation they excrete nitrogen, albeit a low and relatively constant amount; this is termed the *obligatory nitrogen loss* and represents the minimum replacement requirement.

Studies using radioactively labelled amino acids indicate that around 300 g of protein is normally broken down and re-synthesized in the body each day – the *protein turnover*. Most of the amino acids released during the breakdown of body protein can re-enter the body amino acid pool and be recycled into new protein synthesis, but a proportion (say 10 per cent) cannot be recycled and becomes the obligatory nitrogen loss. Several amino acids have additional functions to that of protein building and are irreversibly lost from the body amino acid pool for synthesis of non-protein substances, to maintain acid–base balance, and for conjugation with substances to facilitate their excretion. Amino acids are the nitrogen source for the synthesis of all other N-containing compounds in the body (some examples are shown in Box 11.1).

Box 11.1

Some nitrogen-containing compounds that are synthesized in the body from amino acids

- The purines and pyrimidines (adenine, guanine, cytosine, thymine and uracil) that are key components of DNA and RNA
- Creatine which as creatine phosphate acts as a short-term energy store in muscle
- 5HT (serotonin), a nerve transmitter
- Choline, a component of the nerve transmitter acetylcholine
- The catecholamines (including adrenaline, noradrenaline, dopa and dopamine), an important group of nerve transmitters
- Histamine, a mediator of inflammation
- The thyroid hormones
- Nicotinic acid, vitamin B_3
- Haemoglobin in red blood cells and myoglobin in muscles

→

Box 11.1 *continued*

- Cytochromes that are involved in oxidative phosphorylation
- Carnitine which is important in the metabolism of long-chain fatty acids (see Chapter 13)

Those amino acids that are modified after translation of the protein – such as hydroxyproline and hydroxylysine in collagen and 3-methyl histidine in muscle – cannot be recycled into new protein as there is no specific transfer RNA that recognizes them. These are therefore lost from the body pool of amino acids. When amino acids are lost from the pool for such reasons, some other amino acids are broken down to retain the balance of the body's pool of amino acids. Some protein will be also lost as hair, skin, sloughed epithelial cells and mucus, etc. Such obligatory losses explain why adults have a requirement for dietary protein even though their total body protein content remains constant. Note that perhaps as much as 70 g of endogenous protein is added to gut contents in the form of secreted proteins and sloughed cells, although most of this is normally digested and re-absorbed.

A positive nitrogen balance

A positive nitrogen balance indicates a net accumulation of body protein. Healthy adults do not go into sustained positive nitrogen balance if dietary protein intake is stepped up; they utilize the excess protein as an energy source and excrete the associated nitrogen as urea.

Growing children would be expected to be in positive nitrogen balance, as would pregnant women, those recovering after illness, injury or starvation, and those actively accumulating extra muscle (e.g. body-builders). One would expect these groups, particularly rapidly growing children, to have a relatively higher protein requirement than other adults; that is, they would be expected to require more protein per kilogram of body weight. Lactating women would be expected to have a higher protein requirement because they are secreting protein in their milk. Note that the daily positive nitrogen balance in body-builders is very small and would not of itself indicate a significant increase in their protein requirements.

Dietary adequacy for protein

Table 11.1 shows selected reference nutrient intakes for protein; in addition to the absolute values, the energy yield of the protein RNI is also calculated as a percentage of the estimated average requirement for energy. To put these values into context, the average UK diet has around 17.5 per cent of the energy as protein compared to the 5–10 per cent of energy as protein indicated as maximum requirements in Table 11.1. Note that the RNI is a generous estimate of protein requirement in those who need most, whereas the EAR is a less generous estimate of average requirement. This suggests that primary protein deficiency is highly improbable in the UK (and in other industrialized countries). Some RDAs for protein in the USA are included in the table for comparison.

To give the values in Table 11.1 an international perspective, rice has around 8 per cent of energy as protein and hard wheat around 17 per cent, while most other major cereal staples lie between these two extremes; only finger millet (*Eleusine corocana*) is below this range at 7 per cent. Some starchy roots, which are important staples, do fall substantially below this range for cereals; for example:

- cassava – 3 per cent energy as protein
- plantains (cooked bananas) – 4 per cent
- yam – 7 per cent
- sweet potato – 4 per cent.

Table 11.2 shows the protein content of some common foods. Note that only three of the foods on this list have crude protein contents that are less than that in human milk, and most have more than 10 per cent of their energy as protein.

A comparison of these values with those in Table 11.1 suggests that people meeting their energy needs and eating a varied diet, even a varied vegetarian diet, would seem to run little practical risk of protein deficiency. This is generally true even though fats, oils, alcoholic drinks, soft drinks and sugar-based snacks provide additional energy but little protein so they reduce the nutrient density for protein. Of course, this conclusion might be altered by variations in the quality of different proteins, and this is discussed in the next section.

Table **11.2** Protein content of some foods expressed in absolute terms and as a percentage of energy (values are generally for raw food)

Food	Grams per 100g	As percentage of energy
Whole milk	3.3	20.3
Skimmed milk	3.4	41.2
Cheddar cheese	26.0	25.6
Human milk	1.3	7.5
Egg	12.3	33.5
Wholemeal bread	8.8	16.3
Sweetcorn	4.1	12.9
Corn flakes	8.6	9.3
Beef (lean)	20.3	66.0
Pork (lean)	20.7	56.3
Chicken (meat)	20.5	67.8
Cod	17.4	91.6
Herring	16.8	28.7
Shrimps	23.8	81.4
Peas	5.8	34.6
Broad beans	4.1	34.2
Baked beans (canned)	5.1	31.0
Lentils	23.8	31.3
Potatoes	2.1	9.7
Mushrooms	1.8	55.4
Broccoli	3.3	57.4
Carrots	0.7	12.2
Peanuts	24.3	17.1
Peanut butter	22.4	14.5
Almonds	16.9	12.0
Apple	0.3	2.6
Banana	1.1	5.6
Orange	0.8	9.1
Dried dates	2.0	3.2

Key points

- The nitrogen balance is the difference between nitrogen intake from food and nitrogen losses.
- Positive nitrogen balance indicates a net increase in body protein (e.g. during growth)

→

Key points *continued*

and a negative nitrogen balance indicates a net loss of body protein (e.g. in starvation).

- Adults require protein to replace amino acids lost from the body pool each day. This happens because they are used to synthesize other N-containing compounds, and because amino acids modified after translation cannot be re-used in protein synthesis.
- Protein is lost also as sloughed cells, hair and loss of body fluids and secretions (e.g. blood and nasal mucus).
- Even under conditions of maximal conservation after adaptation to a protein-free diet, there is still an obligatory nitrogen loss.
- When the RNI for protein is expressed as a percentage of the EAR for energy, values of 5–10 per cent energy as protein are obtained for all age groups.
- Diets in industrialized countries typically contain 15 per cent or more of the energy as protein, which makes protein deficiency improbable. Only a few staple foods contain low enough levels of protein to make primary protein deficiency even a theoretical prospect, and in most diets in the developing countries protein is not the limiting nutrient.

PROTEIN QUALITY

The observation that all proteins contain approximately 16 per cent by weight of nitrogen enabled early workers not only to measure the protein contents of diets but also to match them for crude protein content by matching them for nitrogen content. Using such nitrogen-matched diets it soon became clear that all proteins were not of equal nutritional value; that is, both the amount and the quality of protein in foods were variable. For example, pigs fed on diets based on lentil protein grew faster than those fed barley-based diets even though the diets were matched for crude protein (nitrogen) content; lentil protein was apparently of higher nutritional quality than barley protein.

Essential amino acids

It is now known that quality differences between individual proteins arise because of variations in their content of certain of the amino acids. To synthesize body protein, an animal or person must have all 20 amino acids available. If one or more amino acids is unavailable, or in short supply, then the ability to synthesize protein is generally compromised irrespective of the supply of the others. Proteins cannot be synthesized leaving gaps or using substitutes for the deficient amino acids. Each body protein is synthesized with a genetically determined and unalterable, precise sequence of particular amino acids.

About half of the amino acids have carbon skeletons that can be synthesized by people and these amino acids can therefore be synthesized by transferring amino groups from other surplus amino acids – *transamination* (see Chapter 6). The remaining amino acids have carbon skeletons that cannot be synthesized by people and they cannot, therefore, be made by transamination. These latter amino acids are termed the *essential amino acids* and have to be obtained pre-formed from the diet. The protein gelatine is lacking in the essential amino acid tryptophan, and so dogs fed on gelatine, as their sole nitrogen source, do not fare much better than those fed on a protein-free diet. Despite a surplus of the other amino acids, the dog cannot utilize them for protein synthesis because one amino acid is unavailable. Under these circumstances, the amino acids in the gelatine will be used as an energy source and their nitrogen excreted as urea.

The essential amino acids for humans are:

- histidine (in children)
- isoleucine
- leucine
- lysine
- methionine
- phenylalanine
- threonine
- tryptophan
- valine.

The amino acids cysteine and tyrosine are classified as non-essential even though their carbon skeletons cannot be synthesized. This is because they can be made from methionine and phenylalanine, respectively. They may be conditionally essential in premature babies because the enzymes required for their synthesis do not normally develop until late in gestation; and they may also be conditionally essential in patients with liver disease because the ability to synthesize these amino acids in the liver may be compromised. In the hereditary condition *phenylketonuria*, the enzyme phenylalanine hydroxylase that converts phenylalanine to tyrosine is defective and so tyrosine becomes an essential amino acid (see Chapter 17). The terms *non-dispensable and dispensable amino acids* may be used as alternatives to essential and non-essential, respectively.

Establishing the essential amino acids and quantifying requirements

Young rats have been shown to grow normally if synthetic mixtures of the 20 amino acids are given as their sole source of dietary protein. Growth is not affected if one of the non-essential amino acids is left out of the mixture because the rats are able to make this missing amino acid by transamination. Growth ceases, however, if one of the essential ones is left out. In this way the essential amino acids for the rat have been identified and the amount of each one that is required to allow normal growth (when all of the others are in excess) has also been determined.

Such experiments with children are ruled out on ethical grounds. However, adults have been shown to maintain nitrogen balance if fed mixtures of the 20 amino acids and, like the rats, can cope with removal of certain amino acids and still maintain this balance; these are the non-essential amino acids. When one of the essential amino acids is left out then there is a net loss of body nitrogen; that is, a depletion of body protein. The requirement for each of the essential amino acids has been estimated from the minimum amount that is necessary to maintain nitrogen balance when the other amino acids are present in excess. The range and relative needs of the essential amino acids in rats and people are found to be similar, so the rat has been widely used as a model for humans in biological assessments of protein quality.

Limiting amino acid

If the 20 amino acids were distributed evenly throughout proteins, one would expect each of them to make up about 5 per cent in molar terms of each protein. However, some amino acids such as leucine, serine and valine are much more common in proteins than this and each represents 8–10 per cent. Other amino acids including tryptophan tend to be much less common in many proteins. Some of the essential amino acids are present in very low amounts in some vegetable protein sources.

In any given dietary protein, one of the essential amino acids will be present in the lowest amount relative to human requirements; that is, a given amount of the protein will contain a lower proportion of the requirement for this essential amino acid than for any of the others. The availability of this amino acid will 'limit' the extent to which the others can be utilized if that particular protein is fed alone and in amounts that do not fully supply the needs for the amino acid. This amino acid is called the *limiting amino acid*. The amino acid is limiting because if supplies are insufficient then the use of the others for protein synthesis will be limited by its availability – protein cannot be made leaving gaps where this missing amino acid should be. For example, if only half of the requirement for the limiting amino acid is supplied then, in effect, only about half of the protein requirement is being supplied; surpluses of the others will be used as energy sources and their nitrogen excreted.

In many cereals the limiting amino acid is lysine, in maize it is tryptophan, and in beef and milk it is the sulphur-containing amino acids. One of these three is the limiting amino acid in most dietary proteins. In the past, lysine supplementation of cereal-based diets or developing 'high-lysine' strains of cereals has been widely advocated, and sometimes used, as means of improving the protein quality of diets based on cereals.

First- and second-class proteins

Whatever measure of protein quality is used, most proteins of animal origin have high values. Meat, fish, egg and milk proteins contain all the essential amino acids in good quantities; they have been termed *first-class or complete proteins*. Many proteins of vegetable origin, however, have low measured quality; this is true of many staple cereals and starchy roots. These have been termed *second class or incomplete proteins* because they have a relatively low amount of one or more of the essential amino acids. Pulses (peas and beans) are a major exception to this general rule and have good amounts of high-quality protein. Some examples of the relative

quality values of common dietary proteins are shown in Table 11.3.

Table 11.3 Relative qualities (NPU, net protein utilization) of some dietary proteins

	Protein quality (NPU %)
Maize	36
Millet	43
Wheat	49
Rice	63
Soya	67
Cow milk	81
Egg	87
Human milk	94

Mutual supplementation of protein

For the two reasons discussed below, the concept of a limiting amino acid producing large variations in protein quality may have limited practical relevance in human nutrition, especially in affluent countries.

First, the human requirement for protein is low. This is true both in comparison to other species and in comparison to the protein content of many dietary staples.

Second, affluent people seldom eat just single proteins; rather they eat diets containing mixtures of several different proteins. The probability is that the different proteins consumed, over a period of time, will have differing limiting amino acids and thus that any deficiency of an essential amino acid in one protein will be compensated for by a relative surplus of that amino acid in another. Thus the quality of the total protein in different human diets will tend to equalize even though the nature and quality of the individual proteins in those diets may vary considerably. This is called *mutual supplementation of proteins* and it means that any measure of protein quality of mixed human diets tends to yield a fairly consistent value.

Measurement of protein quality

The simplest method of assessing the quality of a protein is to chemically compare its limiting amino acid content with that of a high-quality reference protein; this is called the *chemical score*. Egg protein has traditionally been used as the reference protein in human nutrition, but breast milk protein is another possible reference. In the protein under test, the limiting amino acid is identified and the amount of this amino acid in a gram of test protein is expressed as a percentage of that found in a gram of egg protein:

chemical score (per cent) = (mg of limiting amino acid in 1 gram of test protein *divided by* mg of this amino acid in 1 gram of egg protein) × 100.

This chemical score does not necessarily give an accurate guide to the biological availability of the amino acids in the protein. For example, if a protein is poorly digested then the chemical score could greatly overestimate the real biological quality of the protein.

Net protein utilization (NPU) is a widely used biological measure of protein quality. It is a particularly important measure in agricultural nutrition but is nowadays considered to be of much less significance in human nutrition. To measure NPU, the protein to be tested is fed as the sole nitrogen source at a level below the minimum requirement for growth of the animal (usually weaning rats). The amount of nitrogen retained under these circumstances is corrected for the nitrogen losses that occur even on a protein-free diet and then expressed as a percentage of the intake. NPU can be directly assessed in human adults using nitrogen balance measurements:

NPU = (amount of retained nitrogen *divided by* nitrogen intake) × 100

where

retained nitrogen = intake – (loss – loss on protein-free diet).

The NPU values for some proteins are shown in Table 11.3. The NPU of diets as well as those of individual proteins may be determined and, because of the mutual supplementation effect, the NPU of most human diets come out within a relatively narrow range even though the qualities of the individual constituent proteins may vary widely. An NPU of around 70 would be typical of many human diets and would be not greatly affected by, for instance, the proportion of animal protein in the diet. The NPU is likely to be of significance in human nutrition only if a single staple with low amounts of poor-quality protein makes up the bulk of the diet and is the source of most of the dietary protein.

Key points

- Animal feeding trials using nitrogen-matched diets indicated that proteins vary in their nutritional quality.
- Variation in protein quality is due to variation in their complement of essential or indispensable amino acids.
- Essential amino acids cannot be made in the body but non-essential amino acids can be made by transamination.
- Animals can grow and adults can maintain nitrogen balance if provided with complete amino acid mixtures, but not if one of the essential ones is missing from the mixture.
- Essential amino acids are not equally distributed in all proteins. Some proteins, especially vegetable proteins, have low amounts of some essential amino acids.
- The limiting amino acid is the one present in a food in the lowest amount relative to how much is needed.
- When one essential amino acid is taken in insufficient quantities it limits the extent to which the others can be used for protein synthesis.
- Lysine is the limiting amino acid in most cereals. Lysine, tryptophan or sulphur-containing amino acids are the limiting amino acids in most foods.
- Proteins containing good amounts of all essential amino acids are termed first-class proteins. Examples are meat, fish, egg and pulse proteins.
- Proteins that are low in one or more essential amino acid are termed second-class proteins. Examples are gelatine, cereal proteins and most proteins from starchy root staples.
- When mixtures of proteins are eaten, deficits of essential amino acids in individual proteins will usually be compensated for by relative surpluses in others. This is termed mutual supplementation.
- The protein quality of human diets tends to equalize towards the mean because of mutual supplementation.
- The chemical score is a measure of protein quality. It is the amount of the limiting amino

→

Key points *continued*

acid in a gram of the protein expressed as a percentage of that found in a gram of a high-quality reference protein like egg.

● Net protein utilization (NPU) is a biological measure of protein quality. It is the percentage of the protein that growing animals can retain under conditions where protein intake is limited.

THE SIGNIFICANCE OF PROTEIN IN HUMAN NUTRITION

The change in attitude to protein deficiency as a suspected key cause of human malnutrition represents one of the most striking changes in human nutrition during the second half of the twentieth century. The author has previously reviewed this topic (Webb, 1989), and the book by Carpenter (1994) contains a detailed and thorough review of both the discovery of protein and changing attitudes to protein in nutrition. The following discussion is a development of my earlier review. This topic can serve as a case study to illustrate the three important general points that have been discussed earlier in the book (see below).

● *The potential costs of premature and ineffective 'health promotion' intervention.* These costs may be very real and substantial even if an unhelpful intervention does not do direct physiological harm (Chapter 1). The financial and time costs of all the measures to solve the illusory 'world protein crisis' were enormous and this meant that other more real problems were ignored or deprived of funding.
● *The potential dangers of overestimating dietary standards by 'erring on the safe side'* (Chapter 3). The 'world protein crisis' seems to have been precipitated by a massive overestimation of the protein needs of children.
● *The dangers of hasty and ill-considered extrapolation of results obtained in animal experiments to people* (Chapter 4). Awareness of the very high protein requirements in rapidly growing young animals was probably a factor in creating the illusory belief that the protein needs of children were also very high.

Some expert reviewers of earlier editions of this book have suggested that this section dealing with what is an historical and primarily developing-country issue should not be given such prominence in a book whose main focus is on nutrition for promoting health in industrialized countries. However, it is because this historical example so clearly illustrates the above issues that I continue to include it. These issues are of great relevance to current issues relating to diet and health promotion.

Key points

● Changes in the importance attached to protein illustrate the potential costs of unwarranted health promotion initiatives, the dangers of overestimating dietary standards, and the potential problems of carelessly extrapolating results obtained from laboratory animal studies to people.

Historical overview

For more than two decades (the 1950s and 1960s) the belief that primary protein deficiency was 'the most serious and widespread dietary deficiency in the world' (Waterlow *et al.*, 1960) dominated nutrition research and education. The consensus of nutrition opinion considered it likely that 'in many parts of the world the majority of young children suffered some protein malnutrition' (Trowell, 1954). The relative protein requirements of young children compared to adults were generally considered to be very high, perhaps five times higher on a weight-for-weight basis. Even where diets contained apparently adequate amounts of total protein, it was believed that protein availability might still be inadequate unless some high-quality protein (usually animal or pulse protein) was taken with each meal. Calculations of the amount of protein required by the world's population when compared with estimates of protein availability gave the impression of a large and increasing shortfall in world protein supplies – *the protein gap*. Jones (1974) suggested that an extra 20 million tons of protein were required each year and this figure implied that many hundreds of millions of people were protein-deficient. This protein gap was so large that a whole new field of research was initiated to try to close it, namely the mass production of protein-rich foods from novel sources such as fishmeal and microbes. An agency of the United Nations, 'The Protein Advisory Group', was set up specifically to oversee these developments. In 1972 the chairman's opening address to an international scientific conference contained the following statements:

> Every doctor, nutritionist or political leader concerned with the problem of world hunger has now concluded that the major problem is one of protein malnutrition. ... The calorie supply [of developing countries] tends to be more or less satisfactory, but what is lacking is protein, and especially protein containing the essential amino acids.
>
> *Gounelle de Pontanel, 1972*

As estimates of human protein requirements were revised downwards, this protein gap disappeared 'at the stroke of a pen' with no significant change in protein supplies. The above quotations from Gounelle de Pontanel contrast very sharply with the conclusions of Miller and Payne (1969) that almost all dietary staples contain sufficient protein to meet human needs and that even diets based on very low protein staples are unlikely to be specifically protein-deficient. In the decades since 1969 this latter view has become the nutritional consensus.

Despite this revolutionary change of mind, the greatly reduced emphasis on protein in human nutrition was slow to permeate beyond the ranks of the specialists. Even among nutrition educators some ambivalence towards protein persisted well into the 1990s. The following quotations from a 1991 edition of a well-respected American nutrition text seems to sum up that ambivalence (Hamilton *et al.*, 1991):

> Most people in the United States and Canada would find it almost impossible not to meet their protein requirements. ... Protein is at the heart of a good diet. Menu planners build their meals around the RDA for protein.

This exaggerated importance attached to protein in the past led to a huge concentration of research effort, physical resources, educational effort and political priority into protein nutrition and into efforts to close the protein gap. It now seems almost certain that much of this effort was wasted and

directed towards solving an illusory problem. McClaren (1974), Webb (1989) and Carpenter (1994) have discussed some of these costs of exaggerating human protein needs, and McClaren was moved to entitle his historically important article 'The great protein fiasco'. Some of the measures taken to try to solve the apparently false protein crisis are summarized below; further extensive details may be found in Carpenter (1994).

- In 1955, the UN set up the Protein Advisory Group to 'advise on the safety and suitability of new protein-rich food preparations'. This group held regular meetings and produced various reports until it was finally terminated in 1977.
- In 1957, UN experts suggested that there was an urgent need to develop cheap, locally produced, high-protein foods that would be safe, palatable and easy to incorporate into existing diets from things like fishmeal, soybeans, peanuts, coconut, sesame and cotton seed. To this was added, in the late 1960s, the development of protein from yeasts and bacteria (single-cell protein, SCP), the production of genetically improved plants and the use of synthetic amino acids to boost the quality of dietary proteins.
- In 1970, the UN approved a programme to implement these recommendations despite initial costs estimated at the equivalent of $500 million at today's prices.
- Numerous problems delayed and increased the development costs of high-protein foods from existing raw materials, such as (a) the need to remove lipids from fishmeal to make it palatable and improve its storage; (b) the presence of 'unhygienic' intestinal contents in meal made from small whole fish; (c) the presence of fungal toxins in peanut products; and (c) rising market prices of some of the raw materials.

Ultimately no cheap and widely used product emerged from these expensive undertakings. The poor did not eat the few products that got beyond the trial stage to full marketing.

- Many expensive projects to produce single-cell proteins were begun but most failed to produce products that were safe and acceptable for human consumption. One fungal product (Quorn) did emerge from these efforts but it is now marketed as a meat substitute for affluent vegetarians rather than a high-protein food for needy children in developing countries.

- Decades of expensive research did produce high-protein quality strains of cereals but these have never been widely grown.
- Chemical production of synthetic lysine for food supplementation was tried but proved ineffective in improving nutritional status in human field trials.

The total costs of these largely unsuccessful and seemingly unnecessary programmes and initiatives must amount to billions of dollars at today's prices.

Key points

- In 1960, protein deficiency was widely regarded as the most serious and widespread form of malnutrition and the majority of children in many developing countries were believed to be protein-deficient.

- In 1960, estimates of protein needs greatly exceeded protein supplies and indicated a large and increasing shortfall in world protein supplies – the protein gap.

- As estimates of children's protein needs decreased, so the concept of a protein gap became discredited.

- The current consensus is that few diets are specifically protein-deficient and, if children eat enough food for their energy needs, they will probably get enough protein.

- During the 'protein gap era', huge amounts of time and money were wasted on projects to solve the protein crisis, examples being the production of high-protein foods from fishmeal, peanuts and microbes, the development of genetically enhanced plants, and programmes to supplement cereals with synthetic amino acids.

Origins of the 'protein gap'

The three assumptions listed below seem to have been critical in creating the illusion of a massive world protein shortage.

- There was the belief that children required a high protein concentration in their diets; in other words, that the proportion of total dietary energy

derived from protein should be substantially higher in children than in adults.

- There was the assumption that the nutritional disease known as *kwashiorkor* was due to primary protein deficiency; that is, to a diet in which the proportion of energy derived from protein was too low.
- Kwashiorkor was believed to be the most prevalent form of malnutrition in the world, and cases of frank clinical kwashiorkor represented only the 'tip of the iceberg' with many more children impaired to some extent by lack of protein.

There are now good grounds for suggesting that each of these three assumptions is either dubious or improbable.

Past exaggeration of protein requirements?

Figure 11.2 illustrates the changes in the RDAs for protein since 1943 in the USA. In 1943, the protein RDA for a 2-year-old child was substantially more than double its current value (also more than double the current RNI in the UK). When expressed as a proportion of the energy allowance, the child's protein RNI was well above the adult value in 1943 but is now well below the adult value (see numerical values in Table 11.4).

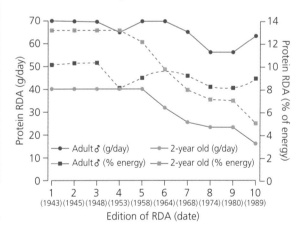

Figure 11.2 Changes in the American recommended dietary amount (RDA) for protein for an adult man and a 2-year-old child over ten editions from 1943 to 1989. Figures are expressed both in absolute terms and as a percentage of the energy RDA. Source: Webb, G.P. (1994) *Journal of Biological Education* 28(1), 104.

Table 11.4 Changing US estimates of protein needs

	1943	1989
Grams per day		
Adult man	70	65
2-year-old	40	18
Per cent of energy		
Adult man	10	8
2-year-old	13	5

The more recent values given above suggest that children can manage on a lower minimum protein concentration in their diets than can adults. This conclusion seems at first sight to be inconsistent with the notion that growing children have higher relative protein needs than adults. It has been and still is assumed that children need more protein on a weight-for-weight basis than do adults, only the assumed scale of this difference has declined. In the past, figures of up to 5 times higher weight-for-weight requirements in children have been suggested (e.g. Waterlow *et al.*, 1960), but nowadays a figure of around double is considered more reasonable.

Table 11.5 shows why this higher relative requirement is not inconsistent with the need for a lower dietary protein concentration, as suggested by Figure 11.2. Children not only require relatively more protein than adults but also more energy. Table 11.5 shows the current RNIs for protein and the EARs for energy in the UK as a multiple of the standard adult value when expressed on a weight-for-weight basis (i.e. expressed per kilogram of body weight). A 2-year-old child requires almost three times as much energy as an adult per kilogram of body weight but only about one and a half times as much protein. The need for increased energy intake (i.e. total food intake) is far greater than the increased relative need for protein. For all ages of children, the increased energy needs cancels out or, in most cases, greatly exceeds the increased need for protein. The 2-year-old child may need 1.5 times as much protein as an adult but needs to eat three times as much food; any diet with enough protein for an adult should therefore provide enough for the child if he or she can eat enough of it to satisfy energy requirements.

Table 11.5 Weight-for-weight estimated average requirements (EARs) and protein reference nutrient intakes (RNIs) as a multiple of the standard adult value at various ages*

Age	Energy EAR	Protein RNI
0–3 months	2.7	2.9
4–6 months	2.7	2.2
7–9 months	2.7	2.1
10–12 months	2.8	2.0
1–3 years	2.9	1.5
4–6 years	2.8	1.5
7–10 years	2.1	1.3
11–14 years	1.5	1.3
15–18 years	1.3	1.2
19–50 years	1.0	1.0
75+ years	0.9	1.0

*Calculated from data in COMA (1991).

Inappropriate extrapolation from animal experiments to humans may have encouraged inflated estimates of protein requirements in children. Primates have slower growth rates than most animals and much lower rates than most common laboratory animals (Table 11.6). The relative protein requirements of these rapidly growing species are thus likely to be higher than those of human infants and children. This seems to be borne out by the comparison of milk composition of the species also shown in the table. Up to 80 per cent of the nitrogen requirements of a growing rat

Table 11.6 Growth rates and milk composition of seven species*

	Days to double birth weight	Protein in milk (g/L)	Energy as protein (%)
Human child	120–180	1.1	6
Calf	47	3.2	19
Sheep	10	6.5	24
Cat	7	10.6	27
Rat	6	8.1	25
Mouse	5	9.0	21
Chimpanzee	100	1.2	7

*Simplified from Webb (1989).

is for growth (Altschul, 1965). Rats were widely used to model humans in protein experiments and so this probably encouraged the belief that children's relative protein requirements were up to five times those of adults. As four-fifths of the requirement of young rats is for growth and only one-fifth for maintenance, by direct analogy it might well suggest a five-fold difference in the requirements of children (for growth and maintenance) compared to those of adults (for maintenance only).

Animal experiments also probably played their part in exaggerating the importance of low protein quality as a practical problem in human nutrition. When a diet containing 10 per cent egg protein as the sole nitrogen source is fed to growing rats under test conditions, then 1 gram of egg protein will bring about an increase in weight of 3.8 grams in the animals. Egg protein is said to have a protein efficiency ratio of 3.8. Around 80 per cent of the consumed protein is retained as body protein. Wheat protein has a protein efficiency ratio of only 1 and just 20 per cent of the wheat protein would be retained as body protein (Altschul, 1965). Under the same test conditions, 1 gram of wheat protein results in only 1 gram of weight gain in the rats. Such experimental demonstrations of the low quality of many cereal and vegetable proteins would have suggested that, unless some high-quality protein was present, protein deficiency would have seemed almost inevitable: 4 grams of wheat protein is equivalent to only 1 gram of egg protein in growing rats.

Of course, most human diets are mixtures of proteins and mutual supplementation can occur. It was for some time thought, however, that this mutual supplementation could occur only within a meal, but it is now thought that such supplementation can occur over an extended time. If a meal lacking in one amino acid is consumed then the liver will donate the deficient amino acid to allow protein synthesis to continue and will replenish its complement of this amino acid at a later meal. Note also the much faster growth rates – and thus protein and amino acid requirements – of young rats compared to children. This makes it rather unlikely that protein deficiency will occur due to unbalanced amino acid composition except under very particular conditions.

Low concentration of dietary protein causes kwashiorkor?

The nutritional disease kwashiorkor was first described in the medical literature in the 1930s and a very tentative suggestion made that it might be due to dietary protein deficiency. Over the next 35 years it became generally accepted that two diseases known as kwashiorkor and marasmus represented different clinical manifestations of malnutrition in children, with differing aetiologies. Marasmus was attributed to simple energy deficit (starvation) whereas kwashiorkor was attributed to primary protein deficiency. Children with marasmus are severely wasted and stunted and the clinical picture is generally consistent with what might be expected in simple starvation. Several of the clinical features of kwashiorkor, however, are not superficially consistent with simple starvation but are consistent with protein deficiency (Table 11.7). Many children suffer from a mixture of these two diseases, so the two conditions were said to represent opposite extremes of a spectrum of diseases with the precise clinical picture depending on the precise levels of protein and energy deficit. The general term *protein-*

Table 11.7 Clinical features of kwashiorkor that are consistent with primary protein deficiency

Symptom	Rationale
Oedema (excess tissue fluid)	Lack of plasma proteins?
Hepatomegaly (liver swollen with fat)	Lack of protein to transport fat?
'Flaky paint' syndrome (depigmented and peeling skin)	Lack of amino acids for skin protein and pigment production?
Mental changes (anorexia and apathy)	Lack of amino acids for transmitter synthesis?
Subcutaneous fat still present	Inconsistent with simple energy deficit?
Changes in colour and texture of hair	Similar causes to skin changes?

energy malnutrition (PEM) was used to describe this spectrum of diseases.

A number of studies over the last 40 years have seriously challenged this assumption that kwashiorkor is necessarily due to primary protein deficiency. When protein needs of children were thought to be high, the protein deficit in the diets of many children in developing countries seemed to be much greater than any energy deficit. When the estimated protein needs of children were reduced then protein no longer appeared to be the limiting factor in these diets and energy deficits exceeded any protein deficits. Comparisons of the diets of children developing kwashiorkor or marasmus have reported no difference in their protein concentrations. Detailed analyses of the diets of children in developing countries have indicated that primary deficiency of protein is uncommon and that protein deficiency is usually a secondary consequence of low total food intake (Waterlow and Payne, 1975).

The symptoms of kwashiorkor listed in Table 11.7 are nonetheless persuasively consistent with protein deficiency rather that energy deficit. Acute shortage of energy would, however, lead to use of protein as an energy source. Thus dietary energy deficit could well precipitate a physiological deficit of amino acids for protein synthesis and to fulfil other amino acid functions. Symptoms consistent with protein deficiency might be triggered by energy deficit. Why starvation should sometimes result in marasmus and sometimes kwashiorkor is still unclear. Some theories have suggested that the symptoms of kwashiorkor may be triggered in an undernourished child by:

- mineral or vitamin deficiencies
- essential fatty acid deficiencies
- infection
- inadequate anti-oxidant response (e.g. due to lack of anti-oxidant vitamins and minerals) to oxidative stress (e.g. exacerbated by infection, toxins, sunlight).

Kwashiorkor: the most common nutritional disease in the world?

McClaren (1974) suggested that the widespread assumption that kwashiorkor was the most prevalent manifestation of protein-energy malnutrition was caused by faulty extrapolation from a World Health Organization survey of rural Africa in 1952. He argued that marasmus was a much more widespread problem than kwashiorkor and that marasmus was becoming increasingly common as breastfeeding declined (marasmus is associated with early weaning). In 1974, even one of the authors of the 1952 WHO report (J F Brock) conceded that there had been a relative neglect of marasmus which was very prevalent even in rural Africa (Carpenter, 1994).

Key points

- The protein gap concept originated because protein needs were exaggerated and because kwashiorkor was assumed to be both the most prevalent form of protein-energy malnutrition (PEM) and the result of a primary deficiency of protein.
- Estimated protein needs of children are now less than half what they were in the 1940s.
- Children were thought to need a much higher proportion of their energy as protein than adults do, but not now.
- Children were thought to need five times more protein per kilogram of body weight than adults do, but today's figure is less than twice as much.
- Young children require three times more energy per kilogram than adults. So, if they get enough energy then any diet with enough protein for an adult should provide ample amounts for a child.
- Most non-primate animals grow much faster than human babies and so require much more protein. This is reflected in much higher protein content in their milk.
- Around four-fifths of a young rat's protein requirement is for growth. This may indicate the origin of the belief that human babies require five times more protein per kilogram than adults.
- Laboratory experiments with rats suggested that many cereal and vegetable proteins were very inferior to animal proteins in supporting

→

Key points *continued*

growth. This probably exaggerated the importance attached to protein quality in human nutrition.

● Many of the symptoms of kwashiorkor are consistent with primary protein deficiency (see Table 11.7), yet there was never any hard evidence to support the belief that kwashiorkor is due to primary protein deficiency.

● Current estimates of protein and energy needs suggest that protein is rarely the limiting nutrient in diets in developing countries.

● Protein deficiency is usually a secondary consequence of inadequate food intake.

● It is now generally accepted that marasmus, not kwashiorkor, is the most prevalent form of PEM.

CONCLUDING REMARKS

Over the last 60 years, opinions about the significance of protein in human nutrition have undergone some dramatic changes. For a time, protein adequacy was top of the list of international nutritional priorities. Nowadays primary protein deficiency is generally considered to be a relatively uncommon occurrence, not because of an improved supply, but rather because of a change of nutritional opinion.

In both the UK and US dietary standards (COMA, 1991; NRC, 1989a) there is even concern voiced about the possible health risks of a high protein intake. It has been suggested, for example, that prolonged excess protein intake may predispose to renal failure in later life. Both of these panels suggested that it would be prudent to regard a value of twice the RNI/RDA as the safe upper limit for protein intake.

12

FATS

Nature of dietary fat	285	Transport of endogenously produced		
Types of fatty acid	287	lipids		303
Sources of fat in the human diet	291	The diet–heart hypothesis		304
Roles of fat in the diet	294	Fish oils		317
Blood lipoproteins	300	Other natural oils used as supplements		322
Digestion, absorption and transport				
of dietary lipids	301			

NATURE OF DIETARY FAT

About 95 per cent of dietary fats and oils are in the form of *triacylglycerol* (note that the alternative term *triglyceride* is still widely used). Most of the storage fat in the body is also in the form of triacylglycerol. Triacylglycerols (TAGs) are composed of three fatty acids linked to the simple three-carbon molecule *glycerol*. Glycerol is a carbohydrate moiety which is called a *tri-alcohol* and has one hydroxyl (alcohol) group on each of its three carbons. Each of these alcohol groups in glycerol can form an ester linkage with the carboxyl (acid) group of a fatty acid. The three fatty acids in a triacylglycerol can be the same (simple TAG) or different (mixed TAG). A triacylglycerol molecule is represented diagrammatically in Figure 12.1. Note that the term 'fat' is often used to imply a solid substance but oils and solid fats are collectively termed fats in this book.

If the third (bottom) fatty acid in Figure 12.1a is replaced by a phosphate group, then this compound is known as *phosphatidic acid*, the parent compound for a group of compounds known as *phospholipids*. Phospholipids make up most of the dietary lipid that is not triacylglycerol, and they have important physiological functions as components of membranes and in the synthesis of a range of important regulatory molecules called the *eicosanoids* (e.g. *prostaglandins*). The phosphate group of phosphatidic acid can link with various other compounds to produce a series of these phospholipids; examples are phosphatidyl choline (lecithin), phosphatidyl inositol and phosphatidyl serine.

Lipids are usually defined on the basis of their solubility – those components of the body or food that are insoluble in water but soluble in organic solvents like chloroform or ether. Using this definition, the term lipids would encompass not only triacylglycerols and phospholipids but also the sterols (e.g. cholesterol) and waxes. Waxes are esters of monohydroxyl alcohols (one OH group) and a long chain saturated fatty acid; they are very insoluble and very inert chemically (e.g. beeswax and carnauba wax from a South American pine tree).

Key points

- Lipids are organic materials that are insoluble in water but soluble in organic solvents. They include triacylglycerols, phospholipids, sterols and waxes.
- Ninety-five per cent of dietary fat (including oils) is triacylglycerol and most of the rest is phospholipid.
- Triacylglycerol comprises three fatty acids attached by ester linkages to each of the three hydroxyl (OH) groups of glycerol.
- If one fatty acid of triacylglycerol is replaced by a phosphate-containing moiety this becomes a phospholipid.

(a) Schematic representation of a triacylglycerol

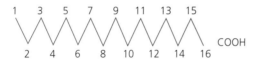

glycerol

(b) General chemical formula of a saturated fatty acid

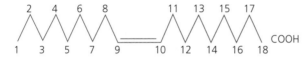

(c) Diagrammatic representation of a saturated fatty acid (palmitic acid – 16:0)

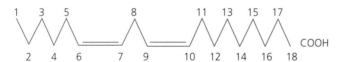

(d) Diagrammatic representation of a monounsaturated fatty acid (oleic acid – 18:1n-9)

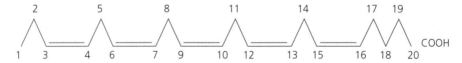

(e) Diagrammatic representation of linoleic acid (18:2n-6)

(f) Diagrammatic representation of eicosapentaenoic acid (EPA, 20:5n-3)

(g) Diagram to illustrate the *cis* and *trans* configurations of unsaturated fatty acids

cis configuration   *trans* configuration

Figure 12.1 The chemical nature of fats.

TYPES OF FATTY ACID

Fatty acids are of three major types: saturated, monounsaturated and polyunsaturated. All consist of a hydrocarbon chain of varying length with a carboxyl or acid group at one end. The only difference between these three types of fatty acid is in the number of carbon–carbon double bonds present in the hydrocarbon chain.

Saturated fatty acids

Carbon atoms have the potential to each form four covalent bonds (i.e. they have a valency of four). In saturated fatty acids, all the carbon atoms in the hydrocarbon chain are joined together by single bonds and all the remaining valencies (bonds) of the carbon atoms are occupied by bonding to hydrogen atoms, as shown in Figure 12.1b. These fatty acids are called saturated because all the available bonds of the carbon atoms are occupied or 'saturated' with hydrogen atoms. No more hydrogen atoms can be added to this hydrocarbon chain.

The chemical structure of fatty acids is often represented schematically as shown in Figure 12.1c. Each angle represents a carbon atom and the carbon atoms in this book are numbered starting with the carbon furthest away from the carboxyl or acid group. The fatty acid depicted in this diagram is called *palmitic acid*, which has 16 carbon atoms and no double bonds (so it can be written in shorthand notation as 16:0).

Monounsaturated fatty acids

Monounsaturated fatty acids have a single point of unsaturation: two of the carbons in the chain are joined together by a double bond, so there are two fewer hydrogen atoms than in a saturated fatty acid of the same length. *Oleic acid* is depicted in Figure 12.1d, which is an 18-carbon monounsaturated fatty acid widely found in nature in both animals and plants (it is the principal acid in olive oil). The double bond in oleic acid is between carbons 9 and 10 in the sequence; the shorthand notation for this acid is 18:1n-9 (i.e. 18 carbons; 1 double bond; and n-9 meaning the double bond is between carbons 9 and 10). In many popular and older sources the 'n' is replaced by the Greek letter omega (ω) so that oleic acid becomes 18:1ω-9.

Polyunsaturated fatty acids

Polyunsaturated fatty acids have two or more double bonds in the carbon chain: they have more than one point of unsaturation. Figure 12.1e shows *linoleic acid*, which has 18 carbons, two double bonds, and the first of these double bonds is between carbons 6 and 7; its shorthand notation is therefore 18:2n-6. Knowing the position of the first double bond makes it possible to predict the position of any further double bonds because they are normally separated by a single saturated carbon atom (i.e. are 'methylene interrupted'). In linoleic acid, the first double bond is between carbons 6 and 7, carbon 8 is saturated, and the second double bond lies between carbons 9 and 10.

Figure 12.1f shows a slightly more complicated example. *Eicosapentaenoic acid* (EPA) has 20 carbons, five double bonds, and the first double bond is between carbons 3 and 4; hence its shorthand notation is 20:5n-3. In EPA, carbon 5 is saturated and the second double bond is between carbons 6 and 7; carbon 8 is saturated and the third double bond is between 9 and 10, the fourth between 12 and 13 and the fifth between 15 and 16. Each of the double bonds in EPA is separated by a single saturated carbon atom, and so knowing the position of the first double bond (given by the 'n' or 'ω' notation) one can predict the position of all of the others.

Note that there is an alternative numbering system in which the carbons are counted from the *carboxyl end of the molecule* (the Δ or delta system). That system is used particularly by organic chemists. Eicosapentaenoic acid (20:5n-3) in Figure 12.1f thus has double bonds at Δ positions 5, 8, 11, 14 and 17. The 'n' system is now the primary nomenclature used in this book and has replaced the 'ω' system used in previous editions.

Cis/trans isomerization

Different geometric isomers (as shown in Figure 12.1g) are possible wherever a fatty acid has a carbon–carbon double bond. When represented in two dimensions, either both hydrogen atoms can be on the same side (the *cis* form), or the hydrogen atoms can be on opposite sides (the *trans* form). Most naturally occurring fats contain almost exclusively *cis* isomers, although small amounts of *trans* fatty acids are found in butter (4–8 per cent) and other natural fats, especially those from ruminating animals where they are produced by bacteria in the animal's rumen. Whether a double bond is in the *cis* or *trans* configuration makes a considerable difference to the three-dimensional shape of the molecule. A *cis* double bond causes the molecule to bend back on itself into a U-shape, whereas a *trans* double bond remains in the more linear form characteristic of saturated fatty acids.

It is possible to chemically convert unsaturated fatty acids to saturated ones if the fat is reacted with hydrogen in the presence of an activating agent or catalyst. This process is called *hydrogenation* and it causes oils to solidify. Partial hydrogenation was the traditional method used in the production of margarine and solid vegetable shortening, particularly hydrogenated vegetable oils and hydrogenated fish oil. The process of hydrogenation can result in the production of relatively large amounts of *trans* fatty acids in the final product. Many of the early, cheap, 'hard' margarines were made from hydrogenated fish oil and were particularly high in *trans* fatty acids (up to 30 per cent of fatty acids) but these have been superseded by soft margarines made from vegetable oil which have little or no *trans* fatty acids. Heating of cooking oils also produces some *trans* isomers and they accumulate if the oil is used repeatedly, for example to cook multiple batches of chips (French fries).

Effects of chain length and degree of unsaturation on fatty acid melting point

The chain length and degree of unsaturation of a fatty acid affect its melting point. In general, the longer the chain length the higher is the melting point, and the more unsaturated it is (i.e. the more *cis* double bonds it has) the lower will be its melting point. The examples below illustrate these points:

- lauric acid (12:0): melting point 44°C
- palmitic acid (16:0): 63°C
- stearic acid (18:0): 70°C
- lignoceric acid (24:0): 84°C
- oleic acid (18:1n-9): 13°C
- elaidic acid (*trans* equivalent of oleic acid): 45°C
- linoleic acid (18:2n-6): –5°C

- linolenic acid (18:3n-3): –10°C
- arachidic acid (20:0): 75°C
- arachidonic acid (20:4n-6): –49°C
- eicosapentaenoic acid (20:5n-3): –54°C.

The first four on this list are all saturated and the melting points increase with the increasing chain length; all are solids at room temperature. Compare the four 18-carbon acids (stearic, oleic, linoleic and linolenic) which have 0, 1, 2 and 3 *cis* double bonds, respectively; the melting points of these decrease with each double bond, and all three of the unsaturated fatty acids would be liquids at room temperature. The *trans* equivalent of oleic acid (elaidic acid) has a much higher melting point than oleic itself; it would be solid at room temperature, illustrating the earlier point that *trans* fatty acids are closer in their three-dimensional configuration and physical properties to saturated fatty acids.

Eicosapentaenoic acid (20:5n-3) has a lower melting point than arachidonic acid, the corresponding acid in the n-6 series, and in Figure 12.2 (later in the chapter) every fatty acid in the n-3 series has a lower melting point than the corresponding n-6 acid because of the extra double bond. This also means that melting point and physical form of triacylglcerols will be dependent on their fatty acid profiles. Those triacylglycerols with lots of saturated and monounsaturated fatty acids tend to be solids at room temperature (e.g. butter and lard) while those with high levels of polyunsaturated fatty acids will be liquids (e.g. corn oil, sunflower oil and fish oil).

Conjugated linoleic acid

Conjugated linoleic acid (CLA) is the collective name given to a group of isomers of linoleic acid found principally in dairy fat and meat fat, especially meat from ruminants. In CLA the double bonds are contiguous (not separated by a methylene group) and they can be in either the *cis* or *trans* configuration. The two most prevalent acids that make up 80–90 per cent of the dietary CLA are *trans* 7 *cis* 9 and *cis* 6 *trans* 8, using the 'n' numbering system counting from the end furthest from the carboxyl group. (Using the Δ nomenclature counting from the carboxyl end, these are designated *cis* 9 *trans* 11 and *trans* 10 *cis* 11, respectively.)

Conjugated linoleic acid is produced from linoleic acid by bacteria in the rumen of cattle and other ruminants – hence its presence in dairy fat and beef fat. Cattle that graze on pasture have higher amounts of CLA in their meat and milk than those that are fed grain and commercial cattle foods. Average intake of CLA by an omnivorous man in the UK was estimated at 150 mg/day in 1995 and more than two-thirds of this came from dairy fat.

Conjugated linoleic acid has been marketed as a dietary supplement. It is argued that, because of modern animal husbandry practices, the amounts of CLA in our diets have decreased; and decreased consumption of dairy and meat fat would also decrease intakes. Studies using animals and in-vitro systems have given rise to a number of claims for potential benefits from consuming supplemental amounts of CLA, some of which are listed here.

- CLA has anti-mutagenic properties in bacterial tests and may reduce the formation of chemically induced experimental tumours in laboratory animals.
- It has been claimed that it moderates the inflammatory response and could thus have beneficial effects in treating chronic inflammatory conditions.
- It may have beneficial effects on blood lipoprotein profiles.
- It may increase lean body mass and reduce body fat content.

The animal studies that have led to most of these claims used large amounts of CLA that are way beyond what would be consumed in any normal diet – the equivalent of several grams per day in human diets (cf. the average 150 mg/day consumed by an omnivorous man). Roche *et al.* (2001) reviewed several relatively short-term trials (up to 2 months) that had tested the effects of doses of around 3000 mg/day of CLA and found that these failed to consistently produce the effects on weight, body composition and lipoprotein profiles that might have been predicted from the animal trials. They suggested that even these doses of around 20 times the usual intake of male omnivores may be insufficient to produce statistically significant effects. One long-term placebo-controlled trial (Gaullier *et al.*, 2004) used up to 4500 mg/day of CLA for a year in 180 (mainly female) subjects who

were overweight but not obese. They reported that the CLA group lost an average of 2 kg in weight over the year and that they had lost significant amounts of fat compared to no significant changes in the placebo group. Some very small adverse effects on blood lipoprotein levels were recorded in the CLA group.

Even if these results are confirmed, the effects were relatively modest and took a year of using a very large dose of CLA. There is as yet no clear mechanistic explanation for the proposed effects of CLA. Under such circumstances the prolonged use of pharmacological doses of a substance without any clear idea of how it might act seems at best imprudent. It should also be borne in mind that high intakes of dairy fat and meat fat are normally associated with negative health implications.

Distribution of fatty acid types in dietary fat

All fat sources contain mixtures of saturated, monounsaturated and polyunsaturated fatty acids but the proportions vary considerably from fat to fat. Table 12.1 shows the variation in proportion of these three types of fatty acids in several common dietary fats.

Table 12.1 Typical proportions of saturated (S), monounsaturated (M) and polyunsaturated (P) fatty acids in several dietary fats

Fat	% S	% M	% P	P:S ratio
Butter	64	33	3	0.05
Lard	47	44	9	0.2
Sunflower oil	14	34	53	4
Soybean oil	15	26	59	4
Rapeseed (canola)	7	60	33	5
Olive oil	15	73	13	0.8
Coconut oil	91[1]	7	2	0.02
Palm oil	48	44	8	0.2
Oil in salmon	28	42	30	1
Oil in mackerel	27	43	30	1

[1] Includes large amount of medium- chain saturates (less than 16 carbons).

The two animal fats in Table 12.1 are high in saturates and low in polyunsaturates and this is typical of fat from farm animals. Fat from ruminating animals (e.g. milk, beef and lamb) is the most saturated and the least amenable to manipulation by alterations in the diet of the animal. The fatty acid composition of the fat from other animals (e.g. pigs) can be manipulated more readily by altering their diets, although this may affect the palatability and the texture of the meat.

Soya oil and sunflower oil are two vegetable oils that are typical of many vegetable oils in that they are low in saturates and high in polyunsaturated fatty acids. In most vegetable oils, the n-6 polyunsaturated fatty acids predominate. Olive oil and rapeseed (canola) oil are the most widely eaten examples of fats that are particularly high in monounsaturates and low in saturates. Rapeseed oil also has a relatively high proportion of n-3 polyunsaturated acids. The composition of the two tropical oils shown in Table 12.1 (coconut and palm oil) show that there are exceptions to the general observation that vegetable oils are low in saturates and high in unsaturated fatty acids. On the simple basis of the proportions of the three main types of fatty acid, palm oil is quite similar in its make-up to lard. Coconut oil contains a particularly high proportion (around 78 per cent) of medium-chain saturated fatty acids (less than 16 carbons) that make up only a small proportion of the fatty acids in most fats. Palmitic acid (16:0) is the dominant saturated fatty acid in most types of fat.

The two fish oils shown in the table are typical of oil in most fish, shellfish and even the fat of marine mammals such as seals and whales. These marine oils are relatively high in polyunsaturates and low in saturates, and are particularly rich in n-3 polyunsaturated fatty acids. Fish oils are the principal dietary source of n-3 polyunsaturated fatty acids that contain 20 or more carbon atoms (long-chain n-3 polyunsaturates), especially eicosapentaenoic acid (EPA) and docosahexaenoic acid (DHA). DHA is also found in the phospholipid lecithin present in egg yolks and in the phospholipids present in muscle meat, and particularly in organ meat like liver and brain. When fish are farmed then there may be some differences in the fatty acid composition of their oil compared to wild fish and this reflects the quite different diets of farmed and wild fish.

The P:S ratio

The P:S ratio of a fat is the ratio of polyunsaturated to saturated fatty acids. In the examples shown in Table 12.1 this ratio ranges from 0.02 in coconut oil to around 5 in rapeseed (canola) oil. The P:S ratio has traditionally been used as a shorthand guide to the likely effect of a fat or a diet on the plasma cholesterol concentration. For many years it has been generally accepted that saturated fatty acids tended to raise and polyunsaturates to lower plasma cholesterol concentration.

This would suggest that fats and diets with higher P:S ratios would have the most favourable (lowering) effects on plasma cholesterol. Current views on the effects of various fatty acid fractions on plasma cholesterol are more complex and are discussed later in the chapter. Despite this, the simple P:S ratio is still a useful indicator of the likely effect of a fat or diet on plasma cholesterol level.

Key points

- Fatty acids are composed of a hydrocarbon chain with a single carboxyl (COOH) or acid group at one end.
- Fatty acids in biological systems usually have between 2 and 22 carbon atoms. In this book the carbons are numbered from the methyl end (furthest from the carboxyl group). Note that chemists may use an alternative Δ numbering system counting carbons from the carboxyl end of the molecule.
- In saturated fatty acids, all of the carbons in the hydrocarbon chain are joined by single bonds.
- Monounsaturated fatty acids have a single carbon–carbon double bond in the hydrocarbon chain.
- Polyunsaturated fatty acids have between 2 and 6 double bonds.
- The n-3 (or ω-3) series of polyunsaturated fatty acids have their first double bond between carbons 3 and 4. The n-6 (or ω-6) series have their first double bond between carbons 6 and 7.
- A single saturated carbon atom (methylene group) separates each double bond in a polyunsaturated fatty acid.

→

Key points *continued*

- The shorthand notation for fatty acids indicates the number of carbons, the number of double bonds and the position of the first double bond. Thus 18:2n-6 (or 18:2ω-6) has 18 carbons, 2 double bonds, and the first double bond is between carbons 6 and 7.

- *Trans* fatty acids are those in which the hydrogen atoms at either end of a carbon–carbon double bond are on opposite sides. In *cis* fatty acids they are on the same side.

- In most natural fats the *cis* configuration predominates but butter, hydrogenated oils, and repeatedly heated oils contain significant amounts of *trans* fatty acids.

- The presence of a *cis* double bond causes the carbon chain to bend back on itself, whereas *trans* fatty acids have a linear configuration that is closer to saturated fatty acids.

- In general, the longer the chain length of a fatty acid, the higher is its melting point. The presence of *cis* double bonds greatly lowers the melting point; *trans* double bonds have a smaller effect on melting point.

- The presence of *cis* double bonds increases the fluidity. Fats with lots of saturated fatty acids tend to be solid at room temperature (e.g. butter and lard), but those with lots of polyunsaturated fatty acids tend to be liquid (e.g. sunflower and corn oils).

- Conjugated linoleic acids (CLAs) are a group of isomers of linoleic acid which have double bonds that are contiguous and may be in either the *cis* or *trans* configuration.

- CLA are taken as supplements although most of the evidence supporting their use comes from studies in animals that have used doses many times that which could be consumed in a normal diet.

- All dietary fats contain a mixture of saturated, monounsaturated and polyunsaturated fatty acids, but the proportions vary enormously.

- Meat fat and milk fat are usually high in saturates and low in polyunsaturates.

- Many vegetable oils are low in saturates but high in polyunsaturates. The n-6 series of polyunsaturates predominate.

→

Key points *continued*

- Olive and rapeseed oils are particularly high in monounsaturates.

- Tropical oils from palm and coconut are high in saturates and low in polyunsaturates.

- Fish oil is low in saturates and high in polyunsaturates, and the n-3 series predominate. Fish oil is the major dietary source of the long-chain n-3 polyunsaturates (i.e. those with 20 or 22 carbons), but docosahexaenoic acid (DHA) is also found in egg yolk lecithin, muscle meat phospholipids, and especially in phospholipids from organ meat such as liver and brain.

- The P:S ratio of a fat is the ratio of polyunsaturated to saturated fatty acids in it. This ratio is a useful guide to the likely effect of a fat on plasma cholesterol concentration; those with a high ratio tend to lower it while those with a low ratio tend to raise it.

SOURCES OF FAT IN THE HUMAN DIET

There are four principal sources of fat in the human diet.

- *Milk fat.* This is found in whole milk and yoghurt, cream, butter and cheese. It is almost inevitably highly saturated because it is difficult to manipulate the fatty acid content of cow milk by manipulating the cow's diet. The fatty acid profiles of foods made from milk fat are sometimes altered by blending it with polyunsaturated oil (e.g. to produce a softer butter that is easier to spread).

- *Meat fat.* This source includes not only carcass meat but also (often especially) meat products such as sausages and burgers and cooking fats of animal origin such as lard and beef tallow. This fat also tends to be highly saturated, especially that from ruminating animals (e.g. beef and lamb/mutton). Note that although animal fats are usually referred to as saturated fats they do contain large amounts of monounsaturated fatty acids (44 per cent in lard), particularly oleic acid.

- *Seeds and nuts.* These contain fat/oil which provides a concentrated source of energy for germination. These fats and oils are prominent in many diets because they are the source of the vegetable oils and most margarine. They usually have a relatively high P:S ratio and most of the polyunsaturated fatty acids are predominantly of the n-6 type in many of the most widely used vegetable oils. The tropical oils are clearly an exception to these generalities and have P:S ratios that are typical of those found in meat fat (see Table 12.1).

- *Fish oil.* This source is the flesh of oily fish such as mackerel, herring, trout, mullet and salmon. The flesh of white fish (e.g. cod and haddock) is very low in fat although considerable amounts of fat may be stored in the livers of such fish (hence cod liver oil). Fish oils tend to have a high P:S ratio, the n-3 acids are generally abundant, and they are the only major dietary source of the long-chain n-3 polyunsaturated fatty acids. Partially hydrogenated fish oil was used to make margarine – it was low in DHA and EPA but contained large amounts of *trans* fatty acids. It has been superseded by soft margarine made from vegetable oils that are high in polyunsaturated fatty acids and have little or no *trans* fatty acids.

Any food that contains any of the above as an ingredient will also contain fat. Fat is a major ingredient of cakes, pastries, biscuits (cookies) and chocolate, so these foods contribute significantly to total fat intake. Any foods cooked with the fats listed above will also be rich in fat. Thus, potatoes and most other vegetables contain almost no fat but when fried or roasted with fat they absorb substantial amounts of the cooking fat.

UK fat intakes and their food sources

Table 12.2 shows the food sources of fat and of saturated fat in adult UK diets. Where foods contribute relatively more to the fat and saturated fat columns than to the energy column, these are rich sources of dietary fat. Thus food in the milk group provided only 10 per cent of total energy but 24 per cent of the saturated fat; fat spreads provided only 4 per cent of total energy but 12 per cent of the fat and saturated fat; and foods in the meat group provided 16 per cent of the energy but 24 per cent of the fat and saturated fat. Conversely, the cereals

group provided 31 per cent of the total energy but only 19 per cent of the fat; and foods in the sugar, confectionery and drinks category provided 17 per cent of the energy but only 3 per cent of the fat.

Table 12.2 Percentage contributions of foods to the energy, fat and saturated fat content of UK diets*

Food group	% energy	% total fat	% saturated fat
Cereals and cereal products	31	19	18
Milk and milk products (incl. cheese)	10	14	24
Fat spreads	4	12	12
Egg and egg dishes	2	4	3
Meat and products	16	24	24
Fish and fish dishes	3	3	2
Vegetables (excl. potatoes)	4	4	2
Potatoes and savoury snacks	9	10	7
Fruit and nuts	3	2	1
Sugar, confectionery, preserves, drinks (incl. alcohol)	17	3	6

*Data source: Henderson *et al.* (2003).

Most dairy fat can be avoided by choosing products made from low-fat milk. Likewise with carcass meat, much of the obvious fat can be removed – although in many meat products such as sausages, burgers and pies it is not possible to selectively remove the fat. Cereal foods, normally classified as starchy foods, provide a surprisingly high proportion of both fat and saturated fat, and much of this comes in products such as cakes, pastries, biscuits (cookies) and pizzas.

Up to the mid-1990s, data from the National Food Survey suggested that the contribution of fat to the UK household diet rose during the 1950s and early 1960s as post-wartime shortages eased and rationing was removed but from 1975 to 1990 it had remained practically constant at around 40 per cent of total energy (e.g. Chesher, 1990). Absolute fat consumption did drop very substantially during this later period but only in proportion to the decline in total energy intake that occurred over this period, leaving the proportion of fat unaltered. As noted in Chapter 5 there were great changes in the types of fat consumed in the UK over this period. In 1959, the P:S ratio of the British diet was 0.17, still only 0.23 in 1979, but by 1996 it had risen to its current level of around 0.5. This change in P:S ratio has been brought about principally by replacement of butter, hard margarine and animal-based cooking fats by soft margarine, low-fat spreads and vegetable oils. There has also been a huge decrease in the consumption of whole-fat milk, which now represents less than a quarter of total milk sales compared with almost 100 per cent of the total in 1975. It is estimated that saturated fat now provides about 14.8 per cent of the energy in household food purchases whereas in 1975 it was around 20 per cent. Data from household expenditure surveys also suggest that, between 1994 and 2000, the contribution of fat to the energy in household food dropped from 38.8 to 36.9 per cent but has remained fairly stable since then and was estimated at 37.6 per cent of food energy in 2004–05.

Table 12.3 compares results from the NDNS adult surveys conducted in 1986–7 and 2009–10 which used a weighed inventory of food as eaten rather than household budget surveys which measure what people buy rather than what they eat. These two consumption surveys show a big drop in the percentage of food energy derived from

Table 12.3 Changes in fat and selected fat fractions as a percentage of food energy in the UK diet between 1986 and 2010*

Fat fraction	Men		Women	
	1986–7	2009–10	1986–7	2009–10
Total fat	40.4	35.5	40.3	34.7
Saturated fatty acids	16.5	12.9	17.0	13.2
Trans fatty acids[1]	2.2	0.8	2.2	0.8

* NDNS data.
[1] The recommendation is that no more than 2 per cent of food energy should come from *trans* fatty acids.

fat from over 40 per cent to close to the target figure of 35 per cent in 2010. There was also a 3–4 per cent drop in the percentage of food energy derived from saturated fatty acids; according to Bates *et al.* (2011) the value is now 12.8 per cent for adults.

Table 12.4 compares average intakes of fat and selected fat fractions recorded in the 2000–1 NDNS and compares these with the dietary reference values (DRVs). This table suggests that average intakes of total fat are close to the DRV – slightly above it for men and just below it for women (similar to values recorded by Bates' survey).

Table 12.4 Percentages of food energy from various fat fractions compared to the daily recommended value (DRV), and the percentage of subjects meeting the DRV*

Fat fraction	DRV (% of food energy)	Average (% of food energy)[1]		% meeting the DRV	
		Men	Women	Men	Women
Total fat	35	35.8	34.9	43	50
Saturated fatty acids	11	13.4	13.2	c20	c20
Trans fatty acids	2	1.0	1.0	>98	c >8
Cis n-3	–	1.0	1.0	100	100
Cis n-6[2]	–	5.4	5.3	100	100
Cholesterol (mg/day)	300	304	213	56	83

*Data from Henderson *et al.* (2003); for more recent data on contribution of fat fractions to food energy see Table 12.3.
[1] Note that, in about one-fifth of all subjects, fat contributed >40 per cent of their food energy.
[2] Individual intakes of *cis* n-6 polyunsaturates also did not exceed 10 per cent of food energy in any subjects (the individual maximum set by COMA in 1991).

The proportions of fat and saturated fat recorded in this survey were fairly consistent in different age groups of adults. Intakes of saturated fatty acids, despite being much lower than recorded in earlier surveys, were still significantly above the DRV, and only about 20 per cent of adults were at or below the DRV of saturated fat representing 11 per cent of food energy. Saturated fatty acid intakes have continued their long-term decline since 2001 and now make up 12.8 per cent of food energy in adults. All individuals met the very low minimum requirements for n-3 (0.2 per cent of food energy) and n-6 (1 per cent of food energy) polyunsaturated fatty acids, and no individual exceeded the recommendation that not more than 10 per cent of food energy should come from n-6 polyunsaturated fatty acids.

Trans fatty acid intakes have been declining for several decades as the hard margarines with their high levels of *trans* fats have been phased out. In 1982, average intakes of *trans* fatty acids in the UK were around 7 g/day; in 1986–7 this had declined to 5.6 g/day for men and 4 g/day for women, and in 2000–1 this was down to 2.9 g/day for men and 2 g/day for women. COMA (1991) suggested that there was wide variation in individual intakes of *trans* fatty acids despite the declining average intake. However, Table 12.4 shows that 98 per cent of men and women had intakes that were below the 2 per cent of food energy recommended by COMA, and that intake had almost halved in the period 1986–7 to 2000–1.

In 2007, estimates of *trans* fatty acids from the 2000–1 survey were revised down to 1 per cent of food energy and are now estimated at 0.8 per cent (Bates *et al.*, 2011). This fall in *trans* fatty acids is because of a greatly reduced contribution from artificial (hydrogenated) fats.

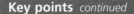

Key points *continued*

- Variation in the fatty acid profiles of dietary fats was summarized at the end of the previous section.
- Table 12.2 shows the contribution of the major food groups to total fat and saturated fat intake in the UK.
- Until the mid-1990s, the proportion of household food energy obtained from fat remained at around 40 per cent for 20 years but has fallen since then.
- Between 1986–7 and 2009–10 the proportion of food energy derived from fat in the UK fell by about 5 per cent.
- Highly polyunsaturated oils and margarine have largely replaced butter, lard and beef tallow in the British diet, and full-fat milk has been largely replaced by lower fat milk.
- The P:S ratio of the British diet has approximately trebled since 1960.
- The proportion of food energy derived from saturated fat has been falling for over 30 years. It is now less than 13 per cent, compared to peak values in the 1970s of around 20 per cent.
- Intakes of *trans* fatty acids have been in long-term decline and reached just 0.8 per cent of food energy in 2009, with almost everyone below the daily recommended value (DRV) of no more than 2 per cent of food energy.

ROLES OF FAT IN THE DIET

Fat as an energy source

A gram of fat yields more than twice as much metabolizable energy as a gram of either carbohydrate or protein. Vegetable oils and animal-derived cooking fats are almost 100 per cent fat and so yield around the theoretical maximum metabolizable energy of any food – 9 kcal (36 kJ) per gram. This compares with less than 4 kcal (16 kJ) per gram for pure sugar which is the most concentrated form of carbohydrate and is generally regarded as an energy-rich food.

Altering the fat content of foods profoundly affects their energy density. Table 12.5 shows some examples of how adding relatively small amounts of

Key points

- Most dietary fat originates from meat, milk, fish, nuts and seeds or from any food that contains these as an ingredient.
- Nuts and seeds are the source of most cooking oils and margarine.

→

fat to portions of food produces disproportionately large increases in the energy yield of the food.

Table 12.5 Effects of adding typical portions of fats to typical portions of some foods*

Food	kJ	% increase	% fat by weight	% energy as fat
Slice of bread	315		2.5	11
+ butter or margarine	563	80	17	61
Jacket potato	617		Trace	0.5
+ butter or margarine	928	50	5.5	34
Potatoes, boiled	504		Trace	1.5
chips (French fries)	1592	215	11	39
Pork chop, lean only	756		6.5	43
lean and fat	1462	95	19	66
Milk, skimmed milk	267		Trace	3
whole	542	100	4	53
Chicken, meat only	508		4	25
meat and skin	773	50	23	58
Fruit pie	937		8	38
+ double cream	1596	70	17	62
Mixed salad	118		Trace	3
+ oil and vinegar	365	210	5	70
+ mayonnaise	697	500	6.5	82.5

*Portion sizes and composition are from Davies and Dickerson (1991).

- Adding 8 g of butter or margarine to a slice of bread increases the energy content by around 80 per cent.
- Adding a 35 g portion of double cream to a slice of fruit pie increases the energy content of the dish by 70 per cent.
- Adding 20 g of mayonnaise to a 210 g mixed salad results in a six-fold rise in the energy yield.

Even in the fat-enriched foods in Table 12.5, fat still accounts for a relatively small proportion of the food's weight and yet in most cases it accounts for a high proportion of the energy yield. Thus fat accounts for:

- 4 per cent of the weight of whole milk but over half the energy
- 6 per cent of the weight of the salad and mayonnaise but over 80 per cent of the energy
- 6 per cent of the weight of the lean pork chop but well over 40 per cent of the energy
- 11 per cent of the weight of the chips (French fries) but 40 per cent of the energy
- 17 per cent of the weight of the buttered bread but 60 per cent of the energy.

Consumers should be very wary of claims that a product is low in fat simply because the percentage of fat by weight is low. A 90 per cent fat-free product has 10 per cent of fat by weight and this may still account for a high proportion of the food's energy. One could, for example, accurately describe whole milk as 96 per cent fat-free despite the fact that more than half its energy comes from fat.

Altering the fat content of a diet profoundly affects its energy density. A high-fat diet is a concentrated diet and a low-fat diet inevitably bulkier. It may be desirable for people expending lots of energy in prolonged heavy physical work to eat a reasonably concentrated diet so that they do not have to eat inordinate quantities of food (particularly people like explorers who also have to carry their food). For relatively sedentary adults, low-fat low-energy density diets are considered desirable because they may reduce the risk of excessive weight gain (see Chapter 9). Very low-fat and low-energy-density weaning diets are, in contrast, considered undesirable because they may precipitate protein-energy malnutrition (PEM) because children cannot eat enough of the dilute food to meet their energy needs.

Palatability

Fat increases the sensory appeal of foods; it enhances the flavour, colour, texture and smell. Many volatile flavour compounds are fat soluble and so are concentrated in the fat fraction of unprocessed foods. Flavour compounds develop when food is cooked in fats and oils even if the oil itself is bland. Fat also changes the texture of solid foods and the viscosity of liquids; butter or margarine spread on bread not only changes the taste but also the texture; full-fat milk has a noticeably higher viscosity than low-fat milk. Fat also affects the appearance of some foods. For example, skimmed milk has noticeably less colour than whole milk and less whitening effect when used in tea or coffee. Volatile, fat-soluble materials contribute to the smell of food as well as its taste. In the foods in Table 12.5, the addition of fat generally increases the sensory appeal of a food as well as the energy yield. Boiled potatoes are essentially bland whereas chips (French fries) have much more sensory appeal to most people. Adding butter to boiled mashed potatoes enhances their flavour, texture, smell and appearance. Adding oily dressings to salads or cream to fruit pie is usually considered to enhance the sensory appeal of these foods. Although some people find the concentrated surface fat on meat nauseating, a moderate amount of intrinsic fat (e.g. 'marbling' of fat in beef) greatly improves the taste and texture; very lean meat may seem dry and stringy.

These effects of fat on the palatability of food mean that as populations become richer they tend to increase the proportion of their dietary energy that is derived from fat. When affluence increases the availability of fatty foods, people tend to consume them in amounts that are probably detrimental to their long-term health prospects. This effect of fat on palatability also explains why it proved difficult to persuade affluent populations to reduce the proportion of fat in their diets. Despite intensifying health education exhortations to reduce fat intake that began well over three decades ago, significant changes in the proportion of energy derived from fat have changed significantly only since the mid-1990s.

Fat is important in the production of weaning foods of appropriate viscosity and energy density for young children (Church, 1979). Children require food of appropriate viscosity for their stage of development. In the immediate postnatal period they require a liquid feed, then after weaning (say 6–12 months) they need to be fed with a semi-solid gruel followed by a gradual transition to a standard adult diet. They may require a lower viscosity when unwell. After cooking, low-fat, starchy, staple foods require the addition of large amounts of water in order to produce foods of suitable viscosity for newly weaned children. They may become edible only if 70–80 per cent of their total weight is water and they may require 95 per cent water to make them liquid. Their viscosity may increase sharply as they cool. Thus thick family pap made from maize may yield 1000 kcal (4.2 MJ) per kilogram but as much as 4 kg of a typical maize gruel suitable for a newly weaned child might be required to supply the same amount of energy. Fat not only adds concentrated energy to weaning foods but also affects their viscosity such that they become palatable to young children over a wider range of water contents. For example, milk remains drinkable even when evaporated to only 20 per cent water.

Satiation

It has traditionally been said that fat delays stomach emptying and so extends the period of satiation after consumption of the meal. Many more recent studies suggest that, in fact, quite the opposite seems to be true; carbohydrate rather than fat may have the greater satiating effect. Not only does fat increase the palatability and energy density of the diet but, calorie for calorie, fat may also have less satiating effect than carbohydrate – thus favouring weight gain and obesity still further (see Chapter 9 for further discussion).

Fat-soluble vitamins

The fat-soluble vitamins (A, D, E and K) are found mainly in the lipid fraction of fat-containing foods and they are also absorbed along with dietary fat in the gut. Dietary deficiency of vitamin A is a major international nutritional problem even today (see Chapter 14). Vitamin A (*retinol*) is found only in certain fats of animal origin, although humans can convert the pigment β-carotene, from brightly coloured fruits and vegetables, into retinol. Dietary fat facilitates the absorption of carotene, so extreme fat deprivation increases the risk of vitamin A deficiency in children even when the diet contains marginally adequate amounts of carotene. Medical conditions that lead to impaired fat digestion or absorption can precipitate fat-soluble vitamin deficiencies (see Chapter 14).

Essential fatty acids

In the 1920s, a deficiency disease was induced in rats by feeding them on a fat-free diet and this disease was cured by the addition of small amounts of fat to the diet. Fatty acids of the linoleic acid series (n-6) cured all of the symptoms of this deficiency disease, whereas those of the linolenic acid series (n-3) gave only partial relief of symptoms. Saturated and monounsaturated fatty acids were not effective in relieving the symptoms. The symptoms of this deficiency disease are scaly dermatitis, poor growth, increased food intake and reduced immune responses.

We now know that there is an essential dietary requirement for polyunsaturated fatty acids; these are the *essential fatty acids*. They have certain structural functions (e.g. in membranes) and they are necessary for the synthesis of a key group of regulatory molecules, the *eicosanoids*, which include the prostaglandins, thromboxanes and leukotrienes. Although humans can synthesize fatty acids from other substrates we do not have the biochemical capability to insert double bonds between any of the first seven carbons of fatty-acid molecules. Thus we cannot synthesize either linoleic acid or α-linolenic acid, neither can we interconvert acids of the n-3 and n-6 series. The minimum human requirement for these essential fatty acids is extremely small (around 1 per cent of energy) and it has not been possible to reproduce the symptoms of this deficiency disease of rats in deprivation studies with human volunteers. The practical risk of overt fatty-acid deficiency in humans is normally remote; COMA (1991) recommend that, to prevent essential fatty acid deficiency, linoleic acid (18:2n-6) should provide at least 1 per cent of dietary energy and that α-linolenic acid (18:3n-3) should provide at least 0.2 per cent of dietary energy for all age groups.

The extremely low requirement for these essential fatty acids, the presence of considerable reserves of polyunsaturated fatty acids in body fat, and the difficulty of eliminating all traces of fat from the diet, compound to make this disease difficult to induce experimentally in people. Even fruits, vegetables and cereals that are regarded as essentially fat-free do contain small amounts of polyunsaturated fat. There have, however, been some reports of

essential fatty acid deficiency in humans. In the 1950s, some low-birth-weight babies fed on skimmed milk developed eczema and other symptoms of essential fatty acid deficiency that were cured by small amounts of essential fatty acids. In the 1970s, dermatitis caused by essential fatty acid deficiency was reported in several patients maintained on intravenous fat-free nutrition (Rivers and Frankel, 1981). The inability to safely infuse a source of fat hindered the development of long-term total parenteral nutrition (TPN) (see Chapter 17). It took more than four decades after the first demonstration in the rat to demonstrate essential fatty acid deficiency in an adult human, and then only under very unusual circumstances.

Fatty acids of both the n-6 and n-3 series may be metabolized to longer chain and more highly polyunsaturated acids as shown in Figure 12.2. The linoleic acid (18:2n-6) or linolenic acid (18:3n-3) first has a double bond inserted at the carboxyl end of the existing sequence of double bonds by an enzyme known as a *desaturase*. The product of this desaturation reaction then has an extra 2-carbon acetate unit added to the carboxyl end by an enzyme system known as an *elongase*. The rest of the pathway involves two further desaturation reactions and one further elongation (i.e. addition of two more double bonds and one more 2-carbon unit).

The fatty acids at the end of these sequences in Figure 12.2 are essential components of cell membranes. The EPA and DHA of the n-3 series predominate in the membranes in the brain and retina while n-6 fatty acids predominate in the membranes of liver cells and platelets. Their concentration in brain and retinal membrane phospholipids is one reason why it is thought that n-3 acids are essential in very small quantities in their own right, not just as partial substitutes for n-6 acids. Abnormal EEG readings and retinal activity have been reported in animals with lowered levels of n-3 fatty acids in these tissues. Adequate availability of n-3 fatty acids is probably critical for brain development in infants. The presence of n-3 fatty acids in the diet is certainly considered to be nutritionally desirable. The major dietary source of the long-chain n-3 fatty acids EPA and DHA is fish oil, or in some populations the fat of marine mammals. In theory these long-chain n-3 acids can be made from α-linolenic acid (ALA, 18:3n-3); it is,

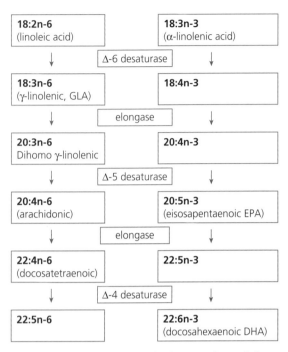

18:2n-6 (linoleic acid)		18:3n-3 (α-linolenic acid)
↓	Δ-6 desaturase	↓
18:3n-6 (γ-linolenic, GLA)		18:4n-3
↓	elongase	↓
20:3n-6 Dihomo γ-linolenic		20:4n-3
↓	Δ-5 desaturase	↓
20:4n-6 (arachidonic)		20:5n-3 (eisosapentaenoic EPA)
↓	elongase	↓
22:4n-6 (docosatetraenoic)		22:5n-3
↓	Δ-4 desaturase	↓
22:5n-6		22:6n-3 (docosahexaenoic DHA)

Figure 12.2 The production of other members of the n-6 (ω-6) and n-3 (ω-3) series of fatty acids from linoleic acid (18:2n-6) and α-linolenic (18:3n-3).

however, now clear that in humans there is only limited conversion of ALA to EPA and very little conversion to DHA (Burdge, 2004). High intakes of n-6 acids will tend to competitively inhibit the conversion of shorter chain n-3 acids to their longer chain derivatives, and vice versa. Almost 30 years ago, Sanders *et al.* (1984) showed that high intakes of n-6 fatty acid reduce the amount of EPA and DHA in rat cell membranes despite the presence of significant amounts of linolenic acid in the diet. This might be of particular significance in vegans consuming very large amounts of n-6 polyunsaturates (from margarine and vegetable oil) because, as was noted earlier, long-chain n-3 acids are not found in plant foods.

The growth in the use of vegetable oils for cooking and vegetable-based spreading fats means that current US and UK diets have at least 10 times more n-6 fatty acids than n-3, and this ratio may be as high as 30 times in some instances. This compares to an n-6 to n-3 ratio of more like 2:1 to 4:1 in hunter-gatherer societies. Most authorities agree that the current n-6 to n-3 ratio is too high although opinions vary as to what is an optimum level; it should be less than 10:1 and a very tentative optimal ratio of between 4:1 and 5:1 has been suggested. Rapeseed oil noted for being high in monounsaturated fatty acids also has a relatively high n-3 to n-6 ratio for a vegetable oil. A number of natural oils are marketed as dietary supplements on the basis of their high concentration of particular polyunsaturated fatty acids, and some are listed below.

- Fish oil and fish liver oil are rich sources of n-3 polyunsaturated fatty acids including EPA and DHA, the long-chain derivatives. (Pregnant women are advised to avoid fish liver oils because they contain vitamin A which in excess can cause birth defects.)
- Evening primrose oil, starflower/borage oil and blackcurrant seed oil are marketed as rich sources of γ-linolenic acid (18:3n-6), the second fatty acid on the n-6 pathway in Figure 12.2.
- Flaxseed oil is a rich source of α-linolenic acid (18:3n-3), the parent compound of the n-3 series. It is marketed as a good vegetarian source of n-3 fatty acids but there is limited conversion of this to EPA and little conversion to DHA in humans.
- Algal extracts containing significant amounts of DHA are marketed as a vegetarian source of DHA.

Essential fatty acids and eicosanoid production

The eicosanoids are a range of regulatory molecules that are involved in the regulation of most physiological processes, including the initiation of labour, blood platelet aggregation, blood vessel constriction/dilation, inflammation and many secretory processes. They are often referred to as 'local hormones' because they act close to or on the cells that produce them. The prefix 'eico' is derived from the Greek for 20 and these eicosanoids are made from n-6 and n-3 polyunsaturated fatty acids that have 20 carbon atoms: dihomo γ-linolenic acid (DGLA, 20:3n-6), arachidonic acid (20:4n-6) and eicosapentaenoic acid (EPA, 20:5n-3). In general those produced from arachidonic acid are the most potent.

Figure 12.3 illustrates the origins of the different eicosanoids produced from their fatty acid precursors. The enzymes involved in the elongation and desaturation of fatty acids are common to the n-3 and n-6 pathways, so there is competition between n-3 and n-6 substrates for these enzymes. Likewise the eicosanoid precursors also compete for the lipoxygenase and cyclooxygenase pathways shown in the figure. This means that altering the availability of the precursor fatty acids will change the balance of eicosanoid production and thus affect the processes regulated by these eicosanoids. High intakes of n-3 fatty acids would be expected to increase the production of the EPA-derived eicosanoids and decrease the production of those from n-6 precursors, especially arachidonic acid; remember, however, that there is only limited conversion of α-linolenic acid (ALA) to EPA in humans, so flaxseed oil (rich in ALA) will have much less effect than fish oil supplements which contain preformed EPA.

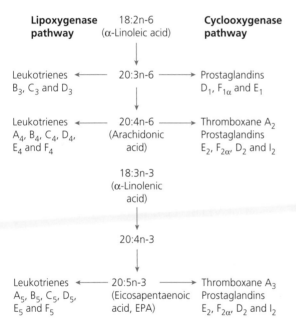

Figure 12.3 Production of eicosanoids from 'essential' n-6 (ω-6) and n-3 (ω-3) polyunsaturated fatty acids.

Certain oils like evening primrose oil and starflower/borage oil are rich in γ-linolenic acid (GLA, 20:3n-6) and this favours the production of eicosanoids made from dihomo γ-linolenic acid. Note that relatively little GLA is synthesized on most human diets because they contain high levels of arachidonic

acid (e.g. from meat) and this inhibits the enzyme that converts linoleic acid to GLA.

Key points

- Fat is the most concentrated source of dietary energy.
- Adding small amounts of fat to a food produces a disproportionately large rise in its energy yield.
- Claims that a food has a low percentage of fat by weight may disguise the fact that fat accounts for a high proportion of its energy yield.
- A relatively high-fat, high-energy-density diet may be necessary for those expending very large amounts of energy and for active and rapidly growing babies and children. For sedentary adults, a high-fat diet probably encourages excessive weight gain and obesity.
- Fat improves the palatability of food. This encourages affluent populations to eat more fat than is good for their long-term health and makes it difficult to persuade them to eat less fat.
- Very low-fat weaning foods may be of such low energy density that babies cannot eat enough of them to meet their energy needs.
- Fat is a concentrated source of energy for weaning foods and produces a suitable viscosity for babies at relatively low water content.
- Calorie for calorie, fat is probably less satiating than carbohydrate.
- Impaired fat absorption or extreme low-fat diets may precipitate fat-soluble deficiencies (especially of vitamin A).
- Polyunsaturated fatty acids are essential nutrients. They have structural functions and are precursors of prostaglandins and other eicosanoids.
- The requirement for essential fatty acids is small and it is difficult to induce overt deficiency in human volunteers.
- The parent compound of the n-6 series of polyunsaturated fatty acids is linoleic acid (18:2n-6) and that of the n-3 series is α-linolenic acid (18:3n-3).

- Linoleic and linolenic acids undergo a series of desaturation and elongation reactions to produce two series of n-6 and n-3 polyunsaturated fatty acids ending with 22:5n-6 and 22:6n-3, respectively.

- Small amounts of n-3 polyunsaturates are almost certainly essential in their own right. The long-chain ones are normal components of brain and retinal membranes and seem to be required for normal brain development.

- Long-chain n-3 polyunsaturates are prevalent in fish oil. They can be made from shorter chain varieties that are prevalent in some vegetable oils (e.g. flaxseed), but in practice there is limited conversion to EPA and very little conversion to DHA in humans.

- Humans cannot interconvert n-6 and n-3 fatty acids.

- Arachidonic acid (20:4n-6) is the precursor of many potent eicosanoids which regulate a multitude of physiological processes, including the inflammatory response, blood coagulation, platelet aggregation and blood vessel tone.

- Eicosanoids made from eicosapentaenoic acid (20:5n-3) and dihomo γ-linolenic acid (DGLA, 20:3n-6) are generally less potent than those made from arachidonic acid.

- Oil of evening primrose and starflower oil contain large amounts of GLA.

- Many omnivorous diets contain large amounts of arachidonic acid which inhibits the enzyme that converts linoleic acid to GLA and thus to DGLA.

- High intakes of long-chain n-3 fatty acids change the balance of eicosanoid production to favour those produced from EPA.

BLOOD LIPOPROTEINS

Fats are, by definition, insoluble in water. To transport them around the body in aqueous plasma they have to be associated with protein carriers and transported as lipid/protein aggregates, the *lipoproteins*. There are several subdivisions of lipoproteins in blood plasma which can be conveniently separated according to their density; the higher the proportion of fat in a lipoprotein, the lower its density because fat has low density. The protein components of lipoproteins are known as *apoproteins*. The subdivisions of the plasma lipoproteins and their approximate compositions are given in Table 12.6.

Chylomicrons are the form in which ingested fat is transported to the liver and tissues after its absorption from the intestine. They are normally absent from fasting blood. Levels of very-low-density lipoprotein (VLDL) should also be low in fasting blood because it is rapidly converted to low-density lipoprotein (LDL) (see below). This means that blood lipid determinations should be measured in fasting blood samples to avoid any distortion due to variable amounts of postprandial chylomicrons and large amounts of VLDL. Intermediate-density lipoprotein (IDL) is a transitory intermediate that normally represents only a very small fraction of total lipoproteins. The principal lipoproteins in normal fasting blood are HDL (high-density lipoprotein), LDL and relatively small amounts of VLDL.

VLDL is rich in triacylglycerol and thus measures of blood triacylglycerols are taken to indicate the amount of VLDL. LDL is the major cholesterol-containing fraction and thus measures of total plasma cholesterol are often taken to indicate the LDL concentration. The normal function of VLDL is to transport triacylglycerol produced endogenously

Table 12.6 Subdivisions of the plasma lipoproteins and their approximate percentage compositions

	Triacylglycerol	Cholesterol	Phospholipid	Apoprotein
Chylomicrons	82	9	7	2
Very-low-density lipoproteins	52	22	18	8
Low-density lipoproteins	9	47	23	21
Intermediate-density lipoproteins	20	35	20	15
High-density lipoproteins	3	19	28	50

in the liver (largely from dietary fat) to the adipose tissue or the muscles where it acts as an energy source. LDL acts as an external source of cholesterol for cells unable to synthesize sufficient for use in membranes or as a precursor for steroid hormone synthesis. The main function of HDL is to transport excess cholesterol from tissues and other blood lipoproteins back to the liver.

Epidemiological evidence and evidence from people with familial hyperlipidaemias suggest that high plasma LDL cholesterol concentrations are causally associated with increased atherosclerosis and increased risk of coronary heart disease (CHD). HDL inhibits atherosclerosis and high HDL cholesterol concentrations are protective against coronary heart disease. The LDL to HDL ratio is a better predictor of coronary heart disease risk than LDL concentration alone. Simple plasma cholesterol measurements do not indicate the distribution of the cholesterol between LDL and HDL, but total cholesterol concentration is used as an indicator of LDL cholesterol concentration. Raised VLDL is associated with obesity, glucose intolerance and high alcohol consumption. High VLDL is certainly an indicator of high risk of coronary heart disease, but whether it is a significant independent risk factor for coronary heart disease is uncertain (Grundy, 1998).

Key points

- Fats are insoluble in water and are transported in blood as lipoprotein complexes.
- Chylomicrons are the lipoproteins that carry absorbed fat from the intestine to the tissues and they are absent from fasting blood.
- Very-low-density lipoprotein (VLDL) is a triacylglycerol-rich fraction that transports fat produced in the liver to the muscles and adipose tissue.
- Low-density lipoprotein (LDL) is rich in cholesterol and acts as an external source of cholesterol for cells.
- LDL is atherogenic. HDL is anti-atherogenic: it removes excess cholesterol to the liver.
- High plasma LDL is associated with increased risk of coronary heart disease, but high HDL is associated with reduced risk.

DIGESTION, ABSORPTION AND TRANSPORT OF DIETARY LIPIDS

A summary scheme for the digestion and absorption of dietary fats is shown in Figure 12.4. Dietary fat is emulsified by the action of bile salts and phospholipids in the intestine. This emulsified fat is then partially digested by the enzyme *lipase*, which is secreted into the gut in the pancreatic juice. Lipase in aqueous solution can digest fat only if it has first been emulsified. Lipase splits off (hydrolyses) fatty acids from the glycerol component of triacylglycerol. *In vivo*, this process does not result in total breakdown of triacylglycerol; the major end-products in the gut are monoacylglycerols and free fatty acids. Lipase does not act on the fatty acid attached to the second (middle) carbon atom of the glycerol component.

Glands at the base of the tongue produce a *lingual lipase*, an enzyme that works at low pH and can readily digest the fat in milk globules before emulsification by bile salts. Lingual lipase is probably only important in suckling babies whose pancreatic function is not fully developed at birth. Churning of fat in the stomach with phospholipids and other digestion products has some emulsifying effect on dietary fat.

The products of lipase action together with bile salts, phospholipids and fat-soluble vitamins form minute molecular aggregates known as *micelles* and this effectively solubilizes them. Fat digestion products and fat-soluble vitamins diffuse from the micelles into the mucosal cells that line the small intestine. Once inside they are re-assembled into triacylglycerol and coated with protein to form the *chylomicrons*. Chylomicrons can be envisaged as droplets or packets of triacylglycerol surrounded by a thin protein coat. These chylomicrons enter the lymphatic vessels that drain the small intestine and pass into venous blood via the thoracic duct, which drains into the right subclavian vein. Most fat is absorbed in the duodenum and jejunum.

In the liver and adipose tissue, the triacylglycerol is removed from the chylomicrons by an enzyme called *lipoprotein lipase* that is located on the inner surface of the capillary. The products of this second digestion are absorbed into the cells and most is again re-assembled into triacylglycerol for storage in adipose tissue or for transport in the liver. Liver

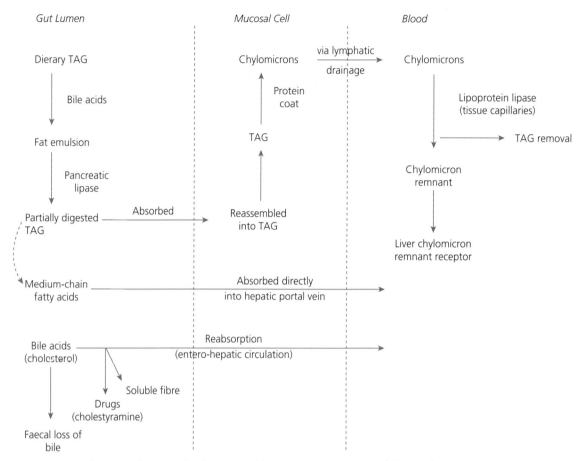

Figure 12.4 A scheme to illustrate the digestion, absorption and transport of dietary fat.

cells clear the fat-depleted chylomicron remnants from the plasma via a specific chylomicron remnant receptor. These chylomicron remnants contain fat-soluble vitamins and these are taken up and stored by the liver along with the chylomicron remnants. Some short- and medium-chain fatty acids are relatively more water soluble and they bypass this process and are absorbed directly from the gut into the hepatic portal vein and transported to the liver bound to plasma albumin.

Large amounts of cholesterol-derived bile salts are secreted into the intestine each day in the bile. Most of this bile salt (*cholesterol*) is reabsorbed in the intestine and recycled to the liver (entero-hepatic circulation). Some substances are thought to exert a lowering effect on plasma cholesterol by interfering with this entero-hepatic recycling, leading to increased faecal losses of cholesterol derivatives.

Soluble fibre and some plant sterols exert such an effect, and the cholesterol-lowering drug cholestryramine is a resin that binds or chelates bile acids in the intestine, preventing their reabsorption.

Key points

- Dietary fat is partly digested by pancreatic lipase in the small intestine. The products of this digestion are absorbed into the mucosal cells and most are re-esterified into triacylglycerol.

- Bile salts emulsify dietary fat so that it can be digested and solubilize fat digestion products so that they can be absorbed.

- Bile salts are re-absorbed in the ileum and returned to the liver (the entero-hepatic circulation).

Key points *continued*

- Chylomicrons carry the absorbed fat into the circulation via the lymphatic system.
- Lipoprotein lipase in tissue capillaries digests the triacylglycerol in chylomicrons so that it can be absorbed into the fat or liver cells and most is again re-assembled into triacylglycerol.
- The chylomicron remnant is removed from the circulation by the liver along with the fat-soluble vitamins that they contain.
- Short- and medium-chain fatty acids can be absorbed directly into the hepatic portal vein and transported bound to plasma albumen.

TRANSPORT OF ENDOGENOUSLY PRODUCED LIPIDS

Figure 12.5 gives a summary of the origins and interrelationship of the non-chylomicron lipoproteins. Triacylglycerol-rich VLDL is produced in the liver by re-assembling dietary fats and by endogenous synthesis of fat (although there is very little *de novo* fat synthesis on most Western diets). VLDL is exported from the liver to tissues and adipose tissue for use in metabolism or storage. The enzyme lipoprotein lipase, in the tissue capillaries, hydrolyses the triacylglycerol in VLDL, enabling it to diffuse into the tissue cells. VLDL that has been depleted of much of its triacylglycerol is called IDL. This IDL is then either rapidly cleared from the plasma by binding with a liver receptor, or some of it is modified within the blood to become LDL. LDL and IDL both bind to a common receptor, called the *LDL receptor*, but this receptor has a higher affinity for IDL than for LDL and so IDL is cleared more quickly (2–6 hours) than LDL (2–3 days). More than 75 per cent of LDL receptors are found in the liver; other tissues are supplied with cholesterol via binding of cholesterol-rich LDL to their LDL receptors (Brown and Goldstein, 1984). Around 80 per cent of LDL leaving the circulation is normally taken up by the liver and just 20 per cent by all other tissues. (The perceived importance of the LDL receptor may be judged by the fact that its discoverers Brown and Goldstein were awarded the Nobel prize for physiology and medicine in 1985.)

Once LDL is absorbed into cells and releases its cholesterol this causes three regulatory responses in the cell.

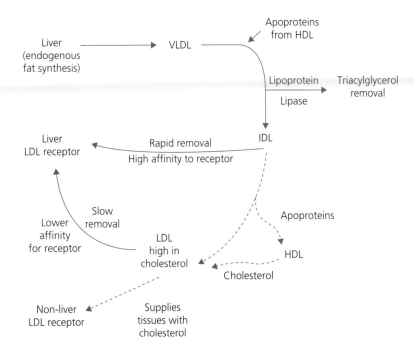

Figure 12.5 The relationship between the various lipoproteins involved in endogenous lipid transport. After Brown and Goldstein (1984).

- It suppresses synthesis of LDL receptors in the cell.
- It inhibits the rate-limiting enzyme in cholesterol synthesis (HMG CoA reductase).
- It activates an enzyme that converts cholesterol to cholesterol esters that can be stored as droplets in the cell.

Key points

- Triacylglycerol produced in the liver is exported as VLDL.
- VLDL is depleted of triacylglycerol by lipoprotein lipase in tissue capillaries. This depleted VLDL is called intermediate-density lipoprotein (IDL).
- Some IDL is cleared rapidly by the liver and some is converted within the circulation to LDL.
- Both IDL and LDL are cleared by LDL receptors, although LDL is cleared much more slowly.
- Three-quarters of LDL receptors are in the liver; the others are spread between the other tissues.
- When cells have surplus cholesterol, they produce less, convert some to cholesterol esters and suppress their synthesis of LDL receptors.

THE DIET–HEART HYPOTHESIS

According to Brown and Goldstein (1984), most people living in the Western industrialized countries have elevated plasma cholesterol concentrations making them prone to atherosclerosis and coronary heart disease. They concluded that this was due to reduced LDL receptor synthesis. This reduced receptor synthesis is one of the mechanisms that protect cells from cholesterol overload but it also leads to elevated levels of circulating cholesterol. They suggested that dietary and other environmental factors that tend to raise the plasma LDL (e.g. high saturated fat and cholesterol intake) induce their effect by suppressing LDL receptor synthesis. Reduced LDL receptor synthesis would be expected not only to increase the lifespan of LDL but also lead to an increased rate of production, because less IDL would be cleared and more would be converted

within the blood to LDL. The elevated level of LDL cholesterol in the blood increases the tendency for it to be deposited in artery walls where it may trigger fibrotic changes (atherosclerosis or 'hardening of the arteries').

When LDL cholesterol levels in blood rise beyond a certain level, it is taken up by macrophages in the blood vessel walls and circulating monocytes, and these LDL-laden macrophages are termed *foam cells* because they have a foamy appearance. These foam cells accumulate in the blood vessel wall giving rise to so-called *fatty streaks* which are an early and relatively benign stage in the process of atherosclerosis. At this 'fatty streak' stage the process is clearly reversible; some fatty streaks disappear but others undergo hardening and fibrosis and become atherosclerotic plaques. HDL is involved in the process of removal of cholesterol from fatty streaks and plaques and returning it to the liver; thus, as noted earlier, high HDL levels are known to be associated with reduced risk of CHD. It is not really clear why some fatty streaks regress and others develop into plaques, but one suggested mechanism is that oxidation of the LDL can make it much more damaging to the artery wall. This theory has also led to suggestions that anti-oxidants, particularly in fruits and vegetables, may inhibit the progress of atherosclerosis (see Chapter 13 for discussion of anti-oxidants).

Reduced LDL receptor synthesis is seen as initiating a chain of events that can lead to increased atherosclerosis and ultimately increased risk of coronary heart disease and other atherosclerosis-linked diseases; this is the diet–heart hypothesis, outlined in Figure 12.6.

There is overwhelming evidence that a raised plasma cholesterol concentration (which indicates a raised LDL cholesterol) is linked to increased risk of coronary heart disease. Not least of this evidence are studies on people with *familial hypercholesteraemia*, an inherited condition in which there is a defect in the LDL receptor gene. Even people who are heterozygous for this condition (i.e. one normal and one abnormal gene) become hypercholesteraemic and they have a markedly increased probability of dying prematurely from CHD, particularly if they are male. Those few people (one in a million) who are homozygous for this condition fail to produce any functional LDL receptors and their plasma

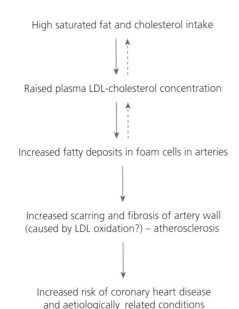

High saturated fat and cholesterol intake

Raised plasma LDL-cholesterol concentration

Increased fatty deposits in foam cells in arteries

Increased scarring and fibrosis of artery wall
(caused by LDL oxidation?) – atherosclerosis

Increased risk of coronary heart disease
and aetiologically related conditions

Figure 12.6 The diet-heart hypothesis.

Table 12.7 Some cut-off points for plasma cholesterol concentration

Plasma cholesterol concentration (mmol/L)	Classification
Below 5.2	Optimal range
5.2–6.5	Mildly elevated
6.5–7.8	Moderately elevated
Over 7.8	Severely elevated

cholesterol concentrations may be up to six times normal. These individuals usually die from CHD in childhood. Injection of radioactively labelled LDL into such individuals confirms that it remains in the circulation about 2.5 times as long as in unaffected people and that the rate of endogenous LDL production is about doubled (Brown and Goldstein, 1984).

This diet–heart hypothesis provides the underlying rationale for many nutrition education campaigns in the UK and elsewhere. Dietary measures that would lead to lowered average plasma cholesterol concentrations are seen as central to nutrition education for health promotion. A figure of 5.2 mmol/L has been widely suggested as a desirable maximum for individual plasma cholesterol levels, yet in 2000 the majority of the UK population exceeded this level. Some frequently used cut-off points for plasma cholesterol concentration are given in Table 12.7.

In Chapter 1 it was noted that in men the individual risk of coronary heart disease increases exponentially as the plasma cholesterol concentration rises above the target value. However, most of the apparent excess population risk from high blood cholesterol seems to be concentrated in men whose blood cholesterol levels are only slightly to moderately elevated. There are vast numbers of men (the

majority of the population) who are apparently at some relatively small increased individual risk due to slight to moderate cholesterol elevation but only a small proportion at greatly increased risk due to very high cholesterol concentrations (Table 12.8). The thrust of nutrition education has been to direct cholesterol-lowering dietary advice at the whole population with the aim of shifting the whole distribution downwards. Additionally, intensive dietary counselling and cholesterol-lowering drugs can be used on those individuals identified as having substantially elevated cholesterol levels or existing coronary heart disease.

The distribution of plasma cholesterol concentrations in the UK adult population in 2000 is shown in Table 12.8. Two-thirds of adults have values that are above the optimal range (i.e. above 5.2 mmol/L). There is a very pronounced trend in both sexes for plasma cholesterol to increase with age; in 19- to 24-year-olds, only 16 per cent of men and 17 per cent of women have values that are above the optimal range and fewer than 1 per cent have values in the moderately or severely elevated ranges. This distribution shifts sharply towards the higher values with each increase in age band, so that, for example, in 65- to 74-year-old men 71 per cent are above the optimum and 22 per cent are over 6.5 mmol/L (76 and 44 per cent, respectively, in women of this age).

In pre-menopausal women, average values for plasma cholesterol level are lower than those of men and the proportion in the higher categories of cholesterol level is also lower. However, this sex difference reverses at the menopause and so, for example, in the 65–74 years category 29 per cent of women have moderately and 15 per cent severely elevated cholesterol levels compared to corresponding values for men of 18 and 4 per cent,

Table 12.8 Distribution of plasma cholesterol concentrations in UK adults by age and sex group (percentages)*

Age group	Serum cholesterol concentrations (mmol/L)			
	Below 5.2	5.2–6.5	6.5–7.8	7.8+
Men				
19–24 years	84	16	–	–
35–49	44	41	14	2
50–64	41	37	20	2
65–74[1]	29	51	18	4
75–84	39	43	15	3
Women				
19–24 years	83	17	–	–
35–49	52	41	6	1
50–64	25	42	24	9
65–74[1]	24	32	29	15
75–84[1]	23	27	36	14

*Data from the NDNS survey of adults aged 19–64 years (Hoare *et al.*, 2004) and the NDNS survey of adults aged over 65 years (Finch *et al.*, 1999).
[1] Free living excludes those living in care homes for the elderly.

respectively. Average plasma cholesterol levels recorded for the whole UK adult population in the 2000–1 NDNS survey (Hoare *et al.*, 2004) were 5.2 mmol/L compared to 5.8 mmol/L recorded in 1986–7 by Gregory *et al.* (1990). The percentage of the sample above the optimal values was around 66 per cent in 1986–7 but only 48 per cent in 2000–1. Almost certainly, therefore, current values would be lower than in Table 12.8.

Key points

- A high saturated fat intake leads to reduced LDL receptor synthesis and to elevated levels of circulating LDL cholesterol.
- LDL is taken up by foam cells in artery walls and forms fatty streaks which may trigger atherosclerosis, perhaps as a result of oxidation.
- Atherosclerosis predisposes to coronary heart disease (CHD).

→

Key points *continued*

- High saturated fat intake (and other environmental influences) triggers a chain of events that can ultimately lead to increased risk of coronary heart disease – the diet–heart hypothesis.
- Risk of CHD rises exponentially with plasma total cholesterol (an indicator of LDL cholesterol concentration).
- People who are genetically prone to have very elevated plasma LDL cholesterol concentrations are at greatly increased risk of CHD.
- 5.2 mmol/L is the ideal upper limit for plasma total cholesterol concentration, but two-thirds of the UK adult population exceeded this level in 2000.
- People with severely elevated cholesterol levels are at greatest individual risk from CHD, but much of the population risk is concentrated in the large numbers of people with mild-to-moderate cholesterol elevation.
- The health promotion priority has thus generally been to reduce average plasma cholesterol concentrations rather than solely seeking to identify and treat those with severely elevated cholesterol concentrations.
- Both average cholesterol level and the number in the elevated categories increase with age.
- Pre-menopausal women have lower average cholesterol levels than men and fewer are in the elevated cholesterol categories, but this situation reverses after the menopause.
- Both average blood cholesterol levels and the percentage of UK adults with elevated levels declined significantly between 1986–7 and 2000–1 and have probably declined since then.

Current 'health images' of various dietary fats

Keys *et al.* (1959) showed, in short-term experiments with young men, that total plasma cholesterol levels were significantly affected by the degree of saturation of the fat in the diet even when the diets were matched for total fat content. As a result of such experiments, saturated fat has acquired a very negative health image. Saturated fat was found to raise plasma cholesterol concentration, and this is associated with increased atherosclerosis and increased risk of coronary heart disease. Polyunsaturated fats were found to lower plasma cholesterol concentration when they replaced saturated fat in the diet. These early experiments suggested that monounsaturated fatty acids were neutral in their effects on blood cholesterol level. Keys and his group concluded that saturated fatty acids were about twice as potent in raising serum cholesterol as polyunsaturated fatty acids were in lowering it. Keys *et al.* (1965) produced an equation that predicted the change in plasma cholesterol of a group in response to specified changes in its dietary fats. Since the 1960s there have been several other attempts to produce such predictive equations (e.g. Yu *et al.*, 1995).

As a result of such observations, some vegetable oils and soft margarines, because of their high P:S ratios, acquired a very positive image and were for a time regarded as 'superfoods' (see Chapter 19). In the early experiments of Keys' team, switching from a diet very high in saturates (P:S 0.16) to one very high in polyunsaturated fat (P:S 2.8) resulted in a rapid, but variable, reduction in an individual's plasma cholesterol concentration even though the total fat intake was kept constant (see Figure 4.4 in Chapter 4).

Effects on LDL and HDL cholesterol

It is now known that the total plasma cholesterol consists of both LDL and HDL fractions. The LDL fraction is atherogenic, and regarded as 'the bad cholesterol' whereas the HDL fraction is antiatherogenic and seen as 'the good cholesterol'. It would thus seem desirable to lower the former and raise the latter. The LDL cholesterol is generally considered to be readily responsive to dietary manipulation but the HDL rather less so. HDL levels do rise in response to regular exercise and seem to be increased by moderate alcohol consumption. Current views on the ways in which the different dietary fat fractions affect these plasma cholesterol fractions and their current 'health image' are summarized below.

Total fat Mangiapane and Salter (1999) concluded that the then published evidence indicated that moderate reductions in total fat consumption without any change in fatty acid composition would not produce any favourable change in blood lipoprotein profiles. There are, of course, several other reasons for reducing our reliance on dietary fats, including improved weight control, better glucose tolerance and perhaps reduced susceptibility to some cancers (see Chapter 5). Better weight control and improved glucose tolerance would be expected to reduce risk of heart disease independently of any effects on plasma lipoprotein profiles.

The saturates These generally raise the LDL cholesterol concentration and so they have been and continue to be viewed negatively. Saturated fats may cause a small compensatory rise in HDL cholesterol, but this is considerably outweighed by the effect on the LDL fraction. Saturated fatty acids vary in their effects on plasma cholesterol. Palmitic acid (16:0) is by far the most common saturated fatty acid in the diet and, together with myristic acid (14:0), the most potent at raising LDL cholesterol. Shorter chain, saturated fatty acids of 12 carbons or less (e.g. found in high amounts in coconut oil) have a smaller cholesterol-raising effect. Stearic acid (18:0) is not atherogenic and may be closer to the monounsaturated fatty acid (oleic acid 18:1n-9) in its effects on plasma cholesterol levels (Yu *et al.*, 1995). Stearic acid is found in large amounts in cocoa butter, which has been found to cause less increase in plasma cholesterol than other saturated fats. In general, if saturated fatty acids in the diet are replaced with either unsaturated fatty acids or with carbohydrate then this leads to a reduction in LDL cholesterol concentration in plasma.

The monounsaturates As a result of the early experiments of Keys *et al.* (1959) and other early workers, monounsaturates were regarded as neutral in their effects on plasma cholesterol concentration. More recent work suggests that, when they replace saturated fatty acids, they have almost as great a lowering effect on the LDL fraction as polyunsaturated fats and are neutral in their effects on the HDL fraction (e.g. Mattson and Grundy, 1985; Yu *et al.*, 1995). At very high intakes they may actually increase HDL concentrations. Some Mediterranean men consume high-fat diets (40 per cent of energy from fat) and yet have very low incidence of CHD, and these Mediterranean diets are rich in olive oil and monounsaturated oleic acid. These monounsaturated fats are very much 'in fashion' at present, partly accounting for the current positive health image of olive oil.

The polyunsaturates Polyunsaturated fatty acids of the n-6 or ω-6 series (the bulk of those in most vegetable oils) are still thought to lower the plasma LDL cholesterol concentration; a beneficial effect. However, some studies suggested that they may also lower HDL cholesterol, a potentially harmful effect (Grundy, 1987). Such studies were widely reported and helped to increase concern about the overall benefits of diets very high in polyunsaturated fat. Results from some of the early intervention trials using diets very high in polyunsaturated fats also suggested that very high intakes of these acids might have other detrimental effects, including an increased cancer risk. Often such studies reported a non-significant decrease in cardiovascular mortality and a non-significant increase in mortality from other causes including cancer (Oliver, 1981). Their high susceptibility to oxidation (see Chapter 13) is one possible mechanism by which high intakes might produce detrimental effects (COMA, 1991). Populations who both consume high-fat diets and have a high proportion of their fat as n-6 polyunsaturated acids have been historically rare because widespread use of large amounts of most extracted vegetable oils is a relatively recent phenomenon. Diets that are high in olive, palm or coconut oils have long been used but none of these contains high levels of n-6 polyunsaturated fatty acids. Safety concerns, together with this lack of historical precedent, have led a number of expert committees (e.g. COMA, 1991) to recommend that it would be prudent not to further raise current average intakes of polyunsaturated fatty acids in the UK and USA. It has also been recommended that individual consumption of polyunsaturated fatty acids should be limited to no more than 10 per cent of total energy. There is little hard evidence of deleterious effects of high polyunsaturated fat intake, but during the early 1990s some health educators viewed them less positively than they did in the 1960s and 1970s. More recent evidence suggests that polyunsaturated fatty acids are probably neutral in their effect on HDL and that

any lowering effect on HDL occurs only at high intakes that are unlikely to be consumed in normal diets (Mangiapane and Salter, 1999).

The n-3 series of acids are found in large amounts in marine oils and in variable amounts in different vegetable oils, for example:

- 11.4 per cent of total fatty acids in walnut oil
- 7 per cent in soya oil
- 10 per cent in rapeseed oil
- 0.29 per cent in sunflower seed oil.

n-3 fatty acids lower blood triacylglycerol concentrations and are generally thought to raise the HDL cholesterol. They are also thought to have other apparently beneficial effects, such as reducing inflammation and the tendency of blood to clot and therefore reducing the risk of thrombosis. Fish oils, the richest dietary source of the long-chain members of this series, are discussed more fully at the end of this chapter. The overall effect of fish oil on LDL cholesterol is minimal at practical levels of consumption.

Trans **fatty acids** Diets containing only naturally occurring fatty acids would normally be low in *trans* fatty acids, but in the past some margarine and vegetable shortening contained quite large amounts of *trans* fatty acids although these have been largely phased out. *Trans* fatty acids are also generated when vegetable oils are heated, so frying adds some *trans* fatty acids to foods especially if the oil is re-heated several times.

There has naturally been concern about whether there are any health implications in consuming relatively large amounts of these *trans* fatty acids because of their low levels in unprocessed foods. In particular, it has been suggested that they may have similar unfavourable effects on blood lipoproteins to saturated fatty acids and they are generally classified as equivalent to saturated fatty acids in their effects on blood lipids. In short-term experiments, using both men and women, Mensink and Katan (1990) compared the effects of diets that were matched except for their *trans* fatty acid content. They concluded that *trans* fatty acids are at least as unfavourable as saturated fatty acids in their effects on blood lipids, tending not only to raise the LDL levels but also to lower HDL levels. Willett *et al.* (1993), in a large cohort study of American nurses, reported a highly significant positive association between risk of CHD and dietary intake of *trans* fatty acids. These results achieved widespread publicity at the time and led margarine manufacturers to change their production methods and produce products that were free of *trans* fatty acids. Other workers have disputed the notion that high consumption of *trans* fatty acids is a major determinant of current risk of CHD. In 1989, average intakes of *trans* fatty acids in the UK were estimated at around 5 g per day (2 per cent of calories) but with very wide variation, some individuals consuming as much as five times this average value (COMA, 1991). Intakes of *trans* fatty acids have decreased substantially in recent years and now represent just 0.8 per cent of total energy, with almost no-one exceeding the maximum of 2 per cent of energy advised by COMA.

Dietary cholesterol In short-term experiments, dietary cholesterol does tend to raise the LDL cholesterol level but, at usual intakes, this effect is small compared to the effects caused by altering the proportions of the various fatty acid fractions in the diet. Some animals (e.g. rabbits) are particularly susceptible to the hypercholesteraemic effects of dietary cholesterol. In these animals, dietary cholesterol suppresses LDL receptor production in liver cells and this reduces LDL clearance. Usual human intake of cholesterol is relatively small when compared to the normal rate of endogenous synthesis (around 10–20 per cent). Keys *et al.* (1965) calculated that a change in cholesterol intake from the top to the bottom of the range in 1960s American diets (i.e. from 1050 mg/day to 450 mg/day) would lower plasma cholesterol by only about 0.23 mmol/L. They concluded that dietary cholesterol should not be ignored in cholesterol lowering but that changing it alone would achieve very little. Dietary cholesterol is usually given low priority in most sets of nutrition education guidelines (see Chapter 5). Note, however, that lowering saturated fat intake will result in a fall in cholesterol intake because cholesterol is found only in animal products. Cholesterol intakes in the UK have fallen in line with the fall in fat and saturated fatty acid consumption (see Table 12.4); the current average cholesterol intake for UK adults is only about 250 mg/day with values of up to 600 mg/day

in the top 2.5 per cent of men. Some individuals are genetically susceptible to the hypercholesteraemic effects of dietary cholesterol, so control of dietary cholesterol is more significant for such individuals (Brown and Goldstein, 1984). Eggs are the single most important source of cholesterol in most Western diets. Average daily cholesterol intake will be greatly affected by changes in egg consumption and those who are particularly sensitive to dietary cholesterol are advised to restrict their egg consumption.

Fifty years ago, dietary cholesterol was widely believed to be of predominant importance in the genesis of high blood cholesterol and atherosclerosis (e.g. Frantz and Moore, 1969). The contribution of experiments with herbivorous rabbits to this belief is critically discussed in Chapter 4. Since the 1960s, the evidence linking high plasma cholesterol levels with increased risk of atherosclerosis has strengthened but the view of dietary cholesterol as the major influence on plasma cholesterol concentration has faded.

Oxidized cholesterol is more toxic to vascular endothelial cells than purified cholesterol (Staprans *et al.*, 2005). In fresh foods, cholesterol oxide concentrations are low, but such oxides would be generated if these foods were subjected to high temperatures or prolonged exposure to air, for example fried foods, powdered egg, some cheeses and, according to Jacobsen (1987), in ghee, the clarified butter used in Indian cooking. Damage induced by oxidation of lipids in LDL may be an important factor in the aetiology of heart disease. How significant oxidized cholesterol and other oxidized lipids in food are to these processes is not yet clear.

Plant sterols Plants do not produce cholesterol but they do produce other sterols such as stigmasterol, ergosterol and β-sitosterol. It has been known for decades that these plant sterols, although poorly absorbed in the gut, do tend to inhibit the absorption of cholesterol. β-Sitosterol and other plant sterols were identified as possible cholesterol-lowering agents more than 40 years ago but their practical effect was small. Several margarines and other dairy-type foods containing phytosterol esters are now available in the UK and are marketed as functional foods that may help lower blood cholesterol (this is discussed in detail in Chapter 19).

Key tenets of the diet–heart hypothesis

The diet–heart hypothesis as summarized in Figure 12.6 can be broken up into the following two key tenets.

- *Total plasma cholesterol concentration causes an increased risk of coronary heart disease.* When the individual lipoprotein fractions in blood are considered, high LDL cholesterol increases atherosclerosis and the risk of coronary heart disease while HDL is thought to be protective against atherosclerosis. High VLDL is associated with increased CHD risk, but this may be an incidental consequence of the link between high VLDL and obesity and diabetes which are both strong risk factors for CHD.
- *The amount and type of dietary fat are important determinants of the plasma cholesterol concentration.* The effects of different dietary fatty acids on blood lipoproteins were summarized earlier in the chapter.

The evidence in favour of both of these propositions is very substantial and many would say overwhelming. However, there are several apparent weak links in the chain of evidence supporting the diet–heart hypothesis and the dietary guidelines that have evolved from it. Some examples are listed here.

- Some populations appear to deviate from the usual trend of increasing saturated consumption associated with increasing average plasma cholesterol concentrations and increasing mortality from CHD.

- There is a lack of correlation between plasma cholesterol concentration and the level of saturated fat in the diet when they are measured in individuals from within a population.
- Many large-scale cholesterol-lowering intervention trials have failed to produce any measurable reduction in overall mortality in the test group.

In the next section, the evidence that underpins the diet–heart hypothesis is briefly summarized and explanations offered for these apparent anomalies.

Key points

- According to the diet–heart hypothesis, an elevated plasma cholesterol concentration causes increased risk of atherosclerosis and coronary heart disease. The LDL fraction of plasma cholesterol is atherogenic whereas the HDL fraction is antiatherogenic.
- Also according to the hypothesis, the composition of dietary fats is a key determinant of total plasma cholesterol concentration and its distribution between the different lipoprotein fractions in plasma.

Review of the evidence for the diet–heart hypothesis

Descriptive epidemiology

Cross-cultural comparisons reveal a general tendency for plasma cholesterol concentration and CHD mortality to rise with increasing saturated fat and cholesterol consumption (e.g. Artaud-Wild *et al.*, 1993). In general, cross-cultural studies tend to support the diet–heart hypothesis, but there are a number of exceptions to these general trends such as those noted below.

- The Masai of East Africa traditionally eat a diet based on milk, meat and blood which is high in saturated fat and cholesterol, and yet they have low blood cholesterol levels and little coronary heart disease. The traditional Masai are a fit and lean population and this could explain their protection from the effects of their apparently atherogenic diet. Their consumption of large amounts of fermented milk (yoghurt) has also been suggested as a possible factor. See McGill

(1979) for a summary of early studies on the Masai.

- Some studies have reported that farmers have lower levels of CHD than non-farmers living in the same locality despite having similar fat intakes and higher plasma cholesterol concentrations. These studies also find farmers to be more active, fitter, and to smoke and drink less than non-farmers (e.g. Pomrehn *et al.*, 1982).
- Recorded rates of coronary heart disease in France are low in comparison to other European countries with similar plasma cholesterol levels and despite saturated fat intake being relatively high in France. This is known as the 'French paradox'. One popular explanation is that high intakes of anti-oxidants in red wine might prevent oxidation of lipid infiltrates into artery walls and thus reduce the development of atherosclerotic lesions (Renaud and de Lorgeril, 1992). Low intakes of vegetables, which are more mundane sources of anti-oxidants, are also found in some of the countries that have unexpectedly high rates of CHD (Artaud-Wild *et al.*, 1993). It is also possible that this paradox is a measurement artefact caused by under-recording of CHD mortality in France. Ferrieres (2004) has written a more recent and readable discussion of this topic.
- McKeigue *et al.* (1985) noted high rates of CHD among British Asians despite their having lower saturated fat and cholesterol intakes and lower blood cholesterol concentrations than the white population. These observations have since been confirmed several times. British Asians also have much higher prevalence of abdominal obesity, insulin resistance and type 2 diabetes than white Britons, and this probably explains their high rates of CHD.

Dietary saturated fat intake is clearly only one of several factors that affect plasma cholesterol concentration, and plasma cholesterol is only one factor that governs the progression of atherosclerosis and the risk of CHD. The study of Morris *et al.* (1980) illustrates this point. In an 8-year cohort study of male British civil servants, they found very low levels of fatal first coronaries in men who did not smoke and who participated in vigorous leisure-time activity. The rates were more than six times higher in cigarette smokers who did not participate in vigorous leisure-time activity. This study took no account of diet or plasma cholesterol and the data were collected before the current nutrition education campaigns aimed at lowering dietary fat intakes had gained much momentum in the UK.

A number of factors that are not part of the diet–heart hypothesis in Figure 12.6 can influence plasma cholesterol concentration, the development of atherosclerotic lesions and the risk of CHD. These factors could obscure the relationship between dietary fats, plasma cholesterol and CHD risk. Some of these factors have been mentioned earlier and selected examples are listed below.

- Plasma total cholesterol is a crude indicator of CHD risk. It is the relative amounts of LDL (causative) and HDL (protective) that are better indicators.
- Being overweight or obese (particularly abdominal obesity) increases the risk of CHD. It is also associated with increased plasma cholesterol levels.
- Insulin resistance and type 2 diabetes (both linked to abdominal obesity) also increase the risk of CHD.
- High levels of physical activity and fitness protect against CHD, perhaps partly mediated by a rise in HDL concentration.
- High blood pressure accelerates atherosclerosis and increases the risk of CHD. The effect of high blood pressure on atherosclerosis is independent of plasma cholesterol level.
- Substances that cause oxidation of LDL accelerate the process of atherosclerosis (e.g. cigarette smoke). According to Steinberg *et al.* (1989), high levels of LDL produce atherosclerosis only if they are oxidized which leads to infiltration and activation of macrophages in the artery wall. Anti-oxidants in fruits and vegetables and perhaps in red wine may reduce this oxidation (see Chapter 13).
- Soluble fibre (NSP) may have a plasma cholesterol-lowering effect.
- Moderate intakes of alcohol may afford some protection against coronary heart disease, perhaps partly mediated by a rise in plasma HDL.
- Long-chain n-3 polyunsaturated fatty acids protect against CHD mortality by reducing

platelet aggregation, blood coagulation and/or cardiac arrhythmias.

From a health promotion viewpoint, undue emphasis placed on the P:S ratio of dietary fats and plasma cholesterol may deflect attention away from other perhaps even more beneficial changes in lifestyle. How significant is a moderately high saturated fat diet or perhaps even moderately elevated plasma cholesterol concentration in lean, active, non-smoking, moderate drinking men who eat good amounts of fruits and vegetables? This question may be even more pertinent for women. How significant are reductions in saturated fat intakes for men who remain overweight, inactive, eat few fruits or vegetables and who smoke and drink heavily? Replacing butter with margarine or frying in oil rather than lard are relatively painless changes that may offer reassurance or salve the conscience but are unlikely to compensate for failure to alter any of these other risk factors.

Some other descriptive epidemiological evidence that supports the diet–heart hypothesis is summarized below.

- Migrants and their descendants who move to areas where saturated fat intake is higher than in their country of origin have increased rates of CHD (e.g. Japanese migrants to the USA and British Asians).
- White vegetarians and Seventh Day Adventists in the USA and UK have lower rates of CHD than the whole population. They also have lower intakes of saturated fat.
- Marked changes in a population's consumption of saturated fat have been associated with corresponding changes in CHD incidence. In Britain, wartime rationing led to decreased saturated fat consumption and decreased rates of CHD. In Japan, marked increases in milk and meat consumption since the 1950s have been associated with marked increases in the prevalence of CHD, although there have also been large increases in life expectancy since the 1950s.

In addition, the observation that atherosclerotic lesions of both animals and humans contain high concentrations of cholesterol adds weight to the belief that high plasma cholesterol helps to precipitate atherosclerosis.

Experimental studies

Numerous short-term experimental studies have shown that plasma cholesterol concentration, primarily the LDL fraction, is alterable by manipulating intake of dietary lipids (e.g. Keys *et al.*, 1959; Mattson and Grundy, 1985; Mensink and Katan, 1990; Yu *et al.*, 1995; reviewed by Mangiapane and Salter, 1999). There is general agreement that increased intake of saturated fat tends to increase the plasma cholesterol whereas replacement of saturated with polyunsaturated fat tends to lower the cholesterol concentration. The probable effects of dietary cholesterol, monounsaturated fatty acids and *trans* fatty acids were discussed earlier in the chapter. Susceptibility to dietary manipulation of plasma cholesterol concentration varies between individuals and there is a general trend for those with the higher baseline levels to be more responsive to dietary change. Despite the absence of any demonstrable effect on total mortality, most of the early cholesterol-lowering, dietary intervention studies did nonetheless produce significant reductions in plasma cholesterol in the test group (Oliver, 1981). However, according to Oliver, plasma cholesterol was usually reduced by less than 10 per cent in free-living subjects despite some very major dietary modification and even drug use in many of these early studies.

'Experiments of nature'

People with several inherited hyperlipidaemias have a high propensity to premature CHD (reviewed by Denke, 2005). In familial hypercholesteraemia the primary genetic defect is in the LDL receptor gene. This genetic defect leads to reduced levels of functional LDL receptors and a marked rise in plasma LDL cholesterol concentration. This condition is associated with marked atherosclerosis and greatly increased risk of premature CHD. This provides persuasive evidence of a direct causal link between high plasma LDL, atherosclerosis and CHD.

Cohort studies

Cohort studies whether within or between populations generally indicate that, at least for young and middle-aged men, high serum cholesterol concentration is predictive of subsequent risk of death from coronary heart disease over the succeeding 5–20 years. In the Framingham study, conducted in Massachusetts, USA, there was a clear progressive increase in CHD mortality in all age groups of men with increasing plasma cholesterol level (see Figure 1.1 in Chapter 1, and Chapter 4 for a summary of the Framingham study). In the famous Seven Countries cross-cultural cohort study, there was a high correlation between dietary saturated fat intake and both plasma cholesterol concentration and incidence of CHD (summarized in Oliver, 1981).

In general, the relationship between total plasma cholesterol and CHD is most convincing in middle-aged men and is much weaker in pre-menopausal women (e.g. Crouse, 1989) and elderly men (Shipley *et al.* 1991). This has caused some editorial writers in medical journals to question whether universal cholesterol lowering was justified, particularly for women (e.g. Dunnigan, 1993; Hulley *et al.*, 1992). The lack of demonstrated holistic benefit in most cholesterol-lowering intervention trials prior to this time was an important reason why these authors recommended such caution. As will be seen below, some more recent intervention trials have provided much stronger evidence that lowering LDL cholesterol can bring substantial net benefits. Total plasma cholesterol is now known to be a relatively crude indicator of CHD risk. Measurement of individual lipoprotein fractions in blood should give a more sensitive indication of CHD risk. In the Framingham study, total plasma cholesterol was only a weak indicator of CHD risk in pre-menopausal women and older men, but there was a very strong negative association (i.e. protective effect) between HDL concentration and CHD risk in these groups.

One of the gaps in the chain of evidence supporting the diet–heart hypothesis has been the failure to find any significant association between measures of dietary fat or saturated fat intake and plasma cholesterol concentration in most within-population studies. Oliver (1981) uses data from the Tecumseh study to illustrate this general finding; dietary intakes of fat, saturated fat, cholesterol and dietary P:S ratio were not significantly different when those in the highest, middle and lowest tertiles (thirds) for serum cholesterol concentrations were compared. Gregory *et al.* (1990) found no significant correlation between any measures of dietary fat and serum LDL cholesterol concentration in men except for a very weak ($r=0.08$) one with dietary cholesterol; all correlation coefficients were less than 0.1. In women they found a weak but significant correlation with percentage of energy from saturated fat and serum LDL cholesterol concentration but only 2 per cent (r^2) of the difference in women's serum cholesterol could be explained by variation in their percentage of dietary energy from saturated fat.

Dietary differences in individual fat consumption do not appear to be an important factor in determining the position of any individual within the population distribution of plasma cholesterol concentrations. As noted in Chapter 4, this may be because other factors affect an individual's serum cholesterol concentration, such as:

• genetic variability in plasma cholesterol concentration, including variation in genetic susceptibility to dietary fats
• other dietary influences on plasma cholesterol
• other lifestyle influences on plasma cholesterol, including exercise, age, smoking, alcohol, and body mass index.

This lack of significant association is thus not incompatible with the proposal that dietary fat composition is a major determinant of a population's average plasma cholesterol concentration. It is still expected that widespread use of a diet with a higher P:S ratio and less cholesterol will lower the plasma cholesterol concentrations of adherents and lead to a downward shift in the distribution for plasma cholesterol of the population – and thus to a reduction in average plasma cholesterol concentration. This general concept is discussed more fully in Chapter 4 using data in Figure 4.4 to illustrate it.

Intervention trials and clinical trials

Numerous trials of a variety of cholesterol-lowering interventions were carried out between 1960 and 1990. None of these produced a significant reduction in total mortality in the test group. Many did not even produce significant reductions in cardiovascular mortality, although most succeeded in reducing plasma cholesterol to some extent. Some reported a non-significant fall in cardiovascular mortality that was offset by a non-significant rise in mortality from 'other causes'. In several of these early trials, the overall incidence of

coronary heart disease was reduced largely as a result of a fall in the number of non-fatal myocardial infarctions (McCormick and Skrabanek, 1988; Oliver, 1981, 1991). Some early intervention trials that involved the use of older cholesterol-lowering drugs actually reported increased mortality in the test group. One of these 'failed' intervention trials was the Multiple Risk Factor Intervention Trial (1982) which is discussed in Chapter 4. This failure to demonstrate measurable benefit from such 'multiple interventions' was confirmed by Ebrahim *et al.* (2011) who conducted a meta-analysis of 55 multiple risk factor intervention trials of at least 6 months' duration. Intervention did achieve some reduction in risk factors, including blood pressure and blood cholesterol, but did not reduce total or CHD mortality or even the number of cardiac events. There was some reduction in mortality in patients identified as hypertensive or diabetic at the outset. It was concluded that counselling and education interventions aimed at behaviour change in the general population were of limited use.

Smith *et al.* (1993) conducted a combined (meta) analysis of 35 randomized, controlled trials of cholesterol-lowering interventions published prior to 1993. They concluded that net benefit (i.e. reduced total mortality) from cholesterol-lowering intervention was confined to those at very high risk of CHD. Only those at greater risk than even asymptomatic patients under 65 years with hypercholesteraemia were reported to derive demonstrable net benefit from cholesterol-lowering interventions that had been used prior to 1993. Cholesterol-lowering drugs were used in more than two-thirds of the trials surveyed by these authors. They concluded that these drugs should be reserved for the small proportion of people at very high risk of death from CHD, perhaps only those with both existing CHD and hypercholesteraemia.

The apparent failure of these early intervention trials was explained by suggesting that the sample sizes were too small to get statistically significant reductions in overall mortality. Dunnigan (1993) estimated that a trial involving 80 000 people over a 5-year period would be necessary to demonstrate whether there was any beneficial effect of cholesterol lowering on all-cause mortality even in patients with asymptomatic hypercholesteraemia under the age of 65 years. This is, of course, another way of saying that, at least within the time-scale of an intervention trial, the difference in risk of dying is only minutely affected by being in the intervention or control group. As a result of such findings many scientists questioned the benefits of many interventions and health promotion campaigns that were aimed at lowering average plasma cholesterol concentrations.

More recent intervention trials using the *statin group of cholesterol-lowering drugs* have given strong evidence that lowering plasma cholesterol can have net beneficial effects both in patients with existing heart disease and in those with asymptomatic hypercholesteraemia. These drugs inhibit the key enzyme in cholesterol biosynthesis (*HMG CoA reductase*) and produce a substantial and sustained reduction in LDL cholesterol with few side-effects. In a 5-year study using over 4000 Scandinavians with existing CHD, the drug simvastatin reduced plasma LDL cholesterol by 35 per cent and reduced total mortality by 30 per cent as a result of reduced cardiovascular mortality (SSSS, 1994). In a study of 6500 Scottish men with asymptomatic hypercholesteraemia, the drug provastatin reduced LDL cholesterol by 26 per cent, heart attacks by a third and total mortality by 22 per cent (Shepherd et al., 1995). These latter authors estimated that treating 1000 healthy but hypercholesteraemic middle-aged men with pravastatin for 5 years would result in 20 fewer non-fatal myocardial infarctions and nine fewer deaths as well as less heart surgery and fewer investigative procedures.

In more recent years it has become clear that lowering the plasma LDL cholesterol concentration by the use of statin drugs lowers the risk of cardiovascular disease across the whole range of LDL levels found in industrialized countries and almost irrespective of the initial cholesterol concentration. This has led to the belief that cholesterol lowering by statins is beneficial for anyone at increased risk of CHD or stroke irrespective of whether or not they have an elevated LDL cholesterol concentration (e.g. if they have diabetes or hypertension). Group (2002) found that adding 40 mg of simvastatin to the existing treatments of high-risk patients with coronary disease, other occlusive arterial disease or diabetes reduced rates of strokes and heart attacks by around a third in those fully complying with the medication

regimen. The size of the benefit was dependent on the patient's initial overall risk rather than the initial cholesterol level. Similarly, Sever et al. (2003) found that 10 mg/day of atorvastatin reduced rates of strokes and CHD in hypertensive patients who had total plasma cholesterol levels that were less than 6.5 mmol/L.

There is thus clear evidence that statins are effective in reducing mortality and cardiovascular events (heart attacks and strokes) in people in high-risk categories, such as those with existing cardiovascular disease, those with hypercholesteraemia, diabetics, and hypertensives.

Taylor et al. (2011) conducted a meta-analysis of primary trials to see whether these benefits could be demonstrated in people without past history of cardiovascular disease. They found 14 trials that met their inclusion criteria, although some of these did include people with established cardiovascular disease. All the trials reported a reduction in total cholesterol and LDL in blood and, overall, statins reduced all-cause mortality, fatal and non-fatal cardiovascular events (strokes and heart attacks) and the number of bypass operations needed. They found no evidence that statins increased cancer or muscle pain, but they noted that many trials did not report on other possible adverse effects of statin use.

As a result of these shortcomings in the trials, Taylor's team advised caution in the routine use of statins for apparently healthy people without elevated risk factors for cardiovascular disease.

This discussion of the benefits of statin-type drugs might initially seem of limited relevance in nutrition but what they show is that, if changes in the population's diet and lifestyle eventually result in substantially lower average population blood LDL cholesterol concentrations over the whole lifespan, then this should shift the age distribution of death and disability from CHD upwards and lead to increased healthy life expectancy.

As a result of such observations on the apparent wide benefits of cholesterol lowering from statins, together with low recorded levels of serious side-effects, low doses of simvastatin (10 mg) were made available without prescription in the UK. The possible side-effects of statins are headaches, insomnia and digestive problems including abdominal pain, wind and diarrhoea. Less commonly they can cause liver problems, so they need to be used with caution in those with a history of liver disease or in heavy drinkers. They may rarely cause a serious myopathy (muscle wasting), so any unexplained muscular pain or weakness needs to be reported to the doctor and investigated.

Key points

- The evidence supporting the diet–heart hypothesis is both impressive and varied.
- Populations with high saturated fat and cholesterol intakes tend to have higher plasma cholesterol concentrations and higher death rates from coronary heart disease than those with low saturated fat intakes.
- Some vegetarian groups in the UK and USA with low intakes of saturated fat and cholesterol have lower rates of CHD than the rest of the population.
- Marked changes in a population's consumption of saturated fat have been accompanied by changes in coronary heart disease rates that are consistent with the diet–heart hypothesis.
- People who migrate from regions of low saturated fat consumption to regions of high consumption tend also to show increased rates of CHD.
- Short-term experimental or therapeutic manipulations of dietary fat composition produce changes in plasma lipoprotein profiles that are consistent with the diet–heart hypothesis.
- People with genetic disorders that raise their plasma LDL cholesterol are at greatly increased risk of CHD.
- In cohort studies using single or several populations, a high plasma cholesterol concentration is associated with increased risk of CHD.
- Some early cholesterol-lowering trials using drugs or diet resulted in significant reductions in the combined number of fatal and non-fatal coronary events.
- Statins are drugs that inhibit a key enzyme in cholesterol synthesis (HMG CoA reductase) and they have a potent cholesterol-lowering effect.

→

Key points *continued*

- Statins have been shown to produce significant reductions in cardiovascular events (strokes and heart attacks) and both cardiovascular and total mortality.
- Statins have been shown to be effective in those at high risk of cardiovascular disease and more recently in people without any identified high risk factors, and even in people without elevated LDL cholesterol concentrations.
- These statin trials suggest that population-wide reductions in plasma cholesterol concentration over the whole lifespan would increase healthy life expectancy.
- The reported benefits and infrequent incidence of serious side-effects have led to a low-dose statin being made available in the UK without prescription.
- A few anomalous observations are superficially inconsistent with the diet–heart hypothesis.
  - Within populations there is little correlation between plasma cholesterol and saturated fat intakes.
  - Some populations with high saturated fat intakes or high plasma cholesterol concentrations seem to have lower rates of CHD than might be expected.
  - Until 1994, cholesterol-lowering intervention trials with diet and/or drugs failed to produce significant reductions in total mortality.
  - Multiple risk factor intervention trials do not have significantly reduced cardiovascular events, cardiovascular mortality or total mortality in general healthy populations (they do have beneficial effects in high-risk populations including diabetics and hypertensives).
- There are plausible explanations for each of these anomalies.
  - Many factors influence plasma cholesterol and any individual's saturated fat intake is only a minor determinant of where they lie in the population distribution of plasma cholesterol concentrations.
  - High levels of fitness and activity or high intakes of anti-oxidants are some of the factors that have been suggested might protect some populations from CHD.

FISH OILS

A series of papers published in the 1970s by Bang, Dyerberg and their colleagues reported that Greenland Inuit had low rates of coronary heart disease and low rates of inflammatory joint disease when compared to Danes. The Inuit ate a traditional diet high in seal meat, whale meat and fish (e.g. Dyerberg and Bang, 1979). This low rate of CHD was despite a diet with similar total fat content to the Danes and despite the fact that most of the fat came from the animal kingdom. The lipid of the Inuit diet differs from the Danish diet in two major respects: it is much lower in saturated fatty acids, and it has higher levels of n-3 polyunsaturated fatty acids (reviewed by Kromhout, 1990).

Fish oils and other marine oils (e.g. from seals and whales) contain large amounts of long-chain n-3 (or ω-3) polyunsaturated fatty acids. The three longest chain members of this series – eicosapentaenoic acid, EPA (20:5n-3), docosapentaenoic acid, DPA (22:5n-3), and docosahexaenoic acid, DHA (22:6n-3) – account for around 20 per cent of the fatty acids in many oils from marine fish. As noted earlier in the chapter, the n-3 fatty acids, because of their extra double bond, have a lower melting point and have greater fluidity at low environmental temperatures than the corresponding n-6 fatty acids – this may explain their prominence in the fat of coldwater mammals and fish. These acids enter the marine food chain via their synthesis by marine plants and plankton which then serve as food for higher marine organisms. These long-chain n-3 polyunsaturates are believed to be the active agents that reduce risk of CHD and inflammatory joint diseases.

The reports on the health and mortality of Inuits served to focus scientific attention on the protective and therapeutic potential of fish oils and the n-3 polyunsaturates. Research papers on fish oils numbered less than 10 per year in the 1970s but rose sharply during the 1980s to a level of several hundred per year in the early 1990s (Simopoulos, 1991). Fish oils can be made available on prescription in the UK for the treatment of certain hyperlipidaemias and for patients with a history of CHD. Fish oils supplements make up a major part of the total UK market for dietary supplements; in 2009, fish oil (17 per cent) and cod liver oil (22 per cent) made up almost 40 per cent of the total market for natural food supplements, with a rise of almost 50 per cent recorded in sales of fish oil over the period 2007–9 (Mintel, 2009).

Fish oil or fish liver oil

Fish liver oil, usually cod liver oil, has traditionally been taken as a source of vitamins A and D. It is still widely used for this purpose and, given the high prevalence of vitamin D inadequacy in most age groups in the UK, there may well be a case for its wider use (see Chapters 13 and 14). A 10 mL dose of cod liver oil contains up to 1.5 times the RNI for vitamin A and up to 10 μg of vitamin D (the RNI for adults not regularly exposed to sunlight). Halibut and shark liver oil have even higher concentrations of these vitamins. Cod liver oil was traditionally taken in liquid form but because of the unpleasant taste many fish oil products are now taken as oil-filled capsules. Vitamins A and D are the most toxic of the vitamins when consumed in excess, so the recommended dose of fish liver oil should not be exceeded and they should not be taken by pregnant women because of the teratogenic effects of vitamin A.

The high concentration of vitamins A and D in some fish liver oil preparations reduces the dose of the long-chain n-3 fatty acids that they can safely provide. Fish body oil can be safely taken in higher doses than fish liver oil, and the FDA suggest that doses equivalent to 10–20 capsules per day should be generally regarded as safe – although they may exacerbate clotting disorders or enhance the effect of anticoagulant drugs.

A single capsule of fish (liver) oil should contain at least 100 mg of EPA and DHA and may contain up to 400 mg (the exact dose of any preparation should be shown on the label). This means that one capsule per day should provide between 1 g and 3 g of EPA/DHA per week, and this compares with:

- 25 mg in a 100 g serving of cod
- 1.9 g in 100 g of mackerel
- 1.3 g in 100 g of herring
- 1.7 g in 100 g of sardines canned in tomato sauce
- 1.5–3 g in a 10 mL dose of cod liver oil.

COMA (1994a) recommended that average population intakes of long-chain n-3 polyunsaturates should rise from 100 mg/day (0.7 g/week) to 200 mg/day (1.4 g/week), and to achieve this aim they recommended that people should eat two portions of fish per week, one of which should be oily fish. People taking one capsule of fish oil each day should achieve this target dose of n-3 polyunsaturates.

Possible protective mechanisms of fish oil

There are a number of mechanisms by which long-chain n-3 fatty acids have been suggested to reduce the risk of CHD and inflammatory joint diseases, and possibly other conditions. Some of these are discussed below.

Effects on the production of eicosanoids

Taking large doses of long-chain n-3 fatty acids, especially large doses of EPA, leads to an increase in the production of eicosanoids from EPA and their partial replacement of those produced from arachidonic acid. Looking back to Figure 12.3, this would mean a decrease in production of the following eicosanoids produced from arachidonic acid:

- LTB_4, a leukotriene that promotes inflammation
- TXA_2, a thromboxane that promotes platelet aggregation
- PGI_2, a prostaglandin with anti-aggregating effects on platelets.

These would be partly replaced by eicosanoids produced from EPA:

- LTB_5, a leukotriene with low activity
- TXA_2, a thromboxane with low activity
- PGI_3, a prostaglandin with anti-aggregating effects on platelets.

The overall effect of these changes, shown in Figure 12.7, would be predicted to reduce the risk of thromboses forming in blood vessels. This would reduce the risk of occlusive strokes (due to blockage of cerebral vessels with a clot) and myocardial infarction (heart attacks due to clots lodging in the coronary vessels). Traditional Inuits have extended bleeding times and are prone to frequent and longlasting nosebleeds and have high stroke mortality (due to increased levels of cerebral haemorrhage). In short-term human and animal

experiments, high consumption of fish oils have been found to reduce the tendency of blood to clot and to extend the bleeding time (Anon, 1984; Sanders, 1985).

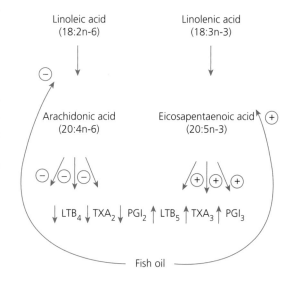

Figure 12.7 Effects of fish oil consumption on the production of eicosanoids that affect platelet aggregation and inflammation.

These changes in eicosanoid production should also lead to a dampening of the inflammatory response and so, for example, may reduce the damage caused by the inflammatory response after a myocardial infarction and may also explain the suggested benefits on inflammatory diseases like arthritis and eczema.

Effects on blood lipoprotein profiles

Fish oils reduce both fasting and post-prandial blood triacylglycerol levels. They also raise the HDL cholesterol concentration, but at normal levels of consumption their effect on LDL cholesterol is negligible.

Effects on heart rhythm

Irregular electrical activity (arrhythmia) in diseased or damaged heart muscle can have fatal consequences. Changes in the balance of n-3 and n-6 fatty acids in the heart resulting from increased intakes of n-3 fatty acids may reduce heart rate variability and arrhythmia, and so the risk of a heart attack being fatal (Buttriss, 1999).

Role in brain functioning

Docosahexaenoic acid is a normal component of brain and retinal membranes. There is evidence that children and animals deprived of n-3 fatty acids *in utero* or during early life may have visual, learning or neurological problems (reviewed by Jones and Kubow, 2006). This suggests that n-3 fatty acids may be essential for normal brain development and probably for optimal brain functioning in later life. This has been used as a rationale for testing fish oil supplements in some behavioural problems with children.

Fish oils and coronary heart disease

In short-term, controlled experiments, fish oils have effects on blood lipoprotein levels, platelet aggregation and blood clotting that could reduce atherosclerosis and the risk of thrombosis. Inuits and other populations consuming very large amounts of fish have a reduced tendency for blood to clot, prolonged bleeding times and a low incidence of coronary heart disease.

The epidemiological evidence that high fatty fish consumption reduces CHD and increases life expectancy is limited. The work on Inuits and other populations consuming very large amounts of fish has been some of the most positive of the epidemiological evidence in favour of fish oils having protective effects against the development of CHD (Kromhout, 1990; Buttriss, 1999). There is little evidence of an independent relationship between fatty fish consumption and reduced risk of CHD in cross-population studies. Comparisons that have been made have generally used total fish consumption as the independent variable (a crude predictor of total n-3 fatty acid consumption); only a weak association was found with CHD mortality and this was dependent on the inclusion of the Japanese. In the Seven Countries study there was no significant association between fish consumption and mortality from CHD; some of those populations with negligible fish consumption in inland Yugoslavia had among the lowest rates of CHD while some with the highest fish consumption in Finland had amongst the highest rates of CHD. Fish consumption was related to subsequent mortality in a 20-year cohort study of 850 men in Zutphen, Holland. In this cohort, death from CHD was inversely related to fish consumption; it was 50 per cent lower in men who ate 30 g of fatty fish per day (equivalent to about two servings per week) compared with those who ate no fish at all. Buttriss (1999) reviewed several other prospective cohort studies published prior to 1999 and concluded that the majority of these studies report a decrease in the risk of heart disease as fish consumption increases. The effects of fish eating were most pronounced in populations that had low habitual fish consumption.

The unconvincing epidemiological evidence relating fatty fish consumption to reduced CHD risk might not be unexpected, because:

- total fish consumption is a crude indicator of n-3 fatty acid intake
- the relationship between saturated fat intake and CHD might well obscure any lesser relationship between fish consumption and CHD.

There is convincing evidence that, in people with established CHD, regular consumption of fatty fish or fish oil supplements produces overall benefits as measured by total mortality in the few years immediately after first infarction. Burr *et al.* (1991) found that, in patients who had previously suffered a myocardial infarction (MI), fish oils significantly reduced both cardiovascular and total mortality whereas their other interventions (low-fat diets or increased cereal fibre) did not. Fish oil patients did not have significantly fewer re-infarcts, but these new infarcts were less likely to be fatal (consistent with reduced post-infarct inflammatory damage). A subsequent intervention trial in Italy found reductions in both total mortality and non-fatal infarction in men receiving large supplements of n-3 fatty acids (GISSI, 1999).

A major review of the effects of omega-3 fatty acids on cardiovascular diseases was commissioned by the Agency for Healthcare Research and Quality, AHRQ (Wang *et al.*, 2004). This review generally confirmed the conclusions that omega-3 fatty acids from fish or fish oil supplements reduce all-cause mortality and various cardiovascular outcomes. Almost all the randomized controlled trials included in that review had used subjects who already had diagnosed cardiovascular disease (i.e. secondary trials). These consistently suggested that fish oil reduced all-cause mortality and other cardiovascular events in this type of subject, although it did not reduce the risk of stroke. With one exception, the studies that had addressed the possible primary preventative role of fish oil (in subjects with no previous clinical history of cardiovascular disease) were epidemiological cohort or case–control studies. Those three cohort studies that had specifically estimated fish oil intake (rather than just fish consumption) all reported a significant reduction in all-cause mortality, cardiovascular deaths and MI associated with high fish oil consumption (average follow-up duration of 10 years). Breslow (2006) concluded from a review of cohort studies that consuming fish or fish oil containing EPA and DHA was associated with decreased cardiovascular death. Breslow also found that fish oil consumption reduced mortality in secondary intervention trials with people who had experienced a heart attack, probably as a result of fewer fatal arrhythmias. He *et al.* (2004) did a meta-analysis of 11 cohort studies relating fish consumption to death from CHD and found a dose-dependent reduction in CHD mortality with increasing fish consumption. These cohort studies had well over 200 000 subjects and the average follow-up time was 12 years. A systematic review by Wang *et al.* (2006) confirmed the beneficial effects of fish oil supplements in secondary intervention trials.

Fish oils and arthritis

Rheumatoid arthritis

Rheumatoid arthritis (RA) is a relatively uncommon autoimmune condition often starting in young people and with rapid progression of symptoms. It was first reported more than 25 years ago that high intakes of EPA appeared to improve the clinical features of RA and reduce the levels of the inflammation-promoting leukotriene LTB-4 (Kremer *et al.*, 1985). It has more recently been reported that very large doses of n-3 fatty acids reduced the dose of anti-inflammatory drugs needed by patients to control their symptoms of RA (Kremer, 2000). These benefits were achieved only after several months and using much more than the usual one or two capsules of fish oil per day.

MacLean *et al.* (2004), in a review of the benefits of fish oils in the management of RA, found only limited evidence to support their use.

Fish oils did not significantly reduce symptoms reported by patients, nor did they have an effect on a more objective outcome measure, erythrocyte sedimentation rate (ESR). Several studies reviewed by Maclean's team did report a reduction in the dose of anti-inflammatory drugs needed in those taking fish oils.

One prospective study found a very slight indication that oily fish might have some effect in reducing the risk of developing RA (Rosell *et al.*, 2009). This result should be treated cautiously as no more than an indication that further investigation may be justified.

Osteoarthritis

Osteoarthritis is a much more common degenerative condition in which damage to and erosion of joints lead to pain and disability. It affects most elderly people to some extent. Many people take fish oils supplements in the hope that they will prevent or alleviate the painful joints and stiffness of osteoarthritis, but there is very little direct evidence that they are effective in this more common form of arthritis.

Some reviewers have suggested that fish oils may be useful in the management of osteoarthritis, but most of the evidence quoted is either from in-vitro studies or from clinical studies using patients with rheumatoid arthritis (e.g. Curtis *et al.*, 2002). Later, Curtis *et al.* (2004) concluded from a more general review that the efficacy of fish oils 'has been demonstrated in several clinical trials, animal feeding experiments and in-vitro models that mimic cartilage destruction in arthritic disease'. Their references do not, however, contain studies that have demonstrated clinical benefits for patients with osteoarthritis. A PubMed search late in 2011 using the terms 'fish oil supplements + osteoarthritis' yielded seven papers and six reviews, and none of these was a clinical trial of fish oils. Most of the evidence for use of fish oils in osteoarthritis is either from animal studies or in-vitro studies or is based on its use in rheumatoid arthritis.

Fish oils, brain and behaviour

Children with the behavioural condition referred to as attention-deficit hyperactivity disorder (ADHD) have lower levels of n-3 fatty acids in their red blood cells than control children, which cannot be explained by differences in their dietary intakes (e.g. Colter *et al.*, 2008). It has been suggested that this might be the result of some differences in n-3 fatty acid metabolism (Burgess *et al.*, 2000). Taken together with the previously noted observations on the importance of n-3 fatty acids in brain development, these reports have led to suggestions that fish oils may be useful in the management of dyslexia, ADHD and some related behavioural disorders in children.

A meta-analysis by Raz and Gobis (2009) found no evidence to support the use of fatty acid supplements to treat ADHD. Richardson and Montgomery (2005), in a clinical trial of a mixture of fish oils and evening primrose oil in children with development coordination syndrome (DCD, a condition with some features of both ADHD and dyslexia), did find some indication that it improved reading, spelling and behaviour (but not motor skills) over 3 months of treatment.

There is no substantial scientific evidence to support claims made in the popular media that fish oils improve behaviour, attention span or examination performance. There have to date been no published scientific trials, but uncontrolled and badly designed 'trials' have been reported in the popular media and have attracted much publicity. In July 2006, the Food Standards Agency concluded that insufficient evidence exists to warrant giving a daily dose of fish oil to all children and that there were 'too many inconsistencies' in the recent studies.

An observational study (Dangour *et al.*, 2009) suggested that elderly people with higher intakes of oily fish have better cognitive functioning and perhaps a reduced risk of developing dementia, but when corrected for confounding variables this became statistically insignificant. Lim *et al.* (2006) found no clinical trials of fish oils on the rate of cognitive decline that met their inclusion criteria for a meta-analysis.

There is thus speculation but as yet no substantial evidence that fish oil taken in food or supplements has any beneficial effect in reducing cognitive decline or reducing the risk of dementia in the elderly.

Conclusions and fish oil recommendations

There is sufficient evidence to recommend that fatty fish be included in healthful and diverse diets. A quantitative recommendation of two portions of fatty fish per week has been suggested by the American Heart Association and COMA (1991). Increases in fatty fish consumption or the use of fish oil supplements are warranted in those with established coronary heart disease or some types of hyperlipidaemia; the American Heart Association recommends that those with existing CHD should eat 1 gram per day of EPA and DHA in food or supplements.

There is limited evidence of clinical benefit from taking fish oils to treat or prevent osteoarthritis, although this is partly because of limited data. Vitamin D deficiency is very prevalent in all age groups of the UK population, so a daily dose of cod liver oil could reduce this problem and provide modest amounts of long-chain n-3 fatty acids. One health authority in the UK (Bradford) has decided to offer free supplements of vitamin D to all children under 2 years old because of high levels of vitamin D deficiency and rickets in the children, especially those of South Asian origin; cod liver oil used as a source of this vitamin D would also provide some n-3 fatty acids.

Some potential dangers of consuming large amounts of fish oil or n-3 fatty acid are listed below, although it must be emphasized that these are theoretical or speculative risks.

- High intake of fish oils reduces blood clotting and increases bleeding time. This should reduce the risk of thrombosis but may not be universally beneficial (e.g. in those at risk of cerebral haemorrhage, those with clotting disorders or taking anticoagulant drugs).
- Fish oils seem to have some immunosuppressive effect because of their effects on eicosanoid production.
- n-3 fatty acids are highly susceptible to oxidation. Foods high in these acids are prone to go rancid, and oxidative damage to them after absorption may have adverse consequences. Fish oil preparations normally have added vitamin E to reduce their oxidative deterioration.

- Some fish liver oil preparations may have too much vitamin A and D for pregnant women. The recommended dose should not be exceeded.

- Fish oils are the major dietary source of long-chain n-3 fatty acids.
- Britons and Americans are advised to eat two portions of oily fish per week and to increase their intake of long-chain n-3 polyunsaturates.
- Low rates of CHD and inflammatory joint disease among Greenland Inuits focused scientific attention on the potential health benefits of eating oily fish and the n-3 polyunsaturates.
- Long-chain n-3 fatty acids alter the balance of eicosanoid production in ways that should reduce platelet aggregation, blood clotting and inflammation.
- Fish oils reduce blood triacylglycerol concentrations and increase HDL levels.
- Increased consumption of n-3 fatty acids may reduce the risk of potentially fatal cardiac arrhythmia.
- n-3 fatty acids are found in membranes in the brain and retina and are probably essential for normal brain development.
- Deprivation of n-3 fatty acids *in utero* or early life leads to visual, learning and neurological impairments in children and animals.
- Inuits and other populations consuming large amounts of fish have reduced blood clotting, extended bleeding times and low risk of CHD.
- Several within-population cohort studies indicate that high fish consumption is associated with reduced risk of CHD.
- Many cohort studies have found that high fish consumption was associated with reduced all-cause mortality, cardiovascular deaths and myocardial infarction in subjects without previous history of cardiovascular disease.
- Secondary intervention trials have reported that fish oil consumption reduces total mortality of patients with existing coronary disease.

→

- Large doses of fish oil reduce inflammatory mediators and may reduce the dose of drugs needed to control rheumatoid arthritis.
- Many people take fish oils to prevent or alleviate osteoarthritis but this usage is mainly supported by animal studies, in-vitro studies or by extrapolation from its use in RA.
- There is almost no direct clinical evidence that fish oils prevent or alleviate symptoms of osteoarthritis.
- There is little evidence that fish oil supplements improve behaviour or academic performance in normal children or improve symptoms in those with behavioural conditions such as ADHD.
- Although high fish oil consumption is associated with better cognitive function and reduced risk of dementia in the elderly, this association becomes insignificant when there is correction for confounding variables.
- Widespread consumption of large doses of fish oils as supplements may have potentially adverse effects for some people; for example, those with impaired blood clotting, immunosuppression and increased susceptibility to oxidative damage by free radicals.

OTHER NATURAL OILS USED AS SUPPLEMENTS

Evening primrose oil supplements contain large amounts (8–11 per cent) of γ-linolenic acid, GLA (18:3n-6), and several other plant oils including blackcurrant oil (15–25 per cent) and starflower oil (20–25 per cent) are also marketed as rich sources of GLA. There have been claims that GLA-rich products may reduce some of the symptoms of premenstrual syndrome, especially breast pain (mastalgia) and may have some benefits for patients with atopic eczema.

It is argued that, on current diets, the production of GLA and thus of dihomo-γ-linoleic acid (20:3n-6) and its associated eicosanoids is low because large intakes of arachidonic acid from meat inhibit the desaturase that converts linoleic acid to GLA (see Figures 12.2 and 12.3).

Until 2002, two evening primrose oil preparations were permitted to be sold as licensed medicines in the UK, but their product licences were withdrawn because it was considered that evidence of their efficacy was not sufficient to meet the standards for a medicine. Srivastava *et al.* (2007) found no evidence from a meta-analysis that evening primrose oil seemed any better than a placebo for treating mastalgia. Van Gool *et al.* (2004) found no evidence from a meta-analysis of clinical trials that any source of GLA was useful in the treatment of atopic eczema. There have been doubts cast on the quality of some of the earlier positive research into this oil and on the impartiality of some of those involved in testing and marketing the substance (Webb, 2011b; see also Williams, 2003).

Flaxseed oil or linseed oil is extracted from the flax plant and contains very high levels of α-linolenic acid (ALA, 18:3n-3), the parent compound of the n-3 series of fatty acids. It has been marketed as a vegetarian alternative to fish oils. However, Burdge (2004) found that there is limited conversion of ALA to EPA and very little conversion to DHA. Wang *et al.* (2006), in their meta-analysis of fish oils discussed earlier, found that n-3 fatty acids consumed as ALA from vegetable sources like flaxseed oil were ineffective in clinical trials aimed at preventing recurrence of coronary heart disease. Algal extracts containing large amounts of DHA are marketed as a source of DHA that is acceptable to vegetarians.

Key points

- Evening primrose oil, blackcurrant oil and starflower oil are rich in γ-linolenic acid (GLA)
- GLA production may be limited on current diets because of large intakes of arachidonic acid, and this might limit production of eicosanoids from dihomo-γ-linoleic acid.
- Claims about the benefits of evening primrose oil for mastalgia or atopic eczema are not substantiated by recent clinical trials.
- Flaxseed oil contains large amounts of α-linolenic acid (18:3n-3) and is sold as a vegetarian source of n-3 fatty acid but there is only limited conversion to long-chain derivatives in humans.
- Vegetarian sources of n-3 fatty acids do not reduce coronary heart disease recurrence in clinical trials.
- DHA is found in some algal extracts which may be an acceptable source for vegetarians.

13

THE MICRONUTRIENTS

Scope of this chapter	324	Anti-oxidants and the oxidant theory of disease	335
Overview of dietary supplements	325	Do high anti-oxidant intakes prevent heart	
Food fortification	329	disease, cancer and other chronic diseases?	341
Assessment of the micronutrient		Use of substances other than essential	
adequacy of British adults	330	nutrients as dietary supplements	346

SCOPE OF THIS CHAPTER

The previous three chapters deal with carbohydrates, proteins and fats which are the energy-yielding nutrients in food. They are present in relatively large amounts in the average diet and so are termed collectively the *macronutrients*. The substances covered in this chapter do not contribute to the body's energy supply and are present in small amounts (milligram or microgram quantities), and so are collectively termed the *micronutrients*. The term micronutrient should strictly be reserved for those substances that are an essential component of the diet – the organic vitamins and the inorganic essential minerals and trace elements.

The vitamins and minerals are specifically covered in Chapters 14 and 15, but in this chapter the general micronutrient adequacy of British adults' diets is overviewed and the use of micronutrient supplements is discussed in the light of these observations about micronutrient adequacy (the micronutrient adequacy of other lifecycle groups is discussed in Chapter 16). Fortification of food with essential micronutrients is briefly discussed as an alternative to the use of micronutrient supplements.

Also discussed in this chapter are several groups of organic substances that are present in micro-quantities in the diet and which, although they are not classified as essential nutrients, may nevertheless have nutritional significance and are widely taken as dietary supplements. Those listed below will be discussed in this chapter.

The anti-oxidants

These are substances that either have inherent anti-oxidant activity or are part of anti-oxidant enzyme systems involved in the disposal of damaging oxygen free radicals. These free radicals are produced as a normal by-product of the oxidative processes in cells and can cause damage to cellular components unless quenched by anti-oxidant systems. It is widely believed that many chronic diseases and perhaps even ageing itself may be partly the result of cumulative damage by free radicals – the oxidant theory of disease. Some anti-oxidants are essential vitamins or minerals, but others are substances that are not recognized as essential nutrients but which may nevertheless have useful anti-oxidant activity. The oxidant theory of disease and the role of anti-oxidants are, for convenience, discussed in this chapter irrespective of which category of substance the anti-oxidant belongs to.

The conditionally essential nutrients

There are several organic substances that are not normally classified as essential micronutrients but which may become essential in certain individuals or in particular circumstances. These are termed conditionally essential.

Other organic substances with vitamin-like cellular functions

There are other organic compounds that are not usually considered to be even conditionally essential nutrients but also have vitamin-like functions in the body (e.g. creatine and co-enzyme Q_{10}). Some of these substances are promoted as dietary supplements on the basis that extra supplies can have some physiologically beneficial effects, it being argued that the endogenously produced supply is insufficient for optimal health or that extra exogenous supplies can ameliorate certain disease states.

Secondary plant metabolites

There are many thousands of so-called secondary plant metabolites that are produced by plants that are additional to those involved in the primary cellular processes of respiration, photosynthesis, growth and development. It is clear that a diet rich in fruits and vegetables is associated with reduced risk of chronic diseases such as cancer and heart disease; and, while conventional nutritional factors in plants like essential micronutrients, dietary fibre and anti-oxidants may explain all or much of this effect, there is also a wide belief that these secondary metabolites may confer particular health benefits. A number of substances in this category are used as conventional drugs or herbal medicines for the treatment or prevention of disease. A brief classification of these factors is included, and the possible ways in which they may influence the development of chronic diseases are considered.

Key points

- This chapter overviews the micronutrients, which are the essential vitamins and minerals required only in small amounts but which do not act as sources of energy.

- The micronutrient adequacy of adult British diets will be overviewed and the case for the use of micronutrient supplements or food fortification discussed and evaluated.

- The anti-oxidant theory of disease and the role of anti-oxidants (both essential nutrients and other plant chemicals) will be discussed in this chapter.

- This chapter also overviews several nutrients that are considered to be conditionally essential – normally synthesized in sufficient quantities to meet physiological needs but which may be essential under certain circumstances.

→

Key points *continued*

- Also discussed are other organic substances which, while having vitamin-like roles in the body, are not classified even as conditionally essential because they are synthesized endogenously. Many of these are used as dietary supplements in the belief that extra supplies can confer specific benefits.

- Plants produce many thousands of so-called secondary metabolites. In this chapter these are classified and possible ways in which they may influence risk of developing chronic age-related diseases will be briefly considered.

- These plant secondary metabolites will be consumed in vegetables and in natural plant extracts sold as food supplements or traditional herbal medicinal products.

OVERVIEW OF DIETARY SUPPLEMENTS

Additional information and references may be found in a recent book by the author (Webb, 2011a), and Webb (2007) gives a more concise review of dietary supplements.

More than a third of UK adults take some form of dietary supplement. Until May 2011, almost anything that was taken in pill or potion form that was not licensed as a medicine was, by default, legally classified as a dietary supplement and was subject to food law rather than the much more stringent rules governing medicines. This is still the case in the USA, but in the UK and EU certain plant extracts that have little or no history of use as foods (e.g. agnus castus, echinacea, milk thistle and St John's wort) can no longer be sold as dietary supplements. As a result of the EU's Traditional Herbal Medicines Directive, products like these which have a long history of safe use within the EU must now be registered as, and sold as, traditional herbal medicinal products. This new regulatory process means that, although the process of registration is much less stringent than getting approval for sale as a 'medicine', there is more scrutiny of their manufacture and the products now need to include information about levels of bioactive ingredients on their labels. There is, however, no need for manufacturers seeking registration to show evidence of efficacy as there would be for approval for sale as a medicine. These products are still readily available for over-the-counter sale in the UK and can also still be legally purchased from foreign internet sites for personal use. Other plant extracts which do have authentic culinary uses may still be sold as food supplements (e.g. garlic, berry fruit extracts, ginger, ginseng and soy extracts).

There are a number of long and all-embracing definitions of dietary supplements, but almost all supplements fall within five major categories.

- *Preparations of vitamins or minerals.* These are sold either singly or in combinations.
- *Organic substances.* These, including creatine and co-enzyme Q_{10}, have vitamin-like roles but are synthesized endogenously and so are not classified as essential nutrients. They may act as co-enzymes or as precursors in synthetic pathways. The distinction between essential and non-essential nutrients is not always clear-cut. As noted earlier, some nutrients are classified as conditionally essential and even some established vitamins only become essential under particular circumstances. Vitamin D is not essential in the diet if the skin is adequately exposed to sunlight, and niacin only if there is not sufficient tryptophan in the diet for endogenous synthesis (see Chapter 14). Some examples of these organic substances are briefly discussed later in the chapter.
- *Natural fats and oils.* Examples are fish (liver) oil, evening primrose oil and flaxseed oil which are discussed in Chapter 12.
- *Natural plant extracts* (or occasionally animal extracts). These contain secondary metabolites that may be bioactive. Some of these must now be registered and sold as traditional herbal medicinal products within the EU.
- *The anti-oxidants.* These span the other categories but are separated out for discussion as a single category in this chapter.

People take supplements for a range of individual reasons but most of these fall under four broad headings:

- to ensure micronutrient adequacy
- to compensate for some (perceived) extra need or defective metabolic handling of a nutrient (e.g. poor absorption, increased need in

pregnancy, increased loss in renal dialysis, an inborn error of metabolism)
- to prevent or treat disease – although only substances registered as medicines can legally make claims to treat or prevent disease
- to improve athletic performance.

There are a number of potential hazards involved in taking dietary supplements, some of which are identified below.

- They may be directly toxic. Some may not be normal dietary constituents, or supplements may contain much greater amounts than would ordinarily be found in food. The larger the dose used and the longer the duration of use, the greater the risk of toxic effects. Even many essential nutrients are very toxic in large excess, for example vitamins A and D and iron. If a micronutrient supplement is taken to ensure adequacy, the dose is likely to be based on the reference nutrient intake (RNI) or recommended dietary allowance (RDA) and unlikely to cause harm, but if taken for other purposes the dose may be many multiples of this.
- Supplements are not always subject to the strict regulation of good manufacturing process that governs the production of medicines. There may be problems with purity, identity, dosage and bio-availability. They may be inadvertently contaminated. There have been cases of medicinal drugs, even withdrawn drugs, having been deliberately added to some products that were in the past sold as dietary supplements. They may contain more or less than is stated on the label and sometimes with natural extracts the 'active' ingredient is uncertain. Some products may not disperse properly when swallowed and so may not be properly absorbed.
- They may divert attention away from more useful dietary and lifestyle changes and used as an easy alternative to such changes. So, an anti-oxidant supplement may be taken as an alternative to stopping smoking; and rather than attempting to moderate alcohol consumption, milk thistle extracts (now a traditional herbal medicine in the EU) may be taken to protect the liver from alcohol abuse; and berry extracts may be taken as an alternative to eating five portions of fruits and vegetables.

- Some people may take supplements rather than their prescribed medication.
- Some supplements could interfere with the action of prescribed drugs. They may increase their metabolic destruction by inducing enzymes in the liver that metabolize 'foreign' substances.

Around a third of British adults aged 19–64 years take a dietary supplement: 29 per cent of men and 40 per cent of women (Hoare *et al.*, 2004). This is almost three times the rate of supplement usage reported in a similar survey conducted 14 years earlier. The percentage of supplement users rises with age, and 55 per cent of women in the highest age category (55–64 years) took supplements. In this and other similar surveys, there is a marked trend for supplement use to be highest in individuals with the highest nutrient intake from food, or to be concentrated in age and social groups with the highest nutrient intakes from food. This means that those most likely to benefit from supplement use are the least likely to take them. In an analysis of the UK supplement market, Mintel (2009) estimated the market then to be worth £396 million, but they suggested that annual growth in the market had been slow since 2004 (<2 per cent a year) and they predicted similar slow market growth up to 2014. Table 13.1 gives a breakdown of the UK supplement market by value. The market in the USA was

estimated to be worth $18.5 billion in 2002 but only growing at a similar low rate to that in the UK; around two-thirds of American adults report using a dietary supplement of some sort.

The Food Standards Agency (FSA, 2003) made recommendations about maximum supplemental doses of all vitamins and minerals. However, in the UK, legal regulation of maximum doses for general sale applies only to vitamins that are also licensed medicines – vitamins A (retinol), D, B_{12} and folic acid. Different regulations apply in different countries even within the EU, ranging from the liberal rules in countries like the UK and Sweden (where it is possible to legally buy large multiples of the RDA for most vitamins) to countries like France (where only doses up to the RDA or a low multiple of it can be sold as food supplements and higher doses must be sold as medicines). High multiples of the RNI of vitamins and minerals are taken in the belief that they may have additional benefits in preventing or alleviating disease or 'optimizing' health in some other way. In countries where only single or low multiples of the dietary standard are permitted, it is clearly implied that supplements should be taken to ensure adequacy and, when high doses of vitamins and minerals are used for some other purpose, this becomes pharmacology rather than nutrition; that is, they are being used as drugs, not foods.

Table 13.1 Approximate breakdown by value of the market for dietary supplements in the UK*

Supplement category	Value	% of total	Change 2007–9 (%)
All vitamins and supplements	396	100	+6.4
All vitamin products	114	29	−5.8
Cod liver oil	62	22	+3.3
Evening primrose/starflower oil	21	7	−16.0
Omega-3 (fish oil)	47	17	+46.9
Glucosamine	48	17	+60.0
Minerals	15	5	–
Garlic	12	4	−14.3
Ginseng	10	4	–
St John's wort[1]	7	2	–
Ginkgo biloba[1]	9	3	–
All others (including tonics)	51	18	+4.1

*Data source: Mintel (2009).
[1] Now classified as a traditional herbal medicinal product within the EU.

In 2004, a voluntary code was established after discussions between the FSA and representatives of the supplements industry. According to this code, manufacturers and suppliers of supplements were encouraged to include advisory notes on labels for products containing more than specified amounts of some vitamins and minerals, and in such cases were encouraged to reformulate their product. Some examples from this voluntary agreement are listed below and a fuller list can be found in Webb (2011).

- Preparations containing more than 1000 mg/day of vitamin C, 20 mg/day of iron or 1500 mg/day of calcium should carry a warning that they might cause mild stomach upsets.
- Preparations containing more than 7 mg/day of β-carotene should carry a warning that they should not be taken by heavy smokers.
- Products containing more than 20 mg/day of nicotinic acid should warn of the possibility of causing skin flushing.
- Preparations containing more than 100 mg/day of vitamin B_6 should warn that long-term consumption of this amount might lead to tingling and numbness.

As part of the general harmonization of EU dietary supplement regulation, the Food Supplements Directive came into force across the EU in August 2005. This legislation contains two positive lists:

- a list of the vitamins and minerals that can be used in the manufacture of food supplements
- a list of the chemical forms of these vitamins and minerals that can be used.

Only substances on these lists are permitted, so anything not included is by default forbidden.

The first positive list did not, for example, contain boron, nickel, silicon, tin or vanadium, all of which had been previously included in some dietary supplements. Silicon and boron have now been added to the list, although that does not imply that they are now considered to be essential nutrients. One of the areas of controversy that still remains is that the only forms of folate permitted in supplements are folic acid (used mostly) and calcium-l-methylfolate. Folic acid is not present in food and the conjugated forms of folate found in food (see Chapter 14) are not listed as permitted forms.

This chapter contains an overview of supplement use and a brief discussion of some substances used as supplements that are not discussed elsewhere in this book. Specific vitamins and minerals and natural oils are discussed in the relevant chapters of the book, and some substances that may be used as functional foods and discussed in Chapter 19 may also sometimes be taken as dietary supplements (e.g. soy extracts and phytosterols).

Key points

- Almost anything taken in medicinal form that is not a licensed medicine is legally classified as a dietary supplement in the USA but in the EU, some plant extracts with limited history of use as foods are now classified as traditional herbal medicinal products and must be registered as such.
- Most dietary supplements are covered by five categories: essential micronutrients; endogenously produced organic substances with vitamin-like roles; natural fats and oils; plant and animal extracts; and the anti-oxidants.
- Supplements are taken to ensure adequacy, to compensate for some (perceived) increase in need, to prevent or treat disease, or to enhance athletic performance.
- Some potential problems of supplement use are:
  - direct toxicity
  - uncertain purity, identity, dosage and bio-availability
  - use as an easy alternative to more useful dietary or lifestyle changes
  - effects on the activity of prescription drugs, or use as an alternative to prescribed medicines.
- A third of British adults and perhaps two-thirds of American adults take dietary supplements.
- Supplements of micronutrients are taken by those with the highest intakes from food and who need them least.
- Micronutrient supplements make a significant difference to average intakes of particular vitamins or minerals, but make almost no difference to the median intakes or the number of people recording unsatisfactory intakes.   →

Key points *continued*

- British regulations are liberal by international standards. For many vitamins and minerals it is legal to sell supplements containing many multiples of the RNI. In some other European countries, only single or low multiples of the RNI may be sold as supplements and higher doses are classed as medicines. There are long-term plans to harmonize permitted maximum doses across the EU.

- The use of high doses of vitamins and minerals could be regarded as a pharmacological (i.e. drug) use rather than a nutritional one.

- In 2004, a voluntary code was introduced in the UK whereby supplements that exceeded an agreed dose should carry an appropriate warning about possible adverse effects. Suppliers were advised to reformulate such products.

- The Food Supplements Directive came into force across the EU in August 2005. This contains a list of permitted vitamins and minerals that can be used in supplements, and a list of the permissible chemical forms that can be used.

FOOD FORTIFICATION

[after a review by Webb, 2011b]

The term food fortification is generally used (and used in this book) to cover the addition of micronutrients for any reason. However, the Codex Alimentarius Commission has given it a more specific definition and identified three reasons why nutrients may be added to food.

- *Restoration.* This is the replacement of nutrients that have been lost during the processing of foods. An example is the addition of B vitamins to white flour to replace those lost during milling.
- *Substitution.* This is the addition of nutrients to a substitute food that are present in the food it is designed to replace. Examples are the addition of vitamins A and D to margarine to match the amounts in summer butter, and the addition of vitamin B_{12} to vegetarian meat substitutes.
- *Fortification.* This is the enrichment of a food with nutrients whether or not they are naturally present in that food, to improve dietary

adequacy. An example is the addition of nutrients to breakfast cereals.

Food fortification is usually deemed to have begun with the addition of iodine to salt in Michigan, USA, in 1924. Widespread use of iodized salt is credited with having played a major part in eliminating endemic goitre due to iodine deficiency in the USA and in Switzerland (see Chapter 15 for further discussion). Fortification of flour and other cereal products with niacin is also credited with helping to eliminate pellagra in southern states of the USA. Prior to 1930 this niacin deficiency disease caused much illness and many deaths in these southern states (see Chapter 14 for further discussion of this example). During the Second World War it became (and remains) a legal requirement in the UK to add vitamins A and D to margarine and to add niacin, thiamin, calcium and iron to most flour. In the USA, the FDA sets standards of identity for enriched foods like breads, flours, corn meals, rice noodles, macaroni and margarine; while it is not a mandatory requirement to fortify foods, any food labelled as enriched must comply with these standards of identity. Thus in order to comply with the standard of identity for bread and flour, these must contain added riboflavin, thiamin, niacin and, since January 1998, folic acid (folic acid fortification is discussed in detail in Chapter 14).

In addition to any mandatory fortification, manufacturers may add micronutrients to a food to improve its marketability. For example, vitamins and minerals are added to many breakfast cereals, vitamins A and D are added to skimmed milk powder, and vitamin B_{12} is added to textured vegetable protein used as a meat substitute by vegetarians. Fletcher *et al.* (2004) estimated that foods subject to mandatory fortification represented about 19 per cent of total UK energy intake and those that were voluntarily fortified a further 3 per cent. Of course, if extra intakes of a nutrient have potential to do harm then the whole population will be exposed to this risk.

Fortification of foods with micronutrients should raise average nutrient intakes and if an almost universally consumed food is fortified it should also raise median intakes and reduce the numbers of people consuming inadequate amounts of the nutrients concerned.

Key points

- The term food fortification can be used to describe the addition of micronutrients to foods for any purpose. More specifically, micronutrients can be added to food to compensate for processing losses (restoration), to make a substitute food nutritionally equivalent to a food it replaces (substitution), or to enrich a food that may or may not normally contain the nutrient (fortification).

- Iodized salt played an important part in eliminating endemic goitre in the USA and Switzerland. Niacin fortification of flour and other grain foods helped to eliminate pellagra in the USA.

- In the UK, most flour must be fortified with niacin, thiamin, iron and calcium and margarine fortified with vitamins A and D. In the USA, bread and flour must be fortified with riboflavin, thiamin, niacin and folic acid in order to meet FDA standards of identity.

- In addition to any mandatory fortification, some manufacturers may choose to voluntarily add micronutrients to their products.

- Foods subject to mandatory fortification account for around 19 per cent of UK energy intake and voluntarily fortified foods a further 3 per cent.

- Fortification of a core food should raise median intakes and raise the intakes of those with low intakes as well as simply increasing average intakes.

ASSESSMENT OF THE MICRONUTRIENT ADEQUACY OF BRITISH ADULTS

A National Diet and Nutrition Survey (NDNS) of adults aged 19–64 years was conducted in 2000–1, reported in summary by Hoare *et al.* (2004). Although since 2006 there has been a rolling programme of NDNS surveys of people aged over 18 months, this is the most recent comprehensive survey of the diets and nutritional status of adults in the UK. This and similar surveys have been used to highlight unsatisfactory intakes and/or poor biochemical status in the UK (Fletcher *et al.*, 2004; Webb, 2007, 2011, and in the previous edition of this book). At other places in this book the latest

NDNS data are used (Bates *et al.*, 2011) – for example, to give estimates of current intakes of macronutrient fractions and dietary fibre to assess compliance with daily reference values (DRVs, e.g. in Chapter 5) and to directly compare the diets of children, adults and elderly adults (e.g. in Chapter 16). At the time of preparing this new edition only limited data have been released from this rolling programme, and it is based on relatively small samples and uses a 4-day food diary rather than a weighed inventory. Other limitations of the data currently available are that:

- it does not subdivide adults within the 19- to 64-year age range into smaller age bands
- there is no published information on biochemical assessment of micronutrient status or salt intake.

While the quantitative details may have changed since this survey was conducted, it is still almost certainly true that many individuals have unsatisfactory intakes or unsatisfactory biochemical status for one or more essential nutrients. This may be true even where average intakes of the nutrient appear to be satisfactory (i.e. above the RNI).

Vitamins

Hoare *et al.* (2004) reported that, for all vitamins, the mean intakes from food were above or very close to the RNI, with the one exception of the vitamin A intakes of men and women in the 19- to 24-year age group. For several vitamins the mean intake was well above the RNI, with the mean being at least double the RNI in men and women for niacin, vitamin B_{12} and vitamin C and also (for men only) for thiamin and vitamin B_6. In general, the average intakes of men were a higher proportion of the RNI than those for women, although this was entirely due to the higher total food intake of men; the nutrient density (amount of nutrient per calorie) of men's diets was actually lower than that of the women. The intakes of the youngest 19–24 age groups were less than those of the total sample for every vitamin and in both sexes.

These high average intakes of most vitamins give a seemingly reassuring picture of the vitamin adequacy of British adult diets. However, when one considers the distribution of individual intakes then the picture is less reassuring. The apparently satisfactory average intakes of most vitamins tended to conceal a substantial number of individuals whose intakes were unsatisfactory (below the lowest RNI); for example:

- 7 per cent of men and 9 per cent of women had unsatisfactory vitamin A intakes, and these rose to 16 and 19 per cent, respectively, in the 19- to 24 year olds
- 3 per cent of men and 8 per cent of women had unsatisfactory intakes of riboflavin, which again rose in the 19- to 24 year olds to 8 and 15 per cent, respectively
- 5 per cent of 19- to 24-year-old women have unsatisfactory vitamin B_6 intake.

Note that these figures apply only to food intake of vitamins, but about 35 per cent of those taking part in the survey were taking dietary supplements. The supplements had little effect on the numbers of people with low vitamin intakes; they tend to be taken by those with the highest intake from food and who need them least. This is a general finding. For example, in an earlier survey of elderly people in the UK, Finch *et al.* (1998) found that supplements increased average intakes of vitamin A and folate but made almost no difference to median intakes. In Chapter 16, data from the latest NDNS survey are presented which show that the percentage of elderly people recording micronutrient intakes below the LRNI is almost exactly the same whether supplements are included in the total intake or not.

It is recommended that all women who could become pregnant take a supplement of 400 μg per day of folic acid in order to minimize the risk of neural tube defects if they become pregnant. However, well over 85 per cent of women of child-bearing age took in less than this value from food and supplements combined. Three per cent of young women (aged 19–24 years) had dietary folate intakes below the LRNI of 100 μg/day.

The nutritional status for vitamins was also assessed biochemically in this survey by analysing *blood samples*. Significant findings included the following.

- Five per cent of men and 3 per cent of women showed biochemical evidence of vitamin C depletion, even though almost none had recorded unsatisfactory intakes of vitamin C and average

recorded intakes were more than twice the RNI. It is possible that the use of food tables overestimated the amount of vitamin C in food as it was eaten.
- Four per cent of men and 5 per cent of women showed biochemical evidence of marginal folate status, with highest prevalence in the youngest age groups.
- Two per cent of men and 4 per cent of women had biochemical evidence of vitamin B_{12} depletion, even though average recorded intakes were 3–4 times the RNI and the number of individuals with unsatisfactory intakes was very low. Vitamin B_{12} deficiency is most often due to poor absorption, including pernicious anaemia.
- Two-thirds of the total sample showed biochemical evidence of riboflavin, although it was noted in the report that this assay is very sensitive to mild depletion of riboflavin in the tissues and thus this almost certainly considerably exaggerates the true extent of riboflavin deficiency in UK adults.
- More than 10 per cent of the total sample had biochemical evidence of vitamin B_6 deficiency.
- Fourteen per cent of men and 15 per cent of women showed biochemical evidence of vitamin D deficiency, with almost double these proportions in the youngest age groups. There is no RNI for vitamin D for adults because it assumed that the endogenous production in the skin when it is exposed to summer sunlight is the primary source of this vitamin for most people. Average dietary intakes of vitamin D were only 3–4 μg/day, which is far less than the 10–15 μg/day recommended for those who do not get regular sunlight exposure. To emphasize this pre-eminence of sunlight as the main source of vitamin D, around 23 per cent of those sampled in the winter had low biochemical status for vitamin D compared to around 3 per cent of those sampled in the summer.

Table 13.2 shows a summary of average vitamin intakes as a percentage of the RNI, the percentage of people recording dietary intakes below the LRNI, and the percentage of those whose blood analysis fell below the value taken to indicate depleted status of the vitamin. It should be borne in mind when viewing Table 13.2, and Table 13.3 later in the chapter, that even where these tables indicate

Table 13.2 Vitamin adequacy of British diets in adults aged 19–64*

Vitamin	Average intake (% RNI)				% below LRNI				% below biochemical threshold			
	Men (aged)		Women (aged)		Men (aged)		Women (aged)		Men (aged)		Women (aged)	
	19–64	19–24	19–64	19–24	19–64	19–24	19–64	19–24	19–64	19–24	19–64	19–24
A (retinol equivalents)	130	80	112	78	7	16	9	19	0	0	0	0
Thiamin	214	160	193	181	1	2	1	0	3	0	1	0
Riboflavin	162	129	146	126	3	8	8	15	66	82	66	77
Niacin equivalents	268	232	257	246	0	0	1	2	–	–	–	–
B_6	204	189	169	165	1	0	2	5	10	4	11	12
B_{12}	431	296	319	266	0	1	1	1	2	0	4	5
Folate[1]	172	151	125	114	0	2	2	3	4	13	5	8
C	209	162	202	170	0	0	0	1	5	7	3	4
D[2]	3.7 (µg)	2.9 (µg)	2.8 (µg)	2.3 (µg)	–	–	–	–	14	24	15	28

*Data from Hoare et al. (2004).
[1] Biochemical value is red cell folate indicating marginal status.
[2] No adult RNI or LRNI for vitamin D – absolute values given.

apparently low percentages of people with inadequate intakes of vitamins or mineral this would still translate into many thousands or even hundreds of thousands of affected individuals if these recorded intakes are truly representative of the usual intakes of British adults.

Minerals

As with vitamin intakes, the findings of Hoare et al. (2004) showed a general tendency for average intakes of essential minerals to be lowest in the youngest 19- to 24-year age group. Male values were also substantially higher than female values, reflecting the higher average food intakes of men. For older men the average intakes of all minerals were at or above the RNI, but for magnesium, potassium, zinc and copper the intakes of men aged 19–24 were significantly below the RNI, as were the potassium intakes of men aged 25–34.

The average iron intakes of all age groups of women were substantially below the iron RNI, except for the oldest group who were assumed to be post-menopausal and thus had the same lower RNI as men. In the youngest age group, the recorded intake was only 60 per cent of the RNI. Average

magnesium, potassium and copper intakes were significantly or substantially below the RNI for all age groups of women, and the average iodine intake of the youngest age group of women was also below the RNI.

Around 25 per cent of women had unsatisfactory recorded iron intakes (below the LRNI), and this figure rose to 42 per cent in the youngest age group of women. Blood analysis indicated that 3 per cent of men and 8 per cent of women were anaemic (haemoglobin concentrations below 13 g/100 mL and 12 g/100 mL, respectively). Serum ferritin concentrations are regarded as a more sensitive indicator of iron status; 4 per cent of men and 11 per cent of women had values indicative of depleted iron stores. The analysis of the distribution of individual intakes of minerals indicates that substantial proportions of men and women, particularly in the youngest age group, had unsatisfactory intakes of some minerals.

A summary of average mineral intakes expressed as a percentage of the RNI, the percentage of individuals with recorded intakes below the LRNI and, for iron only, the percentage with blood values below the threshold value indicating depletion are shown in Table 13.3.

Table 13.3 Mineral adequacy of diets of British adults aged 19–64*

Mineral	Average intake (% RNI)				% below LRNI				% below biochemical threshold			
	Men (aged)		Women (aged)		Men (aged)		Women (aged)		Men (aged)		Women (aged)	
	19–64	19–24	19–64	19–24	19–64	19–24	19–64	19–24	19–64	19–24	19–64	19–24
Iron[1]	151	131	82	60	1	3	25	42	3 (4)	0 (4)	8 (11)	7 (16)
Calcium	144	123	111	99	2	5	5	8	–	–	–	–
Magnesium	103	86	85	76	9	17	13	22	–	–	–	–
Potassium	96	81	76	67	6	18	19	30	–	–	–	–
Zinc	107	95	105	98	4	7	4	5	–	–	–	–
Iodine	154	119	114	93	2	2	4	12	–	–	–	–
Copper	119	95	86	76	–	–	–	–	–	–	–	–

*Data from Hoare et al. (2004).
[1] The two biochemical values are the value for haemoglobin indicative of anaemia and in parentheses the value for serum ferritin indicative of iron store depletion.

Summing up the vitamin and mineral adequacy of adult British diets

With a few exceptions, the average intake of most vitamins and minerals is above the RNI. However, for many nutrients there are significant numbers of individuals, particularly in the younger age groups, who have recorded intakes that are indicative of inadequacy. Even where the percentage of affected individuals is apparently low, it should be noted that a 2 per cent frequency among British adults aged under 65 years would translate into half a million affected people. The errors and uncertainties in measuring habitual food intake and in translating this into nutrient intakes are discussed in Chapter 3 and must be borne in mind when interpreting the results. Another point is that the interpretation of measured values as indicating deficiency or adequacy is very dependent on the validity of the standards against which they are compared. The following are some examples.

- According to the blood analysis, about 66 per cent of adults are classified as having low riboflavin status whereas only 5–6 per cent recorded inadequate riboflavin intakes. Either the biochemical assessment exaggerated the extent of deficiency or perhaps the LRNI is set too low.

- Fewer than 0.5 per cent of adults recorded vitamin C intakes below the LRNI whereas about 5 per cent had plasma vitamin C levels below the threshold value indicating vitamin depletion. This may reflect a problem with the standards used or perhaps with the values used for the vitamin C content of some foods as eaten.

- If American RDA had been used to interpret the values obtained from this survey, the average values for zinc, folate and vitamin E would be below these for both sexes, as would the calcium intakes for women. In general the interpretation would be substantially worse if the generally higher American dietary standards were used rather than the British ones.

Strategies for improving micronutrient adequacy

The information summarized in the previous subsection shows that there is a need to increase micronutrient intakes in British adults, and more especially to raise the intakes of those with the lowest intakes rather than simply raising average intakes. Webb (2011a) discusses three potential ways of raising micronutrient intakes and these are outlined below.

- *Dietary improvement.* Encourage and facilitate consumption of a diverse and nutrient-rich diet.

This seems like the ideal solution from a nutritionist's point of view, but it may be a long and difficult process to get satisfactory intakes of all micronutrients for all sectors of the population even in a generally wealthy industrialized country. In some instances simple dietary improvement may be an impractical solution. For instance, it may be very difficult to achieve good vitamin D status in people not regularly exposed to summer sunlight, and it will be very difficult to raise folate intakes to the extent needed to substantially reduce the incidence of neural tube defects.

- *Use of micronutrient supplements.* This is likely to raise average intakes and supplement advice can be targeted specifically to those likely to benefit. If necessary, high doses can be used without exposing everyone to them. However, supplements are likely to have limited impact because they tend to be taken by those who already have the highest intakes from food and are least likely to need them. It is possible that well-designed and well-targeted campaigns with the provision of free supplements might be effective in raising intakes of those who need them but the general failure of attempts to increase folate intakes in fertile and sexually active women to reduce the incidence of neural tube defects is a discouraging precedent (see Chapter 14).
- *Food fortification.* If a universally consumed food is fortified with a nutrient, this should not only increase average intakes but also raise median intakes and help those with the lowest current intakes from food. It will also further increase the intakes of those with the highest current intakes and greatly increase the intakes of those consuming high amounts of the fortified food. These factors may risk exposing some people to harmful amounts of the micronutrient. It is likely that there will be opposition from some quarters to any attempt to widen the use of food fortification and unequivocal demonstration of safety may be difficult.

The sections on vitamin D and folic acid in Chapter 14 are good examples of case studies that highlight these issues. See also discussion of these examples in Webb (2011a).

Key points

- Average intakes of all vitamins of British adults in 2000 were above the RNI, with the exception of the vitamin A intakes of 19- to 24 year olds.
- Average intakes of a few minerals were below the RNI. This was most pronounced in women and in the lowest age groups (19- to 24 year olds).
- Analysis of the distribution of individual intakes of micronutrients indicates that large numbers of people had intakes of one or more vitamin or mineral that were inadequate (i.e. below the LRNI).
- Many individuals had intakes below the LRNI even where average intakes appeared to be satisfactory.
- The frequency of inadequate intakes was generally higher in women than men and was generally highest in the youngest adults.
- Biochemical assessment of nutritional status for vitamins and for iron also indicated that relatively large numbers of individuals had values that lie on the wrong side of the normal threshold values for adequacy.
- Details of the intakes and measured biochemical status of individual vitamins and minerals are given in Tables 13.2 and 13.3.
- The problem of low micronutrient intakes could be addressed by dietary improvement, use of supplements or fortification of foods with micronutrients.
- Dietary improvement may be a long and difficult process and it may not be practicable to achieve target intakes of some nutrients from diet alone (e.g. for vitamin D and folate in young women).
- Supplements are already widely used. Evidence suggests that they do little to help those with low intakes from food as they tend to be taken by those who need them least.
- Fortification of a core food should raise intakes in those with low intakes, but it may mean that some people are exposed to undesirably high amounts of the micronutrient.

ANTI-OXIDANTS AND THE OXIDANT THEORY OF DISEASE

Nature and effects of free radicals

Free radicals are highly reactive species that have an unpaired electron (e.g. the *hydroxyl* and *superoxide* radicals). The electrons in an atom or molecule orbit the nucleus in shells or layers and the most stable configuration is when these electrons are in pairs that orbit in opposite directions. If an atom or molecule within the body loses or gains an electron then the resulting product is highly reactive and can react with and damage DNA, proteins, lipids or carbohydrates. Cellular damage caused by oxygen-derived free radical species has been implicated in the aetiology of a range of diseases including cancer, atherosclerosis, cataract and age-related macular degeneration (ARMD) and has been suggested as a major contributory factor in the ageing process.

The reactions of free radicals involve the loss or gain of an electron and this can create another free radical, which can initiate a damaging chain reaction unless the free radical is quenched by anti-oxidant systems and the chain reaction halted. This chain reaction has been likened to a line of dominoes: when one is knocked over it falls and knocks over the next, and so on along the line.

- Oxygen free radicals can react with DNA to cause breaks in the DNA chain and alteration of bases (mutation); this could initiate carcinogenesis. The measurement of concentrations of unusual bases like thymine glycol and 8-hydroxy guanine in urine is used as an experimental measure of the oxidative damage to DNA.
- Free radicals can peroxidize polyunsaturated fatty acid residues in *low-density lipoprotein* (LDL). This altered LDL is taken up by macrophages and generates foam cells, which ultimately leads to the scarring and fibrosis of artery walls seen in atherosclerosis. Unoxidized LDL may be relatively benign in its effects on artery walls.
- Free radicals can peroxidize polyunsaturated fatty acid residues in membranes, and this can alter membrane function. In this case, peroxidation of a polyunsaturated fatty acid will generate another unstable compound (the *lipid peroxyl* radical) and this reacts with another fatty acid to produce a

stable lipid peroxide and another peroxyl radical, and so on. This chain reaction would be stopped by vitamin E scavenging the peroxyl residue or by two peroxyl residues interacting to form the stable compound malondialdehyde. The concentration of malondialdehyde in plasma is used as a measure of 'oxidative stress'. Their supposed susceptibility to free radical damage is one of the concerns about diets with very high levels of polyunsaturated fat.

- Free radicals can cause fragmentation of proteins, oxidize sulfhydryl groups on sulphur-containing amino acids, or disrupt sites where metal cofactors bind to proteins.
- Free radicals can degrade the complex polysaccharide *hyaluronic acid* found in synovial fluid and connective tissue and which acts as a viscous lubricant in joints. Neutrophils may generate free radicals in inflamed joints and this inflammation may lead to osteoarthritic damage in the joint.

More than 50 years ago, Denham Harman put forward his free radical theory of ageing in which he postulated that the cumulative effects of free radical damage to macromolecules such as these would make a major contribution to the degenerative changes associated with ageing and to the development of chronic age-related diseases. In Harman (1972), he went on to suggest that the addition of one or more free-radical inhibitors to a good natural diet might increase the average age of death by up to 7 years. Data from clinical trials clearly indicate that this was an optimistic assessment and there is no clear evidence of any holistic benefit from anti-oxidant supplements when given to well-nourished populations.

Oxygen free radicals are a normal by-product of the oxidative processes of the cell. Some of the processes that generate free radicals are listed below.

- Free radicals are a by-product of the electron transport chain.
- Certain environmental factors increase the generation of free radicals. Examples are cigarette smoke, exposure to high oxygen tension, exposure to ionizing radiation including sunlight, some chemicals including excesses of certain anti-oxidant nutrients like iron and perhaps β-carotene.

• Phagocytic white cells generate oxygen free radicals to kill ingested bacteria and fungi and destroy other 'foreign bodies'. They can also secrete these reactive species into surrounding tissues (e.g. to kill large parasites) and this can cause significant damage to surrounding tissues. Injured and diseased tissue thus has high levels of free radicals. This notion that a burst of oxygen free radicals, 'the respiratory burst', generated by neutrophils is responsible for killing tough bacteria and parasites has been used to emphasize their destructive potential and thus their capacity to produce the cellular damage that eventually leads to chronic disease. In the previous edition of this book a paper published in *Nature* (Ahluwalia *et al.*, 2004) was discussed. That paper presented 'evidence' that it is not free radicals produced by neutrophils that kill ingested bacteria, but rather the protease enzymes that they produce, and that an influx of potassium ions via a large-conductance calcium-activated potassium channel (BK channel) was essential for this process. It was implied that these results undermined the oxidant theory of disease because, if free radicals are not as toxic as is generally believed, then they may not play such a prominent role in the aetiology of chronic disease. Several authors have tried unsuccessfully to repeat this work. In an editorial article, DeCoursey (2007) makes a very convincing case for disregarding the paper. He discusses evidence that the key BK channel said by Ahluwalia to be critical in the killing of ingested micro-organisms by neutrophils is not even present on neutrophils. This *Nature* paper was retracted in late 2010 by all of the co-authors except Ahluwalia (see section on scientific honesty in Chapter 4).

Physiological mechanisms to limit free radical damage

Free radicals are normal by-products of the oxidative processes in cells, and there are thus necessarily several physiological mechanisms whose specific role is to neutralize these free radicals and limit their tissue-damaging effects. There are other mechanisms for the repair of the cellular damage induced by free radicals, such as enzymes that repair damaged segments of DNA and selenium-containing enzymes that remove lipid peroxides. Figure 13.1 summarizes some of the mechanisms involved in the disposal of free radicals.

Superoxide dismutase converts superoxide radicals to hydrogen peroxide

$$O_2^{\bullet-} + O_2^{\bullet-} + 2H^+ \xrightarrow{\text{superoxide dismutase}} H_2O_2 + O_2$$

Glutathione peroxidase converts hydrogen peroxide to water

$$H_2O_2 + \text{reduced glutathione} \xrightarrow{\text{glutathione reductase}} H_2O + \text{oxidized glutathione}$$

Glutathione reductase regenerates reduced glutathione

$$\text{Oxidized glutathione} \xrightarrow{\text{glutathione reductase}} \text{reduced glutathione}$$

The enzyme catalase (iron-containing) converts hydrogen peroxide to water and oxygen

$$2H_2O_2 \xrightarrow{\text{catalase}} 2H_2O + O_2$$

Vitamin E can quench free radicals when it is oxidized

$$\text{Free radical} + \text{vitamin E} \longrightarrow \text{water} + \text{oxidized E}$$

$$\text{Lipid peroxyl radical} + \text{vit. E} \longrightarrow \text{stable hydroperoxide} + \text{oxidized E}$$

Vitamin E can be regenerated by a mechanism that involves vitamin C

$$\text{Oxidized E} \xrightarrow{\text{regeneration (vit C)}} \text{vitamin E}$$

Figure 13.1 Some of the mechanisms for the disposal of free radicals.

There are a number of metal-containing enzymes whose function is to scavenge and dispose of free radicals. Several essential nutrients are components of, or cofactors for, enzymes that are involved in free radical disposal, and some examples are listed below.

- Zinc, copper and manganese are components of the enzyme *superoxide dismutase* (SOD), which disposes of the superoxide radical by converting two superoxide radicals to hydrogen peroxide and oxygen. The SOD in the cytoplasm is a copper- and zinc-containing enzyme whereas that found in mitochondria requires manganese.
- Selenium is a component of the enzyme *glutathione peroxidase*, which neutralizes hydrogen peroxide (a powerful oxidizing agent) and converts it to water and oxygen. It also converts peroxidized lipids into stable and harmless products.
- Iron is a component of haem which is a prosthetic group within the enzyme *catalase*. This enzyme converts hydrogen peroxide to water and oxygen.
- The enzyme *glutathione reductase* regenerates the reduced form of glutathione, which is oxidized by the glutathione peroxidase reaction mentioned above. This enzyme is a flavoprotein and utilizes a riboflavin derivative as a prosthetic group.

Defects in these free radical disposal mechanisms can have catastrophic consequences, demonstrating the critical importance of these mechanisms for health.

- Deficiency of the copper–zinc superoxide dismutase in mice leads to skeletal muscle atrophy, the development of liver nodules and liver cancer (Elchuri *et al.*, 2005).
- Deficiency of manganese-dependent superoxide dismutase in mice leads to rapid death with cardiomyopathy and metabolic abnormalities (Li *et al.*, 1995).
- A rare genetic disorder (Takahara's disease) in which there is absence of the enzyme catalase results in oral gangrene (Ogata *et al.*, 2008) and early development of type 2 diabetes due to hydrogen peroxide damage to the pancreatic β cells.
- 'Knockout' mice in which the enzyme glutathione peroxidise 1 had been deleted

showed early cardiac hypertrophy and hypertension (Ardanaz *et al.*, 2010).

In addition to these enzyme systems, some vitamins and other plant pigments have innate anti-oxidant properties and so have the capacity to scavenge free radicals; examples are vitamin E in the lipid phase and vitamin C in the aqueous phase. Vitamin E is used as an anti-oxidant food additive by food manufacturers to prevent fatty foods becoming rancid, and vitamin C is similarly used as a water-soluble anti-oxidant food additive. Some of the substances in food that are known to have or probably have an anti-oxidant effect are:

- the essential minerals selenium, zinc, copper and iron
- vitamins C and E
- β-carotene and other carotenoids including lycopene (abundant in tomatoes), lutein (found in green vegetables), α-carotene, zeathanthin and cryptoxanthin
- other plant pigments including the flavonoids found in some fruits, tea and red wine and the polyphenols found in many herbs and spices, some fruits, tea, chocolate and olive oil
- synthetic anti-oxidants like butylated hydroxytoluene (BHT) and butylated hydroxyanisole (BHA) used as food additives to prevent rancidity of fats.
- other substances with vitamin-like roles are endogenously synthesized in sufficient amounts to meet physiological need and so they are not classified as essential nutrients. Examples are ubiquinone (co-enzyme Q_{10}) from organ meats and yeast extract, lipoic acid from green leafy vegetables, glutathione from yeast extract, and glutamine (an amino acid that acts as a glutathione precursor).

Many natural extracts of fruits and vegetables sold as supplements and many so-called 'superfoods' (see Chapter 19) are marketed on the basis of their high anti-oxidant content; examples are goji berries, pomegranates, green tea, red grapes, acai berries, blueberries, cranberries, bilberries, tomatoes and red peppers. However, some of the extracts of these foods that are sold in pill form as supplements contain very little of the food concerned. The following are examples of claimed amounts in supplement pills:

bilberry extract has the equivalent of 0.5 g of whole fruit and the high-strength version 5 g; goji berry tablets have the equivalent of 1.5 g of berries; and acai berry extract has 2 g of whole berries. (Two blueberries taken from my fridge weighed 3 g.)

Situations that might increase damage by free radicals

The following circumstances may increase the risk of disease due to free radical damage of cellular components.

- *Increased generation of free radicals beyond the capacity of the mechanisms for their safe disposal and repair of the damage that they induce.* This might be due to exposure to noxious environmental stimuli like ionizing radiation (including sunlight), cigarette smoke, high oxygen concentration, and certain toxic chemicals. It might also be caused by any infection or injury that leads to inflammation and the generation of excess free radicals by neutrophils that infiltrate the diseased or injured area.
- *Impaired capacity of the disposal mechanisms to handle any free radicals that are generated.* This might perhaps be due to dietary deficiency of a key anti-oxidant nutrient. Thus it seems highly probable that deficiency of vitamin E, vitamin C or selenium, for example, would slow down the rate of free radical disposal and increase the cellular damage that they cause.

The severe effects of defects in the key enzymes involved in free radical disposal were discussed earlier.

If premature babies are exposed to elevated oxygen concentration in their incubators, this can cause damage to the retina and lead to blindness (*retinopathy of prematurity*). High oxygen concentration is thought to lead to excessive generation of oxygen free radicals, which are responsible for the retinal damage. There is evidence that vitamin E, a free radical scavenger, protects these babies from the damaging effects of oxygen. High oxygen concentration of inspired air also produces lung damage in adults. When water is exposed to ionizing radiations, this generates hydroxyl radicals and they are responsible for much

of the damage to living cells caused by ionizing radiations. There is also evidence that the toxic effects of excess iron may be due to free radical effects; *in vitro*, excess iron in serum stimulates lipid peroxidation and the formation of damaging hydroxyl radicals from hydrogen peroxide. Cigarette smoke and other air pollutants may exert some of their harmful effects by generating free radicals.

In most diseases there is increased formation of oxygen free radicals as a consequence of the disease process. Infiltration of white cells into damaged or diseased tissue will result in excess oxidant load because superoxide generation (the respiratory burst) is used by these cells to kill pathogenic bacteria. Mechanical injury to tissue also results in increased free radical reactions. This means that injured or diseased tissue generates free radicals much faster than healthy tissue, so reports that biochemical indices of free radical damage are raised in disease states should be treated with caution. These raised free radical indices may be a reflection of the disease process rather than an indication that free radical 'attack' is a key factor in initiating the disease; and they do not necessarily indicate that free radical scavengers like vitamin E will prevent or ameliorate the condition. For example, in experimental deficiency of vitamin E in rats there is a muscular atrophy that resembles that seen in the fatal, inherited, human disease of muscular dystrophy. Indices of free radical damage are indeed also raised in the wasting muscles of boys afflicted with muscular dystrophy, but vitamin E does not alter the progress of the disease. In this instance, the free radical damage is almost certainly a result of the disease rather than its primary cause.

The anti-oxidant minerals, together with riboflavin, are essential components of enzyme systems involved in the safe disposal of free radicals. Deficiencies of these micronutrients might be expected to reduce the activity of these disposal mechanisms and thus increase tissue damage by free radicals. However, given this mode of action, it seems unlikely that high intakes would exert any extra protective effects. Selenium or zinc deficiency might be expected to increase free radical damage, but it seems improbable that supplements of these minerals, in well-nourished people, would supply any extra protection against free radicals by increasing synthesis of their dependant enzymes. *Keshan disease* may be an example of a deficiency disease due to lack of one of these anti-oxidant minerals. In this condition there is a potentially fatal degeneration of the heart muscle (*cardiomyopathy*). This disease has been reported in certain areas of China where the soil is very low in selenium. Activity of the selenium-dependent enzyme glutathione peroxidase is low and the condition responds to selenium supplements; and so the disease has been attributed to lack of dietary selenium with consequent failure of the free radical disposal mechanism.

The other anti-oxidant vitamins (E and C) together with the carotenoids and other non-nutrient anti-oxidants have the capacity to react with and quench free radicals without themselves becoming highly reactive. They thus have a free-standing anti-oxidant effect, independent of the enzyme mechanisms. There has, therefore, been considerable speculation as to whether high intakes of these micronutrients and plant pigments might protect against free radical damage and, in particular, reduce the long-term risk of cardiovascular disease and cancer. Epidemiological studies consistently report a negative association between high intakes of fruits and vegetables and risk of cancer and cardiovascular disease, and these foods are the principal dietary sources of carotene, vitamin C and other plant pigments with anti-oxidant activity. This is why many national authorities recommend increased intake of fruits and vegetables – a minimum of five portions a day in the UK.

Figure 13.2 shows a theoretical scheme that seeks to explain how a free radical mechanism might be involved in the development of atherosclerosis. Such a scheme could explain the apparent interaction between several risk factors in the development of cardiovascular disease, and it might also help to explain why plasma LDL cholesterol concentration is an imperfect predictor of cardiovascular risk. A high saturated-fat diet tends to raise the LDL cholesterol concentration; cigarette smoking increases free radical production; and lack of dietary anti-oxidants limits the capacity to scavenge free radicals and thus to minimize the

damage that they can induce. Any unquenched free radicals can react with LDL to convert it to much more atherogenic oxidized forms. Oxidized LDL is taken up very readily by macrophages and these LDL-loaded macrophages become foam cells, which are characteristically found in atheromatous arterial lesions.

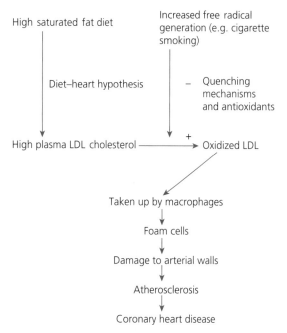

Figure 13.2 A hypothetical scheme to illustrate how free radicals might contribute to the risk of cardiovascular disease.

Figure 13.3 shows a summary scheme for the oxidant theory of disease and how various factors can interact to increase or decrease the cellular damage done by free radicals. Figure 13.4 shows a simplified version of this scheme. Various environmental stimuli, inflammation or disease states can increase free radical generation above its normal level. Deficiencies of anti-oxidant nutrients or defective disposal mechanisms can impair their disposal, while some drugs and non-nutrient anti-oxidants may facilitate their removal. Any surplus free radicals can cause damage to cellular components, and if the damage exceeds the capacity of repair mechanisms this may result in cumulative damage that ultimately leads to degenerative change and chronic disease.

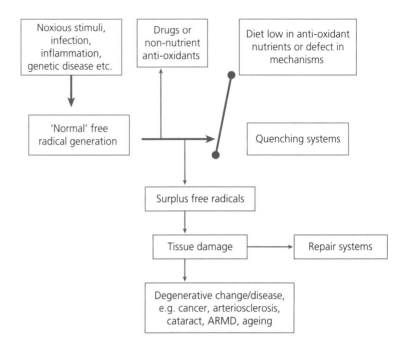

Figure 13.3 The free-radical theory of disease. Reproduced with permission from Webb (2006). ARMD, age-related macular degeneration.

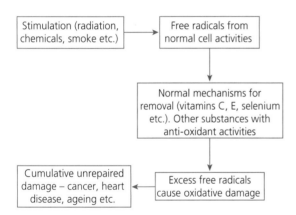

Figure 13.4 Simplified scheme showing the free radical theory of disease. Reproduced with permission from Webb (2007).

Key points

- Free radicals are highly reactive species that are normal by-products of metabolic processes and immune defence mechanisms.
- Free radicals can react with DNA, membrane phospholipids, proteins and other cellular components.
- Oxidative damage caused by reaction of free radicals with cellular components has been

→

Key points *continued*

implicated in the aetiology of several chronic diseases and perhaps even in ageing.

- In 1972 it was claimed that an anti-oxidant supplement would increase life expectancy by up to 7 years in a well-nourished population.
- Free radical reactions generate further free radicals. This can set up a damaging chain reaction leading to extensive cellular damage.
- Several cellular enzymes quench free radicals, and these enzymes have riboflavin or a dietary mineral as essential cofactors.
- Defects in one of these enzymes have major pathological consequences in people or animal models.
- Vitamins E and C and some plant pigments (e.g. the carotenoids) have inherent anti-oxidant and free radical quenching activity.
- Increased free radical damage occurs when there is excess free radical production or impaired free radical disposal.
- Free radical production is increased in injured or diseased tissue and by certain environmental exposures like radiation, sunlight, smoke or high oxygen pressure.

→

Key points *continued*

- Deficiencies of some anti-oxidant nutrients will impair the functioning of free radical quenching enzymes.

- There is much speculation that high intakes of those vitamins and plant pigments with inherent anti-oxidant activity may afford extra protection from free radicals and thus reduce the risk of chronic diseases (including cancer and atherosclerosis).

- Many fruits and vegetable foods are marketed as 'superfoods' on the basis of their anti-oxidant content. Extracts of some of these 'superfoods' are on the same basis sold as dietary supplements, but the tablets may contain very small amounts of the food.

DO HIGH ANTI-OXIDANT INTAKES PREVENT HEART DISEASE, CANCER AND OTHER CHRONIC DISEASES?

Hundreds of compounds in the diet have been claimed to have anti-oxidant activity. Anyone reading a catalogue of dietary supplements will find the term anti-oxidant mentioned for many of the products being promoted. However, relatively few of these potential anti-oxidants have been tested in high-quality clinical trials. In some cases all that has been demonstrated is that a food or supplement contains a chemical that has the potential to act as an anti-oxidant in a test tube. In most cases the claims about the likely long-term health benefits of an 'anti-oxidant-rich' food or supplement are based on extrapolation from observational data or from short-term reductionist studies, for example:

- their effect on some marker of anti-oxidant stress in short-term studies with experimental animals or human volunteers
- their ability to inhibit chemically induced cancers in experimental animals
- their ability to inhibit growth of cultured tumour cells *in vitro*
- their ability to inhibit mutagenesis in bacteria which is used as an indicator of anti-cancer potential
- the epidemiological association between high estimated anti-oxidant intake and lowered risk of heart diseases or cancer.

Many of the trials that have been carried out with human subjects have suffered from one or more of the following limitations:

- they have used small numbers of subjects
- they have been of short duration
- they have used reductionist outcome measures (e.g. a biochemical marker, a single symptom/disease)
- they have been poorly designed (e.g. not properly randomized and/or placebo controlled).

The discussion that follows therefore focuses on some of the anti-oxidants that have been subjected to more holistic testing of their long-term effects, namely:

- β-carotene and the other carotenoids
- vitamin E
- vitamin C
- selenium
- co-enzyme Q_{10}.

The carotenoids

In an influential paper, Peto *et al.* (1981) suggested that high intakes of β-carotene and other carotenoids might reduce the risk of human cancer. This effect was thought to be independent of their provitamin A activity. In the succeeding three decades, hundreds of research papers have addressed the role of carotenoids in the prevention of cancer and other chronic, degenerative diseases.

The carotenoids are a group of over 600 naturally occurring plant pigments and about 10 per cent of these have provitamin A activity. β-Carotene, α-carotene and cryptoxanthin act as provitamin A, but others found in significant amounts in human blood and tissues do not (e.g. lutein and lycopene). All the carotenoids have anti-oxidant activity and are able to quench oxygen free radicals. Lycopene has the most potent anti-oxidant effect. Coloured fruits and vegetables are the richest sources of carotenoids (e.g. carrots, green vegetables, tomatoes, cantaloupe melon):

- carrots are rich in β-carotene
- tomatoes and water melon are rich in lycopene
- green leafy vegetables and red peppers are rich in lutein
- mangoes and sweetcorn are rich in cryptoxanthin.

Details of the chemical mechanisms by which carotenoids are thought to exert an anti-oxidant effect may be found in Ball (2004).

High fruit and vegetable intake is associated with reduced risk of chronic disease

There is a huge body of evidence to suggest that diets high in fruits and vegetables are associated with low risk of cancers and other chronic diseases. This fruit and vegetable group is a major source of the anti-oxidant nutrients and of the many other non-nutrients in the diet with anti-oxidant potential. This therefore means that diets high in carotenoids, vitamin C and other anti-oxidants have been associated with reduced cancer risk and heart disease in many case–control and more reliable cohort studies. It is generally assumed that this association between fruit and vegetable intake is causal – hence the numerous campaigns in different countries to promote a large and varied intake of fruits and vegetables (like the five-a-day campaign in the UK). It is widely believed that their high anti-oxidant content is responsible for much of this reduction in chronic disease risk. If this is correct, then some of these benefits might also be gained by taking anti-oxidants in the form of dietary supplements – hence the prominence given to anti-oxidant effects of supplements in manufacturers' sales catalogues. There are, of course, several potential explanations for this reported association, some of which are noted below.

- The anti-oxidants in fruits and vegetables are directly protective against cancer and degenerative disease because of their anti-oxidant effects.
- Other components of fruits and vegetables might be exerting a protective effect and the raised anti-oxidant intakes are merely coincidental.
- High fruit and vegetable consumption is not directly protective but is merely a marker for a generally healthy diet (e.g. lower in fat, saturated fat or meat protein).
- High fruit and vegetable consumption is a marker for a generally healthy lifestyle – people who eat the most fruits and vegetables are the most affluent, physically active and health conscious.

Other largely observational evidence also supports the notion that anti-oxidants protect against the development of chronic disease. Examples are listed below.

- Low blood levels of β-carotene and other carotenoids (especially lycopene) are also associated with increased risk of some cancers (Ziegler, 1991).
- In some studies, carotenoids have also been reported to protect against experimentally induced cancers in laboratory animals despite the fact that β-carotene is very poorly absorbed by experimental animals.
- In a case–control study of 100 men with previously undiagnosed angina and 400 angina-free controls, Riemersma et al. (1991) found that blood levels of anti-oxidant vitamins were inversely related to risk of angina and that for vitamin E was significant even after correcting for confounding variables.
- Gey et al. (1991) reported an inverse correlation between blood levels of vitamin E and mortality from coronary heart disease in a cross-sectional study of men from 16 European countries (i.e. an apparent protective effect of vitamin E).
- Two large cohort studies in the early 1990s reported that in both women (Stampfer et al., 1993) and men (Rimm et al., 1993) consumption of high levels of vitamin E was associated with reduced risk of coronary heart disease. In both of these studies, the apparent benefit was only observed at doses of vitamin E beyond those consumed in typical US diets and was thus only observed in those taking supplements. Supplements were not associated with any significant reduction in overall mortality. These were not randomized, controlled trials but epidemiological cohort studies, so the subjects using supplements were self-selecting. This means that the supplement users were probably not representative of the total study population in many respects, and despite their best efforts the authors may not have been able to adequately correct for all of these confounding variables.

There is therefore a mass of observational and short-term experimental evidence to suggest a number of anti-oxidant substances may protect against chronic disease when taken in food or supplements. However, despite all of these hundreds of studies spread over more than 30 years there is still little direct holistic evidence that anti-oxidants, when take as supplements, afford any significant long-term protection against any major chronic disease or increase life expectancy in affluent well-nourished populations.

COMA (1994a), in a major report on dietary aspects of cardiovascular disease, concluded that the evidence of a protective effect of the anti-oxidant vitamins E and C against cardiovascular disease was at that time persuasive but not conclusive, and that it would be premature to make specific recommendations about increased intakes of these vitamins until several of the large controlled trials then underway were known. It did warn that the use of pharmaceutical preparations containing high levels of vitamins could not be assumed to be safe. It did, however, feel confident in recommending a diet rich in anti-oxidants – fruits and vegetables, nuts and seeds.

Four years later, when some of the ongoing intervention trials referred to by COMA had been completed or terminated, the COMA (1998) report concluded that, even though there was epidemiological evidence which indicated that high intakes of the anti-oxidant vitamins (β-carotene, vitamin C and vitamin E) were associated with reduced cancer risk, most of the intervention trials conducted had failed to confirm a protective effect of these vitamins against cancer. It also recommended caution in the use of purified micronutrient supplements, and specifically counselled against the use of β-carotene supplements. It concluded also that there was insufficient evidence to reach any conclusions about the relationship between dietary selenium or zinc and cancer risk. There was thus a marked shift of scientific opinion in the later part of the 1990s against the use of anti-oxidant supplements, and this shift has been maintained and strengthened in more recent years.

The Agency for Healthcare Research and Quality (AHRQ) commissioned an extensive report into the efficacy and safety of supplemental anti-oxidants (vitamins C, E and co-enzyme Q_{10}) for the prevention and treatment of cardiovascular disease (Shekelle *et al.*, 2003). The authors of this report identified 144 relevant clinical trials. Their conclusions after reviewing and re-analysing this information are summarized below.

- The evidence available in the literature did not support there being any benefit from supplements of vitamin E (either alone or in combination) on either cardiovascular or all-cause mortality.
- Likewise there was no evidence of any harm caused by vitamin E supplements.
- There was no consistent evidence to suggest a beneficial effect of vitamin E on the incidence of fatal or non-fatal myocardial infarction.
- Vitamin E supplements do not appear to have any significant effects on plasma lipids.
- Their conclusions for vitamin C were similar to those for vitamin E.
- For co-enzyme Q_{10} they found insufficient evidence to convincingly support or refute suggestions that supplements had any beneficial or harmful effects on cardiovascular outcomes.

The AHRQ also commissioned a similar report to investigate the effectiveness of these three anti-oxidants in the prevention and treatment of cancer (Coulter *et al.*, 2003). It also found no evidence to support beneficial effects of vitamin E and/or vitamin C in the prevention of new tumours, the development of colonic polyps or in the treatment of patients with advanced cancer.

One often-cited intervention (experimental) study that did have an apparently positive outcome was conducted in the Linxian province of China. Using 30 000 middle-aged Chinese subjects, Blot *et al.* (1993) found that supplements containing β-carotene, selenium and vitamin E produced a substantial reduction in cancer incidence. However, people living in this area had low baseline intakes of micronutrients, and indeed micronutrient insufficiency was a suspected cause of the very high incidence of certain cancers in this region. Any beneficial effect that might be due to extra β-carotene in this study was perhaps more likely to be related to its provitamin A activity than its anti-oxidant effects.

Over the last two decades there have been several, large controlled trials that have found no indication of benefit afforded by various anti-oxidant supplements and even some indication that β-carotene supplements may be harmful under some circumstances. Several examples are briefly described below.

- In an Italian study of vitamin E and n-3 (ω-3) polyunsaturated fatty acid supplements in 11 000 men who had had a previous myocardial infarction, there was no indication of any benefit from the vitamin E supplements after 3.5 years (GISSI, 1999).
- A 12-year trial of β-carotene supplements in 22 000 American physicians found no benefits of these supplements on either cancer or heart disease incidence (Hennekens et al., 1996).
- A study using male Finnish smokers found no evidence of benefit for either β-carotene or vitamin E. On the contrary, it reported significantly increased deaths from lung cancer, heart disease and strokes and increased total mortality (by 8 per cent) in those taking β-carotene supplements (Group, 1994). Smokers were originally chosen as subjects for this study because it was perceived that they might have most to gain from anti-oxidant supplements.
- The CARET trial tested the effects of combined retinol and β-carotene supplements using 18 000 American men identified as being at high risk of lung cancer because of smoking or work exposure to asbestos. This study was terminated prematurely because rates of lung cancer were higher in the supplemented group than in the placebo group (Omenn et al., 1996).
- Rapala et al. (1997) reported increased death rates from coronary heart disease in those subjects (smokers) given β-carotene supplements compared to those receiving either the placebo or vitamin E supplements.
- A randomized controlled trial of vitamin E supplements using 45 000 healthy women over 45 years compared supplements of natural vitamin E or aspirin to a placebo. After 10 years of follow-up there was no benefit of vitamin E on major cardiovascular events or cancer incidence, nor any effect on cancer, cardiovascular or total mortality (Lee et al., 2005).
- A placebo-controlled trial of vitamin C and E supplements in 2400 women at high risk of pre-eclampsia suggested no benefit from these anti-oxidant vitamins (Poston et al., 2006). A more recent meta-analysis confirmed the lack of any observable benefit of these supplements and the only statistically significant effects were adverse (Rumbold et al., 2008).

Vivekanathan et al. (2003) conducted a meta-analysis of seven large randomized trials of vitamin E supplements and eight trials of β-carotene supplements on long-term mortality and morbidity from cardiovascular disease. The vitamin E trials involved over 80 000 subjects and produced no evidence that these supplements reduced all-cause mortality, death from heart disease or from stroke. There was also no evidence that vitamin E supplements conferred any benefits to patients who had already experienced a cardiovascular event. The analysis of the β-carotene trials suggested a small but statistically significant increase in all-cause mortality and cardiovascular deaths in those receiving supplements (doses were between 15 and 50 mg/day).

Bjelakovic et al. (2008) published a systematic review and meta-analysis of the effects of nutrient anti-oxidant supplements (β-carotene, vitamin A, vitamin C, vitamin E and selenium). They analysed 21 primary prevention trials and 46 secondary prevention trials (i.e. 21 trials with healthy people and 46 that used people with a range of existing illnesses). When all the trials were included in the analysis then they found no effect of the supplements on mortality. However, when they confined their analysis to those studies with a low risk of bias, the supplements increased mortality by a small but statistically significant amount. These low-bias studies found that vitamin A, β-carotene and vitamin E supplements increased mortality by a small amount but that vitamin C and selenium had no statistically significant effect.

There is now a substantial body of high-quality evidence which suggests that supplements of the nutrient anti-oxidants have no significant beneficial effect on total, cardiovascular or cancer mortality in well-nourished populations, and there is some evidence that some of them may cause net harm to some groups of people, especially β-carotene in smokers and asbestos workers. Recent data make it seem unlikely that use of anti-oxidant supplements will substantially delay human death as suggested by Harman (1972).

In the past, β-carotene has generally been regarded as non-toxic even in very high doses of 300 mg/day (used to treat a condition called *erythropoietic protoporphyria*). However, data from these more recent trials seem to suggest that chronic use of doses of β-carotene supplements as low as 15 mg/day may have adverse effects on mortality risk, and especially on risk of lung cancer in smokers and asbestos workers. It is ironic that smokers and asbestos workers were initially chosen as subjects for these trials because it was thought that beneficial effects of anti-oxidant supplements might be more readily demonstrated in these high-risk subjects.

Paolini *et al.* (1999) suggested that β-carotene might exert a co-carcinogenic effect by inducing enzymes that activate certain environmental carcinogens. This was based on short-term experiments with rats. This theory could reconcile the paradox that epidemiological studies are consistent with a protective effect of β-carotene-rich diets on cancer risk whereas large supplements appear to increase lung cancer risk in those considered to be at high risk of developing this disease. Good intakes of anti-oxidants, including β-carotene, might prevent initial oxidative damage to DNA in the initiation of cancer, but high doses might activate carcinogens including those from cigarette smoke in those with high exposure to them.

Wang *et al.* (1999) exposed groups of ferrets (which absorb and metabolize β-carotene in a similar way to humans) to either β-carotene supplements, cigarette smoke, both of these, or neither of them. After 6 months of exposure the lungs of those receiving β-carotene supplements showed evidence of cell proliferation which resembled the early stages of carcinogenesis. These changes were greater in those exposed to cigarette smoke and β-carotene but were not seen in the control group or in the group exposed to just cigarette smoke.

The Food Standards Agency (FSA) (2003) suggested a safe upper level for β-carotene supplements of only 7 mg/day compared to the 15–50 mg/day used in these studies, and supplements with more than this amount should carry a voluntary warning in the UK. The FSA considered that at that time there was no evidence that high intakes of vitamin E were harmful *per se*, and it suggested that prolonged intakes of 500 mg/ day should generally be safe (i.e. around 30 times the maximum UK intake from food sources). Supplements containing 15 mg of β-carotene per tablet are still readily available in the UK (late 2011).

Key points

- The carotenoids are a group of over 600 plant pigments that are found in green and other brightly coloured fruits and vegetables.
- A few carotenoids have provitamin A activity and all of them are anti-oxidants that can quench free radicals.
- Diets high in fruits and vegetables (thus also high in carotenoids and other anti-oxidants) are associated with reduced risk of cancer and chronic disease in both case–control and cohort studies.
- Low blood levels of carotenoids are also associated with increased cancer risk.
- High blood levels and dietary intakes of vitamin E and other anti-oxidants have been associated with reduced risk of cancer and/or coronary heart disease.
- Two large cohort studies have reported that the voluntary taking of vitamin E supplements is associated with reduced risk of coronary disease in men and women.
- On the basis of this observational evidence it was suggested that high intakes of β-carotene or other carotenoids and other anti-oxidant nutrients might protect against cancer and chronic disease.
- There are several other possible explanations for the epidemiological association between high carotenoid intake and low cancer risk. For example, other components of fruits and vegetables may be protective, or a high intake of fruits and vegetables may simply be a marker for a generally healthy diet or lifestyle.
- Large-scale intervention trials of β-carotene containing supplements in industrialized countries have failed to show any beneficial effects and have suggested that they increase lung cancer risk in high-risk groups like smokers and asbestos workers.

→

Key points *continued*

Key points *continued*

- Large supplements of β-carotene may do more harm than good, and this suggests more generally that one should exercise caution in the use of purified micronutrient supplements unless habitual dietary intakes are inadequate.
- Increased consumption of fruits and vegetables is recommended and would increase carotenoid intakes.
- Experiments with rats suggest that large doses of β-carotene may induce certain enzymes that activate environmental carcinogens and thus act as a co-carcinogen.
- A co-carcinogenic action of β-carotene might explain the increased cancer risk in those exposed to high levels of environmental carcinogens and given β-carotene supplements.
- Experiments with ferrets suggest that β-carotene supplements induce proliferative changes in the lung and this is increased by concurrent exposure to cigarette smoke.
- Vitamin E is a potent anti-oxidant.
- Intervention trials of vitamin E supplements suggest that supplements have no effect on risk of cancer or cardiovascular disease, and one recent meta-analysis even suggested a small net harmful effect in the better trials.
- Current evidence does not justify widespread use of vitamin E supplements.
- There is no persuasive evidence that vitamin C supplements confer any benefit in terms of long-term risk of developing cancer or cardiovascular disease.
- Current evidence does not support any benefit of selenium supplements on cardiovascular, cancer or total mortality.
- There is insufficient evidence to make any firm judgements on the risks or benefits of taking co-enzyme Q_{10} supplements but given other evidence of anti-oxidant supplements it would seem that their use cannot be supported and may even be contraindicated.
- At the time of writing, there are no large and convincing clinical trials that suggest a long-term, holistic benefit from taking supplements of any anti-oxidant.

USE OF SUBSTANCES OTHER THAN ESSENTIAL NUTRIENTS AS DIETARY SUPPLEMENTS

Dietary supplements or 'natural medicines'

A medicine is a substance that is used to cure, treat or prevent a disease. Many substances marketed as dietary supplements are taken in the belief that they will offer medicinal benefits, examples being:

- glucosamine and chondroitin sulphate to treat arthritis
- evening primrose oil to treat breast pain (mastalgia) and other symptoms of pre-menstrual syndrome
- fish oils to prevent heart attacks and to treat arthritis
- extracts of saw palmetto (now classified as a traditional herbal medicinal product in the EU) to treat benign prostatic hyperplasia (enlargement of the prostate gland)
- extracts of *Ginkgo biloba* leaves (also now a traditional herbal medicinal product) to treat age-related cognitive deficiency and perhaps to slow the progression of Alzheimer's disease and other forms of dementia.

Despite these medicinal motives, there are considerable commercial advantages for companies to market their preparations as dietary supplements rather than medicines. In the UK, the control and licensing of medicines are the responsibility of the Medicines and Healthcare Products Regulatory Authority (MHRA). Before the MHRA will grant a product licence for a medicine it must receive substantial evidence that the product is both safe and effective. To provide the evidence necessary to achieve licensing may take many years and cost many millions of pounds. However, products marketed as dietary supplements are covered by the less stringent food safety laws. There is no requirement to prove efficacy and safety, although of course it is illegal to sell food that is injurious to health or to dishonestly advertise or describe a food. Enforcement of food safety laws is at the point of sale by local environmental health officers and trading standards officers, and the onus is on the enforcement authorities to 'prove' that a product is *ineffective* rather than on the provider to prove efficacy. The major marketing limitation of selling a substance as a dietary supplement is that medicinal claims cannot be made unless it has a medicinal licence. Thus one cannot claim that a dietary supplement cures or treats a disease, such as:

- 'helps to prevent or treat cancer'
- 'helps to treat or prevent arthritis'
- 'treats eczema'
- 'prevents colds and flu'.

Note that several herbal preparations previously sold as dietary supplements (and still sold as such in the USA) are now sold within the EU as traditional herbal medicinal products. To obtain registration a herbal product must have a long history of safe use within the EU, and it must comply with new quality control requirements, but there is still no requirement for the supplier to provide evidence of efficacy. Products now sold in this way such as agnus castus, echinacea, milk thistle, saw palmetto, *Ginkgo biloba* and St John's wort can make reference to the traditional use of the product.

Despite these restrictions, claims about the disease-treating or disease-preventing properties of foods and supplements can still be brought to public attention by other means, for example:

- by articles in the popular press, usually by unqualified journalists or alternative therapists, extolling the virtues of particular foods or supplements
- by media reports of reductionist scientific studies, often sponsored by companies with a commercial interest in the product being tested and relayed to the media via a press release.

All of the following headlines have been taken from the BBC website www.bbc.co.uk/news, and they certainly imply benefits from the intake of food products:

- Curry spice 'help for arthritis'
- Olive oil 'can cut cancer risk'
- Spice 'may fight cystic fibrosis'
- Watercress 'may cut cancer'
- Pomegranates 'slow tumour growth'
- Berries 'help prevent dementia'
- 'Green tea compound Alzheimer's hope'
- Vitamin D 'slashes cancer risk'
- 'High vitamin D levels cut MS risk'

More sensational headlines can be found in most newspapers. These complete articles from the BBC did give fairly balanced accounts of research findings, usually with comments from independent experts, and they also gave sufficient information to trace the original article. Even so, the headlines themselves make the public aware of health claims and often those claims are based on very limited or preliminary evidence.

For example, the watercress headline refers to some research (sponsored by the Watercress Alliance) which indicates that eating 85 g of watercress (more than most people eat in total over 8 weeks) every day for 8 weeks increases blood anti-oxidant levels, reduces acute measures of oxidant stress and increases resistance of blood to the effect of an oxidizing agent. Dark-green leafy vegetables are well known to be rich sources of substances with anti-oxidant activity, so would it actually not be more surprising if very large supplements of watercress did not have such effects? Even though the scientific data are probably correct, does it really provide significant positive evidence that eating normal amounts of watercress reduces cancer risk? Many similar vegetables taken in this way would probably produce similar effects.

Even though claims relating to disease have not been allowed for substances sold as food or food supplements, some more general health claims have been permitted, such as:

- *helps to maintain healthy joints*
- *helps to mop up damaging free radicals*
- *helps to maintain an effective immune system*
- *helps to maintain a healthy skin.*

In 2007, the European Food Safety Authority (EFSA) began work on compiling a list of health claims that would be permitted on food products. To be approved, a claim must be supported by evidence published in academic journals. In 2009, the EFSA gave its opinions on the first batch of over 500 claims and accepted only about a third of these, mainly relating to the functions of vitamins and minerals, the effects of dietary fibre, the effects of fatty acids on blood cholesterol level, and the benefits of sugar-free gum for dental health. In early 2010, its opinions on a further 400 claims resulted in just nine favourable outcomes. Several high-profile claims were not accepted. For example, it decided that there was insufficient evidence that anti-oxidants, by reducing oxidative damage to cellular components, provided a positive physiological benefit. Similar regulations to those in the UK apply in the USA but note that in the USA there is a list of permitted specific health claims relating to the cure or prevention of disease which can be made on qualifying foods, and there are some so-called 'qualified health claims'.

Health claims are discussed generally in Chapter 19 in the section dealing with food labelling.

Key points

- Many dietary supplements are taken in the belief that they will treat or prevent specific diseases; that is, they are used as medicines.
- There are considerable commercial advantages to marketing a substance as a dietary supplement rather than seeking to license it as a medicine.
- Medicines must be shown to be safe and effective prior to marketing, whereas the onus is on the authorities to show that claims for a supplement are false or that it is unsafe.
- In theory, it is not permitted to claim that supplements or foods alleviate or prevent a specific disease. It is permissible to make a number of more general health claims for dietary supplements.
- Some herbal products previously sold as food supplements must now, within the EU, be registered and sold as traditional herbal medicinal products.
- To be registered as a traditional herbal medicinal product, there must be a long history of safe use within the EU, and the manufacturer must comply with certain quality control requirements but there is still no onus on suppliers to demonstrate efficacy.
- While US regulations relating to health claims are broadly similar to British regulations, there are some permitted health claims relating to prevention or cure of disease that are permitted on foods in the USA (see Chapter 19).
- British and other EU regulations on labelling and sale of supplements can be circumvented by selling them by post from outside British legal jurisdiction.

Conditionally essential nutrients?

In addition to the accepted essential nutrients there are some other substances that may be required only under particular circumstances or by particular groups of people (e.g. required in premature infants, in people with certain genetic defects or in people with certain pathological conditions). Harper (1999) desribes these substances as conditionally essential – 'not ordinarily required in the diet but which must be supplied exogenously to specific groups that do not synthesize them in adequate amounts'. Using this definition, one could classify vitamin D as conditionally essential because a dietary supply is needed only if there is inadequate exposure of the skin to sunlight for the endogenous synthesis of the vitamin.

- Carnitine is a cellular component that is synthesized from the amino acid lysine. It is essential for fatty acid metabolism but healthy people normally synthesize enough carnitine to satisfy their physiological needs, even those who are strict vegetarians and get almost none from their diet. There are several rare inherited disorders of fatty acid metabolism in which carnitine becomes an essential nutrient. It is also widely regarded as essential for infants especially if they are premature.
- The amino acid glutamine may be essential in people with serious illness or injury because utilization exceeds synthesis in such patients and plasma glutamine concentrations drop. Some clinical trials have shown that supplemental glutamine may have beneficial effects in these circumstances.
- The amino acids cysteine and tyrosine are conditionally essential for premature infants because the enzymes for their synthesis do not develop until the end of gestation.

Harper stated three conditions that had to be met before a nutrient could be classified as conditionally essential:

- the level of the substance in plasma must decrease to below the normal physiological range
- this decline must be associated with some biochemical, structural or functional abnormality
- supplements of the nutrient must raise the plasma level and correct the abnormalities.

A number of substances that are normally present in the body but not classified as essential nutrients – or even as conditionally essential nutrients – are widely promoted and taken as dietary supplements. These usually have clear biochemical functions akin to those of vitamins but are not classified as essential because endogenous synthesis is regarded as normally sufficient to meet physiological needs; examples are creatine, glucosamine and s-adenosyl methionine. The implication behind their use as supplements is that endogenous synthesis is not always sufficient to ensure optimal health, or becomes insufficient in certain pathological states, so that they can be considered as potential conditionally essential nutrients. Often it is implicit in their promotion that they may be beneficial in the treatment or prevention of particular diseases.

The biochemical functions and rationale for the use of several of these substances are briefly overviewed below, but no attempt is made to give a reasoned assessment of their effectiveness in preventing or treating disease; fuller referenced accounts may be found in Webb (2011a).

L-Carnitine

A typical adult man synthesizes 11–34 mg/day of carnitine from the essential amino acid lysine. The diet of an omnivore would contain 20–200 mg/day of L-carnitine whereas that of a vegan would contain almost none. Vegans do have slightly lower levels than other adults and this difference is larger in vegan children. Only the L-isomer of carnitine is synthesized in the body, so supplements containing mixture of D- and L-isomers should not be taken. The chemical structure of L-carnitine is shown in Figure 13.5.

$$H_3C - \overset{\overset{\displaystyle CH_3^-}{\textstyle |}}{\underset{\underset{\displaystyle CH_3}{\textstyle |}}{N^+}} - \overset{H_2}{C} - \overset{\overset{}{}}{\underset{\underset{\displaystyle OH}{\textstyle |}}{CH}} - \overset{H_2}{C} - \overset{\overset{\displaystyle O}{\textstyle ||}}{C} - O^-$$

Figure 13.5 The structure of L-carnitine

Fatty acids of 16 carbon atoms or more can only enter the mitochondrion for oxidation when they are in the form of carnitine esters. In the cytoplasm of the cell, co-enzyme A derivatives of fatty acids are converted to carnitine esters and the reduced co-enzyme A released for re-use. Also, when there is a high rate of acetyl co-enzyme A production from β-oxidation of fatty acids then the acetyl moiety can be transferred to carnitine so that co-enzyme A availability for carbohydrate metabolism is maintained.

Certain rare genetic disorders of fatty acid metabolism (e.g. deficiency of the enzyme propionyl CoA carboxylase) can lead to deficiency of carnitine, as can a genetic deficiency in the enzyme that transports carnitine across the plasma membrane. Haemodialysis can increase carnitine requirements, as can certain anticonvulsant drugs and certain antibiotics. Carnitine is added to infant formula – especially soy-based formula (essentially carnitine-free) – to bring its level up to that found in breast milk. There is no evidence that growth is impaired in normal babies fed on unsupplemented soy formula, although their blood levels of carnitine fall and their blood levels of free fatty acids rise. Premature babies have around 10 times less carnitine in their muscles than adults; it is thus widely regarded as a conditionally essential nutrient for babies and especially for premature babies.

Carnitine has been claimed to boost athletic performance and to be beneficial for people with chronic fatigue syndrome and Alzheimer's disease. There is little evidence to support these claims (Webb, 2011a).

Glucosamine and chondroitin sulphate

Polysaccharides known as glycosaminoglycans are major structural components of cartilage, and chondroitin sulphate is one of these. Chondroitin sulphate is obtained commercially from either the cartilage of fish like sharks or from the trachea of farm animals. All of these glycosaminoglycans contain repeating disaccharide units in which glucosamine or galactosamine is combined with glucuronic acid. Glucosamine is synthesized endogenously by substitution of an amino group onto carbon 2 of glucose and it is produced commercially by the acid hydrolysis of the shells of shellfish such as prawns, shrimps and crabs. The chemical structure of glucosamine is shown in Figure 13.6.

Both glucosamine and chondroitin are claimed to be of benefit in the prevention and treatment of osteoarthritis. It is suggested that endogenous glucosamine production is insufficient for optimal

Figure 13.6 The structure of glucosamine.

repair and re-modelling of cartilage in joints, so a supplemental exogenous supply will boost cartilage production and promote the efficient maintenance of healthy joints and encourage repair of eroded arthritic joints. It is also suggested that chondroitin may have anti-inflammatory effects within the joint. Chondroitin is a large polymer and so might not necessarily be expected to pass across the intestinal wall in its polymeric form. However, there is evidence that some chondroitin is absorbed as large-molecular-weight moieties and some absorbed as low-molecular-weight breakdown products.

In-vitro studies suggest that, in high concentrations, glucosamine can increase the rate of cartilage synthesis in cultured chondrocytes – although whether the concentrations used are of relevance to the in-vivo situation is a matter for debate. Evidence from meta-analyses of clinical trials suggests that both glucosamine and chondroitin may confer some positive measurable effects on the symptoms of osteoarthritis and on more objective measures of disease progression. This evidence of benefit is by no means conclusive and there is considerable debate about the clinical significance of any benefits. In general, more recent and probably higher quality studies seem to be less positive than older studies (for more details see Manson and Rahman, 2004; Webb, 2011a; Black *et al.*, 2009).

Co-enzyme Q$_{10}$ or ubiquinone

Co-enzyme Q$_{10}$ or ubiquinone is a key component of the electron transport system in mitochondria which generates ATP from the re-oxidation of reduced NADH$_2$ and FADH$_2$ (oxidative phosphorylation). It is a lipid-soluble substance that has a quinone moiety within its structure; that is, an aromatic ring with two carbonyl (C=O) groups which can be reversibly reduced by the addition of

two hydrogen atoms to hydroxyl (C–O–H) to give the quinol form called ubiquinol:

Ubiquinone (CoQ$_{10}$) + H$_2$ ⟷ Ubiquinone

The reduced quinol form of CoQ$_{10}$ is found in the lipid phase of most membranes where it is believed to have an important role as an anti-oxidant that protects membrane components from oxidative damage by free radicals. CoQ$_{10}$ is synthesized in most tissues and, as the name ubiquinone (ubiquitous quinone) suggests, it is widely distributed in many foods, being especially prevalent in meat, fish, nuts and certain vegetable oils. The structures of ubiquinone and its reduced form ubiquinol are shown in Figure 13.7.

Figure 13.7 The structure of ubiquinone (co-enzyme Q$_{10}$) and its reduced form ubiquinol.

Although supplements of CoQ$_{10}$ are absorbed there is little evidence that they increase tissue levels in young people or animals. It has been suggested that it might be useful as an anti-oxidant that helps prevent chronic disease but, as was discussed earlier, two major reviews (Shekelle *et al.*, 2003; Coulter *et al.*, 2003) found no evidence that supplements of CoQ$_{10}$ conferred any protective benefits against cardiovascular disease or cancer.

It has been speculatively suggested that, because of its pivotal role in cellular energy production, large supplements of CoQ$_{10}$ might improve athletic performance. There is no significant evidence to support this, or even to suggest that supplements increase levels of CoQ$_{10}$ in muscles. Levels of CoQ$_{10}$ decline in some tissues in old age, and so once again it has been speculatively suggested that it might reduce the effects of ageing – but with no significant evidential support.

Creatine

The adult human body typically contains 120–160 g of the amino acid creatine, largely concentrated in muscle. It can be synthesized in the body from other amino acids and so is not considered to be an essential nutrient. The amount synthesized is enough to maintain the normal body pool size and depends on the amount present in the diet; vegetarian diets contain almost no creatine whereas omnivores typically take in around 2 g/day, largely derived from meat and fish. The structures of creatine and creatine phosphate are shown in Figure 13.8.

$$NH_2 \qquad\qquad NH-PO_3H_2$$
$$| \qquad\qquad\qquad\quad |$$
$$C=NH \quad + ATP \rightleftharpoons \quad C=NH \quad + ADP$$
$$| \qquad\qquad\qquad\qquad |$$
$$H_3C-N-CH_2-COOH \qquad H_3C-N-CH_2-COOH$$

Figure 13.8 The structure of creatine and creatine phosphate.

Creatine acts as a short-term energy store in muscle where ATP is used to phosphorylate creatine to phosphocreatine, and this phosphocreatine can then be used to regenerate ATP during periods of intense activity. It is normally taken as a supplement by athletes involved in explosive events requiring short periods of intense maximal activity, or those whose sport involves repeated short bursts of intense activity. Its usefulness as a supplement is discussed further in Chapter 17 in the section dealing with diet and athletic performance.

α-Lipoic acid

α-Lipoic acid is a sulphur-containing compound that is synthesized by both animals and plants and so is widely distributed in foods. It is not considered an essential nutrient because of this endogenous synthesis. The α-lipoic acid in food is covalently bound to lysine residues of the enzymes for which it acts as a cofactor. Human gut enzymes do not break the bonds between lipoic acid and lysine, so dietary lipoic acid from food is absorbed as lipolysine. Free lipoic acid is only present in blood if supplements of pure lipoic acid are being taken.

The amount in supplements is probably at least 10 times that found in normal diets. Only the R-optical isomer of lipoic acid is normally synthesized in cells whereas chemically synthesized supplements often contain a racemic mixture of R and S isomers and the S isomer would not normally be present in the body. The structures of lipoic acid and its reduced form, dihydrolipoic acid, are shown in Figure 13.9.

*Asymmetric carbon atom

Figure 13.9 The strucures of lipoic acid and its reduced form dihydrolipoic acid.

α-Lipoic acid is a cofactor for several important enzymes including pyruvate dehydrogenase (converts pyruvate to acetyl CoA), succinyl CoA dehydrogenase in the Krebs cycle, and some of the enzymes in the metabolism of amino acids. α-Lipoic acid can be reduced to α-dihydrolipoic acid, and this has the potential to act as an anti-oxidant via its oxidation back to α-lipoic acid.

α-Lipoic acid is marketed as a supplement with claims that it can act as an anti-oxidant, and that it can improve memory and energy levels in the elderly – although there is very little evidence to support any of these claims. It is also used in very large pharmacological doses, especially in Germany, to treat peripheral nerve damage in diabetics (peripheral diabetic neuropathy), but such pharmacological use is beyond the scope of this book; see Ziegler et al. (1999) and Singh and Jiala (2008) for further information on this usage.

Lecithin and choline

Lecithin is the term used by scientists to describe the phospholipid phosphatidylcholine. Dietary supplements of lecithin are usually extracted from soybean oil and also contain lesser amounts of two other phospholipids, phosphatidylinositol and phosphatidylethanolamine.

Choline is a component of the important neurotransmitter acetylcholine. Choline can also act as a methyl donor in cellular reactions and it is an important component of the phospholipids in membranes and in plasma phospholipids. The chemical structure of lecithin is shown in Figure 13.10.

Figure 13.10 The structure of lecithin or phosphatidyl-choline.

In the UK, COMA (1991) specifically excluded choline and lecithin from its list of essential nutrients. However, in the USA the Food and Nutrition Board added choline to its list of essential nutrients in 1998 because it could not guarantee that the synthetic pathway was capable of producing adequate amounts of choline at all stages of the lifecycle. Note that choline is found in many foods, especially in soya beans, nuts, eggs, liver, meat, cauliflower and lettuce, so even if there is a dietary requirement deficiency would be very unlikely.

On the basis of its presence in acetylcholine and the low levels of synthesis of this transmitter in the brains of patients with Alzheimer's disease, supplements of choline and lecithin have been tested in patients with dementia, but even in large doses they did not confer any measurable benefit (Higgins and Flicker, 2000). Large doses of lecithin have also been found not to have any cholesterol-lowering effect despite earlier reports to the contrary (Oosthuizen *et al.*, 1998).

s-Adenosylmethionine

s-Adenosylmethionine (SAMe) is synthesized in the body from the sulphur-containing amino acid methionine. SAMe is the most important source of methyl groups for a host of methyl transfer reactions in biochemical pathways, including synthesis of nerve transmitters, synthesis of creatine, glutathione, carnitine, phospholipids, DNA and

RNA. A healthy adult synthesizes several grams of SAMe each day. The chemical structure of s-adenosylmethionine is shown in Figure 13.11.

Figure 13.11 The structure of s-adenosylmethionine (SAMe).

It was not until the late 1990s that a preparation of SAMe that could administered orally was first produced and supplements first went on sale in the USA in 1999. It has become a big selling supplement in just a few years. Many potential benefits have been suggested for SAMe supplements and these implicitly suggest that, despite the high rate of endogenous synthesis, there may be occasions when the supply of SAMe is rate-limiting in one or more of the pathways noted earlier, and thus that additional supplemental SAMe may confer benefits under those circumstances. In a very detailed and thorough evaluation of clinical trials of supplemental SAMe, Hardy *et al.* (2002) concluded that it may:

- have clinically useful effects in the treatment of depression
- have some effect in reducing osteoarthritic pain
- reduce some of the symptoms of liver disease such as severe itching.

More recent reviews have generally not altered these conclusions (Webb, 2011a).

> **Key points**
>
> - Conditionally essential nutrients are normally synthesized in adequate amounts but one might become essential under particular circumstances (e.g. in certain pathological conditions or in certain lifecycle groups).
>
> →

Key points *continued*

- For a nutrient to be conditionally essential, the plasma level must be abnormally low. This must give rise to adverse consequences and supplements must raise the blood level and correct the consequences.
- Examples of conditionally essential nutrients are:
  - vitamin D becomes essential in the diet when there is inadequate exposure to sunlight
  - carnitine is essential for those with some rare, inherited disorders of fatty acid metabolism and probably for premature babies
  - glutamine may become essential during severe illness or injury.
- Some substances that are frequently taken as dietary supplements fulfil vitamin-like biochemical roles but are not normally classified as essential or conditionally essential.
- The biochemical roles and rationale for their use as dietary supplements have been briefly outlined for L-carnitine, glucosamine, chondroitin sulphate, co-enzyme Q_{10}, creatine, α-lipoic acid, lecithin, choline and s-adenosyl-methionine.

Secondary metabolites in plant extracts

Plant secondary metabolites are substances that are additional to those involved in the primary processes of photosynthesis, respiration, growth and development. While the 'primary metabolites' will be widely distributed and common to most or even all plants, they are much more individual in their profiles of secondary metabolites. Some secondary metabolites may be found in only one plant or a group of related plants while others may be widely distributed in plants. These secondary metabolites serve roles such as:

- acting as attractants for pollination and seed dispersal
- imparting an unpleasant taste to a plant or producing unpleasant symptoms when eaten so as to discourage consumption of the key parts of the plant

- protecting the plant from bacterial and fungal damage
- protecting the plant against damage by ultraviolet light.

The total number of these secondary metabolites runs into many tens of thousands but they can be broken down into a small number of categories as below (classification based on Crozier, 2003).

The terpenoids

This is a diverse group of over 25 000 substances composed of varying numbers of five carbon (C5) isoprene units and derived from the precursor substance isopententyl diphosphate:

$$CH_2 = C - CH_2 - CH_2 - O - P - P$$
$$CH_3 \ (\text{isopentyl diphosphate})$$

where P is a phosphate moiety.

The different categories of terpenoids are classified according to the number of isoprene units; these are the hemiterpenes (C5), the monoterpenes (C10), the sesquiterpenes (C15), the diterpenes (C20), the triterpenoids (C30), the tetraterpenoids (C40) and the higher terpenoids (C40+). Several volatile oils that give plants their characteristic odour are monoterpenes, examples being geranial in lemon oil, linalool in coriander oil and menthol in peppermint oil. Ginkgoglide A which is found in *Ginkgo biloba* is derived from a diterpene. Two of the compounds that help give ginger its characteristic smell are sesquiterpenes. The important plant sterols sitosterol and stigmasterol are triterpenoids, as are the saponins which have surfactant properties and which form a stable foam when shaken in aqueous solution. The large group of carotenoid pigments are all tetraterpenoids, and ubiquinone (CoQ_{10}) is a higher terpenoid derivative.

The phenols and polyphenols

These are a group of more than 8000 compounds having at least one aromatic ring and at least one hydroxyl (–OH) group attached to it. They vary from simple compounds with a single aromatic ring, like the phenolic acids and hydroxycinnamates, through the stilbenes and flavonoids with two aromatic rings, and up to complex polymeric forms and complexes of phenols conjugated with other substances. Flavonol glycosides that have an attached sugar residue make up a quarter of the weight of *Ginkgo biloba* leaf extract. Examples of substances in this large grouping include:

- flavonols such as quercetin and kaempferol found in tea, red wine, green vegetables, onions and berries
- simple monomeric flavonols such as the catechins found in green tea and apricots, and more complex polymeric forms found in chocolate and red wines (tannins from tea are complex flavonols)
- isoflavones found particularly in soya beans, some of which (e.g. genisten and daidzein) are termed phyto-oestrogens because they have weak oestrogenic activity in humans – see the section on phyto-oestrogens in Chapter 19.

The alkaloids

These are a group of around 12 000 nitrogen-containing compounds that are mainly synthesized from amino acids, but a few (e.g. theobromine in chocolate and caffeine in tea and coffee) are synthesized from purine bases such as adenine. Many substances in this category have pharmacological activity; some are potent poisons and some are used as medicinal drugs. Examples include:

- atropine from deadly nightshade which blocks acetylcholine receptors at parasympathetic nerve endings
- nicotine from the tobacco plant which stimulates acetylcholine receptors except those at parasympathetic endings
- curare from a vine which grows in South American rain forests (blocks acetylcholine receptors on skeletal muscle and so causes muscle paralysis, including respiratory arrest)
- the anti-cancer drug vincristine extracted from the blue periwinkle
- cocaine from the coca plant, used as an illegal recreational drug and formerly used as a local anaesthetic
- codeine and morphine from the opium poppy which are very important narcotic analgesics
- quinine from the bark of the *Cinchona* tree which was the first effective treatment for malaria.

Sulphur-containing secondary metabolites

These consist of the glucosinolates from members of the cabbage or *Brassica* group of vegetables and the s-alkyl sulphoxides from the onion or *Allium* genus.

All of the cruciferous vegetables contain substances called glucosinolates which contain both nitrogen and sulphur. These are synthesized from the amino acids tyrosine, methionine or tryptophan. The Cruciferae include not only the cabbage family (e.g. sprouts, broccoli and cauliflower) but also rape, horseradish, mustard, turnip, swede, watercress and rocket. It is breakdown products of the glucosinolates produced when the vegetable is cut or chewed that are responsible for the hot or bitter tastes of some of these vegetables (e.g. horseradish and mustard).

Members of the *Allium* or onion family produce sulphur-containing compounds called s-alkylcysteine sulphoxides from the sulphur-containing amino acid cysteine. The side-chain of cysteine is oxidized and alkylated (addition of a hydrocarbon group) to give compounds that have side-chains with the following general formula:

$$- CH_2 - \overset{\overset{\textstyle O}{\|}}{S} - R$$

where R is an alkyl or hydrocarbon group.

Some examples of these compounds are s-methylcysteine sulphoxide found in most *Allium* species, s-propylcysteine sulphoxide found in chives and s-propenylcysteine sulphoxide found in onions (it is metabolites of this compound that irritate the eyes when onions are cut). The compounds found in garlic are of particular interest because of many claims for medicinal properties that have been made for garlic and which are attributed to its s-alkylcysteine sulphoxide content. The predominant compound in garlic is s-allylcysteine sulphoxide or alliin. This compound has little smell and whole undamaged garlic cloves also have little smell, but when they are cut or crushed an enzyme called allinase cleaves off the side-chain of alliin and two of these side-chains condense to produce allicin which is regarded as the 'active ingredient' in garlic:

$$CH_2 = CH - CH_2 - S - S - CH_2 - CH - CH_2$$
(allicin)

Although one 2–4 g clove of garlic can produce around 5–20 mg of allicin, it is degraded to other sulphur compounds during cooking and is relatively unstable even if crushed garlic is not cooked. Some garlic supplements claim to contain as little as 0.05 mg of allicin.

Role of plant secondary metabolites in preventing chronic disease

Many plant extracts are sold as dietary supplements and are implied to be of benefit in the treatment of particular health problems or to produce specific short-term health benefits. It is the plant secondary metabolites that are usually believed to afford these therapeutic effects; a number of conventional drugs are derived from plant secondary metabolites (some examples were listed earlier in the section on alkaloids). Detailed discussion of these issues is beyond the scope of a general nutrition text and is an area that is at the fringes of nutrition *per se*, and there is considerable overlap here with both herbal and allopathic medicine. Use of some of the more popular herbal extracts is discussed more fully in Webb (2011a).

It has already been noted and discussed several times in this book that people with a high fruit and vegetable intake are less prone to chronic diseases like cancer and cardiovascular disease. The exact reasons for this association are still not clear, but it is generally believed that the association is cause-and-effect; that is, high intake protects against chronic disease. This has led to campaigns in many countries to encourage higher fruit and vegetable intake (five-a-day in the UK). If this association is causal then there are several ways in which fruits and vegetables might be protective, such as:

- they contain relatively large amounts of potassium
- they contain relatively large amounts of anti-oxidant vitamins and minerals
- they are rich in (soluble) dietary fibre.

It is also possible that the high and varied intake of secondary plant metabolites in those eating lots of fruits and vegetables may be responsible for some of this apparent protective effect. Listed below are some of the potential ways in which plant secondary

metabolites might afford some protection against chronic disease (after Jackson 2003).

- A number of plant secondary metabolites have anti-oxidant potential (e.g. the carotenoids and many flavonoids). These anti-oxidants might act to prevent DNA damage by carcinogens that add hydroxyl or alkyl groups to bases in DNA and thus induce mutations that may initiate carcinogenesis. LDL cholesterol is much more damaging to arterial walls when it is oxidized, so anti-oxidants might help to reduce the risk of cardiovascular disease by inhibiting this LDL oxidation.

- Potential carcinogens and other foreign chemicals are detoxified in the body by so-called phase I and phase II enzymes. Phase I enzymes convert the foreign substance into a water-soluble metabolite to facilitate its excretion; phase II enzymes convert foreign chemicals to harmless metabolites. In some cases the action of phase I enzymes may convert some environmental carcinogens into a more damaging and more mutagenic form. It has been suggested that certain plant secondary metabolites including the glucosinolates from *Brassica* vegetables might act to prevent this metabolic activation of potential carcinogens. It has been suggested that the sulphur-containing compounds found in garlic and other members of the onion family might activate phase II enzymes and thus speed up the detoxification of foreign and potentially harmful chemicals. High intakes of some plant secondary metabolites, especially if concentrated supplements are used, might therefore affect the metabolism of prescribed drugs (also foreign chemicals) and thus influence their effectiveness; for example people taking extracts of St John's wort (now classified as a traditional herbal medicinal product) have been warned that it may accelerate the breakdown of several prescription drugs and thus reduce their effectiveness (DH, 2000).

- Once cancerous change has been initiated in a tissue then substances called promoters may stimulate the abnormal cells to develop into tumours and spread to other sites. A number of chemicals in food may have such cancer-promoting activity. The female hormone oestrogen promotes many breast cancers and the phyto-oestrogens found particularly in soy foods might inhibit this promotion. The phyto-oestrogens are only weakly oestrogenic, so in women who are producing oestrogen their net effect may be to reduce the oestrogen stimulus by competing with the more potent human oestrogen for binding sites on the cancer and other cells. See Chapter 19 for further discussion of phyto-oestrogens.

- A high plasma LDL cholesterol level is known to be a risk factor for atherosclerosis and cardiovascular disease. Some plant secondary metabolites might reduce plasma LDL cholesterol, a claim widely made for garlic (supplements). An analysis of 37 trials of garlic supplements on plasma total cholesterol found that they produced a small fall in cholesterol level that was statistically but not clinically significant. Even this small fall was only transitory and did not persist if the supplements were taken for 6 months or more (Mulrow *et al.*, 2000). There is much more persuasive evidence that phytosterols do have a cholesterol-lowering effect (see Chapter 19).

- Heart attacks, strokes and pulmonary embolisms are the result of a blood clot or thrombus lodging in and blocking arteries that supply the heart muscle, brain or lungs. Some plant secondary metabolites may reduce blood platelet aggregation and/or the clotting process *per se* and thus lessen the chance of thrombosis. Certain polyphenols and the salicylates (aspirin-type compounds) inhibit platelet aggregation in *vitro* and phyto-oestrogens may also have an anti-clotting effect.

- Some carotenoids are found in the human retina where they may protect it from damage by ultraviolet light and thus inhibit the degenerative changes seen in age-related macular degeneration.

In his discussion of this list, Jackson warns that most of the studies on which these theoretical mechanisms are based are short-term experiments with purified chemicals using laboratory animals or in-vitro systems. Such studies can only be a first step in providing reliable evidence of the protective effect of crude plant extracts or even whole foods in free-living people. They do not justify the use of supplemental extracts or even the consumption of a particular food on purely health grounds; they are interesting observations worthy of further study!

Key points

- Plants produce many thousands of so-called secondary metabolites.
- The complement of secondary metabolites may be unique to a plant or group of plants.
- These secondary metabolites are classified as follows:
  - the terpenoids based on multiple isoprene units
  - the phenols and polyphenols which have at least one aromatic ring and one hydroxyl group attached to it
  - the alkaloids from which many potent drugs and poisons originate and which are nitrogen-containing compounds derived from either amino acids or purine bases
  - sulphur-containing compounds – the glucosinolates from members of the cabbage or *Brassica* group and s-alkyl sulphoxides from the *Allium* or onion family.
- Plant secondary metabolites may contribute to preventing chronic degenerative diseases by the following mechanisms:
  - by acting as anti-oxidants
  - by affecting the phase I and phase II enzymes involved in detoxification of potential carcinogens and other xenobiotics
  - by preventing cancer 'promotion'
  - by favourably affecting the blood lipoprotein profile
  - by reducing platelet aggregation or reducing blood coagulability
  - plant pigments may reduce damage by ultraviolet radiation.
- The evidence that underpins many of these mechanisms is largely derived from reductionist experiments with isolated cells, animals or cell-free systems and can thus only be regarded as preliminary.

14

THE VITAMINS

General concepts and principles	357	Niacin (vitamin B$_3$)	377
Vitamin A (retinol)	361	Vitamin B$_6$ (pyridoxine)	380
Vitamin D (cholecalciferol)	365	Vitamin B$_{12}$ (cobalamins)	381
Vitamin E (α-tocopherol)	371	Folate or folic acid (vitamin B$_9$)	383
Vitamin K (phylloquinone)	372	Biotin	389
Thiamin (vitamin B$_1$)	374	Pantothenic acid	389
Riboflavin (vitamin B$_2$)	376	Vitamin C (ascorbic acid)	390

GENERAL CONCEPTS AND PRINCIPLES

Readers with a limited biochemical background are urged to refer back to Chapter 6 to facilitate their understanding of the significance of particular biochemical lesions that result from a vitamin deficiency. Chapter 3 has a discussion of the methods used to determine vitamin requirements and assess vitamin status, and Table 3.6 contains a summary of some of the biochemical tests of vitamin status.

What is a vitamin?

Vitamins are a group of organic compounds that are indispensable to body functioning. Some vitamins cannot be synthesized in the body. Others cannot be synthesized in sufficient quantity to meet the metabolic needs, or can be synthesized only from specific dietary precursors. Vitamins or their precursors must therefore be provided in the human diet. Vitamins are required in small amounts and they do not serve as sources of dietary energy. Vitamins or their derivatives now have clearly defined roles in particular biochemical pathways or physiological processes, as illustrated by the following examples.

- The active principle of rhodopsin, the light-sensing pigment in the rods of the retina, is a derivative of vitamin A. One of the early consequences of vitamin A deficiency is night blindness.
- *Thiamin pyrophosphate* (TPP) is an essential cofactor for several key enzymes in metabolism, including pyruvic oxidase, the enzyme responsible for the conversion of pyruvic acid to acetyl co-enzyme A in carbohydrate metabolism (see Chapter 6). In thiamin deficiency, the metabolism of carbohydrates is progressively blocked at this step and the function of other TPP-dependent enzymes is similarly impaired.
- Niacin (nicotinic acid) is a component of the important co-enzymes *nicotinamide adenine dinucleotide* (NAD) and the *phosphorylated derivative* (NADP). NAD and NADP serve as hydrogen acceptors and donors in numerous oxidation and reduction reactions. They are essential in many human biochemical pathways.
- Vitamin D (cholecalciferol) is the precursor of a hormone produced in the kidney, 1,25-dihydroxy cholecalciferol (1,25-DHCC) or calcitriol. This hormone stimulates the synthesis of proteins essential for calcium absorption in the gut. In vitamin D deficiency (rickets), children absorb insufficient calcium for normal skeletal development.

Classification

Vitamins are divided into two broad categories according to their solubility characteristics. Vitamins A, D, E and K are not soluble in water, but they are soluble in lipid or lipid solvents and they are thus classified as the *fat-soluble vitamins*. The B group of vitamins and vitamin C are the *water-soluble vitamins*. The term 'B vitamins' actually describes a group of eight different vitamins that were originally grouped together as the *B-complex* because they were found together in, for example, yeast extract. The B vitamins are:

- thiamin (B_1)
- riboflavin (B_2)
- niacin (B_3)
- vitamin B_6 (pyridoxine and related compounds)
- vitamin B_{12} (cobalamin)
- folate (B_9)
- pantothenic acid
- biotin.

In general, the fat-soluble vitamins are stored in the liver, so daily consumption is not required provided that average consumption over a period is adequate. Excesses of these vitamins are not readily excreted so, if intakes are very high, toxic overload is possible (vitamins D and A are the most toxic of the vitamins, but vitamins E and K have very low toxicity). Concentrated supplements are the most likely cause of toxic overload, but some very rich food sources can also produce symptoms of toxicity. For example, the livers of marine mammals and fish may contain toxic amounts of vitamins A or D, and even liver from farm animals may contain enough vitamin A to cause birth defects if eaten by pregnant women. Fat-soluble vitamins are normally absorbed

from the gut and transported along with the fat, so malabsorption of fat or disorders of fat transport can increase the risk of fat-soluble vitamin deficiency. For example, in cystic fibrosis, the lack of pancreatic fat-digesting enzymes may precipitate fat-soluble vitamin deficiency (see Chapter 17).

The water-soluble vitamins leach into cooking water, potentially resulting in substantial losses during food preparation. Stores of these vitamins tend to be smaller than for the fat-soluble vitamins and excesses tend to be excreted in the urine. A more regular supply is required than for the fat-soluble vitamins, and symptoms of deficiency tend to occur much sooner (vitamin B_{12} is a clear exception to this generalization). Toxicity is much less likely because of their water solubility and urinary excretion, and is all but impossible from natural foodstuffs.

Vitamin deficiency diseases

Dietary deficiencies of vitamins give rise to clinically recognizable deficiency diseases that are cured by administering the missing vitamin. Vitamin discoveries in the first half of the twentieth century greatly increased the perception of good nutrition as a vital prerequisite for good health. Common and frequently fatal diseases could be cured by the administration of small amounts of vitamins or vitamin-containing foods. These cures probably unreasonably raised the expectation of the ability of nutrition to cure or prevent other non-deficiency diseases. In many cases, the symptoms of these deficiency diseases, or at least some of them, are readily explicable from knowledge of the cellular functions of the vitamin, as illustrated by the examples below.

- The impaired night division seen in vitamin A deficiency is explained by its role as a component of visual pigments.
- The inadequate bone mineralization seen in rickets is because vitamin D is required to produce the hormone calcitriol that is required for calcium absorption and normal bone mineralization.
- The breakdown of connective tissue seen in scurvy can be explained by the role of vitamin C in the production of the structural protein collagen.
- The megaloblastic anaemia seen in vitamin B_{12} and folic acid deficiency is because these two vitamins are required for DNA synthesis, and thus for cell division and red cell production in bone marrow.
- The haemorrhagic disease seen in vitamin K deficiency in newborn babies is because this vitamin plays an essential role in the synthesis of active prothrombin and several other blood clotting factors.

Several of these deficiency diseases have in the past represented major causes of human suffering:

- beriberi in Japan, China and several other rice-eating countries of the Far East
- pellagra in southern Europe, North Africa, South Africa and southern states of the USA where maize was the dominant staple
- rickets, rife among poor children living in industrial cities of the UK and northern Europe
- scurvy, a major hazard for sailors and others undertaking long sea voyages by sail.

These deficiency diseases are now rare in industrialized countries and are generally confined to people with predisposing medical or social problems, such as alcoholics and the frail elderly. While average intakes of most vitamins appear to be satisfactory, this may obscure the fact that the individual intakes of large numbers of British adults

may be unsatisfactory and substantial numbers may have biochemical indications of unsatisfactory status for some vitamins (see Chapter 13). Even in developing countries, most of the historically important deficiency diseases are now relatively uncommon, but a few vitamin deficiencies still represent important public health problems in parts of the world, such as the examples listed below.

- Vitamin A deficiency is still widespread in children in many parts of the developing countries where it causes blindness and is associated with high child mortality.
- Vitamin D deficiency is an important precipitating factor for osteoporosis and bone fractures in elderly housebound people in the UK and some other industrialized countries. Large numbers of people in all age groups in the UK have poor vitamin D status.
- Lack of folic acid is an important cause of anaemia in several developing countries.
- Pellagra is still endemic in parts of southern Africa.
- Subclinical thiamin deficiency may still be prevalent in some rice-eating populations.

Key points

- Vitamin deficiencies cause clinically recognizable deficiency diseases that can be cured by vitamin therapy.
- Often the symptoms of deficiency diseases are explained by their known functions.
- Some deficiency diseases still represent important public health problems in some areas, although in the industrialized countries they are usually confined to people with predisposing social and medical problems.
- Average vitamin intakes of UK adults are almost always above the current recommended nutrient intakes (RNIs), although many individuals may have less than satisfactory intake of one or more vitamins.

Precursors and endogenous synthesis of vitamins

Vitamins may be present in food in several different forms, and some substances may act as precursors from which vitamins can be manufactured. In a few cases, external supply of the pre-formed vitamin may make a relatively minor contribution to the body supply of the vitamin. Some examples of these 'alternative' sources of vitamins are given below.

- The plant pigment β-carotene and several other carotenoids can be converted to vitamin A (retinol) by enzymes in the intestinal mucosa, liver and other human tissues.
- The amino acid tryptophan can be converted to the vitamin niacin. Niacin can be obtained either directly from the vitamin present in food or indirectly by the conversion of tryptophan in dietary protein to niacin.
- The principal source of vitamin D for most people is endogenous synthesis in the skin. Ultraviolet radiation, from sunlight, acts on the substance 7-dehydrocholesterol, which is produced in the skin, and initiates its conversion to cholecalciferol or vitamin D_3.
- Most mammals can convert glucose to ascorbic acid (vitamin C), but primates, guinea pigs and a few exotic species lack a key enzyme on this pathway and thus they require a dietary supply of this vitamin.

Circumstances that precipitate deficiency

People meeting their energy needs and eating a variety of different types of food seldom show clinical signs of vitamin deficiency. Dietary deficiencies arise when either the total food supply is poor or the variety or nutritional quality of the food eaten is low, or a combination of these factors. Vitamin deficiencies may occur as an added problem of general food shortage and starvation. They may also be associated with diets that are very heavily dependent on a single staple food that is deficient in the vitamin or associated with some other very particular circumstance or dietary restriction. Some examples of circumstances associated with deficiency states are noted below.

- Beriberi (thiamin deficiency) has historically been associated with diets based on white rice. Rice is inherently low in thiamin and most of it is

located in the outer layers of the rice grains, which are removed by milling.
- Pellagra (niacin deficiency) epidemics have usually been associated with diets based on maize (or sometimes sorghum). Maize protein is low in the amino acid tryptophan which can serve as a niacin precursor, and most of the niacin present in maize is present in a bound form (niacytin) that is unavailable to humans. Sorghum and maize contain large amounts of the amino acid leucine, which inhibits the conversion of tryptophan to niacin.
- Scurvy (vitamin C deficiency) is not a disease of famines. It occurred principally among people living for extended periods on preserved foods, such as those undertaking long sea voyages or taking part in expeditions to places where the fruits and vegetables that normally provide our vitamin C were unavailable.
- Vitamin B_{12} is naturally confined to foods of animal origin and micro-organisms, so strict vegetarians (vegans) are theoretically at risk of deficiency unless they obtain supplementary B_{12}. The usual cause of deficiency is poor absorption of the vitamin. An autoimmune disease, pernicious anaemia, results in damage to the parietal cells of the stomach that produce an intrinsic factor that is necessary for the absorption of B_{12} from the gut.
- Inadequate exposure of the skin to sunlight is regarded as the primary cause of vitamin D deficiency (e.g. in elderly people who are immobile and unable to go outside).
- Primary dietary deficiency of vitamin K is almost never seen, but some anticoagulant drugs (e.g. warfarin) exert their effect by blocking the effects of vitamin K and lead to reduced levels of clotting factors in blood and risk of bleeding and haemorrhage. Therapeutic overdose of these drugs or accidental consumption of warfarin-based rodent poisons leads to excessive bleeding and vitamin K acts as an antidote in these circumstances.
- In affluent countries, alcoholics are a group who are at particular risk of vitamin deficiencies, most obviously because high alcohol consumption is likely to be associated with low food and nutrient intake. Poor alcoholics spend

their limited money on alcohol rather than food. High alcohol consumption may also increase the requirement for some nutrients and reduce the efficiency of absorption of others. Several of the deficiency diseases listed earlier do occur in alcoholics in affluent countries, and in many cases there are multiple deficiencies. Some of the harmful effects of very high alcohol intakes may be attributable to dietary deficiency rather than harmful effects of alcohol *per se*. Alcoholics are particularly prone to thiamin deficiency and some neurological manifestations of thiamin deficiency: Wernicke–Korsakoff syndrome.

• The very low-fat diets seen in some developing countries may precipitate fat-soluble vitamin deficiencies. These diets contain low amounts of fat-soluble vitamins and the absorption of the vitamins may also be impaired by the lack of fat. Poor fat absorption (e.g. in cystic fibrosis and coeliac disease) may also be associated with fat-soluble vitamin deficiencies.

Key points

- Vitamin deficiency diseases can be a secondary consequence of general food shortages.
- Vitamin deficiencies are usually associated with very specific dietary or other lifestyle circumstances, such as consumption of a restricted range of foods, high alcohol consumption, lack of exposure to sunlight, or low absorption of fat from the diet.

A note about sources of information

The relevant chapters in Gropper *et al.* (2008), Geissler and Powers (2010) and Shils *et al.* (2006) are recommended as sources of factual information about the vitamins and the pathological consequences of deficiency, and Ball (2004) has written a substantial monograph on the vitamins and their functions. Chapters in those texts dealing with individual vitamins will not be specifically referenced here. Figures related to high UK intakes and recommendations for maximum safe intakes are taken from FSA (2003). Figures for average UK adult intakes and numbers with low intakes or low biochemical status for vitamins are largely taken from NDNS data, usually from Hoare *et al.* (2004).

VITAMIN A (RETINOL)

Key facts

- *Names and dietary forms.* Retinol; β-carotene and other carotenoids; vitamin A activity is expressed as retinol equivalents.
- *Dietary standards.* UK RNI M/F is 700/600 µg/day of retinol equivalents; LRNI is 300/250 µg/day; American RDA is 900/700 µg/day.
- *Dietary sources.* Retinol in dairy fat, eggs, liver, fatty fish and supplemented foods like margarine; Carotene in many dark-green, red or yellow fruits and vegetables.
  - 1 cup whole milk – 110 µg retinol equivalents
  - 40 g Cheddar cheese – 150 µg
  - 1 portion (90 g) fried lamb liver – 18 500 µg
  - 1 egg – 110 µg
  - 1 tomato – 75 µg
  - 1 serving (95 g) broccoli – 400 µg
  - 1 serving (65 g) carrots – 1300 µg
  - 1 banana – 27 µg
  - one-half cantaloupe melon – 700 µg.
- *Biochemical functions.* Precursor of 11-*cis* retinal, a component of visual pigments; maintains integrity of epithelial tissues and immune system; synthesis of glycoproteins. Retinoic acid plays an important role in the regulation of gene expression.
- *Effects of deficiency.* Night blindness; xerophthalmia leading to permanent blindness; poor growth; thickening and hardening of epithelial tissue; reduced immunocompetence.
- *Risk factors for deficiency.* Poor diet, based on starchy staple and unsupplemented with dairy fat, fatty fish or fruits and vegetables; very low-fat diet or fat malabsorption.
- *Biochemical measure of nutritional status.* At normal levels of dietary intake plasma retinol concentration is homeostatically regulated and only correlates well with dietary intake when it is very low or very high. For adults, plasma retinol concentrations below 0.35 µmol/L are considered severely deficient and concentrations between 0.35 and 0.7 µmol/L indicate marginal status.
- *Prevalence of deficiency.* Common in some developing countries and a major factor in child mortality and blindness in these areas. In 2000,

→

average UK intakes from food of men and women aged 19–24 years were below 80 per cent of the RNI; 7 per cent of UK men and 9 per cent of UK women below the LRNI, rising to 16 per cent and 19 per cent, respectively, in those aged 19–24 years.

- *Toxicity.* Retinol is teratogenic in high doses. Acute vitamin A poisoning occurs with doses of around a hundred times the RNI and produces abdominal symptoms, blurred vision, anorexia and headaches. Chronic toxicity leads to cracked lips, dry hard skin, conjunctivitis, liver damage, headaches, bone mineral loss and joint pain.

- *Recommendations on high intakes.* Supplements may not contain more than 2400 µg/day in the UK. Pregnant women should not take vitamin A-containing supplements without medical supervision. A maximum daily retinol intake of 1500 µg/day is recommended. β-Carotene has low acute toxicity with doses of 300 mg/day well tolerated, but it is recommended that supplements should not exceed 7 mg/day because of adverse outcomes noted in long-term clinical trials.

- *Typical highest UK intakes.* These are estimated at 6000 µg of retinol per day from food for the top 2.5 per cent of consumers, and this is usually associated with regularly eating liver. The highest consumers take in around 7 mg/day of β-carotene from food and, according to a voluntary agreement, supplements in the UK should contain no more than 7 mg/day.

Nature and sources of vitamin A

The chemical structure of vitamin A is shown in Figure 14.1. If the alcohol (CH_2OH) group at carbon 15 is oxidized to an aldehyde group (CHO) then this is *retinal*, and if oxidized to a carboxyl group (COOH) then this is *retinoic acid*. All the double bonds in the side-chain of retinol are in the *trans* configuration. Retinol is fat soluble and found only in the fat fraction of some foods of animal origin, examples being butter and milk fat, liver, egg yolk, oily fish or fish liver oil. There is very little

retinol in muscle meat or white fish, but margarine, some breakfast cereals, some processed milks and infant foods are fortified with the vitamin.

Figure 14.1 The structure of vitamin A (all *trans* retinol).

Humans can also make retinol from β-carotene and several other members of the carotenoid group of pigments, although 90 per cent of the 600 carotenoids do not have vitamin A activity. β-Carotene can be cleaved by humans to yield two units of vitamin A (retinol). Absorption of carotene is less efficient than that of retinol, so 6 µg of carotene (12 µg of other carotenoids with vitamin A activity) is by convention taken to be equivalent to 1 µg of retinol. Note that in practice the absorption of carotene varies from food to food (e.g. less than 10 per cent from raw carrots but over 50 per cent when dissolved in palm oil). The vitamin A content of the diet is expressed in *retinol equivalents* (RE):

$$1\,\mu g\ RE$$
$$= 1\,\mu g\ \text{of retinol}$$
$$= 6\,\mu g\ \text{of β-carotene}$$
$$= 12\,\mu g\ \text{of other provitamin A carotenoids.}$$

β-Carotene, and any other similar plant pigments with vitamin A activity, must all be converted to retinol equivalents to give the total vitamin A activity of foods or diets. Dark-green vegetables, orange and yellow fruits and vegetables and palm oil are rich plant sources of vitamin A.

Functions of vitamin A

Rhodopsin is the light-sensitive pigment in the rod cells of the retina. It comprises 11-*cis* retinal (the chromophore) and a protein called *opsin*. Within the eye, all *trans* retinol (vitamin A) is converted by enzymes to 11-*cis* retinal and this binds spontaneously with opsin to form rhodopsin. Light induces isomerization of the 11-*cis* retinal in rhodopsin to all *trans* retinal, and this causes the opsin and retinal to dissociate and the pigment to become bleached. It is this light-induced *cis* to *trans* isomerization that generates the nervous impulses that we perceive as vision. Enzymes in the eye then regenerate 11-*cis* retinal and thus rhodopsin (summarized in Figure 14.2).

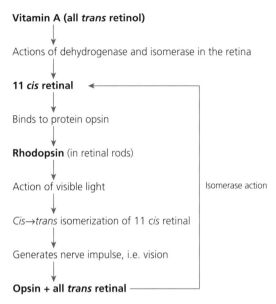

Vitamin A (all *trans* retinol)

↓

Actions of dehydrogenase and isomerase in the retina

↓

11 *cis* retinal ←

↓

Binds to protein opsin

↓

Rhodopsin (in retinal rods)

↓

Action of visible light   Isomerase action

↓

Cis→trans isomerization of 11 *cis* retinal

↓

Generates nerve impulse, i.e. vision

↓

Opsin + all *trans* retinal ─────

Figure 14.2 Schematic of the visual function of vitamin A in the rods of the retina.

Rhodopsin is the most light sensitive of the human visual pigments and is responsible for our night vision. In bright light, rhodopsin is completely bleached and other less sensitive pigments in the cones of the eye are responsible for day vision. During dark adaptation, rhodopsin is being regenerated. Note that 11-*cis* retinal is the chromophore in all known visual pigments including those in the cones of the eye. The light-absorbing characteristics of the chromophore are modified by binding to different proteins, but the essentials of the light response are as described for rhodopsin.

Vitamin A maintains the integrity of epithelial tissues in the eye, respiratory tract, gut and elsewhere. In vitamin A deficiency there are pathological changes in the integrity of epithelial tissues. Normal epithelial tissue has columnar or cuboidal cells and goblet cells produce mucus, which moistens the epithelial surface. In vitamin A deficiency there is overgrowth of undifferentiated flat cells, which are dry and keratinized (hard). Retinoic acid acts as a hormone, which binds to specific receptors within epithelial cells and controls

the expression of numerous genes; these receptors are similar to those that mediate the actions of steroid and thyroid hormones. This control of gene expression and protein synthesis regulates the proliferation and differentiation of epithelial cells. Retinol also plays a role in the synthesis of cell surface glycoproteins, which contain the sugar *mannose*.

Vitamin A is essential for proper functioning of the immune system. It is well established that vitamin A deficiency is associated with reduced resistance to infection and increased child mortality. In experimental vitamin A deficiency in rats, both antibody and cell-mediated immune responses are impaired and they improve when vitamin A is administered. In vitamin A deficiency there is reduced antibody production, reduced numbers of natural killer cells in the circulation, and neutrophils show a reduced ability to ingest and kill pathogens and tumour cells. Loss of integrity of epithelial surfaces, which normally act as a primary barrier to infection, also increases vulnerability to infection.

Vitamin A is necessary for normal fetal development. Fetal abnormalities occur both in vitamin A deficiency and in vitamin A overload, and this has been confirmed by experimental studies with animals. These effects on development are mediated by the effects of retinoic acid on gene expression in the fetus.

Requirements and assessment of vitamin A status

The estimated adult requirements for vitamin A are given in the key facts box and the origin of these values is discussed in Chapter 3. In practice, the biochemical assessment of individual vitamin A status using plasma retinol concentration is insensitive because plasma levels change only after prolonged deprivation or oversupply. Healthy adults have large stores of vitamin A in the liver, which take many months to deplete. Poor dark adaptation and lack of goblet cells and other histological changes in smears of corneal epithelium are often used as clinical indicators of inadequate vitamin A status.

Vitamin A deficiency states

The most obvious effects of deficiency are on the eye. A reduced ability to see in low-intensity light (night blindness) due to reduced production of rhodopsin is an early indication of vitamin A deficiency. The corneal epithelium is also affected. There is drying and hardening of the cornea and the appearance of *Bitot spots* (white clumps of keratinized epithelial cells on the surface of the cornea). In the early stages these changes in the eye can be reversed by vitamin A intake, but as they progress they become irreversible and permanent blindness results. Infection and necrosis of the cornea may eventually result in the extrusion of the lens. The clinical terminology used to describe the various levels of ocular pathology in vitamin A deficiency is complex, but the term *xerophthalmia* is used to cover all the manifestations. Other consequences of vitamin A deficiency are:

• impaired growth
• depressed immune function and increased susceptibility to infection
• overgrowth and keratinization of other epithelial tissues (e.g. in the trachea).

Vitamin A deficiency is very prevalent in South East Asia, the Indian subcontinent and several developing countries in Africa and South America. It is the major cause of child blindness in these regions and also causes high child mortality from infections. The World Health Organization has estimated that there may be up to 7 million new cases of xerophthalmia each year, with around one-tenth of these being severe enough to cause corneal damage. More than half of this 10 per cent with ocular damage die within a year and three-quarters of the survivors are totally or partially blind. In a recent meta-analysis of 43 studies that involved over 200 000 children, Mayo-Wilson *et al.* (2011) estimated that as many as 190 million children under 5 years old may be deficient in vitamin A. Providing supplements reduced mortality rates by around a quarter in countries known to be deficient. The WHO estimated that, if supplements could be provided to all deprived children, this would have the potential to save 600 000 child deaths each year as well as reducing blindness, measles and diarrhoea.

Risk factors for vitamin A deficiency

A diet that is almost entirely composed of starchy roots or cereals (e.g. rice or cassava) has no significant source of either retinol or the provitamin A carotenoids. Such a diet is also very low in fat and this reduces the absorption of any carotene that is present in the diet. Vitamin A deficiency can also be a secondary consequence of poor fat absorption in cystic fibrosis, coeliac disease, obstructive jaundice or cirrhosis of the liver (because of inability to store the vitamin). Deficiency does not usually manifest while children are being breastfed even if it is only partial breastfeeding.

Benefits and risks of high intakes

It has been claimed that the carotenoids may have protective effects against cancer and other chronic diseases because of their anti-oxidant properties and independent of their provitamin A functions. This is discussed in Chapter 13.

Retinol is relatively toxic when taken in excess but carotene is not. Chronic consumption of ten times the RNI (RDA) of retinol causes:

• loss of hair
• dry itchy skin
• swollen liver and spleen, with permanent liver damage possible.

Very large single doses can also be acutely toxic. Excess retinol in pregnancy is *teratogenic* (causes birth defects).

The epithelial changes seen in vitamin A deficiency resemble some of those seen in the early stages of *epithelial carcinogenesis*. Some prospective case–control studies published in the 1970s and early 1980s (e.g. Wald *et al.*, 1980) reported that low plasma retinol concentrations were associated with increased risk of cancer. There are many reasons why the results from such studies might not necessarily indicate a protective effect of dietary vitamin A on cancer risk (see Chapter 3 for fuller discussion of this example). Two very obvious criticisms of such studies are:

• changes in plasma retinol concentration may be an early consequence of cancer rather than a cause
• plasma retinol concentration is not a sensitive indicator of individual vitamin A intake and is affected by hormonal and other non-dietary factors.

Many epidemiological studies have found that a low intake of vitamin A is associated with an increased risk of cancers of epithelial origin and experimental vitamin A deficiency is associated with increased cancer incidence.. There are overwhelming grounds, unrelated to cancer risk, for measures to ensure adequacy of vitamin A intake in areas of the world where deficiency exists. There is, however, no convincing evidence that supplemental intakes of retinol, well in excess of the RNI/RDA, are likely to be beneficial; given the known toxicity and teratogenicity of vitamin A, they are undesirable.

Natural and synthetic retinoids have been widely and successfully used in the treatment of skin diseases including acne, psoriasis and skin cancer. They have been used as topical applications and orally. When given orally these retinoids have toxic effects like those described for vitamin A, and this limits the doses that may be used. Pregnancy is a contraindication for the use of these retinoids because of their teratogenic effects.

VITAMIN D (CHOLECALCIFEROL)

Key facts

- *Names and dietary forms.* Cholecalciferol (D_3) is the normal form found in animal foods; calciferol (D_2) from irradiated yeast is sometimes used in supplements and supplemented foods.
- *Dietary standards.* None for white young and middle-aged adults and school-aged children in the UK if they are regularly exposed to sunlight. For younger children, those with pigmented skin and elderly people the RNI ranges from 7.5 to 10 µg/day. In the USA, the RDA has recently been raised to 15 µg/day for those aged 1–70 years and to 20 µg/day for those aged over 70. Note that 1 µg/day is equivalent to 40 International Units for vitamin D.
- *Dietary sources.* Dairy fat, eggs, liver, fatty fish and supplemented foods like margarine and some breakfast cereals.
  - 1 cup whole milk (UK unsupplemented) – 0.03–0.06 µg
  - 1 egg – 1.2 µg
  - 40 g Cheddar cheese – 0.1 µg
  - 5 g cod liver oil – 10.5 µg →

Key facts *continued*

  - 1 portion (90 g) fried lamb liver – 0.5 µg
  - 100 g fatty fish: herrings (most), salmon, tuna, pilchards, sardines (least) – 6–22 µg
  - 5 g pat of butter/margarine – 0.04/0.4 µg.
- *Biochemical functions.* A precursor of 1,25 dihydroxycholecalciferol (calcitriol), a hormone produced in the kidney which increases the capacity of gut and kidney tubule to transport calcium; it regulates deposition of bone mineral. It is becoming increasingly clear that it also plays a role in regulating immune responses.
- *Effects of deficiency.* Rickets/osteomalacia with skeletal abnormalities; increased risk of osteoporosis in the elderly; low plasma calcium; muscle weakness, possibly tetany; growth failure; increased risk of infection and increased susceptibility to several autoimmune conditions such as type 1 diabetes and multiple sclerosis.
- *Risk factors for deficiency.* Inadequate exposure to sunlight for a variety of reasons such as dress customs, being housebound, working indoors for long hours, a heavily polluted atmosphere. Lack of back-up from the limited range of vitamin D-rich animal foods or supplemented foods exacerbates the problem. Risk is increased in elderly people and people with heavily pigmented skin.
- *Biochemical assessment of nutritional status.* Plasma concentration of 25-hydroxycholecalciferol (25-OHD), a metabolite of vitamin D which is the main circulating form. A plasma 25-OHD concentration of less than 25 nmol/L has traditionally been taken as an indicator of poor vitamin status, but a figure of less than 60 nmol/L or even more may indicate suboptimal status.
- *Prevalence of deficiency.* In 2001, 15 per cent of UK adults (aged 19–64 years) had plasma 25-OHD levels below the threshold, with values worst in the younger age groups. Evidence of widespread poor vitamin D status has also been reported in UK children and elderly people (see Chapter 16). Note that the threshold value of 25 nmol/L is now regarded by most international authorities as much too low; the Institute of Medicine (IOM) in the USA suggests a minimum threshold value at least twice this number.

Key facts *continued*

- *Toxicity.* The most acutely toxic of the vitamins. Overdose leads to elevated calcium concentrations in blood and urine with calcification of soft tissues and high risk of kidney stones.

- *Recommendations on high intakes.* Long-term intakes of up to a maximum of 25 µg/day from all sources should be generally safe (FSA, 2003), but this limit is conservative by European and other international standards; the IOM in the USA has recently set an upper limit of 100 µg/day.

- *Typical highest UK intakes.* Those people in the UK with highest intakes may get 9 µg/day from food. The maximum permitted dose in supplements in the UK is 10 µg/day; note, fish liver oil supplements also contain vitamin D.

Nature, sources and requirements for vitamin D

Vitamin D_3 is formed in the skin of animals by the action of UV light (sunlight) on 7-dehydrocholesterol. This latter compound is made by a skin enzyme that inserts an extra double bond into cholesterol (in the B ring of the steroid nucleus). The chemical structures of 7-dehydrocholesterol and cholecalciferol are shown in Figure 14.3.

Almost all the vitamin D found naturally in food is vitamin D_3 and it is, like retinol, obtained only from foods of animal origin such as eggs, butter, liver, oily fish and fish liver oil. Irradiation of the plant sterol *ergosterol* (e.g. from yeast) yields vitamin D_2, which has similar activity to cholecalciferol in mammals. Vitamin D_2 is often used in the production of vitamin tablets and to supplement foods like margarine, milk in the USA, baby foods and breakfast cereals.

For most people, endogenous synthesis of cholecalciferol in the skin is the primary source of the vitamin, so a dietary supply has not been considered necessary if someone is regularly exposed to summer sunlight. Dietary supply of the vitamin becomes much more important in people who do not get adequate exposure to sunlight, including the housebound elderly. Vitamin D does not strictly satisfy the criteria of Harper (1999) for an essential

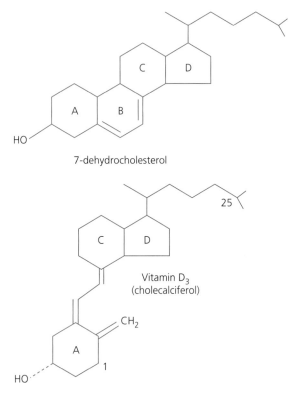

Figure 14.3 The structures of 7-dehydrocholesterol and cholecalciferol (vitamin D_3).

nutrient if the skin is adequately exposed to sunlight, but could be classified as conditionally essential in people without adequate exposure to summer sunlight. In the UK, winter sunlight does not contain the correct UV wavelengths for vitamin D production, but production and storage during the summer months should be adequate to last through the winter. In British adults, the proportion recording low biochemical status for vitamin D was around five times higher in those sampled in the period January to March than those sampled in July to September. For those with white skins, short periods of exposure of the hands and face to summer sunlight is sufficient to maintain adequate vitamin D status.

Holick and Chen (2008) suggest that the capacity to produce vitamin D in the skin may be reduced by as much as 75 per cent in those who are aged over 70. Sunscreens also reduce the production of vitamin D and if applied properly to all exposed skin a sunscreen of SPF15 or more may reduce vitamin D production by up to 99 per cent. When levels of solar radiation are low, skin pigmentation also reduces vitamin D production; those people of African descent with the darkest skin may have their capacity to produce vitamin D in the skin reduced by up to 99 per cent. One theory suggests that the evolution of white races in northern latitudes and those with darker skins near the equator might have been due to differences in ability to produce vitamin D.

Fair-skinned people who are prone to sunburn may need supplements to safely achieve the serum concentrations of 25-hydroxyvitamin D of 60 nmol/L regarded by many as minimum threshold values for satisfactory vitamin D status. Only in individuals reporting lengthy periods of sunlight exposure that risked sunburn and increased risk of melanoma were these levels achieved in the UK (Davies *et al.*, 2011).

As noted in the key facts box, there is no RNI given for vitamin D in the UK for most adults and school-aged children because it was assumed that they would normally manufacture sufficient of the vitamin in their skin during the summer to last the whole year. RNIs of 7–10 μg/day are given for babies and younger children, the elderly, and for pregnant and lactating women, but average UK dietary intake is only around 2–3 μg/day. Clearly anyone whose skin is not regularly exposed to summer sunlight is therefore unlikely to obtain enough vitamin D to meet their expected needs. The Chief Medical Officers for England and Scotland issued advice in February 2012 that all pre-school children should be taking vitamin D drops after weaning and that pregnant and breastfeeding women should take supplements of 10 μg/day.

In the USA, the RDA is 15 μg/day for most adults and children and 20 μg/day for elderly people aged over 70. Holick and Chen (2008) suggest even higher supplementary intakes of 20–25 μg of vitamin D for both adults and children where production from sunlight cannot be assured. These recommendations imply that anyone not regularly exposed to summer sunlight needs to obtain extra vitamin D from supplements or fortified foods. The RDA for children and adults were raised to their current levels in 2010 by the Institute of Medicine and for many people this represents a tripling of the older value; the aim is to achieve serum levels of 25-OH vitamin D of 50 nmol/L. This target value is double the threshold taken to indicate unsatisfactory status in NDNS

surveys in the UK. These new US recommendations have caused considerable controversy and debate, not because they are considered too high but because many experts and expert groups think that they should be even higher. The Endocrine Society in the USA has classified people with plasma levels of 25-OH vitamin D of <50/nmol/L as 'vitamin D deficient' and levels in the range 50–72.5 nmol/L as being insufficient. This organization suggests an optimal serum level of 100–150 nmol/L which would require a daily intake/production of 50 μg/day. See Maxmen (2011) for a full discussion of these issues and opinions.

Vitamin D must undergo two hydroxylation reactions to convert it to its active form. First a hydroxyl group is added to carbon 25 in the liver and a second hydroxyl added at carbon 1 in the kidney to give 25-hydroxyvitamin D and 1,25-dihydroxyvitamin D, respectively (see Figure 14.3). The 25-hydroxyvitamin D is the main circulating form of the vitamin and measures of its level in blood are used as a biochemical indicator of vitamin D status. A plasma concentration of <25 nmol/L 25(OH) D (25-hydroxycholecalciferol) is taken as the cut-off point for vitamin D deficiency in the UK NDNS (Hoare *et al.*, 2004). Holick and Chen (2008) suggest that a level of <50 nmol/L should be the criterion for deficiency and that values of <75 nmol/L indicate some degree of insufficiency, because in postmenopausal women these levels are necessary to minimize parathyroid hormone (PTH) levels (an elevated level of PTH is an indicator of vitamin D insufficiency). Even the high estimated prevalence of vitamin D deficiency for most adults noted in Chapter 13 and those for children and older people noted in Chapter 16 may be substantial underestimates of the real prevalence of some degree of vitamin D insufficiency.

Functions of vitamin D

The 1,25-dihydroxycholecalciferol or calcitriol produced in the kidney acts like a steroid hormone. The activity of the renal hydroxylase that converts the circulating 25-hydroxycholecalciferol into calcitriol is regulated by parathyroid hormone – a key hormone involved in calcium homeostasis. Calcitriol binds to receptors within the nucleus of its target tissues and affects gene expression (the synthesis of particular proteins). In the intestine, it increases the synthesis of several proteins that are involved in the absorption of calcium. In vitamin D deficiency the gut absorbs calcium very inefficiently.

In the bone, calcitriol has several effects. It induces undifferentiated bone cells to become osteoclasts, and these cells release calcium and phosphorus from bone when plasma calcium is low and they are activated by parathyroid hormone. It also stimulates bone resorption by osteoclasts. Calcitriol also induces the synthesis of some of the proteins that are prominent in the bone matrix (e.g. osteocalcin) and it is necessary for normal bone development, mineralization and remodelling. Calcitriol is also necessary for the efficient reabsorption of filtered calcium in the renal tubule.

Some cells that are not considered to be involved in maintaining calcium homeostasis have cellular receptors for calcitriol. These include T- and B-lymphocytes, monocytes, skin cells and many cultured tumour cells. Calcitriol reduces proliferation in these cultured tumour cells which have calcitriol receptors. The presence of calcitriol receptors on cells of the immune system has led to suggestions that it may have a role in regulating immune responses, and thus that poor vitamin D status may be a significant aetiological factor in the development of some autoimmune diseases including multiple sclerosis and type 1 diabetes. It has also been suggested that calcitriol which is produced in the kidney reduces the output of renin from the kidney and this would lead to reduced blood pressure. The status of these more recent claims for non-bone roles of vitamin D may be judged by the conclusions of an EFSA expert panel set up to decide whether such claims were sufficiently supported by published scientific data to merit their being made allowable claims for food labelling. It concluded that:

> a cause and effect relationship has been established between the dietary intake of vitamin D and contribution to the normal function of the immune system and healthy inflammatory response, and the maintenance of normal muscle function. ... a cause and effect relationship has not been established between the dietary intake of vitamin D and maintenance of normal cardiovascular function.

As noted in Chapter 13, a high proportion of such claims considered by the EFSA are rejected.

Acute deficiency states

Rickets in children and *osteomalacia* in adults are due to lack of vitamin D. During the late nineteenth century and early twentieth century, rickets was extremely prevalent among poor children living in the industrial cities of the UK. The symptoms arise from a failure to absorb calcium from the gut, which leads to reduced plasma calcium concentration, and reduced calcification of bones. Muscle weakness, gastrointestinal and respiratory infections are general symptoms of rickets. There are a series of skeletal abnormalities that are characteristic of the disease, such as:

- bowing of the legs or 'knock knees'
- swelling of the wrist
- beading of the ribs at the normal junction of cartilage and bone ('rickety rosary')
- pelvic deformities which may cause problems in childbirth in later years.

In severe rickets, plasma calcium concentration may fall low enough to induce uncontrolled convulsive muscle contractions (*tetany*).

Inadequate exposure of the skin to sunlight is regarded as the primary cause of vitamin D deficiency. Poor dietary supply of the vitamin is usually regarded as an exacerbating factor. Dietary intake of vitamin D is almost always inadequate for people who do not get enough access to sunlight. The risk of vitamin D deficiency is increased by any factor that reduces exposure of the skin to the correct ultraviolet wavelengths, such as:

- living in northern latitudes
- atmospheric pollution
- skin pigmentation
- some traditional costumes
- being housebound because of illness or immobility
- working indoors for very long hours, and other cultural or social factors that prevent people getting outside during the daytime.

Many adults, children and elderly people in the UK have low biochemical status for vitamin D, with a much higher proportion in those sampled in the winter months compared to those sampled in the summer. In the 1970s, relatively high levels of rickets and osteomalacia were a problem in Asian women and children who had recently migrated from the Indian subcontinent. This problem had largely disappeared by the 1990s, but there has been a resurgence of rickets in British Asians (see section on racial minorities in Chapter 18).

Vitamin D and osteoporosis

Poor vitamin D status is a risk factor for osteoporosis in elderly people (Lips et al., 2006). Lack of vitamin D leads to a compensatory increase in secretion of parathyroid hormone and this maintains the plasma calcium level by increasing breakdown of bone mineral (Chapuy et al., 1996). This means that prolonged vitamin D deficiency, as seen in elderly housebound people, will lead to bone loss and increased fracture risk (i.e. osteoporosis). Not only are elderly and largely housebound people less exposed to the sunlight that is vital for production of vitamin D in the skin, they are also less efficient at synthesizing the precursor substance in their skin, and declining kidney function may also impair their ability to produce the active compound calcitriol from its vitamin D-derived precursor. Holick and Chen (2008) suggest that the capacity to produce vitamin D in the skin may be reduced by as much as 75 per cent in those aged over 70 years.

Several clinical trials have suggested that supplements of vitamin D and calcium can reduce fracture risk in elderly people. For example, Chapuy et al. (1994) reported that calcium and vitamin D supplements given to elderly institutionalized women in France over a period of 3 years substantially reduced the risk of fractures, including hip fractures, compared to a placebo. There was biochemical evidence of widespread vitamin D deficiency among these women prior to the supplementation. Dawson-Hughes (2006) summarized trials of oral supplements of vitamin D in elderly people and found that there was up to 50 per cent reduction in non-vertebral fracture risk in four studies that used 17.5–20 µg/day whereas those that used lower doses of 7.5–10 µg did not find a significant effect. Three of the four high-dose trials gave supplemental calcium along with the vitamin D. Dawson-Hughes also discussed a Finnish study that used annual injections of vitamin D (eliminating the issues of patient compliance and poor intestinal absorption). This achieved a substantial reduction in fracture risk. In a large trial

(RECORD Trial Group, 2005), neither vitamin D nor calcium supplements alone or in combination were effective in preventing new fractures in elderly people who had already experienced a low-trauma fracture. Avenell et al. (2009) conducted a systematic review and meta-analysis of the effects of vitamin D and calcium in preventing post-menopausal fractures. Meta-analysis of nine trials (c25 000 participants) of vitamin D alone found no statistically significant effect on fracture risk but with eight trials (c47 000 participants) that used vitamin D plus calcium they found significantly reduced hip fracture risk, particularly in frail elderly people living in institutions. These reviewers did not report a differential analysis according to dosage, which means that their results may not be inconsistent with the earlier analysis of Dawson-Hughes (2006) discussed above. Given current views on vitamin D requirements and measures of vitamin D status, even the higher levels of supplementation in the four studies discussed by Dawson-Hughes look modest.

This discussion suggests that, on the basis of current evidence, vitamin D supplements of sufficient dose do reduce first-fracture risk in elderly people, especially those who are frail and living in institutions for the elderly. These supplements may also need to include calcium to be most effective. There is no evidence that supplements reduce fracture recurrence in those with established osteoporosis and previous fracture history.

There is further background information on osteoporosis in the section covering calcium in Chapter 15.

Vitamin D and non-bone conditions

It is generally accepted that vitamin D has important roles in regulating the immune system and inflammatory responses (note the earlier quote from the EFSA). There is a rapidly growing body of evidence to suggest that poor vitamin D status may be a significant aetiological factor in the development of some autoimmune diseases, including multiple sclerosis (MS) and type 1 diabetes. It has also been suggested that calcitriol which is produced in the kidney reduces the output of renin from the kidney and this would lead to reduced blood pressure. Observations such as these have led to numerous claims that vitamin D deficiency or suboptimal status may increase the risk of type 1 diabetes, MS, infections, hypertension and certain cancers, and conversely that vitamin D supplements may help in the prevention of – or even the treatment of – some of these conditions. Some of the evidence supporting these suggestions is briefly summarized here.

- The incidence of some cancers, type 1 diabetes, MS and hypertension increases with increasing latitude – which could be linked vitamin D insufficiency.
- Some epidemiological studies have reported a reduced risk of some cancers in people with good vitamin D status or those taking vitamin D supplements. A major international report (WCRF/AICR, 2007) concluded that there is limited (but inconsistent) evidence that good vitamin D status protects against colorectal cancer.
- Vitamin D or calcitriol reduced the incidence of diabetes in a mouse model of type 1 (autoimmune) diabetes, the non-obese diabetic (NOD) mouse (e.g. van Etten *et al.*, 2002).
- Some epidemiological studies suggest an association between poor vitamin D status and the risk of type 1 diabetes. Zipitis and Akobeng (2008) reviewed several studies which provided some evidence that early childhood vitamin D supplementation may offer protection against the development of type 1 diabetes.
- In an analysis of 28 previous studies, Parker *et al.* (2010) found that the highest levels of 25-OH vitamin D in serum were associated with a substantial reduction (about 40 per cent) in cardiometabolic disorders, including cardiovascular diseases, type 2 diabetes and metabolic syndrome – suggesting that improved vitamin D status in middle-aged and elderly people could reduce the prevalence of these conditions.
- Several cross-sectional studies have reported that low vitamin D status is associated with increased risk of hypertension. Forman *et al.* (2008) found levels of 25-hydroxyvitamin D were significantly lower in previously collected blood samples from obese women who developed hypertension in the following few years than in a matched women who did not become hypertensive.
- A majority of clinical studies supported the hypothesis that vitamin D sufficiency lowered blood pressure in vitamin D-deficient hypertensive patients (Pilz *et al.*, 2009).

- Multiple sclerosis incidence is lower in areas where solar radiation is higher, even where genetically similar populations living in the same country but at different altitudes are compared. Changes of MS rates in migrant populations are consistent with a protective effect of solar radiation. Most MS patients exhibit long-term vitamin D deficiency. Calcitriol reduces development of symptoms in experimental murine models of MS induced by immunizing mice with spinal cord homogenates (from reviews by Hayes, 2000, and Smolders *et al.*, 2008). Scotland has one of the highest rates of MS in the world and, because of lack of sunlight and low oily fish consumption, one of the highest rates of vitamin D deficiency. Professor George Ebers and some other experts attending a conference in Scotland advised the Scottish government in 2011 that they should fortify foods with vitamin D to reduce the toll of multiple sclerosis. Professor Ebers is a senior member of an Oxford University-based research group who, along with international collaborators in Canada, have published a series of papers about the role of genetic and environmental factors in the aetiology of multiple sclerosis (e.g. Banwell *et al.*, 2011; Ramagopalan *et al.*, 2011). People who are homozygous for a rare gene develop an inherited form of rickets, and in a Canadian survey of families, the presence of one (heterozygous) copy of this gene was very strongly linked to developing MS. This Oxford group also found a strong association between infectious mononucleosis (caused by the Epstein–Barr virus), sunlight exposure and MS. It concluded that the sunlight exposure was probably exerting an effect via its vitamin D-generating effect.
- Calcitriol inhibits proliferation and increases differentiation in human epithelial cells (note its anti-proliferative effect in cultured tumour cells). Oral supplements of vitamin D have been used in the treatment of psoriasis, although creams containing less toxic analogues of vitamin D are now an accepted mode of treatment.
- Sunlight exposure has in the past been used to treat tuberculosis, and rachitic children are generally prone to infections. Vitamin D may increase innate immunity responses and reduce susceptibility to infection (Liu *et al.*. 2006; Holick and Chen 2008).

Safely improving the vitamin D status of the population

Poor vitamin D status is common in most age groups in the UK, particularly during the winter months. If the higher thresholds of adequacy suggested by many experts were used, this already high estimated prevalence of insufficiency would rise sharply. Vitamin D deficiency leads to adverse effects on calcium homeostasis, bone growth and strength, and functioning of the immune system. Small numbers of clinical cases of rickets that are starting to re-emerge in parts of the UK represent the extreme consequence of vitamin D deficiency. However, these cases of rickets are just the tip of the iceberg because it is clear that vitamin D deficiency is implicated in the development of osteoporosis and the hundreds of thousands of bone fractures caused annually by this condition. There is also a growing body of evidence that poor vitamin D status:

- increases infection risk
- may increase the risk of developing an autoimmune condition such as multiple sclerosis or type 1 diabetes
- may increase the risk of some cancers
- may increase the risk of developing hypertension.

There is thus a very strong case for taking measures aimed at improving the vitamin D status of the UK population.

However, vitamin D is also the most acutely toxic of the vitamins. Overdose causes hypercalcaemia and this can lead to anorexia, nausea, vomiting, hypertension, kidney stones, renal failure and possibly calcification of soft tissues. It may have fatal consequences if severe and prolonged. In the 1950s, some British babies developed a vitamin D-induced hypercalcaemia because of excessive fortification of milk and other foods. This means that measures to improve vitamin D status must do so without causing toxic overdose in some people.

Four possible strategies for improving population vitamin D status are discussed briefly below.

Increase sun exposure
Encourage outdoor activity in children and improve access to sunlight for the elderly. However, excessive sunlight exposure, especially where it causes burning, is associated with increased risk of skin cancer and melanoma, so a difficult balance needs to be struck. Morning or late-afternoon exposure may be good for vitamin D production without causing skin damage, and even *short periods* of exposure to the midday sun may be encouraged. Detailed discussion of this issue is beyond the scope of this book. Vitamin overdose is not possible from sunlight exposure, perhaps because vitamin D_3 is sensitive to photo-degradation.

Targeted supplementation
As in the past, free supplements of vitamin D or cod liver oil to pregnant women, children and elderly residents of residential homes could be useful. Without such active measures, supplements tend to be ineffective because they are taken by those who need them least.

Food fortification
Fortification of milk or bread with moderate amounts of vitamin D would lead to a general improvement in status of all sections of the population. Even the maximum intake of vitamin D from food in the UK (9 μg/day) is below estimated physiological needs and is well short of the safe long-term intake (25 μg/day suggested by the FSA in the UK, but 50 μg/day suggested by EU and US experts). This means that moderate levels of fortification would not expose higher intake consumers to potentially toxic amounts.

The high prevalence of vitamin D insufficiency among British Asians, discussed in Chapter 18, might lead to reconsideration of a proposal to fortify chapatti flour, which was first suggested in the 1970s.

VITAMIN E (α-TOCOPHEROL)

Key facts

- *Names and chemical forms.* α-Tocopherol; other tocopherols have vitamin activity; vitamin E activity expressed as α-tocopherol equivalents.
- *Dietary standards.* UK 'safe intake' M/F is 4/3 mg/day; American RDA is 15 mg/day.
- *Dietary sources.* Vegetable oils, wheat-germ and whole-grain cereals, dark green leaves of vegetables, seeds and nuts.

Key facts *continued*

- 1 egg – 1 mg
- 5 g pat of butter/polyunsaturated margarine – 0.1/1.25 mg
- 1 slice wholemeal bread – 0.05 mg
- 5 g sunflower/olive/rapeseed oil – 2.5/0.26/1.2 mg.

- *Biochemical functions.* Anti-oxidant in the lipid phase; scavenges free radicals and prevents lipid peroxidation.

- *Effects of deficiency.* Progressive degeneration of nerves, muscle atrophy and retinopathy. In rats, deficiency produces infertility and reabsorption of fetuses in pregnant animals.

- *Risk factors for deficiency.* Overt deficiency is almost never seen and is usually confined to people with a medical disorder that impairs fat and/or fat-soluble vitamin absorption.

- *Biochemical measure of nutritional status.* Plasma tocopherol, often expressed as the ratio of α-tocopherol to total cholesterol in plasma. The lower limit of normality is deemed to be a tocopherol to cholesterol ratio of at least 2.25 µmol/mmol.

- *Prevalence of deficiency.* Overt deficiency is rare. In 2000, only 1 per cent of UK men aged 19–64 years had plasma tocopherol to cholesterol ratios below the satisfactory level (2 per cent of women).

- *Toxicity.* There is little evidence of toxicity even at very high intakes.

- *Recommendations on high intakes.* Prolonged intakes of as much as 500 mg/day generally regarded as safe and little indication of ill-effects at double this value.

- *Typical highest UK intakes.* Estimated that highest 2.5 per cent of UK adults take in around 18 mg/day from food; supplements (which are widely used) may contain up to 670 mg/day.

Overview

There are several compounds synthesized by plants that have vitamin E activity and the most active and important is α-tocopherol, whose structure is shown in Figure 14.4. Vitamin E is widely distributed in plant foods and is particularly concentrated in plant oils that typically contain 10–50 mg of vitamin E per 100 g. Animal fats contain small amounts of vitamin E.

The estimated requirements for vitamin E are given in the key facts box.

Figure 14.4 The structure of vitamin E (α-tocopherol).

Vitamin E is readily oxidized and so acts as an anti-oxidant. Its primary function is to prevent oxidative damage by free radicals to polyunsaturated fatty acids in membrane phospholipids. The requirement for vitamin E is increased by high intakes of polyunsaturated fatty acids because of their susceptibility to peroxidation by oxygen *free radicals*. Free radicals and anti-oxidants including vitamin E are discussed more fully in Chapter 13.

Overt deficiency of vitamin E is rare and is usually associated with some disorder of fat absorption or fat transport. As discussed in Chapter 13, there is considerable debate about whether low intakes of vitamin E may allow increased oxidative damage to membranes and thus increase the risk of chronic disease. Nerve degeneration, muscle atrophy and retinopathy are seen in both animals and people with prolonged vitamin E deficiency. Early studies of experimental vitamin E deficiency in rats found that it produced sterility, and this is the origin of its ineffective use in preparations that are claimed to increase sexual potency or act as aphrodisiacs. Many people take very large supplements of vitamin E, but doses up to 800 mg/day seem to produce no acute toxic effects.

VITAMIN K (PHYLLOQUINONE)

Key facts

- *Names and chemical forms.* Phylloquinone (K_1) from plants; menaquinone (K_2) produced by intestinal bacteria. The synthetic water-soluble forms menadione (K_3) and menadiol (K_4) are not permitted to be used in supplements under EU regulations.

- *Dietary standards.* UK 'safe intake' is 1 µg/kg of body weight per day; American RDA is M/F 120/90 µg/day.

→

- *Dietary sources.* Liver, green leafy vegetables, some vegetable oils, milk.

- *Biochemical functions.* A cofactor for the enzyme γ-glutamyl carboxylase which carboxylates glutamic acid residues in the synthesis of several clotting factors including prothrombin. May play a role in bone metabolism; there are several proteins with carboxylated glutamic acid residues found in bone.

- *Effects of deficiency.* Excessive bleeding, especially brain haemorrhage in the newborn.

- *Risk factors for deficiency.* Normally confined to newborns, especially premature infants; in adults it is usually a secondary result of poor fat absorption. Overdoses of warfarin and other coumarin-type drugs may precipitate symptoms of vitamin K deficiency.

- *Toxicity.* Few reports of any toxic effects, although it will interfere with anticoagulant therapy because coumarin-type drugs act as antimetabolites to vitamin K.

- *Recommendations on high intakes.* Intakes of 1 mg/day of natural vitamin K should be safe.

- *Typical highest UK intakes.* There is little information. Supplements may contain up to 200 μg/day.

Overview

Phylloquinone (vitamin K_1) is found largely in plant foods, particularly green leafy vegetables although it is found in smaller amounts in many foods. An alternative form of the vitamin, menaquinone, is produced by bacteria. Human gut bacteria produce significant amounts of vitamin K, which probably contribute to vitamin K intakes. The structure of phylloquinone is shown in Figure 14.5.

Figure 14.5 The structure of vitamin K (phylloquinone).

Several clotting factors, including prothrombin, only become functional when several residues of the amino acid glutamic acid within their structures are carboxylated (addition of COOH group); this carboxylation occurs after translation. The enzyme responsible for this carboxylation (γ-glutamyl carboxylase) requires vitamin K as a co-enzyme. These proteins with carboxylated glutamic acid residues are know as *Gla proteins* and they bind calcium much more readily than the non-carboxylated form. This binding of calcium to clotting factor proteins produces the conformational changes that make them biologically active.

Vitamin K deficiency leads to a reduced efficiency of the blood clotting system and thus to a tendency to bleed. Primary dietary deficiency of vitamin K is almost never seen, but malabsorption (e.g. in untreated coeliac disease) can precipitate deficiency and lead to bleeding. The coumarin group of anticoagulant drugs (e.g. warfarin) exert their effect by blocking the effects of vitamin K and lead to reduced levels of clotting factors in blood. Therapeutic overdosage of these drugs or accidental overdose from warfarin-containing rodent poisons leads to bleeding and vitamin K acts as an antidote to warfarin.

Some newborn babies, especially if premature, may develop intracranial haemorrhages shortly after birth. This tendency can be prevented by prophylactic administration of vitamin K, and the routine administration of vitamin K is common in maternity units. Golding *et al.* (1992) reported that vitamin K injections in the newborn were associated with an increased risk of childhood cancer. This report naturally raised concerns about the safety of this prophylactic use of vitamin K, but subsequent studies (e.g. Eklund *et al.*, 1993) have suggested that these concerns were probably unwarranted.

Similar carboxylated Gla proteins are found in other tissues although the significance of these proteins is not clear. There are, for example, three Gla proteins in bone: osteocalcin, matrix Gla protein and protein S. The presence of these proteins in bone has led to suggestions that vitamin K may play an important role in bone metabolism and thus that vitamin K insufficiency may be a contributory factor in the cause of osteoporosis. Ball (2004) has summarized evidence that provides some preliminary support for an association between vitamin K insufficiency and osteoporosis risk, and this is summarized below. It would be premature to assume that there is a cause-and-effect relationship.

- On a normal diet with normal blood clotting, the osteocalcin that circulates in the blood is not fully carboxylated and substantial supplements are needed to achieve full carboxylation.
- In very elderly women there is reduced carboxylation of circulating osteocalcin.
- High levels of under-carboxylated osteocalcin in elderly women are associated with reduced bone density at the hip and increased risk of fracture.
- Low intakes of vitamin K have been associated with increased hip fracture risk.
- Women in the lowest quartile of vitamin K intakes have been reported to have lower bone density than those in the highest quartile.

THIAMIN (VITAMIN B₁)

Key facts

- *Names and chemical forms.* Thiamin (vitamin B₁).
- *Dietary standards.* UK adult RNI is M/F 1.0/0.8 mg/day; UK LRNI is 0.6/0.45 mg/day; American RDA M/F is 1.2/1.1 mg/day.
- *Dietary sources.* Found in all plant and animal tissues but only whole cereals, nuts, seeds and pulses are rich sources.
  - 1 slice wholemeal bread (UK) – 0.12 mg
  - 1 egg – 0.04 mg
  - 1 pork chop – 0.7 mg
  - 1 cup whole/skimmed milk – 0.06 mg
  - 30 g peanuts – 0.27 mg
  - 1 serving (165 g) brown/white rice – 0.23/0.02 mg
  - 1 serving (75 g) frozen peas – 0.18 mg
  - 1 serving (200 g) baked beans – 0.14 mg
  - 1 teaspoon (5 g) yeast extract – 0.16 mg.
- *Biochemical functions.* Gives rise to thiamin pyrophosphate, a co-enzyme for pyruvic oxidase (carbohydrate metabolism), transketolase (pentose phosphate pathway) and α-oxyglutarate oxidase (Krebs cycle).
- *Effects of deficiency.* Beriberi and the neurological disorder Wernicke–Korsakoff syndrome.

→

Key facts *continued*

- *Risk factors for deficiency.* A diet very heavily dependent on polished rice; alcoholism.
- *Biochemical measure of nutrient status.* Erythrocyte transketolase activation coefficient (ETKAC) with values greater than 1.25 indicative of deficiency.
- *Prevalence of deficiency.* Average UK intakes around double the RNI with around 1 per cent recording intakes below the LRNI; 3 per cent of men and 1 per cent of women had ETKAC above the threshold value for thiamin deficiency.
- *Toxicity.* Few reports of any toxic effects.
- *Recommendations on high intakes.* Daily doses of 100 mg/day regarded as safe but doses well in excess of this may well be safe.
- *Typical highest UK intakes.* Thiamin-only supplements may contain as much as 300 mg/day but normal multinutrient supplements contain 1–5 mg/day.

Nature and sources of thiamin

The chemical structure of thiamin is shown in Figure 14.6. Thiamin is water soluble and so can leach into cooking water. It is oxidized when heated in alkaline solution. It is found in wholegrain cereals where it is concentrated in the bran and germ layers. Much of the thiamin is removed from cereals when they are refined (e.g. when milled to produce white flour or white rice). White rice is particularly low in thiamin but white flour is fortified with thiamin in the UK and the USA (see food fortification in Chapter 13). Thiamin is present or added to many breakfast cereals and is found in pulses, vegetables, milk, organ meat and pork.

Figure 14.6 The structure of thiamin.

Functions of thiamin

Thiamin is the precursor of the important co-enzyme thiamin pyrophosphate (TPP). TPP is formed by addition of pyrophosphate (two phosphate groups) at the position marked by an asterisk in Figure 14.6. TPP is an essential co-enzyme in several key reactions in metabolism, including those listed below (see also Chapter 6):

- conversion of pyruvate to acetyl CoA in carbohydrate metabolism
- conversion of α-ketoglutarate to succinyl CoA in the Krebs cycle
- reactions catalysed by transketolase in the pentose phosphate pathway.

In thiamin deficiency there is a progressive block at these steps in metabolism. The pyruvate dehydrogenase enzyme that converts pyruvate to acetyl CoA seems to be particularly sensitive to thiamin deficiency. Thiamin deficiency leads to an inability to metabolize carbohydrate aerobically, so pyruvate and lactate accumulate in the blood and tissues. The block in the pentose phosphate pathway restricts the production of reduced NADP which is essential for lipid biosynthesis, including the synthesis of *myelin* (the fatty sheath that surrounds many nerves).

Requirements of thiamin and assessment of status

The estimated adult requirements for thiamin are given in the key facts box. The requirement for thiamin increases as energy expenditure increases, the RNI is set at 0.4 mg per 1000 kcal (4.2 MJ) and the LRNI is set at 0.23 mg per 1000 kcal. The erythrocyte transketolase activation coefficient is used to assess thiamin status with values of greater than 1.25 taken as an indication of thiamin deficiency. The theoretical basis of these enzyme activation tests is discussed in Chapter 3.

Thiamin deficiency states

Beriberi and Wernicke–Korsakoff syndrome are caused by thiamin deficiency. The major symptoms of beriberi are:

- lactic acidosis
- peripheral neuropathy – degeneration of peripheral nerves with tingling and loss of

sensation at the extremities followed by gradual loss of motor function, muscle wasting and paralysis (dry beriberi)
- heart failure and oedema (wet beriberi).

Wernicke–Korsakoff syndrome is the neurological and psychiatric manifestation of thiamin deficiency that is often associated with alcoholism. This syndrome is characterized by paralysis of eye movements or rapid jerky eye movements (nystagmus), unsteadiness when walking or standing, and mental derangements including loss of memory and the ability to learn. Post-mortems on such patients show lesions in various parts of the brain ranging from loss of myelin to complete necrosis.

The clinical manifestations of beriberi can be largely explained by the known biochemical functions of TPP. Under conditions of normal eating, nervous tissue relies on carbohydrate metabolism for its energy generation, and the metabolism of heart muscle also relies heavily on the aerobic metabolism of glucose. Thiamin deficiency impairs carbohydrate metabolism, so it is not surprising that many of the symptoms of beriberi are associated with changes in nerve and cardiac function. Production of the fatty sheath (myelin) covering nerve fibres is dependent on the enzyme transketolase in the pentose phosphate pathway; this enzyme requires thiamin pyrophosphate as a co-enzyme and demyelination of nerves is a feature of beriberi and Wernicke–Korsakoff syndrome. The accumulation of lactic acid in blood and tissues that results from impaired pyruvic oxidase functioning may exacerbate the oedema of wet beriberi.

Beriberi has been known in China and the Far East for several thousand years, but large-scale epidemics occurred in the late nineteenth and early twentieth centuries and were probably precipitated by the introduction of machine milling for rice. Epidemics of beriberi are associated with diets that are based on white (polished) rice. Rice is low in thiamin and if rice is efficiently milled then most of this thiamin is removed with the bran. The high carbohydrate content of rice may also increase requirements. The poorest members of these eastern societies often escaped beriberi because they ate the cheaper brown rice with its thiamin still present. Only those who could afford the more expensive and higher prestige white rice were vulnerable to this condition, including the armed forces of Japan and China.

In the late nineteenth century, a Japanese naval surgeon noted that many supplementary foods were effective in curing and preventing beriberi and he proposed that it might be caused by protein deficiency. In 1890, Eijkman noted that beriberi among patients at a military hospital in Java seemed to be associated with eating polished rice but not brown rice. He induced similar symptoms to human beriberi in chickens when he fed them with boiled polished rice. These symptoms could be prevented by feeding them rice bran. In 1926, Jansen and Donath, working in Eijkman's lab in Java, purified thiamin from rice bran. Most parts of India escaped epidemics of beriberi because of different milling practices. The rice was soaked and then steamed or boiled prior to milling (parboiled), and this greatly increases the retention of B vitamins within the rice grain after milling. Introduction of less harsh milling practices, fortification of white rice with thiamin, and diversification of the diet have all contributed to the decline in beriberi. Intakes of thiamin are, however, still low in many rice-eating countries and offer little margin of safety.

It is very common for alcoholics to be thiamin deficient and Wernicke–Korsakoff syndrome is largely confined to alcoholics. There are several reasons for this:

- the diet of alcoholics is poor and thiamin intake is low
- high alcohol intake impairs the absorption of thiamin
- alcohol may increase the requirement for thiamin
- high alcohol intake may impair the activity of the enzyme that converts thiamin to the active co-enzyme thiamin pyrophosphate.

Thiamin deficiency may contribute to *fetal alcohol syndrome*, a syndrome seen in some babies born to alcoholic mothers and described more fully in Chapter 16. Given the frequent association of manifestations of thiamin deficiency in those with very high alcohol consumption, there are some grounds for suggesting that those who cannot be persuaded to reduce their alcohol intake might gain some benefit from additional thiamin intake in the form of a supplement.

RIBOFLAVIN (VITAMIN B$_2$)

Key facts

- *Names and chemical forms.* Riboflavin, vitamin B$_2$.
- *Dietary standards.* UK adult RNI M/F is 1.3/1.1 mg/day; LRNI is 0.8 mg/day in both sexes; American RDA M/F is 1.3/1.1 mg/day.
- *Dietary sources.* Small amounts in many foods; rich sources are liver, milk, cheese and egg.
  - 1 slice wholemeal bread (UK) – 0.03 mg
  - 1 egg – 0.21 mg
  - 1 cup whole milk – 0.33 mg
  - 40 g Cheddar cheese – 0.16 mg
  - 1 portion (90 g) fried lamb liver – 4 mg
  - 1 teaspoon (5 g) yeast extract – 0.55 mg
  - 1 serving (95 g) broccoli – 0.19 mg.
- *Biochemical functions.* Component of flavin nucleotides which are cofactors for several enzymes involved in oxidation–reduction reactions.
- *Effects of deficiency.* Cracking at the corners of the mouth; raw red lips; enlarged nasal follicles plugged with sebaceous material.
- *Risk factors for deficiency.* Absence of milk from the diet.
- *Biochemical measure of nutrient status.* The erythrocyte glutathione reductase activation coefficient (EGRAC). A value of 1.3 has traditionally been taken as the upper limit of normality; this value may now need to be reconsidered (see later in this section).
- *Prevalence of deficiency.* Mild to moderate deficiency regarded as common. Around 3 per cent of UK men and 8 per cent of women have measured intakes below the LRNI, with much higher numbers in the youngest age group. Around two-thirds of UK adults have an EGRAC above the 1.3 threshold level.
- *Toxicity.* Little evidence of toxicity in humans; its low solubility may prevent absorption of sufficient amounts to cause toxicity.
- *Recommendations on high intakes.* Regular intakes of 40 mg/day should be safe but no evidence that values well in excess of this produce any adverse effects.
- *Typical highest UK intakes.* Maximum from food sources around 4 mg/day. Supplements may contain up to 100 mg/day.

Nature and sources of riboflavin

The structure of riboflavin is shown in Figure 14.7. Dairy products, meat, fish, eggs, liver and some green vegetables are rich sources, but it is widely distributed in many foods. Milk is an important contributor to total riboflavin intakes in the UK. Cereals are generally a poor source unless they are fortified, as in the USA.

Figure 14.7 The structure of riboflavin.

Functions of riboflavin

Riboflavin gives rise to *flavin mononucleotide* (FMN) and *flavin adenine dinucleotide* (FAD). These flavin nucleotides are essential components (prosthetic groups) of several key flavoprotein enzymes involved in oxidation–reduction reactions. They are involved in both the Krebs cycle and oxidative phosphorylation, so riboflavin deficiency leads to a general depression of oxidative metabolism. Glutathione reductase, an enzyme involved in disposal of free radicals, also has a flavin prosthetic group.

Requirements and assessments of status

The adult requirements for riboflavin are given in the key facts box. Riboflavin status may be assessed by the erythrocyte glutathione reductase activation coefficient (EGRAC) and a value in excess of 1.3 is taken to indicate poor status. Around two-thirds of British adults had EGRAC values in excess of 1.3, with the frequency rising to around 80 per cent of those aged 19–24 years. The theoretical basis for these enzyme activation tests is discussed in Chapter 3. The very high proportion of adults recording values in excess of the threshold value for the EGRAC may indicate the need to re-evaluate the suitability of this threshold value, especially as relatively few have recorded unsatisfactory intakes of riboflavin.

Riboflavin deficiency

Mild riboflavin deficiency has long been considered to be relatively common even in industrialized countries, but no severe and characteristic deficiency disease has been described for this vitamin. This may be because the wide distribution of small amounts of the vitamin in food prevents mild deficiency progressing to major life-threatening illness. Also, riboflavin deficiency is usually associated with concurrent beriberi and the severe symptoms of beriberi mask the symptoms of riboflavin deficiency. In volunteers deliberately made riboflavin deficient, the symptoms were chapping at the corners of the mouth (angular stomatitis), raw red lips (cheilosis) and enlarged follicles around the sides of the nose which become plugged with yellow sebaceous material (nasolabial seborrhoea).

NIACIN (VITAMIN B₃)

Key facts

- *Names and chemical forms.* The generic term niacin (designated vitamin B₃) covers nicotinic acid, its amide form nicotinamide, and the co-enzymes NAD and NADP found in animal and plant tissue. It may also be synthesized from the amino acid tryptophan. The amount in food is expressed as niacin equivalents.
- *Dietary standards.* UK RNI M/F is 17/13 mg niacin equivalents/day; LRNI M/F is 11/9; American RDA M/F is 16/14.
- *Dietary sources.* Widely distributed in small amounts in many foods but good amounts in meat, offal, fish, wholemeal cereals and pulses. In some cereals, especially maize, much of the niacin may be as unavailable niacytin. The tryptophan in many food proteins is also a potential source of niacin.
  - 1 slice wholemeal bread (UK) – 1.4 mg + 0.6 mg from tryptophan
  - 1 portion (90 g) lamb liver – 13.7 mg + 4.4 mg
  - 1 pork chop – 6.1 mg + 4.9 mg
  - 1 serving (95 g) canned tuna – 12.3 mg + 4.1 mg
  - 1 egg – 0.04 mg + 2.2 mg

→

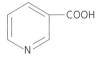

Figure 14.8 The structure of niacin (nicotinic acid).

Key facts *continued*

- 1 cup whole milk – 0.16 mg + 1.5 mg
- 1 portion (75 g) frozen peas – 1.1 mg + 0.7 mg.
- *Biochemical functions.* Component of nicotinamide adenine dinucleotide (NAD) and NADP which are co-enzymes involved in many oxidation–reduction reactions.
- *Effects of deficiency.* Pellagra.
- *Risk factors for deficiency.* A diet that is heavily dependent on maize (or sorghum) and not supplemented by high-protein foods.
- *Biochemical measure of nutrient status.* Urinary N′ methyl nicotinamide excretion: milligrams per gram of creatinine. Values above 1.6 mg/g indicate normality and values less than 0.5 indicate frank deficiency.
- *Prevalence of deficiency.* Given the high protein content of current diets, deficiency is unlikely in industrialized countries.
- *Toxicity.* High doses of nicotinic acid have been used to lower plasma cholesterol. This led to reports of adverse symptoms associated with these high pharmacological doses, such as flushing, itching, and nausea and vomiting.
- *Recommendations on high intakes.* Doses of the amide form nicotinamide of up to 500 mg/day should not have any adverse effects.
- *Typical highest UK intakes.* The highest consumers will take in around 60 mg/day from food (as tryptophan and niacin). Multivitamins may contain up to 150 mg/day and single niacin preparations up to 250 mg/day.

Nature and sources of niacin

Niacin is designated vitamin B_3. The chemical structure of nicotinic acid is shown in Figure 14.8. If the OH of the carboxyl group is replaced by an amine group ($-CONH_2$) then this gives rise to the amide, nicotinamide. Pre-formed niacin is found in red meat, liver, pulses, milk, whole-grain cereals and fish and it is added to white flour and many breakfast cereals. Much of the niacin naturally present in cereals may be in a bound form that is not readily available to humans.

The amino acid tryptophan can also act as a source of niacin. Niacin can therefore be obtained from the diet either directly as the pre-formed vitamin or indirectly by the conversion of tryptophan in dietary protein to niacin. This means that early suggestions that pellagra was due to protein deficiency were partly correct because high-protein foods, by providing tryptophan, could permit endogenous niacin synthesis and cure or prevent deficiency.

The niacin content of foods and diets is expressed in milligrams of niacin equivalents. In the calculation, 60 mg of tryptophan is usually taken to be equivalent to 1 mg of niacin. In the typical British or American diet, tryptophan would make up just over 1 per cent of the total dietary protein.

1 mg niacin equivalent =
1 mg niacin or 60 mg tryptophan.

Functions of niacin

Niacin is a component of the important co-enzymes nicotinamide adenine dinucleotide (NAD) and the phosphorylated derivative (NADP). NAD and NADP serve as hydrogen acceptors and donators in numerous oxidation and reduction reactions in all human biochemical pathways. It is during the re-oxidation of the reduced NAD, produced during the oxidation of foodstuffs, that most of the ATP yielded by aerobic metabolism is produced in the mitochondria of human cells (see Chapter 6).

Dietary requirements and assessment of status

The adult dietary standards for niacin are given in the key facts box. The requirement for niacin varies with energy expenditure and the UK RNI is set at 6.6 mg of niacin equivalents per 1000 kcal (4.2 MJ). There is no ideal method for assessing niacin status, but the urinary excretion of N′ methyl nicotinamide is one method that can be used. This is usually expressed as milligrams of nicotinamide per gram of creatine in the urine, because this value is more meaningful than simple urinary concentration which obviously fluctuates according to fluid intake.

Niacin deficiency

Niacin deficiency causes the disease *pellagra*. The symptoms of the disease are often referred to as the 3Ds – dermatitis, diarrhoea and dementia. If prolonged and severe then the fourth D is death. An early sign of pellagra is itching and burning of the skin which becomes roughened and thickened. Skin exposed to sunlight is most liable to show dermatitis, and a ring of affected skin around the neck (Casal's collar) is a common manifestation. Gastrointestinal symptoms, including diarrhoea, are a characteristic manifestation of pellagra. Early neurological symptoms are weakness, tremor, anxiety, depression and irritability and, if there is severe prolonged deficiency, eventually dementia. The disease has high mortality and caused many thousands of deaths in the USA in the first half of the twentieth century.

Pellagra has usually been associated with diets based on maize. Maize protein is low in tryptophan and the pre-formed niacin present in maize is present in a bound form (niacytin) that is unavailable to humans. Introduction of maize from the Americas has been associated with major epidemics in those parts of the world where it became established as the dominant staple (e.g. southern Europe, North Africa and South Africa).

Epidemics of pellagra began in the southern states of the USA in the early decades of the twentieth century, and by 1950 there had been more than 3 million cases and 100 000 deaths. It was so prevalent in these parts of the USA that it was thought to be an infectious disease and was one of the top 10 causes of death in some southern US states. It affected largely subsistence farmers in these southern states whose diets were based on fat pork, molasses and cornmeal (the so-called 3M diet: meat, molasses, maize). According to Davies (1964), the first recorded outbreak of pellagra in southern USA was in 1907 and Davies attributes this to changes in the way the corn was milled. At the turn of the twentieth century, large-scale machine milling replaced the old inefficient water-driven mills and this harsher milling produced a finer and more palatable cornmeal but it also removed the germ of the corn grain and reduced its vitamin content. Note that introduction of machine milling may have been an important factor in precipitating epidemics of both beriberi and pellagra. Harsh machine milling is very efficient at removing the nutrient-rich outer layers of the cereal grain. Traditional hand-milling methods were less efficient in removing these outer layers and left more of the vitamins in the final product.

Davies considered that the decline in cotton prices which led to a departure from the cash-crop monoculture was important in the decline of this disease. As cotton growing became less viable so many farmers began to cultivate gardens and smallholdings to produce food crops, leading to a diversification of the diet and less reliance on maize. Park et al. (2000) looked at the influence of food fortification on the eradication of pellagra. They identified two periods of rapid decline in pellagra mortality in the USA. The first period of decline (1928–32) occurred before niacin was identified as the pellagra-preventing vitamin and was probably due to better treatment with foods by then known to be curative (e.g. fresh meat, eggs, milk and yeast) and the distribution of yeast and other high-protein foods in high pellagra areas, notably by the American Red Cross. The second major decline in both mortality and morbidity from pellagra started in 1939 after US bakers started to enrich flour with high-vitamin yeast. Following mandatory enrichment of several foods with niacin in Mississippi, pellagra morbidity rates fell 100-fold between 1946 and 1947. Thus Park et al. (2000) considered that fortification of food with niacin played a significant role in eliminating pellagra in the USA. Rajakumar (2000) has written a historical review of pellagra in the USA.

Among the people of Central America, where maize originated, its consumption was not associated with pellagra. The traditional method of tortilla preparation resulted in the release of niacin from its bound state; the maize grains were mixed with slaked lime (calcium hydroxide) and subjected to prolonged heating prior to grinding and cooking.

Sorghum consumption is associated with pellagra in some parts of India and China despite the fact that sorghum contains reasonable amounts of tryptophan (almost as much as rice which is not pellagragenic). Bender (1983) concluded that this is because of the high content of another amino acid (leucine) in sorghum, which inhibits key enzymes in the conversion of tryptophan to niacin. The high leucine content of maize may also increase its potential to cause pellagra.

VITAMIN B₆ (PYRIDOXINE)

Key facts

- *Names and dietary forms.* Pyridoxine and related compounds are collectively termed vitamin B_6.
- *Dietary standards.* UK RNI M/F is 1.4/1.2 mg/day; UK LRNI M/F is 1.0/0.9 mg/day; American RDA is 1.3 mg/day for both sexes.
- *Dietary sources.* Liver is a rich source, cereals, meats, fruits and vegetables all contain moderate amounts.
- *Biochemical functions.* Precursor of pyridoxal phosphate, a co-enzyme involved in amino acid metabolism and other important metabolic pathways.
- *Effects of deficiency.* Overt deficiency rare, convulsions reported in infants fed on B_6-depleted formula.
- *Risk factors for deficiency.* Overt deficiency is rare.
- *Biochemical measure of nutrient status.* The erythrocyte aspartate aminotransferase activation coefficient (EAATAC), with values >2.0 indicative of vitamin B_6 deficiency.
- *Prevalence of deficiency.* Five per cent of young women (19–24 years) in the UK have recorded intakes that are below the LRNI. More than 10 per cent of adults have EAATAC values >2.0 (i.e. biochemical indication of deficiency).
- *Toxicity.* In animal studies, high doses of vitamin B_6 have been shown to be neurotoxic, producing abnormalities in gait and balance and histological evidence of peripheral nerve damage. There have been some reports of sensory neuropathy in people taking large supplemental doses, early symptoms being tingling sensations in the hands and feet.
- *Recommendations on high intakes.* A lifetime dose of 10 mg/day should pose no risk, but there are insufficient data to judge whether doses well in excess of this are safe.
- *Typical highest UK intakes.* Food may contain up to 4 mg/day. Although most supplements contain up to 10 mg/day a few provide as much as 100 mg/day.

Nature and sources of vitamin B₆

Vitamin B_6 is present in food as pyridoxine, pyridoxal or pyridoxamine, which are all biologically active and interconvertible. The structures of these are shown in Figure 14.9.

The various forms of vitamin B_6 are widely distributed in both plant and animal foods. Liver, eggs, meat, fish, green leafy vegetables, pulses, fruits and whole-grain cereals all contain significant amounts.

Functions of vitamin B₆

Vitamin B_6 is a precursor of the important co-enzyme pyridoxal phosphate. This co-enzyme is essential in many biochemical reactions, particularly those involving the metabolism of amino acids. The following are some of the reactions/pathways where pyridoxal phosphate acts as a co-enzyme:

- transamination reactions – transfer of amino groups to produce non-essential amino acids (see Chapter 6)
- decarboxylation of amino acids, for example to produce the nerve transmitters GABA, histamine, dopamine and 5HT (serotonin)
- synthesis of niacin from tryptophan
- breakdown of glycogen by the enzyme glycogen phosphorylase
- synthesis of the haem component of haemoglobin.

Requirements and assessment of status

The adult requirements for vitamin B_6 are given in the key facts box. A wide range of tests of vitamin B_6 status have been developed, including the measurement of pyridoxal phosphate concentrations in blood or erythrocytes. Erythrocyte enzyme reactivation tests (see Chapter 3) using the enzymes aspartate aminotransferase (EAATAC) or alanine aminotransferase are used as measures of long-term B_6 status, and the critical value for the EAATAC is 2.0.

Deficiency and toxicity

Overt primary dietary deficiency of vitamin B_6 is rare. In the 1950s, deficiency was seen in some

Figure 14.9 The structures of the three forms of vitamin B$_6$.

babies in the USA who had been fed formula depleted of its vitamin B$_6$ by a fault in the processing. These babies suffered from convulsions and had abnormal EEGs. Symptoms of deficiency in adults include anaemia, raw red lips, smooth inflamed tongue, lesions at the corners of the mouth, dermatitis and fatigue. Note that, although overt symptomatic deficiency is rarely seen, many British adults have unsatisfactory biochemical status for this vitamin.

Certain drugs used in the treatment of tuberculosis, rheumatoid arthritis and epilepsy increase the requirement for B$_6$, so supplements of the vitamin are normally given with these drugs.

There has been much speculation about whether vitamin B$_6$ alleviates the symptoms of pre-menstrual syndrome, primarily because of its involvement in the synthesis of nerve transmitters. It has been widely used as a self-medication for this purpose. A systematic review by Wyatt *et al.* (1999) found limited evidence to support the view that doses of up to 100 mg/day may have some beneficial effect on the symptoms of pre-menstrual syndrome but the trials were generally small and of low quality. Some cases of B$_6$ toxicity have been reported in women who chronically consume very large doses of this vitamin. The symptoms are sensory neuropathy of the hands and feet. The FSA (2003) suggested a safe lifetime dose of 10 mg/day, largely on the basis of animal studies which have found that high doses of the vitamin can be neurotoxic. Although there are reports of sensory neuropathy in people taking higher doses (up to 200 mg/day), the FSA felt that there was insufficient information to judge the risk posed by such doses.

VITAMIN B$_{12}$ (COBALAMINS)

Key facts

- *Names and chemical forms.* Cyanocobalamin and related compounds are collectively termed vitamin B$_{12}$.

- *Dietary standards.* UK RNI is 1.5 µg/day; UK LRNI is 1 µg/day; American RDA is 2.4 µg/day.

- *Dietary sources.* Meat (especially organ meat), fish, milk, eggs and fermented foods or foods contaminated with mould or other micro-organisms. Note that the algal product *Spirulina* is not a source of active vitamin B$_{12}$ despite having been promoted as such, although another algal product *Chlorella* does contain the active vitamin.

- *Biochemical functions.* Interacts with folate in methylation reactions necessary for DNA synthesis and cell division; required for production of the myelin sheath around many nerves.

- *Effects of deficiency.* Megaloblastic anaemia; demyelination and degeneration of the spinal cord leading to progressive paralysis and to neuro-psychiatric effects if demyelination occurs in the brain.

- *Risk factors for deficiency.* A vegan diet; poor vitamin absorption, as in pernicious anaemia due to inadequate production of intrinsic factor by the parietal cells of the stomach.

- *Biochemical measure of nutrient status.* Serum B$_{12}$ concentration with a value of 118 pmol/L taken as the lower limit of normality in adults.

- *Prevalence of deficiency.* Average intakes are 3–4 times the RNI and very few adults have

→

unsatisfactory intakes. Two per cent of men and 4 per cent of women had blood levels indicative of deficiency suggesting that inadequate absorption is the main factor causing deficiency. In 1999 it was reported that 6 per cent of free-living elderly UK adults and 9 per cent of those living in institutions had blood levels below the threshold value.

- *Toxicity.* High oral intakes are poorly absorbed. Excessive amounts in blood are excreted in urine so potential for toxicity is low.

- *Recommendations on high intakes.* Long-term consumption of 2 mg/day should not produce any adverse effects.

- *Typical highest UK intakes.* Some UK adults may get as much as 20 μg/day from food, and supplements may provide up to 3 mg/day.

Figure 14.10 The structure of cyanocobalamin (vitamin B_{12}).

Nature and sources of vitamin B_{12}

Vitamin B_{12} comprises a group of complex molecules which contain the element cobalt. The structure of cyanocobalamin is given in Figure 14.10. All of the vitamin B_{12} ordinarily present in the diet is in foods of animal origin. The ultimate source of the cobalamins is their synthesis by microorganisms and any foods contaminated by microorganisms will contain B_{12}.

Functions of vitamin B_{12}

Together with folic acid, vitamin B_{12} is essential for the synthesis of the nucleotide thymidylate. This nucleotide is found exclusively in DNA and so its production is essential for DNA synthesis and cell division. This means that cell division – including the production of red blood cells – will be impaired by lack of B_{12} or folic acid. Vitamin B_{12} is also required as a co-enzyme for a reaction that is essential for the metabolism of fatty acids with odd numbers of carbon atoms (methylmalonyl CoA conversion to succinyl CoA).

Requirements and assessment of status

Human requirements for vitamin B_{12} are only 1–2 μg/day and healthy omnivorous adults have

several years' supply stored in their liver. Vitamin B_{12} status is assessed by measurement of serum B_{12} concentration. Quantitative details are given in the key facts box.

Deficiency of vitamin B_{12}

Lack of vitamin B_{12} or folic acid causes a macrocytic (large-cell) or megaloblastic anaemia. In this type of anaemia, red blood cells are large, irregular and fragile. In severe cases the blood haemoglobin concentration may fall to less than one-third of the normal level. Dietetic lack of B_{12} is rare and usually associated with a strict vegetarian (vegan) diet. Folic acid deficiency is, on the other hand, common in some developing countries and high intakes of folic acid can compensate for lack of B_{12} and mask the haematological consequences of B_{12} deficiency.

Prolonged vitamin B_{12} deficiency also leads to irreversible damage to the spinal cord and neurological changes. This nerve damage manifests initially as loss of sensation or tingling sensation in the fingers and toes which leads to progressive paralysis. These consequences of B_{12} deficiency on the nervous system are not corrected by folic acid, so misdiagnosis and treatment of B_{12} deficiency with folic acid may mask the haematological consequences but allow the insidious progression of the irreversible spinal cord damage. This is a theoretical risk if common foods are supplemented with folic acid.

Vitamin B_{12} is naturally confined to foods of animal origin and to micro-organisms, although meat substitutes usually contain added B_{12}. This means that strict vegetarians (vegans) may avoid all foods that naturally contain B_{12} and thus be at risk of dietary deficiency of the vitamin unless they eat supplemented foods or take B_{12} supplements. In practice, even among those theoretically at risk, dietary deficiency is uncommon because requirements are very small and an omnivore has stores that represent several years' turnover of the vitamin. Contamination of food with micro-organisms, insects, faecal matter or perhaps synthesis by gut bacteria may contribute significant amounts of B_{12} to the diet of even the strictest vegetarian (e.g. mould on nuts, insects or insect droppings on fruit or vegetables). Algal preparations like *Spirulina* and *Chlorella* have been marketed as sources of vitamin B_{12} that are suitable for vegans but the form of the vitamin found in *Spirulina* is almost certainly not active in humans (Watanabe *et al.*, 1999) although that in *Chlorella* is bio-available (Kittaka-Katsura *et al.*, 2002). Some lactovegetarian Asian women in the UK develop signs of deficiency despite the presence of B_{12} in milk, and this is explained by suggesting that the traditional practice of boiling milk with tea may destroy the B_{12} in the milk.

It may take many years of dietary deficiency of vitamin B_{12} before clinical symptoms of deficiency manifest in adults. The usual cause of B_{12} deficiency is not dietary lack but *inadequate absorption*. An autoimmune disease, *pernicious anaemia*, results in damage to the parietal cells of the stomach that produce an intrinsic factor that is necessary for the absorption of B_{12} from the gut. Until the 1920s, pernicious anaemia was an inevitably fatal condition, but nowadays the effects of the resulting B_{12} deficiency can be alleviated by monthly injections of the vitamin.

The efficiency of absorption of vitamin B_{12} declines in the elderly, so insufficiency becomes more prevalent in older age groups. Probably because of the neurological consequences of B_{12} deficiency, it has been suggested that supplements may be beneficial in elderly people with cognitive impairment or dementia, but there are very few data from clinical trials to back up this suggestion (Malouf and Sastre, 2003).

FOLATE OR FOLIC ACID (VITAMIN B₉)

Key facts

- *Names and chemical forms.* Folate/folic acid (folacin) is also designated vitamin B_9. Note that folate is the generic name for all dietary forms but folic acid refers to the parent compound used in most supplements and fortified foods but not naturally present in food.
- *Dietary standards.* UK RNI is 200 µg/day, but all sexually active women of child-bearing age are currently recommended to take supplements of 400 µg/day; UK LRNI is 100 µg/day; American RDA is 400 µg/day.
- *Dietary sources.* Liver, nuts, green vegetables, whole-grain cereals are good sources.
  - 1 portion (90g) lamb liver – 220 µg
  - 1 slice wholemeal bread (UK) – 14 µg
  - 30g peanuts – 33 µg
  - 1 portion (95g) broccoli – 100 µg
  - 1 banana – 30 µg
  - 1 orange – 90 µg
  - 1 teaspoon (5g) yeast extract – 50 µg.
- *Biochemical functions.* Involved with B_{12} in methylation reactions necessary for DNA synthesis and thus important in cell division.
- *Effect of deficiency.* Megaloblastic anaemia.
- *Risk factors for deficiency.* Poor diet – deficiency common in tropical countries; prolonged heating (e.g. of pulses) destroys folate; poor absorption, e.g. in coeliac disease; some drugs (e.g. anticonvulsants) may interfere with folate functioning.

- *Biochemical measure of nutritional status.* Red cell folate concentration with values <230 nmol/L are considered to indicate severe deficiency. Values <345 nmol/L are indicative of marginal deficiency.

- *Prevalence of deficiency.* In 2000, 4–5 per cent of UK adults had red cell folate levels indicative of marginal status but fewer than 1 per cent had values indicating severe deficiency. In elderly UK adults, 8 per cent of free-living subjects and 16 per cent of those living in institutions had red cell folate concentrations indicative of severe deficiency and a further 20 per cent had marginal values.

- *Toxicity.* Direct toxicity is very low. High doses can mask the haematological effects of vitamin B_{12} deficiency but do not prevent the damage to the spinal cord. It may also reduce the effectiveness of drugs that work by affecting folate metabolism.

- *Recommendations on high intakes.* Doses of up to 1.5 mg/day should not have any adverse effects, but note the previous bullet point.

- *Typical highest UK intakes.* The highest consumers may get in excess of 500 μg/day from food. Supplements aimed at women may provide up to 800 μg/day.

Nature and sources of folate

Folic acid or pteroylmonoglutamic acid is the parent compound for a group of substances known collectively as folate. This is the form used in supplements and fortified foods. Folic acid is made up of three components: pteridine, para-amino benzoic acid (PABA) and glutamic acid (Figure 14.11). Most of the folate in food is conjugated with 5–7 glutamic acid residues linked to the glutamic acid residue shown in the figure. In food folate, there is usually also reduction of one or two of the double bonds in the pteridine ring and the addition of single carbon units to one or more of the nitrogen atoms. These conjugated forms of folate must be deconjugated in the intestine before they can be absorbed, so they may be less bioavailable than folic acid. Details of the different forms of folate, their presence in different foods and their bioavailability may be found in Ball (2004).

Free folic acid is not normally present in blood but it can be detected in the serum of those taking supplements of folic acid or eating fortified food. In the USA, where flour is fortified with folic acid, it has been found that 40 per cent of older adults now have free folic acid in their plasma (Bailey *et al.*, 2010). There has been speculation that this free folic acid could increase cancer risk. Free folic acid has been shown to reduce the ability of natural killer (NK) cells of the immune system to kill emerging tumour cells (Troen *et al.*, 2006). A number of anti-ancer drugs like methotrexate work by reducing folic acid availability to tumour cells, so extra folic acid might accelerate tumour growth. Food folate is normally transformed in the intestine to 5-methyl tetrahydrofolic acid, but when folic acid is consumed this transformation takes place relatively slowly in the liver after absorption and so free folic acid appears in the circulation.

Folates are found in good amounts in green vegetables, liver, yeast extract, mushrooms, nuts and whole grains. It has been a source of considerable controversy that the conjugated forms of folate naturally present in food are not permitted to be

Figure 14.11 The structure of folic acid.

used in supplements or food fortification within the EU.

Functions of folate

Folate interacts with vitamin B$_{12}$ in the transfer of methyl groups. The synthesis of thymidylate, the nucleotide necessary for DNA synthesis, involves methyl transfer and requires both folate and B$_{12}$. As with B$_{12}$, deficiency of folic acid limits DNA synthesis and thus cell division.

Requirements and assessment of status

The estimated adult requirements for folate are given in the key facts box. Long-term folate status can be assessed by measurements of red cell folate concentrations and the critical values are also given in the key facts box. Serum folate concentration is used as a measure of recent folate consumption.

Folate deficiency

Megaloblastic or macrocytic anaemia is a symptom of both folic acid and B$_{12}$ deficiency. The bone marrow's ability to produce blood cells is affected by the reduced ability to synthesize thymidylate and thus DNA. Large, immature and unstable red cells are found circulating in the blood in megaloblastic anaemia as well as abnormal white cells and platelets. Other rapidly dividing tissues are also affected, including the gut lining. High doses of folic acid will mask the haematological consequences of B$_{12}$ deficiency but will not prevent the neurological consequences, so it is important that the cause of megaloblastic anaemia be determined before treatment is undertaken.

Some degree of folate deficiency is relatively common in people living on a poor diet in developing countries; that is, a diet lacking in green vegetables and pulses and made up largely of a low-folate starchy staple. Several drugs including some anti-epileptics increase folate requirements, and alcoholics often have poor folate status. Folate deficiency may be precipitated also by diseases that affect absorption of folate, such as coeliac disease and tropical sprue.

Folic acid and birth defects

There is now very persuasive evidence that, under clinical trial conditions, consumption of folic acid supplements by women immediately prior to conception and in the first 12 weeks of pregnancy greatly reduces the risk of the baby developing a *neural tube defect* (NTD). The collective term NTD is used to describe a group of conditions (most commonly anencephaly and spina bifida) in which the brain, spinal cord, skull and/or vertebral column fail to develop properly early in embryonic life. In anencephaly there is almost complete absence of the brain and skull and these babies die *in utero* or shortly after birth. In spina bifida, the spinal canal in the vertebral column fails to close and in severe cases the spinal cord bulges out of the back. Babies affected by this condition suffer from a range of physical disabilities that in severe cases include paralysis, bladder and bowel incontinence and neurological damage caused by hydrocephalus (accumulation of fluid around the brain).

About 1 in 250 pregnancies in the UK are affected and, despite screening and termination of affected pregnancies, around 1 in 4000 babies born in the UK have a neural tube defect. In the 1970s, before widespread screening and termination, 1 in 700 births were affected. The risk is 10 times higher in women who have already had an affected pregnancy, but most babies born with these defects are nevertheless first occurrences.

Studies published in the 1960s indicated that women who had taken a folic acid antagonist during pregnancy had an increased risk of having a baby affected by an NTD. Others had shown that women who gave birth to NTD-affected babies showed biochemical evidence of defective folic acid metabolism. In 1965, Hibbard and Smithells put forward the hypothesis that folic acid supplements might reduce the risk of neural tube defects by compensating for some defect in folic acid absorption or metabolism. The MRC (1991) conducted a randomized, double-blind prevention trial using around 2000 women identified as being at high risk of delivering an NTD baby because of a previous affected pregnancy. Half of these women were given supplements of 5 mg/day of folic acid (with or without other B vitamins) and half received no folic acid (although half of these received other B vitamins). There were only six affected babies in the folic acid-supplemented groups but 21 in the same number of women not receiving folic acid supplements – a 72 per cent protective effect. This study convincingly demonstrated the benefits of supplements for such high-risk women.

Subsequent studies confirmed the protective effect of folic acid both in preventing the recurrence of NTDs in previously affected women and also in preventing primary occurrence in women with no history of an NTD-affected pregnancy (e.g. Czeizel and Dudas, 1992). Doses that are an order of magnitude less than those used by MRC (1991) have been shown to be effective in greatly reducing occurrence of NTDs. There now seems to be a general acceptance that increased peri-conceptual intake of folic acid reduces the incidence of NTDs. In a review of experience in Hungary of using supplements containing 800 μg of folic acid it was found that the rate of primary NTDs fell by up to 90 per cent (Czeizel, 2009). In a meta-analysis of five published studies involving over 6000 women, De-Regil et al. (2010) found a substantial and highly significant effect of peri-conceptual folic acid supplements in preventing both first occurrence and recurrence of NTDs. There were insufficient data to properly evaluate the effect on other birth defects such as cleft lip and cleft palate, but they found no significant effect on these and other birth defects.

There is also increasing evidence that folic acid supplements may reduce the incidence of other birth defects. Czeizel (2009) suggests that the incidence of other congenital defects had decreased significantly in Hungarian women receiving large folic acid supplements, especially congenital defects of the heart and urinary tract. A large case–control study of Norwegian women concluded that folic acid supplements in early pregnancy reduced the incidence of cleft lip by around a third (Wilcox et al., 2007). In the Canadian province of Quebec, there was a significant and sustained decrease in the incidence of severe congenital heart defects in the years immediately after fortification of flour and pasta with folic acid was made mandatory (Ionescu-Ittu et al., 2009).

In 1992, an expert advisory group in the UK recommended that all women in the high-risk category should take supplements of 5 mg of folic acid daily if they planned to become pregnant and during the first 12 weeks of pregnancy. All other women were recommended to take a more modest 400 μg extra folic acid when planning to become pregnant and in the first 12 weeks of pregnancy

(DH, 1992b). However, as many as half of all pregnancies may be unplanned so, to have maximum impact on the incidence of NTDs, all women of reproductive age would need to substantially increase their intake of folic acid. Note that average intakes of UK women are about 250 μg/day and more than 85 per cent of women of child-bearing age take in less than 400 μg/day when their intakes from food and supplements are combined. Since 1998 there has been fortification of all cereal grain products with 140 μg/100 g in the USA. About 50 other countries have since followed the American lead and implemented mandatory fortification of flour with folic acid. More than a decade ago, an expert report in the UK (COMA, 2000) also recommended that there should be universal fortification of flour with folic acid. In 2006 the FSA also made a recommendation that in the UK there should be mandatory fortification of flour, but at the start of 2012 these recommendations had not been implemented.

There is no doubt that where food fortification with folic acid has been introduced it has been effective in substantially reducing the incidence of neural tube defects, as the examples below illustrate.

- Fortification has reduced NTD frequency in the USA by 25–30 per cent (Pitkin, 2007) and increased levels of fortification have been advocated for optimal NTD prevention.
- Spina bifida prevalence is now 53 per cent lower in seven Canadian provinces than prior to the introduction of mandatory fortification (De Wals et al. 2008).
- Mandatory fortification programmes in Chile, Argentina and Brazil reduced the incidence of NTDs by up to 50 per cent (Lopez-Camelo et al., 2010).

Folic acid supplements do not eliminate neural tube defects completely; a small residue of cases that are not responsive to supplements will remain even with large doses (Heseker et al., 2008). In the USA, it has been estimated that current levels of fortification prevent about half of the folate-responsive cases (Pitkin, 2007).

In contrast to the confirmed effectiveness of food fortification, recommendations that women 'at risk' of pregnancy take supplements have not been effective in measurably reducing the incidence of NTDs. Botto *et al.* (2005) found that the incidence of NTDs in Europe and Israel did not change significantly between 1988 and 1998 despite the fact that in some countries (UK and Ireland) supplement recommendations had been made since 1992. Most pregnancies are not specifically planned, so many women will not take supplements until they realize they are pregnant – and this is after the time when folate is most effective (in the first month after conception). It is also a general observation that supplements are rarely taken by those with low nutrient intakes from food but are taken by those least likely to need them.

As already stated, folate is required for methyl transfer reactions involved in DNA synthesis, so rapidly dividing cells (as in bone marrow) are susceptible to any folate deficit. The rapidly dividing cells of the developing neural tube of the fetus would also be susceptible to folate deficit and result in an NTD. It is not thought that maternal folate deficiency *per se* is a major reason why NTDs occur, but it seems that extra folic acid probably compensates for some genetic variation in folate-dependent enzymes or receptors involved in folate metabolism (van der Linden *et al.*, 2006).

Food fortification with folic acid exposes several hundred thousand people to the folic acid for each case of NTD prevented. Regulators must therefore be confident that there are no significant hazards from the extra folate.

Possible other benefits of high folate intake

If there were wider benefits of folic acid fortification of food then this would strengthen the case for the introduction of mandatory fortification. Poor biochemical status for folate is relatively common in the UK especially among elderly institutionalized people, so one benefit of fortification would be to improve folate status of the UK population as it has done in the USA. There is epidemiological evidence that a high intake of natural food folate is associated with a reduced incidence of *bowel cancer* (WCRF/AICR, 2007). Roswall *et al.* (2010), in a large cohort study of middle-aged Danes, found that high intake of food folate but not folic acid supplements was

associated with reduced risk of bowel cancer. Mathers (2009) speculated that low folate status would reduce thymine production and perhaps lead to uracil incorporation into DNA; this and other abnormalities of methylation might lead to cancerous changes in the bowel.

Folate deficiency can lead to moderate elevation of homocysteine levels in the blood as folate is necessary for its methylation and conversion to methionine. It is known that greatly elevated homocysteine levels in people with the inherited condition predisposes people to premature *vascular disease*, and there is some epidemiological evidence that moderate elevation of homocysteine levels due to folate deficiency may increase cardiovascular risk. However, there is no evidence that supplements of folic acid have any benefit on cardiovascular disease in primary or secondary intervention trials, even though they significantly reduce plasma homocysteine levels (Marti-Carvajal *et al.*, 2009; SEARCH Collaborative Group, 2010).

There is some epidemiological evidence that high folate intake is associated with reduced risk of *Alzheimer's disease*, but clinical trials have not found evidence of any benefit of folic acid supplements (Malouf and Grimley Evans, 2008).

Potential hazards of high folic acid intake

The FSA (2003) concluded that total intakes of folate of 1.5 mg/day would not be expected to have any adverse effects, and this is well below what would be consumed from food even if mandatory fortification occurs. The main concerns that have been voiced about mandatory fortification of bread with folic acid are noted below.

- High folic acid intake could mask the haematological consequences of vitamin B$_{12}$ deficiency and thus delay its diagnosis. This might increase the spinal and neurological damage caused by B$_{12}$ deficiency.
- High folate intake could reduce the effectiveness of certain drugs like methotrexate that work by interfering with folate metabolism.
- High folic acid intake might increase the growth of existing bowel cancers or increase the risk of benign bowel adenomas developing into cancers.

- As noted earlier, there are suggestions that the folic acid used in supplements and for fortifying food might pose risks not posed by natural conjugated forms of folate found in food.

Cases of serious neurological damage due to vitamin B_{12} deficiency are extremely rare, with fewer than 30 cases per year in the UK. As supplements of well in excess of 1 mg/day are needed to mask the anaemia of vitamin B_{12} deficiency, this seems to be probably only a theoretical risk. According to FSA (2003), even if UK flour were fortified with 240 μg/100 g (cf. current US level of 140 μg/100 g), only 0.6 per cent would have a total folate intake of 1 mg/day; many more would have their currently poor folate status improved by supplements.

Methotrexate is used in cancer chemotherapy and in the treatment of rheumatoid arthritis (RA). It is taken up very efficiently by cancer cells and, because it is structurally similar to folic acid, it acts as an anti-metabolite to folic acid and reduces the availability of folate co-enzymes necessary for DNA synthesis – and thus reduces cancer cell proliferation. Supplements of folic acid might make methotrexate and a number of drugs that work by a similar mechanism less effective or increase the dose needed. There is some evidence that, since the introduction of folic acid fortification in the USA in 1998, there has been an increase in the doses of methotrexate used to manage patients with RA (Arbelovic et al., 2007). When used to treat RA, methotrexate results in gastrointestinal and haematological side-effects that limit its use in many patients. A meta-analysis by Ortiz et al. (1999) found that concurrent provision of folic acid supplements substantially reduced these side-effects of methotrexate.

Despite epidemiological evidence that diets rich in folate are associated with reduced risk of bowel cancer, it has been paradoxically suggested that high intakes of folic acid from supplements or fortified food might increase the risk of bowel cancer. Mason et al. (2007) reported that recorded rates of colorectal cancer rose slightly in both the USA and Canada in the period immediately after the introduction of folic acid fortification of flour. Even though rates then resumed their previous downward tendency, they remained slightly above those that would have been predicted from pre-fortification

trends, and they estimated that this 'blip' resulted in between four and six 'extra' cases per 100 000 people. Even though this is a very small number of possible extra cases, the fact remains that several hundred thousand people are exposed to folic acid in fortified food for every case of NTD prevented. More recently, Stevens et al. (2011) have conducted a specific and detailed analysis of the relationship between colorectal cancer risk and both natural folate intake and supplemental folic acid intake in a cohort of 100 000 American men and women. They found that high levels of neither natural folate nor folic acid were significantly associated with risk of colorectal cancer, but total folate intake was associated with a significantly lower risk.

Summing up

The foregoing observations on the risks and benefits of fortification of food with folic acid would suggest the following, on the basis of current evidence.

- Folic acid fortification of flour in the UK would reduce the number of pregnancies affected by neural tube defects and probably reduce the incidences of several other birth defects.
- Several hundred thousand people would be exposed to folic acid in fortified flour for every case of NTD prevented.
- Fortification would improve population status for folate and reduce the currently large prevalence of poor folate status especially in older people.
- It seems improbable that the amount of extra folic acid in fortified flour would pose any practical danger to elderly people by masking the anaemia of vitamin B_{12} deficiency.
- There seems very little hard evidence to support suggestions that increasing folate intakes by fortification would reduce rates of cardiovascular disease or dementia.

There are conflicting views about the likely effect of extra folic acid on colorectal cancer risk. First, epidemiological studies suggest that folate-rich diets are associated with *reduced* risk. Second, some preliminary evidence from North America suggested that rates of colorectal cancer *rose* very slightly in the period immediately after fortification of flour with folic acid was introduced. Third, the latest evidence from a large cohort study found no evidence that folic acid intake increased colorectal cancer risk but that high total folate intake was associated with reduced risk of colorectal cancer.

BIOTIN

Key facts

- *Names and chemical forms.* Biotin.
- *Dietary standards.* UK 'safe intake' is 10–200 µg/day; USA 30 µg/day.
- *Dietary sources.* Widely distributed in many foods at low concentrations but good amounts in liver and organ meat, egg yolk, whole-grain cereals and yeast.
- *Biochemical functions.* A cofactor for several carboxylase enzymes that add carboxyl or – COOH groups.
- *Effects of deficiency.* Dermatitis and other symptoms.
- *Risk factors for deficiency.* Simple dietary deficiency is rare. It can occur as a side-effect of certain treatments including dialysis and total parenteral nutrition (TPN) or in some rare genetic abnormalities.
- *Biochemical measure of nutritional status.* Plasma biotin with values below 1.02 nmol/L are thought to indicate deficiency – rarely measured.
- *Prevalence of deficiency.* Nutritional deficiency is rare.
- *Toxicity.* Little evidence of toxicity associated with oral biotin consumption.
- *Recommendations on high intakes.* Doses up to 0.9 mg/day should not have any adverse effects, but doses 10 times higher than this have no reported adverse effects.
- *Typical highest UK intakes.* The highest UK consumers may get around 70 µg/day from food. Over-the-counter supplements may contain up to 2 mg/day.

Overview

Biotin was originally known as the 'anti-egg white injury factor' because it cured a dermatitis induced in rats by feeding them large amounts of raw egg white. A protein present in raw egg white inhibits the absorption of biotin but this is denatured when eggs are cooked. Biotin deficiency in humans is rare and usually associated with eating large amounts of raw egg or other bizarre diets. It has been reported in the past in patients being fed by total parenteral nutrition for long periods. Human milk is relatively low in biotin and some cases of biotin-responsive dermatitis have been reported in babies breastfed by poorly nourished mothers.

Biotin functions as a co-enzyme for several important carboxylase enzymes; that is, enzymes that add a carboxyl (COOH) group via fixation of carbon dioxide. The enzyme pyruvate carboxylase is important in gluconeogenesis (production of glucose from pyruvate and amino acids – see Chapter 6). Other carboxylase enzymes are important in fatty acid synthesis (acetyl CoA carboxylase) and the metabolism of branched-chain amino acids.

Biotin requirements have not been clearly established, partly because gut bacteria may make some indeterminate contribution to biotin supply. Current dietary standards are given in the key facts box. Biotin is present in good amounts in liver, cooked eggs, cereals and yeast.

PANTOTHENIC ACID

Key facts

- *Names and chemical forms.* Pantothenic acid; it is present as co-enzyme A (CoA) in food.
- *Dietary standards.* UK 'safe intake' is 3–7 mg/day; USA 5 mg/day.
- *Dietary sources.* Present as CoA in most animal and plant cells, so widely distributed in foods.
- *Biochemical functions.* It is the precursor of CoA, and CoA-containing compounds are key intermediates in many biochemical pathways (e.g. acetyl CoA and succinyl CoA).
- *Effects of deficiency.* 'Burning feet' syndrome (abnormal skin sensations induced by warmth) has been associated with deficiency of pantothenic acid.
- *Biochemical measure of nutritional status.* A plasma pantothenic acid concentration of less than 100 µg/L is indicative of low intake but it is rarely measured.

→

Key facts *continued*

- *Prevalence of deficiency.* Overt dietary deficiency is rarely seen.
- *Toxicity.* No reports of toxic effects.
- *Recommendations on high intakes.* Supplemental doses of 200 mg/day should not have any harmful effects; no harmful effects have been reported with doses over 10 times this amount.
- *Typical highest UK intakes.* Food may provide up to 12 mg/day. Over-the-counter supplements may contain 550 mg/day.

Overview

Pantothenic acid is a precursor of co-enzyme A which is essential for many metabolic processes – note the acetyl CoA in carbohydrate and fatty acid metabolism and the succinyl CoA of the Krebs cycle. The vitamin is widely distributed in food and clinical deficiency is rare. A 'burning feet' syndrome has been reported in severely malnourished prisoners of war and in experimental deficiency. Requirements for pantothenic acid are difficult to estimate accurately.

VITAMIN C (ASCORBIC ACID)

Key facts

- *Nature and chemical forms.* Ascorbic acid.
- *Dietary standards.* UK RNI is 40 mg/day; UK LRNI is 10 mg/day; American RDA M/F is 90/75 mg/day.
- *Dietary sources.* Fruit, fruit juices, salad and leafy vegetables are good sources.
  - 1 serving (95 g) broccoli – 30 mg
  - 1 serving (75 g) frozen peas – 10 mg
  - 1 portion (150 g) boiled potatoes – 14 mg
  - 1 portion (45 g) sweet pepper – 45 mg
  - 1 tomato – 15 mg
  - 1 orange – 95 mg
  - 1 banana – 8 mg
  - 1 serving (100 g) strawberries – 60 mg
  - 1 apple – 2 mg
  - 1 glass (200 g) orange juice – 70 mg.
- *Biochemical functions.* Important in synthesis of collagen; promotes non-haem iron absorption;
  →

Key facts *continued*

cofactor in synthesis of carnitine, synthesis of several nerve transmitters and peptide hormones. An important water-soluble anti-oxidant.

- *Effect of deficiency.* Scurvy.
- *Risk factors for deficiency.* Living on preserved foods, absence of fruits and vegetables from the diet.
- *Biochemical measure of nutritional status.* Plasma vitamin C concentrations <11 µmol/L are indicative of biochemical depletion.
- *Prevalence of deficiency.* In 2000, 5 per cent of UK adult men and 3 per cent of women had plasma concentrations below the threshold value. Around 14 per cent of free-living elderly UK adults had plasma levels below the threshold, and this rose to around 40 per cent in those living in institutions.
- *Toxicity.* Several grams of vitamin C can cause diarrhoea owing to unabsorbed vitamin entering the large bowel. There are claims that high doses can increase the risk of calcium oxalate kidney stones because oxalate is a metabolite of the vitamin, but the data are conflicting.
- *Recommendations on high intakes.* Doses of 1 g/day are unlikely to have any significant adverse effects even in susceptible groups. Doses well in excess of this are widely used without any apparent ill-effects.
- *Typical highest UK intakes.* The highest consumers may get 200 mg/day from food. Supplements may provide as much as 3 g/day.

Nature and sources of vitamin C

The structure of vitamin C or ascorbic acid is shown in Figure 14.12. Most species are able to make ascorbic acid from glucose, but primates, guinea pigs, bats and some birds lack a key enzyme (gulanolactone oxidase) on this synthetic pathway. Ascorbic acid is water soluble and in solution is readily oxidized to dehydroascorbic acid; thus it acts as an anti-oxidant. It is sometimes used in food processing as an anti-oxidant.

Fruits and vegetables (including potatoes) are the classical sources of vitamin C. Significant amounts are present in offal and fresh cow milk. There may

Figure 14.12 The structure of vitamin C (ascorbic acid).

even be traces in fresh raw meat and fish. Because of its use as an anti-oxidant additive, it may also be present in foods like ham, sausages and pâté.

Functions of vitamin C

Vitamin C or ascorbic acid is necessary for the functioning of the enzyme proline hydroxylase. This enzyme hydroxylates residues of the amino acid proline to hydroxyproline once it has been incorporated into the important structural protein *collagen*. Collagen is a major structural protein. It has the capacity to form strong insoluble fibres and is the most abundant protein in mammals and serves to hold cells together. It is a structural component of bones, skin, cartilage and blood vessels, and indeed fulfils a structural role in most organs. The hydroxylation of proline residues occurs after incorporation of the amino acid into pro-collagen (the precursor of collagen) and the hydroxylation is necessary for the structural properties of collagen; hydroxyproline is almost exclusively confined to collagen. A similar vitamin C-dependent hydroxylation of lysine residues in pro-collagen also occurs. Some other functions of vitamin C are listed below.

- It acts as an anti-oxidant in the aqueous phase and this was discussed in Chapter 13.
- It is a cofactor in the synthesis of the important nerve transmitter noradrenalin (norepinephrine).
- It is a cofactor in the synthesis of carnitine, which is necessary for the transfer of long-chain fatty acids into the mitochondrion where β-oxidation occurs (see Chapter 13).
- Large doses of vitamin C increase the absorption of non-haem iron from the gut.
- It is involved in the synthesis of several peptide hormones and transmitters, including oxytocin, gastrin, calcitonin and antidiuretic hormone. These hormones all have a glycine residue at their C-terminals which has to be converted to an amide to make the active hormone.

Requirements and assessment of status

The dietary standards for vitamin C are shown in the key facts box. Vitamin C status can be assessed by measurement of plasma vitamin C concentration. Values below 11 μmol/L are taken as indicative of biochemical depletion.

Deficiency states

Scurvy is the disease caused by lack of vitamin C. Most of the symptoms of scurvy can be attributed to impaired synthesis of the structural protein collagen – bleeding gums, loose teeth, subdermal haemorrhages due to leaking blood vessels, impaired wound healing and breakdown of old scars. Large areas of spontaneous bruising occur in severe scurvy, and haemorrhages in heart muscle or the brain may cause sudden death. Sudden death from haemorrhage or heart failure may occur even when the outward manifestations of scurvy do not appear particularly severe. Anaemia is usually associated with scurvy, almost certainly because vitamin C is an important promoter of iron absorption from the gut. The organic bone matrix is largely collagen and so osteoporosis may also occur in scurvy.

Scurvy occurs in people deprived of fresh foods for extended periods, especially diets lacking in both fruits and vegetables. Outbreaks of scurvy commonly occurred among people living for extended periods on preserved foods (e.g. those undertaking long sea voyages or taking part in expeditions to places where fresh foods were unavailable). The curative and preventative effects of fresh vegetables, fruits and fruit juices were documented almost two centuries before the discovery of vitamin C. In 1795, the regular provision of lime juice (or some suitable alternative) to British naval personnel resulted in the 'limey' nickname for British sailors. This nickname is still sometimes used to describe the British.

Benefits and risks of high intakes

Around 10 mg/day of vitamin C is enough to prevent scurvy but some sources recommend intakes of several grams per day for 'optimal health'. The role of vitamin C as an anti-oxidant was discussed in Chapter 13 where it was concluded there that there is no convincing evidence to support the suggestion that high supplemental intake of vitamin C (or any other anti-oxidant) reduces the long-term risk of developing cancer or cardiovascular disease.

The UK panel on dietary reference values (COMA, 1991) listed at least eight benefits that have been suggested for intakes of vitamin C that are well in excess of those needed to prevent or to cure scurvy. It was nevertheless not persuaded to allow any of these suggested benefits to influence its decisions about the reference values. The size of the body pool is maximized at intakes of 100–150 mg/day. At higher intakes, the absorption of vitamin C from the intestine becomes saturated and there is increased renal excretion.

One of the best known and most persistent of the claims for vitamin C is that intake of more than 10 times the RNI/RDA might help prevent the development of the common cold. This view was popularized by a book published in the early 1970s that was written by the double Nobel Prize winner Linus Pauling (Pauling, 1972). The original bases for advocating very high intakes were either extrapolations of the amounts synthesized by the rat, or the amounts consumed by non-human primates requiring vitamin C, such as gorillas. Since 1970 there have been dozens of controlled trials on the efficacy of vitamin C in preventing colds and/or reducing their duration. Despite this plethora of research effort there remains no convincing evidence that high vitamin C intake affects the frequency of colds. In a meta-analysis of 30 trials involving over 11 000 participants, Hemila et al. (2007) found no evidence that vitamin C prophylaxis (at least 200 mg/day) reduced the risk of developing a cold. A subgroup of six trials involving participants who were marathon runners, skiers or soldiers on sub-arctic exercises did find evidence of preventative benefit under these circumstances. These reviewers concluded that 'routine mega-dose prophylaxis is not rationally justified for community use'. There was evidence from these prophylaxis studies that vitamin C has a small but statistically significant effect in reducing the duration of cold symptoms, but these authors concluded that this small effect may be of little clinical value. Four trials using up to 8 g/day of vitamin C found no significant evidence that it had any benefits when it was taken at the onset of cold symptoms.

Many millions of people (maybe a third of Americans) are unconvinced by arguments against the efficacy of vitamin C supplements and continue to take sometimes large vitamin C supplements. Such widespread consumption of doses that are far in excess of those that can be obtained from normal human diets means that the potential toxicity of these preparations needs to be considered.

Many people take very large doses (1–5 g/day) without any obvious toxic effects. When the body pool of the vitamin exceeds 1500 mg then it starts to be excreted in the urine along with its metabolites because the reabsorption system for vitamin C in the kidney becomes saturated. The only reasonably well-established hazard of taking substantial doses of vitamin C is that it may lead to diarrhoea and gastrointestinal symptoms because the absorption system is saturated and vitamin C remains in the gut. Other theoretical hazards such as increased risk of kidney stones and risk of precipitating iron overload in genetically susceptible people are discussed in FSA (2003), who concluded that doses of up to 1 g/day can probably be tolerated for very long periods with no obvious ill-effects in most people, and doses several times higher than this are frequently taken without obvious ill-effects.

Use of gram quantities of vitamin C – or any other vitamin – is the province of the pharmacologist rather than the nutritionist.

15

THE MINERALS

Introduction	393	Selenium	399
Chromium	394	Zinc	400
Copper	395	Iodine and iodine-deficiency diseases	402
Fluoride	396	Iron and iron-deficiency anaemia	405
Magnesium	396	Calcium storage and uptake	410
Manganese	397	Calcium and bone health	414
Molybdenum	398	Sodium and disease	421
Phosphorus	398	Review of evidence for a salt–	
Potassium	398	hypertension link	427

INTRODUCTION

In the UK, dietary reference values (DRVs) are given for 11 minerals and safe intakes are listed for a further four (COMA, 1991). These same 15 minerals are also deemed to warrant a recommendation of some type in the USA. There is, therefore, international acceptance that at least 15 dietary minerals are essential. Several of these essential minerals are required only in trace amounts and in some cases requirements are difficult to establish with confidence. COMA considered the possible essentiality of a further 19 minerals. Most of these it classified as non-essential or of unproven essentiality, while a few it regarded as probably essential in trace amounts.

The original version of the European Union's Food Supplements Directive allowed 15 minerals to be used in supplements:

calcium, chloride, chromium, copper, fluoride, iodine, iron, magnesium, manganese, molybdenum, potassium, selenium, zinc, phosphorus and sodium.

This original list was criticized by some pressure groups because it did not contain several minerals that had previously been used in supplements, such as boron, vanadium and silicon. After an appeals process, boron and silicon were added to this list in 2009 – although it was made clear that this did not mean that the review group considered them to be essential nutrients.

The incidence of clinically recognizable, acute dietary deficiency states is extremely rare for most essential minerals. Only two such deficiency diseases have either historically been seen or are currently seen as anything other than extremely rare or localized; they are *iodine-deficiency disease*, manifested most obviously by a goitre (swelling of the thyroid gland), and *iron-deficiency anaemia*. This has not prevented very active debate about whether suboptimal intakes and subclinical deficiencies of other minerals are widespread, particularly for calcium, selenium and zinc.

What this chapter covers

The first sections of the chapter present brief reviews of several of the essential minerals, each section starting with a key facts box. Later sections discuss four mineral-related issues that have been singled out:

- iodine-deficiency diseases
- iron-deficiency anaemia
- calcium, diet and osteoporosis
- salt (sodium chloride) and hypertension.

Note that the role of dietary fluoride in dental health is discussed in Chapter 10 and so is mentioned only briefly here. Fluoride has *not* been proven to be an essential nutrient, so in both the UK and the USA only 'safe intakes' are given. In the UK, even this safe intake is restricted to infants. The roles of zinc, selenium, iron and copper as prosthetic groups for anti-oxidant enzyme systems are discussed in Chapter 13 in the section dealing with free radicals and anti-oxidants. Average intakes of several minerals are below the *reference nutrient intake* (RNI) in some sections of the UK population (especially in young women), and many individuals across all age groups have recorded intakes of one or more that are below the *lower reference nutrient intake* (LRNI).

Further information on individual minerals can be found in Geissler and Powers (2010) and Gropper *et al.* (2008), and particularly recommended is Shils *et al.* (2006). The chapters in these texts dealing with particular minerals are not individually referenced here.

Key points

- There are at least 15 essential minerals.
- Iodine and iron deficiencies are the most prevalent micronutrient deficiencies in the world.
- Acute, clinical deficiency of most other minerals is rare or localized.
- Whether intakes of several other minerals are suboptimal has been a topic of active debate in nutrition.
- Data presented in Chapters 13 and 16 indicate that average intakes of several minerals are below the RNI in some groups, especially young women; many individuals across all age and sex groups have recorded unsatisfactory intakes of at least one mineral.

CHROMIUM

Key facts

- *Dietary standards.* UK 'safe intake is >25 μg/day; American RDA M/F is 35/25 μg/day.   →

Key facts *continued*

- *Dietary sources.* Relatively large amounts in processed meats, whole-grain cereals and pulses. Only the trivalent form is present in food and this is the only form permitted in supplements within the EU.
- *Biochemical functions.* It potentiates the actions of insulin. A chromium-containing oligopeptide called chromomodulin stimulates the tyrosine kinase activity of the insulin receptor and this amplifies mechanisms in insulin signalling.
- *Effects of deficiency.* Impaired glucose uptake, increased fat utilization and other signs of reduced insulin action seen in TPN patients not given chromium in their infusions.
- *Risk factors for deficiency.* Overt deficiency only seen in TPN patients.
- *Biochemical measure of nutritional status.* No reliable indicator available.
- *Prevalence of deficiency.* Overt deficiency almost never seen.
- *Toxicity.* Compounds permitted for use in supplements have very low toxicity.
- *Recommendations on high intakes.* Doses of 10 mg/day should not have any adverse effects.
- *Typical highest UK intakes.* The highest consumers may get 200 μg/day from food. Supplements may provide a further 600 μg/day.

Overview

Chromium-responsive symptoms of reduced insulin response have been reported in isolated cases of patients undergoing long-term total parenteral nutrition (TPN) where their infusion solution was not supplemented with chromium. These symptoms included weight loss, peripheral neuropathy, reduced glucose utilization, hyperglycaemia and a low respiratory quotient (indicative of high fat utilization). Reduced insulin response has also been reported in experimental chromium deficiency in animals. It is suggested that chromium is a component of a factor called *chromomodulin* that enhances the response to insulin. A tyrosine kinase enzyme is a component of the insulin receptor and plays a key role in insulin signalling. Chromomodulin stimulates the activity of this tyrosine kinase and is necessary for a normal response to insulin. Vincent (2000) has published a review of the biochemistry of chromium.

Early studies of chromium supplementation in patients with impaired glucose tolerance and type 2 diabetes (insulin resistant) suggested that these supplements did have measurable beneficial effects. More recent analyses do not support these findings and there seems to be no case for widespread use of chromium-containing supplements. In a meta-analysis of randomized controlled trials, Althuis *et al.* (2002) found no evidence of a significant effect of chromium supplements in healthy subjects or those with impaired glucose tolerance. Their analysis of trials with diabetic subjects did suggest that the supplements may have increased insulin responses, but the subjects were almost all from a single Chinese trial, so it was concluded that the results were not without doubt. High doses of permitted supplemental forms seem to have no harmful effects, but this might be due partly to its poor absorption.

COPPER

Key facts

- *Dietary standards.* Adult RNI in the UK is 1.2 mg/day but there were insufficient data to set an LRNI; American RDA is 0.9 mg/day.

- *Dietary sources.* Nuts, seeds, shellfish, offal, cocoa powder and chocolate are good sources of copper but it is widely distributed in plant and animal foods.

- *Biochemical functions.* There are several copper-containing enzymes and other proteins in the body involved in transmitter synthesis, iron metabolism, electron transport and disposal of free radicals.

- *Effects of deficiency.* Experimental deficiency in animals results in anaemia, low white cell count and osteoporosis.

- *Risk factors for deficiency.* Overt deficiency is rarely seen in humans but has been reported in patients receiving TPN and in premature babies fed on milk diets.

- *Prevalence of deficiency.* Only seen in special circumstances.   →

Key facts *continued*

- *Toxicity.* Acute copper poisoning is rare because copper compounds have an unpleasant taste and an emetic effect; they cause abdominal pain and diarrhoea. The risk of chronic overload is reduced because of homeostatic regulation of gut absorption.

- *Recommendations on high intakes.* An upper safe limit for lifetime consumption has been set at 10 mg/day.

- *Typical highest UK intakes.* The highest intakes from food in the UK are around 3 mg/day. Over-the-counter supplements may contain up to 2 mg/day.

Overview

Copper has clearly been established as an essential nutrient but overt deficiency of the mineral is rarely seen. As noted in the key facts box, copper requirements of adults are of the order of 1 mg/day and several rich food sources contain between 0.3 and over 2 mg/100 g, including shellfish, nuts, seeds, cocoa powder, legumes, the bran and germ component of cereals, liver and other organ meats. Many other foods have intermediate amounts of copper (0.1–0.3 mg/100 g), including many fruits and vegetables (including potatoes), chocolate products, most meats, and most grain products. Drinking water may also contain significant amounts of copper. While estimates of current copper intakes are below those recorded in the past, this largely reflects improved analytical procedures and reduced use of Bordeaux mixture, a fungicide applied in horticulture which contains copper sulphate. Its wide distribution in food and low requirement make overt dietary deficiency of copper improbable. Note that cow milk is particularly low in copper.

Experimental copper deficiency has been induced in animals. It resulted in anaemia, low neutrophil count, osteoporosis and skeletal abnormalities. In humans, there have been isolated reports of copper deficiency in patients receiving TPN which was not supplemented with copper and in premature babies fed on milk diets. The symptoms in humans are similar to those induced by experimental deficiency in animals. There is a rare hereditary disorder called *Menkes' disease* which is associated with reduced copper uptake but this condition is not alleviated by copper administration and the sufferer dies in early childhood. It has been proposed but not established that marginal copper deficiency might lead to raised blood cholesterol, reduced skin pigmentation and impaired glucose tolerance.

There are a number of important copper-containing proteins in the body, including:

- some types of superoxide dismutase which is involved in free radical disposal (discussed in Chapter 13)
- enzymes involved in the synthesis of the catecholamine group of nerve transmitters from tyrosine (e.g. adrenalin, noradrenalin and dopamine)
- enzymes involved in the synthesis of the pigment melanin responsible for, among other things, skin pigmentation
- cytochrome *c* oxidase involved in the electron transfer system in mitochondria
- ceruloplasmin, involved in the transport and oxidation of iron that is necessary for haemoglobin synthesis.

Acute copper poisoning is rare because copper compounds have an unpleasant taste and cause gastrointestinal symptoms when consumed in excess. There is homeostatic regulation of copper absorption from the gut which reduces the risk of chronic poisoning. There are two rare inherited conditions called *Wilson's disease* and *Indian childhood cirrhosis* that lead to excessive accumulation of copper in the body; in both cases the excess copper causes cirrhosis of the liver, and in Wilson's disease it accumulates in the brain and causes neurological damage. Both conditions can be treated with chelating agents that hasten copper excretion, and by preventing the consumption of copper-rich diets.

FLUORIDE

It is generally agreed that fluoride is not strictly an essential nutrient but that it can be a beneficial dietary substance that reduces the risk of dental decay, especially if consumed in optimal amounts by young children. A level of 1 mg per kilogram of drinking water is regarded as optimal for dental health. In the USA, more than half of the population drink water that has been fluoridated up to this optimal level but fluoridation is much less widespread in the UK. In the

UK, a daily 'safe intake' of 0.05 mg/kg is recommended but only for infants; in the USA, there are 'adequate intakes' for all age groups ranging from 0.5 mg/day for children aged 6–12 months up to 4 mg/day for adult men. Tea and seafood are the richest sources of fluoride in the British diet – tea may provide up to 70 per cent of the total fluoride intake.

Fluoride supplements are sold in the UK as medicines rather than dietary supplements and the amount recommended to be taken varies with the concentration in the local water supply. The British Dental Association (BDA) recommends that supplements should not be given before 6 months of age, and not used at all if the water concentration exceeds 700 μg/L. The BDA further recommends that if the water concentration is below 300 μg/L then supplement doses are as follows:

- 250 μg/day from age 6 months to 3 years
- 500 μg/day at 3–6 years
- 1 mg/day from 6 years until puberty.

If the water concentration is between 300 and 700 μg/L, then the following supplement doses should be used:

- 200 μg/day for 3- to 6 year olds
- 500 μg/day for those over 6 years.

The role of fluoride in dental health is discussed more fully in Chapter 10.

MAGNESIUM

Key facts

- *Dietary standards.* Adult UK RNI M/F is 300/270 mg/day; UK LRNI is 190/150 mg/day; American RDA is 400/310 mg/day.
- *Dietary sources.* Leafy vegetables, wholegrains, nuts, seafood and legumes are good sources. Some drinking water may contain 50 mg/L in hard water areas.
- *Biochemical functions.* Many magnesium-dependent enzymes exist and most biochemical pathways have magnesium-dependent enzymes.
- *Effects of deficiency.* Induced magnesium deficiency leads to muscle weakness, spasms, personality changes, anorexia, nausea and vomiting.

→

Overview

As noted in Chapters 13 and 16, many children, adults and elderly people have recorded intakes of magnesium that are below the LRNI. Several enzymes such as DNA and RNA polymerase contain magnesium which binds to the enzyme and makes it active. Magnesium can also affect enzyme activity by binding to the substrate and increasing its affinity for the enzyme; for example, it complexes with ATP which increases its affinity for kinases. About 60–65 per cent of body magnesium is present in bone, 1 per cent is in extracellular fluids, and the rest is found within soft tissues, especially muscle. There are over 300 enzyme reactions where magnesium is important, including many kinases and enzymes involved in glycolysis, the Krebs cycle, the pentose phosphate pathway, β-oxidation of fatty acids, creatine phosphate formation in muscle and nucleic acid, (RNA and DNA) synthesis.

Although many people across the age groups have low or inadequate intakes of magnesium, primary symptomatic deficiency of magnesium is rare. Deficiency may occur as a secondary consequence of several conditions listed in the key facts box. There are claims that magnesium supplements may lower blood pressure in healthy people or those with moderate hypertension (e.g. Sacks *et al.*, 1998). Dickinson *et al.* (2006a) in a meta-analysis of 12 published trials found that magnesium supplements given for at least 2 months resulted in a small but statistically significant reduction in diastolic blood pressure. However, some of these trials were of low quality and the results were heterogeneous, making bias a likely cause of the observed effect.

Chronic low magnesium status has been linked to increased risk of coronary heart disease and this has been used to explain the slightly lower incidence of CHD in hard water areas. There is, however, little substantial evidence to support this or other claims that magnesium supplements enhance athletic performance or help to prevent osteoporosis.

MANGANESE

Overview

Although experimental manganese deficiency can be induced in animals and has been reported in individual cases of patients receiving TPN, it is almost never seen. Average intakes are high in relation to estimated requirements. Most plant foods contain reasonable amounts, but the concentrations in animal tissues are low and thus the amounts in meat, fish and milk are low. Two manganese-containing enzymes are listed in the key facts box and a number of other enzymes are activated by manganese, although many of these are activated also by magnesium.

MOLYBDENUM

Key facts

- *Dietary standards.* UK 'safe intake' is 50–400 µg/day. In the USA it is 45 µg/day.
- *Dietary sources.* Widespread in foods and the amount depends on soil content.
- *Biochemical functions.* At least three molybdenum-requiring enzymes exist: xanthine oxidase, aldehyde oxidase and sulphite oxidase.
- *Effects of deficiency.* Reduced activity of the above enzymes.
- *Risk factor for deficiency.* Total parenteral nutrition.
- *Biochemical measure of nutritional status.* Not usually measured.
- *Toxicity.* Has low toxicity and symptoms may resemble copper deficiency.
- *Recommendations on high intakes.* Few data, but may require >10 mg/day to produce any ill-effects
- *Typical highest UK intakes.* Highest UK intakes from food may be 250 µg/day. Supplements may contain further 330 µg/day. Highest total intake is usually at least an order of magnitude below the toxic effect amount.

Overview

Although experimental molybdenum deficiency can be induced in animals, just one verified case of deficiency has been reported in a single TPN patient. Molybdenum is a cofactor for:

- xanthine oxidase, an enzyme involved in purine breakdown
- aldehyde oxidase, an enzyme involved in nucleotide breakdown from nucleic acids
- sulphite oxidase involved in breakdown of sulphur-containing amino acids.

Reduced excretion of sulphate and uric acid was recorded in the one confirmed case of human molybdenum deficiency.

PHOSPHORUS

Around 80 per cent of the body's phosphorus is in bone mineral as the calcium salt hydroxyapatite. Phosphorylation and dephosphorylation reactions are an important feature of biochemical reactions (note ATP and creatine phosphate). Phosphorus is a component of phospholipids which are important in membranes and is important in some buffering systems. In the UK, the RNI for phosphorus is set at 550 mg/day which is the molar equivalent of the calcium RNI; in the USA the RDA is 700 mg/day. Phosphate is a major component of all plant and animal cells and so is found in all natural foods.

POTASSIUM

Key facts

- *Dietary standards.* Adult UK RNI is 3500 mg/day; adult LRNI is 2000 mg/day; American RDA is 4700 mg/day.
- *Dietary sources.* Fruits and vegetables are the best sources although there is some in milk and flesh foods.
  - 1 orange – 490 mg
  - 1 banana – 470 mg
  - 1 apple – 145 mg
  - 1 portion (95 g) broccoli – 210 mg
  - 1 portion (75 g) frozen peas – 100 mg
  - 1 tomato – 220 g
  - 1 portion (265 g) chips (French fries) – 2700 mg
  - 1 glass (200 g) canned orange juice – 260 mg.
- *Biochemical functions.* Potassium is the major cation in intracellular fluid; nerve impulse transmission; contraction of muscle and heart; acid–base balance.   →

Overview

The richest sources of potassium are fruits and vegetables, but it is present in all animal and plant tissues and in milk. The body of an average man contains around 135 grams of potassium, and the actual amount in any person's body is a reflection of his or her lean tissue mass. All but 5 per cent of the body's potassium is found within cells and it is the principal cation in intracellular fluid. Measures of total body potassium have been used to estimate lean tissue mass and thus body composition.

Potassium is the principal cation in intracellular fluid and sodium the principal cation in extracellular fluid. This differential distribution of these two ions on each side of the cell membrane is maintained by active cellular pumps which use energy to pump sodium out of the cell in exchange for pumping potassium in. This differential distribution is crucial for many cellular processes, including the generation and propagation of nerve impulses, active transport processes, and the maintenance of acid–base balance.

Potassium is present in most foods and so overt dietary deficiency is improbable. However, many people in all age groups have intakes of potassium that are considered unsatisfactory, and this is likely to be due to low consumption of fruits and vegetables. The low recorded intake of potassium in many British people adds weight to the campaigns to increase fruit and vegetable intake up to five portions per day. Low blood potassium may be a secondary consequence of other conditions or situations such as prolonged diarrhoea, vomiting, laxative abuse or excessive secretion of the hormone aldosterone by the adrenal cortex. This low blood potassium leads to a range of symptoms listed in the key facts box.

Later in this chapter there is an extended discussion of the influence of dietary factors, especially dietary salt intake on blood pressure and the incidence of hypertension. Reduced *sodium* intake and reducing the prevalence of obesity are the primary focus of attempts to reduce the average population blood pressure (BP), and so reduce the adverse consequences of high BP. Regardless of that, there is a substantial body of evidence to suggest that high *potassium* intake may also have some effect in reducing blood pressure (Cappuccio and MacGregor 1991; COMA, 1991, 1994a). A meta-analysis of six randomized controlled trials of potassium supplements found that they did not have any significant benefit in treating high blood pressure (Dickinson *et al.*, 2006b). These trials were small and of short duration, and there was a big disparity between the results of individual trials, so the results are not conclusive.

COMA (1994) recommended that average potassium intake should be increased to 3.5 g/day from the then current level of around 2.8 g/day by increasing the consumption of fruits and vegetables.

SELENIUM

Key facts *continued*

- *Biochemical functions.* Component of enzyme system glutathione peroxidase, involved in disposal of free radicals. There are other selenium-containing enzymes, including one that is involved in converting the thyroid hormone thyroxine into its more active form triiodothyronine.
- *Effects of deficiency.* Keshan disease, a progressive cardiomyopathy.
- *Risk factors for deficiency.* Low levels of selenium in the soil.
- *Biochemical measure of nutritional status.* Plasma or serum selenium is regarded as a good short-term indicator of selenium intake, and red cell selenium a more long-term measure.
- *Prevalence of deficiency.* Estimates of selenium intake are not reliable because the food database is incomplete for this mineral. There are probably substantial numbers of people in the UK with values below the LRNI, although symptomatic deficiency does not occur.
- *Toxicity.* Selenosis leads to skin lesions and changes to the hair and nails and is followed by a range of neurological symptoms. It occurs in areas of the world where soil levels of selenium are particularly high.
- *Recommendations on high intakes.* A safe intake for lifetime consumption is set at 450 μg/day.
- *Typical highest UK intakes.* It has been estimated that highest intakes from food in the UK are around 100 μg/day. Supplements may provide up to a further 300 μg/day.

Overview

Selenium is present in food largely as the selenium-containing amino acids selenomethionine and selenocysteine, where selenium replaces the sulphur present in the parent amino acids cysteine and methionine. The selenium content of the soil in any particular region will have a major effect on the selenium content of food grown there, and thus on the dietary intake of the local people. Affluent populations tend not to be so reliant on food grown locally and may eat selenium-rich seafood – and so are

to some extent protected from these localized problems. Thomson and Robinson (1980) give figures for the blood selenium concentrations of people living in different regions which vary from around 0.22 mg/L in people sampled in the USA where selenium soil content is reasonably high down to around 0.06 mg/L in some areas of New Zealand where the selenium content of the soil is low. Areas of China have low intakes of selenium in the soil, and this is where a progressive cardiomyopathy (*Keshan disease*) attributed to selenium deficiency has been reported.

A number of seleno-proteins are important enzymes. The best known of these are the enzymes (including glutathione peroxidase) that are involved in free radical disposal mechanisms – discussed in Chapter 13.

Despite its apparent role in protecting against free radical damage, COMA (1998) found no substantial evidence to support the suggestion that supplements of selenium might have cancer-preventing effects. As discussed in Chapter 13, Bjelakovic *et al.* (2008) found no evidence that selenium supplements reduced mortality in healthy people or those with existing disease.

ZINC

Key facts

- *Dietary standards.* UK adult RNI M/F is 9.5/7 mg/day; LRNI is 5.5/4 mg/day; RDA in the USA is 11/8 mg/day.
- *Dietary sources.* Meats, whole-grain cereals, pulses and shellfish.
  - 1 slice wholemeal bread – 0.7 mg
  - 1 pork chop – 2.8 mg
  - 1 portion (75 g) frozen peas – 0.5 mg
  - 1 portion fried lamb liver – 4 mg
  - 1 serving (70 mg) canned crabmeat – 3.5 mg.
- *Biochemical functions.* Numerous zinc-containing enzymes are involved in DNA synthesis (and so cell division) and in the synthesis and metabolism of fats, carbohydrates and proteins. Superoxide dismutase involved in disposal of free radicals is a zinc-containing enzyme. Insulin is stored as a complex with zinc in the pancreas. →

Key facts *continued*

- *Effects of deficiency.* Experimental zinc deficiency leads to anorexia and growth reduction, reduced immune function, slow healing, hypogonadism and delayed sexual maturation, skin lesions and hair loss.

- *Risk factors for deficiency.* Diets with lots of unleavened bread – and thus high in phytate – may reduce zinc absorption

- *Biochemical measure of nutritional status.* Serum or plasma zinc concentration <700 µg/L is indicative of deficiency.

- *Prevalence of deficiency.* Average intakes in the UK are around the RNI, but 4 per cent of adults have intakes below the LRNI, with higher prevalence in older children and the elderly.

- *Toxicity.* Excess zinc interferes with copper absorption and precipitates symptoms of copper deficiency, and may also interfere with iron absorption. Excess zinc can also depress the activity of superoxide dismutase in red cells (an enzyme involved in free radical disposal). Zinc supplements can cause gastrointestinal symptoms.

- *Recommendations on high intakes.* The safe upper limit for lifetime supplemental zinc is 25 mg/day.

- *Typical highest UK intakes.* The highest UK consumers may get around 17 mg/day from their food, and occasionally water may contain up to 10 mg/day. Supplements in the UK may contain as much as 50 mg/day.

Overview

Zinc was clearly established as an essential nutrient for experimental animals in the 1930s and in humans in 1961. Zinc is found in all living tissue, where it is concentrated in the cell nuclei. Good food sources are whole-grain cereals, pulses, meat and shellfish. Overt symptomatic dietary deficiency of zinc is uncommon although it may be a contributory factor to low growth rates in some children. Zinc deficiency can be precipitated by high intakes of phytate from unleavened bread which impairs zinc absorption. Some cases of zinc deficiency associated with high consumption of such bread were reported in Egypt and Iran in the

1960s. Note that the phytate in cereals is destroyed when bread dough is raised by yeast.

More than 200 zinc-containing enzymes have been recorded. These are involved in DNA synthesis and metabolism and synthesis of the three major macronutrients. Zinc is important in cell division. The role of the zinc-containing enzyme superoxide dismutase in free radical disposal is discussed in Chapter 13. When animals are fed on zinc-deficient diets there is rapid onset of anorexia and growth retardation. Response to zinc deficiency is classified as a type II response where there is rapid reduction in growth and conservation of body zinc for essential metabolic functions (in the more common type I response there is depletion of body stores to maintain normal functions followed by reduced functioning of the nutrient-dependent functions when stores become depleted).

Studies conducted in the USA have suggested that marginal zinc deficiency may be a contributory factor in low growth rates of children. Healthy children selected because of their low weight-for-height showed increased growth when given small zinc supplements compared to those given a placebo; zinc supplements given to random samples of children had no effect on growth rates. Brown *et al.* (2009) conducted a series of meta-analyses of the effects of zinc supplements in different age groups around the world. In children over 1 year old they found that supplements reduced the risk of diarrhoea and the incidence of respiratory tract infections, resulted in fewer deaths, and led to small increases in linear growth and weight gain. They concluded that there was sufficient evidence to warrant international programmes to improve zinc status in children.

Zinc deficiency occurs also in a rare inherited condition *acrodermatitis enteropathica* as a result of impaired zinc absorption, and the condition can be controlled by zinc supplements.

As well as its effects on growth, zinc deficiency also causes reduced immune function, slow healing, delayed sexual maturation and hypogonadism, and skin lesions.

Given the effects on the immune system and wound healing, it might seem prudent to ensure that people with injuries, those at high risk of infection and those undergoing surgery have good zinc status, and small zinc supplements might well be an appropriate way of ensuring this. Of course, proper evaluation of the effectiveness of these supplements would require assessment of prior zinc status; that is, whether the zinc has an effect in those who are deficient and whether it confers any additional benefits in those whose zinc status is normal. In a wide-ranging review of the effects of zinc on wound healing, Lansdown *et al.* (2007) concluded that deficiency can lead to delayed wound healing and that there is evidence that oral supplements may be beneficial in treating leg ulcers in people who are zinc deficient. They review possible benefits of topical application of zinc to wounds and conclude that they have important benefits; topical use rather than oral supplements is more appropriate in most of these situations.

A recent well-publicized meta-analysis of 13 therapeutic trials suggested that zinc supplements taken within 24 hours of the onset of cold symptoms might significantly reduce the severity and duration of the symptoms (Singh and Das, 2011). Some adverse effects were also reported, including nausea. Evidence from just two prevention trials suggested that long-term use (at least 5 months) might have some effect in reducing the incidence of colds.

It is much too early to recommend zinc preparations as a cold remedy, and it would be unwise to recommend long-term use of zinc supplements as a preventative measure on the basis of the limited data. The key facts box indicates that some people who are already taking zinc supplements may have intakes that are significantly above the safe upper limit for lifetime consumption.

Zinc supplements have also been promoted as being of benefit in the treatment of anorexia nervosa, and in treating male infertility, but this is based on the symptoms of zinc deficiency and there is no evidence that they are effective.

IODINE AND IODINE-DEFICIENCY DISEASES

Key facts

- *Dietary standards.* Adult UK RNI is 140 μg/day; LRNI is 70 μg/day; American RDA is 150 μg/day.
  →

Key facts *continued*

- *Dietary sources.* The richest natural sources are seafood. Amounts in fruits, vegetables and meat depend on soil content of iodine. Modern farming and processing methods increase the amounts in milk and some bakery products; iodized salt.
- *Biochemical functions.* A component of the thyroid hormones thyroxine and triiodothyronine.
- *Effects of deficiency.* Goitre and the iodine-deficiency diseases including cretinism and myxoedema.
- *Risk factors for deficiency.* Living in inland areas where soil iodine content is low and no seafood is eaten.
- *Biochemical measure of nutritional status.* Usually based on clinical assessment.
- *Prevalence of deficiency.* Worldwide, some 2 billion people and 266 million school-aged children are iodine deficient. Four per cent of UK adult women have estimated intakes below the LRNI, but average intake is well above the RNI and symptomatic dietary deficiency is not seen in developed countries.
- *Toxicity.* High intakes can lead to disturbances of thyroid function which usually manifest as hyperthyroidism and toxic nodular goitre.
- *Recommendations on high intakes.* Supplements of up to 500 μg/day should cause no problems.
- *Typical highest UK intakes.* The highest consumers may get up to 450 μg/day from their food and drinking water may provide a further 30 μg/day. Supplements may provide up to 490 μg/day.

Distribution and physiological function of body iodine

Iodine is a component of the thyroid hormones, *thyroxine* and *triiodothyronine*. The thyroid gland traps and concentrates absorbed iodine very efficiently; if radioactively labelled iodine is taken in, this radioactivity can be shown to be rapidly concentrated within the thyroid gland. The ability of the thyroid to concentrate 'labelled' iodine is used diagnostically as a measure of thyroid functioning. High doses of radioactive iodine may be used also as an alternative to surgery to selectively destroy thyroid tissue in some cases of *hyperthyroidism* or *thyroid carcinoma*, especially in the elderly. Nuclear emissions released after accidents or explosions contain large amounts of relatively short-lived radioactive iodine and this accumulates in the thyroid where it can ultimately cause thyroid carcinoma. Administration of iodine-containing tablets can be used as a public health measure after nuclear accidents, to compete with and competitively reduce the uptake of the radioactive iodine into the thyroid.

Iodine deficiency

Goitre is a swelling of the thyroid gland. This swelling ranges from being detectable only by the trained eye to massive and sometimes nodular overgrowth. The thyroid swells because of excessive stimulation by the pituitary hormone, thyrotrop(h)-in. Thyrotropin output is normally inhibited by circulating thyroid hormones, so any reduced output of thyroid hormones caused by iodine deficiency leads to compensatory increases in thyrotropin output and consequent thyroid growth (Figure 15.1). In some cases the swelling of the thyroid is the only apparent symptom of iodine deficiency. Women and girls are more susceptible to goitre than males.

In severe iodine deficiency there are symptoms of thyroid hormone deficiency. In children, iodine deficiency can lead to *cretinism*, a condition characterized by impaired mental and physical development. In adults, iodine deficiency not only causes goitre but can also lead to impaired mental functioning, low metabolic rate, hypotension, weight gain and other symptoms of thyroid hormone deficiency. In places where goitre is endemic it causes increased rates of spontaneous abortion and stillbirth and the birth of large numbers of children with congenital physical and neurological abnormalities including deaf-mutism, spasticity and mental deficiency. There is a general impairment of intellectual performance and psychomotor skills in children from iodine-deficient areas. If a goitre is very large it may lead to problems with breathing or swallowing that may require surgery, and occasionally large nodular goitres may become malignant.

The link between iodine deficiency and goitre was established early in the twentieth century by trials conducted by David Marine in the USA. Iodine fortification of salt is generally acknowledged as the first example of a successful (voluntary) food fortification programme. It began in Michigan in 1924 and within a year almost all Michigan homes used iodized salt. Between 1924 and 1936, the incidence of goitre in Michigan schools dropped from 38.6 to 8.2 per cent. Likewise, in those Swiss

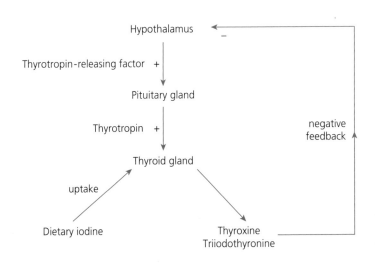

Figure 15.1 Regulation of thyroid hormone output and the origins of goitre. Lack of dietary iodine reduces negative feedback and leads to overproduction of thyrotropin, which causes over-stimulation and swelling of the thyroid.

cantons with universal use of iodized salt, incidence of goitre dropped rapidly and had almost disappeared by 1945. David Marine in 1915 proclaimed that 'endemic goitre is the easiest known disease to prevent', yet 2 billion people and 266 million school-aged children are still iodine deficient and it is still the leading cause of preventable mental retardation in children (de Benoist *et al.*. 2008a). Historical accounts of the local eradication of endemic goitre can be found in Kimball (1953) and Lowenstein (1960).

Causes and scale of the problem

The richest sources of dietary iodine are seafoods. The smaller amount of iodine in other foods varies according to the iodine level in the soil. The iodine content of drinking water gives a good indication of the general iodine level in the soil in an area. In many regions of the world the soil iodine content is low – especially in mountainous regions and flooded river valleys where glaciation and run-off from melting snow and heavy rain have leached much of the iodine from the soil. Switzerland, the area around the Great Lakes in North America, and Derbyshire and the Cotswold areas of England were once 'goitre areas'. The Himalayas, Andes, Alps and the mountains of China together with the Ganges valley and other river valleys in Asia are all areas where soil iodine content is inadequate. In areas where the soil iodine content is low and where seafood is not consumed, the iodine-deficiency diseases, manifesting most apparently as goitre, have been and often still are endemic.

Iodine deficiency is one of the most common nutrient deficiencies in the world and is the most common cause of preventable mental deficiency in children. Two billion people in the developing countries are deficient, with around 200 million suffering from goitre and around 20 million of these suffering from some degree of resultant mental defect. More than 5 million people suffer from gross cretinism and mental retardation. Iodine deficiency is endemic in large parts of Central and South America, large parts of India, China and South East Asia, some regions of Africa and the Oceanic islands; around 85 per cent of those suffering from overt cretinisn are in Asia. De Benoist *et al.* (2008a) have written a detailed review of current levels of iodine deficiency around the world and, although they found that progress had been made, the problem was still very widespread. Nowadays, few affluent communities rely solely on food produced in their locality and this reduces the risk of goitre. Zimmerman and Delange (2004) have argued, however, that two-thirds of people in western Europe live in areas that are iodine deficient, and they go on to suggest that most women in Europe are deficient during pregnancy so that all pregnant women in Europe should receive supplements containing 150 µg/day.

In both the UK and USA the iodine content of cow milk is high because of supplementation of feed and the use of iodine disinfectants. In some regions, iodized salt has been effectively used as a prophylactic measure to prevent goitre. Kelp is a form of seaweed that is marketed as a dietary supplement partly on the basis of its high iodine content, and the suggested dose typically contains up to twice the adult RNI/RDA. Note that people with thyroid disorders should not take this supplement as it may interfere with the management of their condition. In some iodine-deficient areas, injections of iodized oil have been used and a single injection gives protection for 2–3 years. Iodized oil can be administered orally but the duration of effectiveness is reduced to about a year.

One important problem with assessing iodine intakes and levels of dietary adequacy is that food tables may not always be a totally reliable guide to the iodine content of food grown in a particular locality.

Requirements and intake of iodine

The adult daily RNI (or RDA) for iodine is 140 (or 150) µg, but intakes are typically double this in the UK and more than double in the USA. Very high intakes can cause toxic nodular goitre and hyperthyroidism. De Benoist *et al.* (2008a) found that iodine intake was more than adequate or even excessive in 34 countries, and they suggested that susceptible groups within these populations are exposed to risk of iodine-induced hyperthyroidism. The FSA (2003) suggested a safe upper limit of 500 µg/day from supplements, which equates to a total maximum intake of around 1000 µg/day. Some Japanese populations who habitually consume seaweed have intakes many times this suggested maximum with no apparent ill-effects, and Hetzel and Clugston (1999) suggested that populations that have been iodine deficient may be much more sensitive to the toxic effects of excess iodine.

Certain foods of the cabbage (*Brassica*) family and cassava contain goitrogenic substances that either block the uptake of iodine by the thyroid gland or block the synthesis of thyroid hormones. The presence of such goitrogens may precipitate deficiency where intakes of iodine are at the borders of adequacy. Cassava, in particular, may be a significant factor in precipitating iodine deficiency in some tropical areas where it is the principal energy source for around 200 million people. Intakes of iodine should be doubled to 200–300 μg/day where there is high intake of these goitrogens.

Key points

- Iodine is essential as a component of the hormones thyroxine and triiodothyronine.
- In iodine deficiency, reduced thyroid hormone output causes increased thyrotropin output from the pituitary, which stimulates the thyroid and causes it to swell (goitre).
- Severe iodine deficiency in children causes impaired mental and physical development (cretinism) and leads to symptoms of thyroid insufficiency in adults.
- In goitre areas there is general impairment of mental performance and increased numbers of abortions, stillbirths and birth of children with mental and physical defects.
- Iodine deficiency occurs in mountainous areas and frequently flooded river valleys where melting snow and floodwater have leached the iodine from the soil.
- Around 2 billion people and 266 million school-aged children in the world are iodine deficient, and up to 20 million suffer some degree of mental defect as a result of iodine deficiency.
- Iodine deficiency is the most common cause of preventable mental deficiency in children.
- Access to seafood and food from various geographical regions reduces the risk of iodine deficiency.
- Iodized salt and injections of iodized oil have been used to prevent and treat iodine deficiency.

→

Key points *continued*

- Very high intakes of iodine may cause toxic goitre and hyperthyroidism. People with chronically low iodine intake may be particularly susceptible.
- Certain foods (e.g. cabbage and cassava) contain goitrogens that increase the requirement for iodine.

IRON AND IRON-DEFICIENCY ANAEMIA

Key facts

- *Dietary standards.* UK adult RNI M/F is 8.7/14.8 mg/day; LRNI is 4.7/8 mg/day; American RDA is 8/18 mg/day.
- *Dietary sources.* Meat (particularly offal); fish; cereals; green vegetables. Biological availability of iron is much higher from meat and fish than from vegetable sources.
  - 1 pork chop – 1 mg
  - 1 portion (90 g) fried lamb liver – 9 mg
  - 1 egg – 1.1 mg
  - 1 serving (80 g) peeled prawns – 0.9 mg
  - 1 serving (85 g) canned sardines – 3.9 mg
  - 1 portion (75 g) frozen peas – 1.1 mg
  - 1 portion (95 g) broccoli – 1 mg
  - 1 bar (50 g) dark plain chocolate – 1.2 mg
  - 1 serving (130 mg) spinach – 5.2 mg
  - 1 slice wholemeal bread – 1 mg.
- *Biochemical functions.* Component of haemoglobin, myoglobin and cytochromes; there are several iron-containing enzymes such as catalase.
- *Effects of deficiency.* Iron-deficiency anaemia which, especially in developing countries, leads to: poor pregnancy outcome including increased risk of maternal death; impaired physical and mental development in children; high rates of child ill-health; reduced work capacity in adults.
- *Risk factors for deficiency.* Chronic blood loss arising from heavy menstrual bleeding, malignancy, intestinal parasites or repeated pregnancies. A vegetarian diet that is low in iron has low bioavailability and lacks promoters of absorption such as vitamin C.

Features of iron nutrition

Distribution of body iron

An average well-nourished male body contains about 4 grams of iron. Around 70 per cent of this total will be present in the respiratory pigments – *haemoglobin* in blood (67 per cent) and *myoglobin* in muscle (3–4 per cent). Most of the body's non-haem iron will be stored as the iron-protein complex, *ferritin*. Small amounts of iron will also be found in a variety of important iron-containing enzymes and proteins and bound to the protein *transferrin* in plasma that is responsible for the transport of iron around the body. The first effect of iron deficiency is depletion of iron stores and this is followed by reduced levels of the iron-containing respiratory pigment haemoglobin – leading to iron-deficiency anaemia.

Requirement for dietary iron

Iron is very efficiently conserved by the human body, with a daily loss in a typical healthy male amounting to around 1 mg (i.e. only 0.025 per cent of normal body iron content). This tiny net loss compares with around 20 mg of iron in the ageing red blood cells that are removed from the circulation and destroyed each day. The iron released from broken-down red cells is recycled and the small amount of iron lost from the body is that present in lost skin, nails, hair, body fluids and sloughed cells from the alimentary and genito-urinary tracts. In pre-menopausal women, losses of menstrual blood and the losses of iron at parturition and during lactation also contribute. Average menstrual blood loss represents an additional increment of around 80 per cent to the general iron losses of women, but in some women (say 10 per cent) these extra menstrual losses may represent an addition of 150 per cent or more to the general iron loss. Any condition that results in chronic blood loss will deplete body iron stores and increase the risk of anaemia; examples are ulcers, intestinal parasites and intestinal cancer.

Average intakes of iron in the UK are about 13.2 mg/day in men and 10.0 mg/day in women, so are around 13 times the average daily loss in men and, even in those women with particularly high menstrual losses, still around four times estimated loss. The iron RNI is 8.7 mg/day for men and 14.8 mg/day for pre-menopausal women. According to COMA (1991), even this RNI may be insufficient for those women with particularly high menstrual losses.

The very large differences in estimated requirements for iron and estimated losses are because only a small and variable proportion of dietary iron is absorbed. The proportion varies with several factors listed below.

- *The iron status of the individual.* Inorganic iron absorption is 2–3 times higher in subjects who are iron deficient compared with those with good iron stores. There is also a substantial increase in the efficiency of iron absorption during pregnancy.

- *The form in which the dietary iron is present.* Haem iron from meat and fish and organic iron in milk are much better absorbed than inorganic iron from vegetable foods. Most of the inorganic iron in food is in the trivalent or ferric state whereas that in most supplements is in the divalent ferrous state which is better absorbed.
- *The presence of promoters of inorganic iron absorption* – for example, vitamin C, alcohol and meat protein.
- *The presence of inhibitors of inorganic iron absorption* – such as phytate (e.g. from unleavened bread), tannin (e.g. from tea) and perhaps even large amounts of dietary fibre.

Haem iron from meat and fish is far better absorbed (10–30 per cent) than the iron in vegetable foods (2–10 per cent). Absorption of haem iron is also unaffected by the presence of inhibitors and promoters. Vitamin C, stomach acid and the presence of meat and fish all promote iron absorption. Vitamin C is a major factor in promoting the absorption of iron from vegetable foods. Fibre, phytate (from unleavened bread) and tannin in tea all tend to hinder iron absorption. Alcohol increases gastric acid secretion and facilitates iron absorption.

COMA (1991) assumed an average efficiency of absorption of iron of about 15 per cent when making calculations of dietary reference values.

Regulation of iron balance and iron overload

The principal physiological mechanism for regulating body iron balance is by controlling the efficiency of absorption. When iron stores are low then iron is absorbed more efficiently than when the stores are full. The efficiency of iron absorption may more than double when iron stores are depleted. This regulatory system is usually sufficient to prevent iron toxicity from dietary sources, and even when moderate doses of therapeutic iron are consumed chronically by people who do not need them. Chronic iron overload can lead to cirrhosis of the liver. Single very high doses of iron can cause diarrhoea, vomiting, gastro-intestinal bleeding, circulatory collapse and liver necrosis. Iron poisoning resulting from children consuming pharmaceutical preparations of iron is one of the most common causes of accidental poisoning.

Alcohol also promotes iron absorption and consumption of alcoholic drinks containing large amounts of iron can precipitate iron overload and contribute to liver cirrhosis. White *et al.* (1995) found a positive association between alcohol consumption and level of iron stores in both men and women.

As there is no physiological mechanism for excreting excess iron, iron overload and toxicity is a major problem for those with certain conditions that require repeated blood transfusions (e.g. *thalassaemia*, an inherited blood disorder, and *aplastic anaemia* from bone marrow failure). Drugs that bind or chelate iron and facilitate its excretion can be used to treat or prevent iron overload. Hereditary *haemochromatosis* is an inherited condition in which there is chronic over-absorption of iron which can lead to liver and other tissue damage unless it is treated by regular therapeutic bleeding.

Determination of iron status

Iron deficiency will eventually impair the ability to synthesize haemoglobin. Iron status has traditionally been diagnosed by measurement of blood haemoglobin concentration. Iron-deficiency anaemia is characterized by reduced blood haemoglobin concentration and reduced red blood cell size – a *microcytic anaemia* (small cell) as compared to the *macrocytic anaemia* (large cell) of vitamin B_{12} or folic acid deficiency. A blood haemoglobin concentration of <12 g/100 mL has traditionally been taken as 'the level below which anaemia is likely to be present' and the prevalence of anaemia has usually been established by use of a cut-off value like this. Currently the World Health Organization suggests a value of <13 g/100 mL for men and <12 g/100 mL for women at sea level (because living at altitude increases red cell count and haemoglobin concentration).

Other measures of iron status have been increasingly used in recent years. The *plasma ferritin level* indicates the state of body iron stores, and these stores may become depleted without any fall in blood haemoglobin concentration. Plasma ferritin is a more sensitive measure of iron status than blood haemoglobin concentration. Normal ranges for plasma ferritin are given in the key facts box; a value below 15 μg/L is indicative of iron depletion in women, and a level below 25 µg/L may indicate that iron stores are suboptimal. In iron deficiency, the concentration of the iron-transport protein (transferrin) in the plasma rises but the amount of iron in plasma drops; so a low ratio of iron to transferrin in plasma – the *transferrin saturation* – indicates low iron status. When the percentage saturation of transferrin with iron is below 15 per cent, the ability to synthesize haemoglobin is impaired.

The symptoms of anaemia result from the low haemoglobin content of blood leading to impaired ability to transport oxygen. They include general fatigue, breathlessness on exertion, pallor, headache and insomnia.

Key points

- An adult male body contains about 4 grams of iron, with 70 per cent in haemoglobin and myoglobin, small amounts in iron-containing enzymes, and the rest stored as the iron-protein complex ferritin.
- A healthy male loses less than 1 mg of iron per day. Menstrual losses, pregnancy and lactation increase the average losses of younger women.
- Iron requirements greatly exceed iron losses because only a proportion of dietary iron (c15 per cent) is absorbed.
- The efficiency of iron absorption increases in iron deficiency and decreases when iron stores are full. The gut is the main site of regulation of body iron balance.
- Haem iron is absorbed more efficiently than inorganic iron from vegetable sources.
- Substances such as phytate and tannin inhibit inorganic iron absorption, whereas alcohol, gastric acid and vitamin C promote its absorption.
- There is no route for excreting body iron. Chronic high consumption of iron can lead to cirrhosis of the liver and other tissue damage due to iron overload.
- Single high doses of iron can cause acute poisoning, typically in children accidentally consuming iron tablets prescribed for an adult.
- Iron deficiency eventually impairs haemoglobin synthesis and the capacity of blood to transport oxygen – iron-deficiency anaemia.

→

Key points *continued*

- Iron-deficiency anaemia is a microcytic (small red cell) anaemia and leads to pallor, fatigue, breathlessness on exertion and headache.
- Iron status may be assessed by measuring blood haemoglobin concentration, plasma ferritin concentration or plasma transferrin saturation. Plasma ferritin indicates the level of the body's iron store and is a more sensitive indicator of iron status than blood haemoglobin concentration, because iron stores become depleted before anaemia occurs.

Features of iron deficiency

Prevalence of iron deficiency and anaemia

The prevalence of iron deficiency will vary according to the criterion used to define it. Functional impairment due to iron deficiency (as measured by plasma ferritin) may occur in the absence of anaemia (COMA, 1991). Reduced work capacity and changes in certain brain functions that adversely affect attention span, memory and learning in children are some of these suggested adverse consequences of iron deficiency without anaemia.

Iron deficiency is considered to be the most common nutrient deficiency in the world. A WHO report used low blood haemoglobin level to define anaemia and estimated that over 1.6 billion people (25 per cent of the world's population) were anaemic (de Benoist *et al.*, 2008b). The highest prevalence was in young children, the lowest in men, and the highest number of people affected by anaemia were pre-menopausal women. More than 40 per cent (56 million) of pregnant women were classified as anaemic (Hb <11 g/100 mL of blood) and this increases the risk of maternal death, premature labour and low-birthweight babies. Anaemia in children impairs their development and it reduces work capacity in adults.

In the developed countries, the condition is considered to be uncommon in young men. The low iron intakes and poor iron status of many British women are discussed in some detail in Chapter 13, and many British children and elderly people also have intakes of iron that are below the LRNI, and many have biochemical evidence of iron depletion or iron-deficiency anaemia (see Chapter 16).

Preventing iron deficiency

In people consuming the same type of diet, iron intake is likely to be directly related to total energy intake. On a good mixed European or American diet, iron intake will be around 5–7 mg per 1000 kcal (4.2 MJ). This means that if the diet provides enough iron for women to meet their dietary standard then men consuming the same type of diet are likely to take in around double theirs. Young vegetarian women who restrict their food intake to control their weight are clearly at increased risk of iron deficiency. Any food fortification programme that seeks to eliminate iron-deficiency anaemia in women who have particularly high needs will increase still further the surplus intake of men.

Some possible risk factors for iron deficiency are considered below.

- *A diet that is low in available iron.* Vegetarians (10 per cent of adolescent girls) are an obvious high-risk group because they exclude the most available form of iron (haem iron) from their diet.
- *Lack of inorganic iron absorption.* High intake of substances like phytate (unleavened bread) and tannin (tea) taken with meals will reduce the efficiency of inorganic iron absorption. So will low intake of promoters of inorganic iron with meals, especially vitamin C. High vitamin C intake may help prevent anaemia in some vegetarians.
- *Menstrual blood loss and pregnancy.* High menstrual blood loss, repeated pregnancies or prolonged lactation are risk factors.
- *Any other condition that leads to chronic blood loss.* Such a state will increase the risk of iron depletion. An example is infestation of the gut with parasites that cause blood loss; hookworm infestation is a major precipitating factor in many tropical countries.
- *Stomach acid depletion.* Any condition that reduces production of stomach acid reduces iron absorption, from surgical gastrectomy through to simple age-related decrease in gastric acid production (*achlorhydria*).
- *Haemodilution.* Athletes have been said to be at increased risk because of suggestions that endurance training increases iron losses. This perception of increased iron deficiency in athletes arises because endurance training has a haemodilution effect; it leads to increases in plasma volume that are greater than the increase in circulating haemoglobin, thus causing a fall in the measured concentration of haemoglobin in blood even though the total circulating mass of haemoglobin is increased. True anaemia in athletes is usually due to low iron intake in the diet (Maughan, 1994).

Strategies

There are essentially three strategies that can be used to try to prevent and treat iron deficiency:

- selective use of iron supplements and even provision of free supplements to those with, or at high risk of, deficiency
- fortification of a core food(s) with iron
- education aimed at general improvement in the dietary iron content or increasing its bio-availability.

Of course, where chronic blood loss is identified as a precipitating factor then this problem should also be appropriately dealt with.

It is possible for public health campaigns to make an impact on iron-deficiency anaemia. In Sweden, the prevalence of iron deficiency was reduced by around three-quarters between 1965 and 1975. This was achieved by increased levels of fortification of flour, increased vitamin C intakes, and the widespread use of iron supplements (Anon, 1980). Indiscriminate use of pharmaceutical preparations leads to risk of minor side-effects, accidental poisoning, and chronic iron overload in susceptible people. In the UK, all flour other than wholemeal must be fortified with iron, and there is also iron fortification in the USA. The iron added to British and American flour is in a form that is very poorly absorbed and so it is not very effective in preventing anaemia.

Any fortification programme designed to eliminate anaemia in women with high iron needs inevitably results in men, and even many women, receiving iron intakes greatly in excess of their needs. This excess iron might cause harm, particularly to subjects inherently sensitive to iron overload. It seems unlikely that in the foreseeable future there will be any increase in the mandatory fortification of UK food with iron.

If pre-menopausal women and other groups at increased risk of anaemia are advised to eat a diet containing more available iron, then such a diet would probably contain more meat (and/or fish). This could lead to increased intake of saturated fat and might not be entirely consistent with other nutrition education guidelines. It might also be unacceptable or impractical for many women. Nevertheless, lean meat and fish are important sources of iron and other nutrients and moderate amounts should be promoted as important components of a healthy diet especially for those at high risk of anaemia. Many young women mistakenly view red meat as particularly fattening, so nutrition education should aim to correct this misconception. Current advice to increase consumption of fruits and vegetables would increase vitamin C intake and thus increase iron absorption. Several fruits and vegetables are also good sources of available iron, examples being tomatoes, cabbage and broccoli. Large increases in consumption of cereal fibre might tend to reduce iron availability.

In developed countries, iron supplements are clearly appropriate for those with poor iron status. The case for higher levels of intervention (supplements or increased food fortification) will clearly be much stronger in developing countries where the scale and severity of iron deficiency are much greater than in developed countries.

Key points

- Some symptoms of iron deficiency may occur in the absence of anaemia.
- Iron deficiency is the most common micronutrient deficiency in the world and an estimated 1.6 billion people worldwide suffer from anaemia.
- Even in the UK, a third of pre-menopausal women may have relatively low iron stores and half of these are iron depleted.
- Children, adolescents, pregnant women and the elderly may all be regarded as at increased risk of anaemia. It is generally uncommon in young men.

→

Key points *continued*

- Risk of anaemia is increased by chronic blood loss, lack of available iron in the diet, repeated pregnancies, prolonged lactation and lack of stomach acid.
- Strategies for tackling iron deficiency include increased use of iron supplements, food fortification, and nutrition education aimed at improving iron availability in the diet.
- On a normal mixed diet, iron intake will be roughly proportional to energy intake.
- Any fortification programme aimed at increasing iron intakes of high-risk women will lead to some men consuming large excesses of iron.
- Iron from fortified bread (UK and USA) is often poorly absorbed.
- Increased use of prophylactic iron preparations may result in some women taking supplements they do not need.
- Excess iron from fortified food or supplements may cause harm, particularly to people who are inherently sensitive to iron overload.
- Increased consumption of meat is the most obvious way of improving iron availability. Modest amounts of lean meat are consistent with a healthy diet. Nutrition education should counteract the view of many girls and young women that red meat is very fattening.
- Increased consumption of fruits and vegetables would increase vitamin C intake and thus increase inorganic iron uptake. Several fruits and vegetables are also good sources of available iron.

CALCIUM STORAGE AND UPTAKE

Key facts

- *Dietary standards.* Adult UK RNI is 700 mg/day; LRNI is 400 mg/day; American RDA is 1000 mg/day with higher values for the elderly and adolescents.
- *Dietary sources.* Milk and milk products are rich sources with high biological availability; fish, especially if the bones can be eaten as in

→

canned fish; green vegetables; pulses; nuts; whole-grain cereals (brown and white flour is supplemented in the UK); the calcium in vegetables and in cereals may have relatively low biological availability.

- 1 cup (195 g) milk – 225 mg
- 1 slice (40 g) Cheddar cheese – 290 mg
- 1 serving (20 g) almonds – 50 mg
- 1 slice wholemeal bread – 19 mg
- 1 serving (95 g) broccoli – 72 mg
- 1 serving (75 g) cabbage – 40 mg
- 1 portion (85 g) canned sardines – 390 mg
- 1 serving (80 g) peeled prawns – 120 mg
- 1 portion (130 g) grilled cod – 13 mg.

- *Biochemical functions.* Ninety-nine per cent of body calcium is in bone mineral, but the other 1 per cent plays vital roles in nerve and muscle functioning, release of hormones and nerve transmitters, blood clotting and acts as an intracellular regulator of metabolism.

- *Effects of deficiency.* Overt, primary calcium deficiency is rare. Vitamin D deficiency leads to poor absorption of calcium.*

- *Risk factors for deficiency.* Vitamin D deficiency and lack of sunlight exposure lead to secondary deficiency through poor absorption. Low calcium intake is associated with lack of dairy products in the diet.*

- *Biochemical measure of nutritional status.* No routine method available.

- *Prevalence of deficiency.* In 2000, 5 per cent of British women had unsatisfactory calcium intakes. Higher prevalences were reported in older children and older British adults living independently.

- *Toxicity.* At high doses, gastro-intestinal symptoms may occur. In those taking medicinal calcium supplements, a milk alkali syndrome sometimes occurs and results in hypercalcaemia, calcification of tissues, alkalosis, hypertension, neurological symptoms and renal impairment.

- *Recommendations on high intakes.* Supplemental doses of 1500 mg/day should have no adverse effects.

- *Typical highest UK intakes.* The highest UK consumers may get 1700 mg/day from food, with up to a further 600 mg/day supplied by drinking water in some hard water areas. Over-the-counter supplements may provide up to 2400 mg/day.

* The role of vitamin D in calcium absorption from the gut and its requirement for bone health are discussed in Chapter 14, as is the role of vitamin D deficiency in the aetiology, prevention and treatment of osteoporosis.

Distribution and functions of body calcium

A typical adult human body contains more than 1 kg of calcium and 99 per cent of this is in the skeleton. The skeletal calcium is present as the calcium phosphate substance *hydroxyapatite*, which gives bone its mechanical strength. The small amount of calcium that is outside the skeleton has a multitude of other vital functions such as those listed below.

- Calcium plays a major role in the release of hormones and neurotransmitters.
- It is an important intracellular regulator.
- It is an essential cofactor for some enzymes and is necessary for blood clotting.
- It is involved in nerve and heart functioning.
- Electrical excitation of muscle cells leads to release of calcium from intracellular storage sites, and this calcium release triggers muscle contraction.

Any variation in the calcium concentration of body fluids can thus have diverse effects on many systems of the body and the calcium concentration in extracellular fluids is under very fine hormonal control. The skeletal calcium not only strengthens bone, it also serves as a reservoir of calcium. The skeleton can donate or soak up excess calcium and thus enable the concentration in extracellular fluid to be regulated within narrow limits. A fall in blood calcium concentration, as seen after removal of the parathyroid glands or in extreme vitamin D deficiency, leads to muscle weakness and eventually to tetany and death due to asphyxiation when the muscles of the larynx go into spasm. A rise in plasma calcium is seen in vitamin D poisoning and in hyperparathyroidism. This hypercalcaemia can lead to gastro-intestinal symptoms, neurological symptoms and formation of kidney stones. In some cases it might lead to death from renal failure.

Hormonal regulation of calcium homeostasis

The hormone *1,25-dihydroxycholecalciferol* (1,25-DHCC or *calcitriol*) is produced in the kidney from vitamin D and is essential for the active absorption of dietary calcium in the intestine. Calcitriol promotes the synthesis of key proteins involved in active transport of calcium in both the gut and kidney. Some passive absorption of calcium occurs independently of vitamin D and this passive absorption increases with increasing dietary intake. Parathyroid hormone and calcitonin (from the thyroid gland) regulate deposition and release of calcium from bone and also the rate of excretion of calcium in the urine. Parathyroid hormone also indirectly regulates the intestinal absorption of calcium by activating the renal enzyme that produces calcitriol. Typical daily fluxes of calcium and the hormonal influences on these fluxes are summarized in Figure 15.2.

Requirement and availability of calcium

The adult RNI for calcium in the UK is 700 mg/day for both men and women, significantly less than the

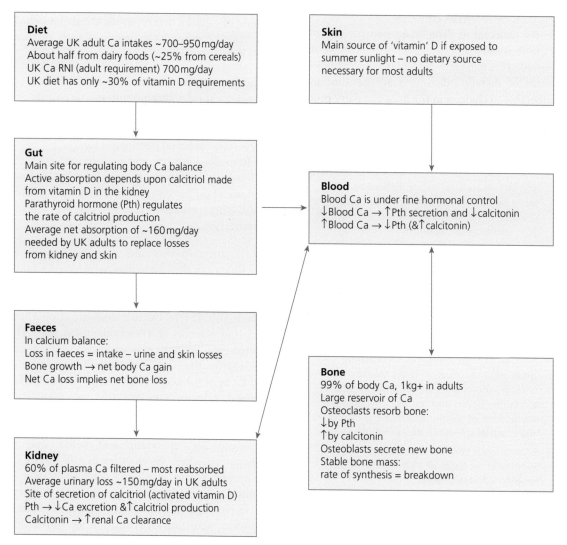

Figure 15.2 Typical calcium fluxes in UK adults with summary of the main dietary and hormonal influences on calcium homeostasis.

American RDA of 1000 mg/day. The extra increments allowed for growth and pregnancy are also generally higher in the USA than the UK. Probably two-thirds of non-pregnant women in the USA consume less than the current RDA. A very substantial minority of British women also take in less than the RNI and about 5 per cent take in less than the LRNI; many older children and independently living elderly people also take in less than their LRNI.

In the UK, COMA arrived at the dietary standards by calculating the amount needed to replace typical urinary and skin losses (c160 mg/day), assuming that around 30 per cent of the dietary intake is absorbed. In Western countries, 50–70 per cent of dietary calcium is from dairy produce and the calcium in dairy produce tends to be well absorbed. This predominance of dairy produce as the major source of dietary calcium makes calcium intake vulnerable to changes in the image of dairy produce induced by health education messages. In the UK, daily calcium intake fell by 20 per cent over the period 1975–95 as a result of reduced total food intake and milk consumption. This trend was most pronounced in young women and teenaged girls, but more recently Hoare *et al.* (2004) recorded a significant improvement in average adult calcium intake in the preceding decade. Lower fat milks contain just as much calcium as whole milk, so reduced intake of dairy fat does not inevitably lead to reduced calcium intake.

The efficiency of absorption of calcium varies according to the phase of the lifecycle, the food source of calcium and the total intake. Examples are given below.

- The efficiency of calcium absorption increases markedly in pregnancy but is reduced in the elderly.
- Calcium from vegetable sources is generally less well absorbed than that from milk and cheese. Efficiency of absorption from breast milk is higher than from infant formula.
- At low calcium intakes the active, vitamin D-dependent absorption process predominates. At high intakes, the less efficient passive process predominates so that the proportion of the oral load that is absorbed tends to decline with increasing intake.

Many populations who do not consume large amounts of dairy produce as adults have average calcium intakes that are less than half the current UK reference nutrient intake and thus below even the current LRNI. Despite this, overt symptoms of acute dietary deficiency are not seen. For example, Prentice *et al.* (1993) reported calcium intakes in pregnant and lactating women in rural Gambia in 1979 of only around 400 mg/day. Despite this there were no overt symptoms of calcium deficiency and rates of bone fractures in the Gambia are low. There is evidence that individuals who consume chronically low calcium amounts of calcium can adapt to these low intakes by increasing efficiency of absorption and by reducing their urinary losses of calcium.

Key points

- An adult body contains over 1 kg of calcium and 99 per cent of this is in the bone mineral.
- Calcium has numerous functions in addition to being a component of bone mineral.
- Large fluctuations in the calcium concentration of extracellular fluid have adverse effects on several systems and it is subject to fine hormonal control.
- Bone mineral acts as a large reservoir of calcium.
- Calcitriol, produced from vitamin D, induces key proteins necessary for the active absorption of calcium.
- Parathyroid hormone and calcitonin control the flow of calcium into and out of bone and the rate of calcium excretion in the urine.
- Parathyroid hormone indirectly controls the intestinal absorption of calcium by regulating the renal enzyme that produces calcitriol.
- The UK RNI for calcium is 700 mg/day for men and women. Substantial numbers of women in the UK do not take in this much, and 5 per cent take in less than the LRNI.
- The RNI is calculated as the amount needed to replace daily losses assuming that 30 per cent of the dietary intake is absorbed.
- More than half of the calcium in Western diets is from milk and dairy products.

→

- UK intakes of calcium fell during the 1970s and 1980s as total food intake and milk consumption dropped, but more recently this trend seems to have been reversed.

- Low-fat milk has just as much calcium as full-fat milk.

- Calcium from dairy products is much better absorbed than that from vegetable sources.

- The efficiency of calcium absorption increases in pregnancy but declines in the elderly.

- At low calcium intakes the active vitamin D-dependent process predominates but at high intakes this becomes saturated and passive absorption becomes increasingly prominent.

- Calcium intakes of many populations are much lower than in the UK and well below the current LRNI. However, those populations show no overt signs of calcium deficiency and often have very low rates of bone fractures.

CALCIUM AND BONE HEALTH

The nature of bone

The skeletal calcium is present as *hydroxyapatite*, a crystalline complex of calcium, phosphate and hydroxide ions. These crystals are laid down on an organic matrix that is largely composed of the protein *collagen*. Hydroxyapatite makes up around half the weight of the bone and is responsible for conferring its mechanical strength. There are two types of mature bone: 80 per cent is cortical or compact bone and 20 per cent is trabecular bone. Cortical bone is on the outside. Trabecular bone has a honeycomb structure with marrow filling the spaces and is located at the centre of the pelvis, vertebrae and the ends of the long bones.

Effects of age and sex on bone density and fracture risk

Bones are not fixed and inert but living dynamic structures. The processes of bone deposition and bone breakdown continue throughout life. Bones are continually being remodelled by cells that synthesize new bone (osteoblasts) and cells that reabsorb bone and cartilage (osteoclasts). Thus if a bone's weight remains constant this is the result of a dynamic equilibrium, a balance between synthesis and breakdown. Bone mass increases throughout childhood as the skeleton grows and the rate of bone deposition exceeds the rate of breakdown. A newborn baby has 25–30 g of calcium in its skeleton, and by the time the peak bone mass (PBM) is reached the skeletal calcium content has risen to well over 1 kg in an adult male. People reach their peak bone mass in their thirties and for a few years bone mass remains fairly constant. During middle and old age, the rate of breakdown exceeds the rate of bone formation and there is a steady decline in bone mass, involving loss of both organic matrix and mineral matter (Figure 15.3).

As people age, their bones become thinner, less strong and increasingly prone to fracture when subjected to trauma. This may take them below a threshold so that they become liable to fracture

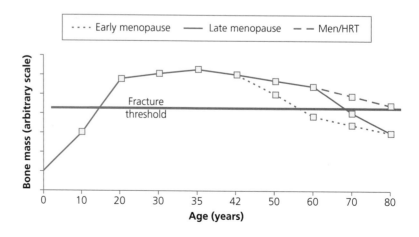

Figure 15.3 Changes in bone mass throughout life. After Webb and Copeman (1996).

during minor trauma such as a fall from a standing position. This thinning of the bones and consequent increase in fracture risk is termed *osteoporosis*.

In healthy men and pre-menopausal women, the age-related decline in bone mass is relatively slow – around 0.3–0.4 per cent a year. In women, the decade immediately after the menopause sees a marked acceleration in the rate of bone loss. This is due to the decline in oestrogen production and means that women usually reach the 'fracture threshold' bone density long before men. Osteoporosis-related fractures are much more common in women than men. Spector *et al.* (1990) recorded a 4:1 female to male ratio in the age-specific incidence of hip fracture in the UK. This high ratio is seen only in countries where rates of osteoporosis are high.

Bone density can be measured in living subjects by techniques such as dual-energy X-ray absorptiometry, and these measurements are regarded as reliable indicators of bone strength. However, although a subthreshold density is a necessary permissive factor for osteoporotic fracture, bone mineral density measurements are imperfect predictors of individual susceptibility to fracture, especially for fractures of the hip (Smith, 1987; Cummings *et al.*, 1985). Leichter *et al.*, (1982) measured bone density and the shear stress required to fracture the femoral neck using isolated human bones obtained from cadavers. As expected, they found a high statistical correlation between shear stress at fracture and both bone density and bone mineral content. Breaking stress, bone density and bone mineral content all declined with the age of the subject. However, they found that breaking stress declined with age much faster than either bone density or bone mineral content. They concluded that changes in bone strength are apparently influenced too by other factors, such as changes in the micro-architecture of the bone.

The imperfect association between fracture risk and measured bone density needs to be borne in mind when evaluating reports of weak associations between environmental/lifestyle variables and bone density. This also means that evidence that interventions can have acute effects on bone density need to be treated with caution. Will any short-term increase be maintained in the longer term?

Will small measured increases in bone density significantly reduce fracture risk?

Key points

- Bone consists of crystals of the calcium phosphate salt, hydroxyapatite, deposited on an organic matrix consisting largely of the protein collagen.
- Hydroxyapatite makes up half of the bone weight and increases its mechanical strength.
- Bones are living dynamic structures that are continually being broken down and re-synthesized.
- Cells called osteoblasts synthesize new bone and osteoclasts cause bone breakdown.
- During childhood the rate of bone synthesis exceeds breakdown as the skeleton grows.
- In early adulthood the peak bone mass is reached and for a few years the rates of synthesis and breakdown are matched. In middle and old age there is a net loss of bone and they become thinner.
- Thinning of bones weakens them and can take them below a 'fracture threshold' where they break in response to relatively minor trauma. This is called osteoporosis.
- There is a marked acceleration in bone loss in women around the menopause that is due to decreased oestrogen production. Women usually reach their 'fracture threshold' before men and so elderly women are more prone to bone fractures than elderly men.
- Non-invasive bone density measurements are indicators of bone strength.
- Bone strength decreases more rapidly than bone density, probably owing to age-related changes in bone micro-architecture. Bone density is thus an imperfect measure of fracture risk, and this should be borne in mind when assessing the results of studies where bone density has been used as the measured outcome.

The incidence of osteoporosis

In this section, unreferenced facts and figures relating to the UK are taken from a freely downloadable booklet produced by the National

Osteoporosis Society: see www.nos.org.uk/page.aspx?pid=328&srcid=328 (accessed April 2012).

Thinning of the bones in osteoporosis is responsible for increased rates of bone fracture in older people, especially fractures of the vertebrae, wrist and the neck of the femur (hip fracture). Rates of osteoporotic fractures increased very substantially in many industrialized countries during the second half of the twentieth century. Since adult bone mass declines with age, the increased prevalence of osteoporosis can be accounted for partly by the larger numbers of people surviving into old age. Wickham *et al.* (1989), in a prospective study of 1400 elderly British people, found that the incidence of hip fracture was four times higher in women aged over 85 years than in women in the 65- to 74-year age band.

Figure 15.4 shows the age and sex distribution of hip fractures in one region of England. The proportion of fractures in each age group rises exponentially with increasing age and the higher prevalence in females is also illustrated. The number of people aged over 85 years doubled in the UK in the final two decades of the last century and this group now represents 2 per cent of the population. There has, however, also been a real increase as demonstrated by the large increases in age-specific incidence of fractures seen in the UK (Spector *et al.*, 1990). The incidence of hip fractures doubled in the UK in the 27 years up to 1983 and is projected to increase from 46 000 in 1985 to 117 000 in 2016.

Up to 3 million people in the UK may currently be affected by osteoporosis, which results in around 70 000 hip fractures, 50 000 wrist fractures and 120 000 vertebral fractures annually. As many as one in two women and one in five men in the UK over the age of 50 will have a fracture caused by poor bone health. Fractures of the hip are currently considered to be the major public health priority. A significant proportion of those affected die within a few months of the initial fracture, and many more are permanently disabled or never regain full mobility. Around 15 000 deaths each year in the UK may be consequences of hip fracture or the associated surgery. A third of all orthopaedic beds in UK hospitals are occupied by patients with osteoporosis, which probably costs the National Health Service almost 2 billion pounds each year. In the USA there are over a 200 000 hip fractures each year that are attributable to osteoporosis. Johnell *et al.* (1992) published comparative rates of osteoporotic fracture in different countries.

General and lifestyle risk factors for osteoporosis

Box 15.1 lists some of the known or possible risk factors. It is clear that one should expect the risk of osteoporosis and fractures to increase with age and elderly women to be at increased risk compared to elderly men. Projected increases in the elderly populations make it likely that the number of people affected will rise over the coming decades unless prevention and treatment become more effective. The over-85 age group has been and will continue to increase more rapidly than the total elderly population. Women outnumber men by three to one in the over-85 age group.

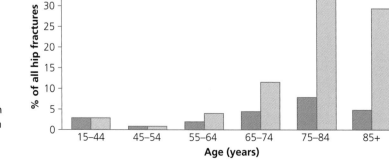

Figure 15.4 Age distribution of hip fractures in the Trent region of England, 1989–90. Data from Kanis (1993), after Webb and Copeman (1996).

Box 15.1

Risk factors for osteoporosis

- Old age – risk of osteoporosis increases with age and accelerates in women when they reach the menopause
- Being female – rates are higher in women than men in western Europe and North America
- Lack of sex hormones – factors that reduce sex hormone secretion (e.g. early menopause or ovarian removal) increase risk, and hormone replacement therapy (HRT) reduces risk
- Being white – there are distinct racial differences in bone density and considerable genetic variations within races
- Never having borne a child
- Sedentary lifestyle
- Smoking
- High alcohol consumption
- Being small or underweight
- Inadequate calcium intake in childhood?
- High consumption of carbonated, cola drinks?
- Being an omnivore – vegetarians have lower rates of osteoporosis

The accelerated bone loss associated with menopausal oestrogen loss suggests that anything that diminishes sex hormone output might be likely to increase bone loss and fracture risk. Many conditions in which there is reduced sex hormone output are indeed associated with reduced bone density, including:

- early menopause or surgical removal of the ovaries
- cessation of menstruation due to starvation or anorexia nervosa
- amenorrhoea due to extremely high activity and low body fat content in women athletes
- hypogonadism in men.

Hormone replacement therapy (HRT) in post-menopausal women prevents or reduces the acceleration in rate of bone loss and reduces the risk of osteoporotic fracture. HRT is widely accepted as being effective in the prevention of osteoporosis. The controversy about the treatment is over whether this and other benefits are sufficient to outweigh any possible risks, such as increased risk of uterine cancer or perhaps of breast cancer.

Until about 2002, many older women were being prescribed HRT for the long-term prevention of osteoporosis, and many family doctors routinely encouraged their older female patients to use it. Then, a study by Nelson *et al.* (2002) suggested that HRT might increase the risk of heart disease in post-menopausal women whereas in the past it had been thought to be cardioprotective. That study has been criticized because most of the subjects were elderly and had existing heart disease and so were unlikely to benefit from any cardioprotective effects of HRT. The critics have suggested that if started in younger women when menopausal symptoms first appear it may still have these benefits. Beral *et al.* (2003) looked at the relationship between breast cancer and HRT in a study that involved over a million women. They seemed to confirm what had long been suspected, that long-term HRT is associated with a small increase in breast cancer risk.

Family doctors are now advised that they should not routinely prescribe HRT to post-menopausal women to prevent osteoporosis, although its use for alleviation of acute menopausal symptoms like 'hot flushes' is still recommended. Phyto-oestrogens from soy products have been marketed as an alternative to HRT for alleviation of menopausal symptoms and prevention of osteoporosis in older women (discussed in Chapter 19).

There are clear racial differences in bone density. People of European and Asian origin have bones that are less dense than those of African origin. In the USA, white women are much more likely to suffer from osteoporotic fractures than black women. Even within racial groups there is almost certainly a very large inherited variability in bone density and susceptibility to fracture. Prentice (1997) estimated that 80 per cent of the variation in bone mineral status can be attributed to genetic factors.

The increasingly sedentary lifestyle of those living in the industrialized countries is widely believed to be a major factor in the increased age-specific incidence of osteoporotic fractures. There are numerous observations that suggest inactivity reduces bone density and that weight-bearing exercise increases it. Some examples are listed below.

- Immobilization or extreme inactivity (e.g. confinement to bed or the weightlessness experienced by astronauts) results in loss of bone mass.
- When bones are repeatedly mechanically stressed they thicken and become stronger. Tennis players have much thicker bones in their racket arm, and runners have higher than average bone density in their vertebrae. Experimental studies have shown that jumping up and down or use of a small trampoline increases bone density in pre-menopausal women although not in post-menopausal women (Bassey *et al.*, 1998).
- Increased activity in childhood and adolescence increases the peak bone mass. Children who spent more than 2 hours daily in weight-bearing activity were reported to have greater bone mineral density than those who spent less than an hour daily in such activity (Cooper and Eastell, 1993).
- Weight-bearing exercise in older people slows down the rate of age-related bone loss. In a cross-sectional study of 600 post-menopausal women, Coupland *et al.* (1999) were able to show that reported levels of stair-climbing and brisk walking was positively associated with bone density at the hip and over the whole body. In 1400 elderly British people sampled by Wickham *et al.* (1989), the risk of hip fracture was reduced in those people with higher levels of outdoor physical activity.
- Pocock *et al.* (1986) found a significant correlation between measured fitness level and bone mineral density in healthy women. In the post-menopausal women in this sample, fitness was the only measured variable that correlated significantly with bone mineral density.

Being underweight is associated with a higher risk of osteoporotic fracture, and in the elderly this is often as a result of low lean body mass caused by inactivity. More active and fitter elderly people may also be less prone to osteoporotic fracture because they are better coordinated and stronger and therefore less prone to falling or less liable to injury if they do fall.

Many studies have suggested that cigarette smoking is associated with reduced bone density and increased fracture risk. In their sample of elderly British people, Wickham *et al.* (1989) reported a strong association between cigarette smoking and risk of hip fracture. Smoking is associated with:

- lower body weight
- reduced physical activity
- early menopause
- reduced blood oestrogen concentration (even in women receiving HRT).

These all have known associations with higher fracture risk.

High alcohol consumption has also been widely reported as a risk factor for osteoporosis. Heavy drinking is associated with extensive bone loss even in relatively young adults (Smith, 1987). High alcohol consumption might also be expected to increase the risk of falling.

Dietary risk factors for osteoporosis

The emerging consensus is that there is little evidence of a relationship between bone density and dietary calcium intake in young and middle-aged adults, but that calcium supplements may slow the rate of bone loss in post-menopausal women – especially those whose habitual intakes from food are low (Phillips, 2003). Cross-cultural comparisons indicate that it is unlikely that low calcium intake *per se* is a major causative factor for osteoporosis or a major determinant of bone density. Osteoporosis is uncommon in some populations with low calcium intakes but prevalence is high in many populations with relatively high calcium intakes (e.g. in the USA, UK and northern Europe). For example, rural Bantu women suffer only one-tenth the fracture incidence of Western women despite taking in only half as much calcium (Rolls, 1992), and the similar findings of Prentice *et al.* (1993) in rural Gambia were discussed earlier. Hegsted (1986) found a positive correlation between calcium intake and incidence of hip fracture in nine countries in Europe, the Far East, Australasia and North America. International comparisons may be of limited usefulness in proving cause-and-effect relationships but if high calcium intake is associated internationally with high rates of osteoporosis this makes it improbable that calcium deficiency is a major cause. High calcium intakes or calcium supplements might still offset an increase in osteoporosis risk even though it is primarily due to other causes. Double-blind placebo-controlled trials of calcium supplements in childhood suggest that for the first few months they do cause a small increase in measured bone density, but this effect disappears once the supplements are stopped (Prentice, 1997; Phillips, 2003).

Good vitamin D status is essential for the efficient absorption of calcium from the intestine, and biochemical evidence of widespread vitamin D inadequacy has been found in children, adults and elderly people in the UK. Some of the beneficial effects of calcium supplements in slowing the rate of bone loss in older people may be because they compensate for poor vitamin D status; at high calcium intakes, more calcium is absorbed by mechanisms that do not depend on vitamin D.

Prevention of osteoporosis and its consequences

There are several strategic approaches that may be employed to try to reduce the number of fractures attributed to osteoporosis.

- Promote changes in diet and lifestyle of children and young adults that increase the PBM. This would increase the amount of bone that can be lost in later life before the fracture threshold is reached.
- Encourage dietary and lifestyle changes that slow the rate of bone loss in older people, particularly post-menopausal women. This would mean that it would take longer to reach the fracture threshold from any given PBM.
- Try to reverse the process of osteoporosis in older people. Promote dietary, behavioural and pharmacological measures that increase bone density in those with low bone density or frank osteoporosis.
- Try to reduce the risk of bones being subjected to the traumas that cause them to fracture. Fractures of the hip usually occur during a fall, and the high risk of falling contributes towards the increased risk of all fractures in the elderly. In someone with advanced osteoporosis, measures that reduce the tendency to fall or to protect the faller from injury may offer the greatest potential. Design and maintenance of accommodation for

the elderly should pay particular attention to the risks associated with a fall. Measures designed to improve muscle strength may reduce the risk of falling. In contrast to the enormous amount of work done looking at factors that affect bone density, there has been relatively little work done on the causes of falls in the elderly.

A good intake of calcium in childhood together with ensuring good vitamin D status may increase peak bone mass and thus reduce the later risk of osteoporosis. Calcium intakes substantially below the dietary standard during childhood may limit peak bone mass and poor vitamin D status certainly has adverse effects on skeletal development. However, in observational studies there is little or no correlation between calcium intake and bone density in children. According to Prentice (1997) and Phillips (2003), studies in children suggest that calcium supplements can have a small effect on bone density. This effect seems to be greatest in the first few months of supplementation and the effect disappears quickly once the supplements are stopped. In contrast, there is clear evidence that active children have denser bones than those who do little load-bearing exercise. Increasing the outdoor activity levels of children can be promoted on many grounds and would seem to be the most effective long-term strategy for improving bone health. Good intakes of milk and cheese in growing children will, in most cases, be necessary for children to achieve calcium intakes that reach dietary standard values. Vitamin D is produced by the action of sunlight on the skin and so outdoor activity is the preferred option.

As noted earlier, there is little evidence that normal variation in dietary calcium intake has any major effect on bone density in adults. Supplemental calcium in women during the menopause is generally ineffective at preventing oestrogen-related bone loss, but supplements in the elderly may reduce the rate of bone loss at the hip (Prentice, 1997; Phillips, 2003). As discussed in Chapter 16, many elderly Britons, especially those living in residential homes, have poor vitamin D status primarily due to lack of sunlight exposure and this will reduce calcium absorption. Evidence that vitamin D and calcium supplements reduce fracture risk in elderly people, especially those living in residential homes, is also discussed in Chapter 14. There is a sound case for taking measures to increase access to summer sunlight and/or for the use of vitamin D and calcium supplements in elderly housebound people. Inactivity is a cause of osteoporosis and so there is an overwhelming case for encouraging increased amounts of load-bearing exercise in all age groups. There are many other reasons for encouraging increased activity and physical fitness (see Chapter 18).

There is compelling evidence that the administration of oestrogen to menopausal women prevents or reduces the post-menopausal acceleration in rate of bone loss and reduces fracture risk. There is some discussion of the effects of phyto-oestrogens on bone density and their use as possible 'natural' alternatives to HRT in Chapter 19.

Treatment of osteoporosis

The treatments for osteoporosis include the following:

- administration of sex hormones or synthetic analogues – oestrogen replacement therapy in women and testosterone injections in men
- supplements of vitamin D and calcium (but, as noted in Chapter 16, there is as yet no evidence that these are effective in people who have already had a fracture)
- calcitonin injections or the bisphosphonate group of drugs which both inhibit bone breakdown by osteoclasts.

A drug called teriparatide has become available for those women most severely affected by osteoporosis. It is a synthetic analogue of part of the parathyroid hormone molecule. It can be administered only by injection and at the moment its use is restricted to 18 months, but the benefits last beyond that period. It stimulates new bone formation, and so, unlike other treatments, it does reverse the process of osteoporosis.

Conclusions on promoting bone health

An active lifestyle (preferably including outdoor weight-bearing exercise), absence of cigarette smoking, moderate alcohol consumption and a diet that meets the standards for essential nutrients is both consistent with general health education guidelines and offers expectation of reducing the risk of osteoporosis and bone fractures. There seems to be no convincing evidence that calcium supplements *per se* will prevent osteoporosis or be effective in its treatment. Good intakes of calcium in childhood and early adulthood may contribute to increased peak bone mass, but other lifestyle factors (e.g. activity level) are probably more significant and the case for calcium supplements seems unconvincing. Widespread vitamin D deficiency in the elderly is probably an important cause of increased fracture risk, so increased exposure to sunlight and/or supplements of vitamin D and calcium should be encouraged; sunlight exposure needs to be balanced to ensure adequate vitamin D production but not cause sunburn and increase the risk of skin cancer.

Key points

- The risk factors for osteoporosis are listed in Box 15.1.
- Osteoporotic fracture rates are increasing with the rise in numbers of the elderly population and because of increased age-specific incidence.
- In the UK, up to 300 000 fractures each year are attributed to osteoporosis.
- Many of the 80 000 people who annually suffer hip fractures die within a few months of the initial fracture or never regain full mobility.
- Up to 15 000 people die annually as a result of osteoporosis and it costs the NHS around £2 billion annually.
- A third of all orthopaedic beds in the UK are occupied by people with osteoporosis.
- Menopausal oestrogen loss and vitamin D deficiency are major precipitating factors in elderly women.
- Lack of sex hormones in men or women increases bone loss and oestrogen replacement therapy slows bone loss.
- There are inherent racial and individual differences in bone density, and perhaps 80 per cent of the variation in bone mineral status can be attributed to genetic factors.

→

- Bones thicken when exposed to repeated stress and they become thinner when immobilized. Experimental and epidemiological studies suggest that weight-bearing exercise:
  - increases bone deposition in children and increases peak bone mass
  - slows the rate of bone loss in older adults
  - increases bone density in older adults.
- Cigarette smoking and high alcohol consumption reduce bone density.
- Osteoporosis is often most prevalent in those countries with the highest calcium intakes – which makes it unlikely that low calcium intake is a primary cause of osteoporosis.
- Calcium intake seems to have a small positive effect on bone density in children but only while the supplements continue to be taken.
- Calcium supplements slow the rate of bone loss in elderly women especially in those whose intake from food is low; they may be compensating for poor vitamin D status. Many elderly people have little exposure to sunlight and low vitamin D status.
- Combined supplements of vitamin D and calcium have been shown to reduce fracture risk in very elderly housebound women.
- Osteoporosis would be reduced by the following:
  - increased weight-bearing activity in children and ensuring they have good vitamin D and calcium status
  - increased participation in (outdoor) load-bearing activity in all adults
  - ensuring the vitamin D status of elderly people by increasing access to sunlight or the provision of supplements
  - measures to reduce the risk of falling in the elderly or to decrease the risk of injury in elderly fallers
  - increased use of hormone replacement therapy by post-menopausal women
  - less tobacco use and alcohol abuse.
- A class of drugs (e.g. teriparatide) which are analogues of parathyroid hormone seem to reverse the process of osteoporosis and result in new bone synthesis.

SODIUM AND DISEASE

Key facts

- *Dietary standards.* Sodium adult RNI is 1.6 g/day, chloride 2.5 g (these are equivalent in molar terms and represent 4.1 g of salt); sodium LRNI is 575 mg/day, chloride 888 mg/day (c1.5 g/day of salt). USA values are: sodium 1.5 g/day, chloride 2.3 g/day.
- *Dietary recommendations.* Average population salt (sodium chloride) intake should be reduced to around 6 g/day.
- *Dietary sources.* Processed foods are the major source, plus small amounts in natural foods, and some discretionary salt is added at the table and during home cooking. The salt content of some typical food portions:
  - 2 medium slices bread – 1 g
  - 1 serving (60 g) Cheddar cheese – 1.1 g
  - 1 serving (60 g) Danish blue cheese – 2.1 g
  - 4 fish fingers – 0.9 g
  - 1 portion corn flakes (25 g) – 0.7 g
  - 1 portion All-Bran (45 g) – 1 g
  - 1 portion (90 g) prawns – 3.7 g
  - 1 gammon steak (120 g) – 6.5 g
  - 2 slices (60 g) corned beef – 1.5 g
  - 2 large sausages – 1.5 g
  - 1 packet crisps – 0.4 g
  - 1 bowl (220 g) canned tomato soup – 2.3 g
  - 1 portion baked beans (200 g) – 2.4 g
  - 1 portion (100 g) sardines in tomato sauce – 0.9 g
  - 1 takeaway cheeseburger – 2.2 g
  - lime pickle (15 g) – 0.2 g
  - takeaway vegetable curry – 2 g
  - beef chow mein – 5.5 g
- *Biochemical functions.* Sodium is the major cation in extracellular fluid. It maintains fluid and electrolyte balance, is important in nerve transmission and in acid–base balance. Chloride is the major anion in the body and is important in maintaining fluid and electrolyte balance.
- *Effects of deficiency.* Dietary deficiencies do not normally occur.
- *Risk factors for deficiency.* Unaccustomed heavy physical activity in a warm environment can lead to substantial salt losses in sweat. This can cause short-term increases in salt requirement, but adaptation occurs and results in the production of a much more dilute sweat.

Overview of salt (sodium chloride)

Historical importance

Salt has been prized throughout history for its ability to flavour and preserve foods. Roman soldiers used to be paid partly with salt (their 'salarium'), which is the origin of the word salary and of the common expression 'to be worth one's salt'. Salt has been an important trading commodity with whole empires built on the revenues derived from it. Salt has also been attributed with mystical and purifying properties by many cultural groups and it certainly does have useful antiseptic properties. In their excellent monograph on salt, MacGregor and de Wardener (1999) devote a whole chapter to these non-culinary uses – the image of Sumo wrestlers purifying the fighting arena with handfuls of salt is one example that is familiar to many of us. In past times in the USA, salt was left in the room of a dead person to purge their sins, and it was common practice in parts of Britain to sprinkle salt on a corpse or place salt in the coffin. Macgregor and de Wardener even reproduce an ancient woodcut of French women sprinkling salt on their husbands' genitals to enhance their sexual performance! The monograph is entitled *Salt, Diet and Health* and contains a good introduction to work concerning the health consequences of a high salt intake and lists and discusses many of the landmark studies in this field.

Problems with salt

Elevated blood pressure

High salt intake has long been suspected of being involved in the aetiology of essential hypertension (the most common type). Salt (sodium chloride) is made up of the two mineral elements sodium and chlorine. It is the sodium component that has been generally regarded as significant in causing hypertension, but this discussion usually refers to salt rather than to sodium alone. Even in patients with hypertension, sodium balance is very effectively hormonally regulated; if salt intake is raised or lowered then urinary excretion rapidly rises or falls so as to restore the balance between intake and output. This *homeostatic mechanism* is so effective that salt excretion in a 24-hour urine sample is generally regarded as the best way of measuring daily salt intake. Despite this homeostatic mechanism, it is suggested that prolonged excess salt intake can lead to excess salt retention and therefore increased fluid retention and hypertension. Evidence from dialysis patients and those with endocrine disorders confirms that salt retention does indeed lead to increased blood pressure.

MacGregor and de Wardener (1999) suggested that the kidneys of patients with essential hypertension have an impaired ability to excrete salt. When large amounts of salt are consumed by susceptible people their kidney defect means that there is a tendency to retain excess salt, which triggers several compensatory mechanisms which increase salt excretion and restore homeostasis. A rise in blood pressure and consequent increase in renal filtration of salt is one of these compensatory mechanisms. As evidence for this theory they cite cross-transplantation studies in rats. When the kidneys of genetically hypertensive and normal rats were surgically swapped, the blood pressure rose in the normal rats with hypertensive-strain kidneys but remained normal in the hypertensive-strain rats with normal kidneys. They claimed that limited observations on patients receiving therapeutic kidney transplants showed a similar trend.

Affluent populations have generally been advised to substantially reduce their dietary salt intake. The World Health Organization has suggested a move towards a population average salt intake of 5 g/day. In both the UK and the USA it is recommended that salt intake should be limited to 6 g/day. The principal aim of such recommendations is to reduce the 20–25 per cent incidence of essential hypertension in the adult populations of affluent countries and thus to reduce the morbidity and mortality from diseases precipitated by high blood pressure, namely strokes, myocardial infarction, renal failure and retinopathy.

Adults can be classified into four categories when trying to assess the prevalence of high blood pressure:

- *normotensive and untreated* – systolic <160 mmHg, diastolic <95 mmHg
- *hypertensive and untreated* – systolic >160 mmHg and/or diastolic >95 mmHg

- *normotensive and treated* – systolic <160 mmHg, diastolic <95 mmHg, taking drugs to control BP
- *hypertensive and treated* – systolic >160 mmHg and/or diastolic >95 mmHg, taking drugs to control BP.

All except those in the first category are people who have developed elevated blood pressure and they represent about 22 per cent of all adults in the UK.

The prevalence of hypertension rises steeply with age:

- 1 per cent at 16–24 years
- 3 per cent at 25–34 years
- 7 per cent at 35–44 years
- 18 per cent at 45–54 years
- 38 per cent at 55–64 years
- 57 per cent at 65–74 years
- 70 per cent at over 75 years.

A wide variety of drugs are available that are effective in lowering blood pressure, at least in the short term. These drugs also seem to be effective in reducing the renal and cerebrovascular complications of hypertension, and the modern ones also reduce the risk of coronary conditions. As with any drugs, there may be acute side-effects. Possible long-term problems are of particular concern because antihypertensives may need to be taken for the rest of the patient's life. There have been suggestions that use of some of the older antihypertensives was associated with increased overall mortality (e.g. MRFIT, 1982).

Despite the availability of this wide range of antihypertensive drugs, the proposition that moderation of dietary salt intake might prevent hypertension – or be a useful alternative to drug treatments – is still attractive. Salt restriction may also be used in conjunction with the drugs to increase their effectiveness or to reduce the dose needed. High intakes of potassium and possibly calcium have also been suggested as having possible protective effects against the development of hypertension.

Gastric cancer

High salt intake has been implicated also in the aetiology of gastric cancer. One theory suggests that salt acts as a gastric irritant and that continued irritation leads to atrophy of the acid-secreting glands in the stomach. Reduced acid secretion in the stomach then allows proliferation of bacteria and they produce carcinogenic substances (*nitrosamines*) from some components of food. Again there is considerable support for the latter part of the hypothesis: patients with pernicious anaemia who produce less gastric acid have markedly increased rates of gastric cancer. In recent years it has become clear that infection with the bacterium *Helicobacter pylori* is the most important predisposing factor for gastric cancer. Chronic infection with this organism leads to atrophic gastritis and eventually to cancer. Most early studies on the relationship between diet and cancer have taken no account of the presence or absence of this organism.

There is some evidence that diets rich in salted meats and fish and salted pickled vegetables consumed in some countries are associated with increased risk of gastric cancer (COMA, 1998).

Osteoporosis

MacGregor and de Wardener (1999) have reviewed limited evidence that high salt intake may be a factor in the aetiology of osteoporosis. A positive correlation between rates of bone loss and urinary salt excretion in older women has been reported.

Key points

- High salt intake is considered to be an important cause of essential hypertension.
- High blood pressure increases the risk of strokes, myocardial infarctions, renal failure and retinopathy.
- One theory suggests that the kidneys of hypertensives have an impaired ability to excrete salt and that a rise in BP is a compensatory mechanism that increases renal filtration and salt excretion. There is very effective renal regulation of daily salt balance even in hypertensives.
- Salt has been implicated also in the aetiology of gastric cancer and, less convincingly, in the aetiology of osteoporosis.
- In the UK and the USA, a maximum salt intake of 6 g/day has been recommended – compared to the current average of around 10 g/day.

→

Key points *continued*

- Reduced salt intake is expected to reduce the prevalence of hypertension and thus ultimately the risk of linked diseases. Salt restriction may be a useful adjunct to or alternative to antihypertensive drug therapy.
- Up to 25 per cent of all UK adults may be hypertensive and the proportion rises steeply with age.

Assessing the requirement for salt

What the body neeeds

The sodium and chloride in salt are both essential nutrients. Sodium is the principal cation in extracellular fluid; the average 70 kg man has around 92 grams of sodium in his body, equivalent to about 250 grams of salt. Around half of total body sodium is in the extracellular fluid, 38 per cent in bone and the remaining 12 per cent in the intracellular fluid; potassium is the dominant cation in intracellular fluid.

Despite the undoubted essentiality of sodium, the habitual intake of most affluent populations greatly exceeds minimum requirements. Almost all ingested salt is absorbed in the intestine and the homeostatic control of salt excretion by the endocrine system enables individuals, even those with hypertension, to remain in salt balance over a huge range of intakes. Some populations, such as the Kalahari bushmen and New Guinea highlanders, manage on habitual salt intakes of around 1 g/day whereas other populations (e.g. in some regions of Japan and Korea) habitually take in more than 25 g/day. Average urinary excretion of salt in a sample of adult Yanomamo indians in Brazil was found to be only 50 mg per day, which is less than 1 per cent of that excreted by an average Briton. MacGregor and de Wardener (1999) listed comparative salt intakes of different populations.

The NRC (1989a) estimated that minimum requirements for sodium chloride were only around 1.25 g/day. This minimum figure did not provide for large prolonged losses from the skin through sweat. Individuals adapt to salt restriction during heavy exercise or in a hot environment by producing very dilute sweat.

The reference nutrient intakes for sodium and chloride in the UK amount to a salt intake of around 4 g/day. The panel felt that this value allowed for losses in sweat during exercise and high temperatures once adaptation had occurred, but that, in the short term, extra intake might be required under these circumstances.

Dietary sources and amounts

It is generally accepted that *discretionary salt*, used in cooking and on the plate, makes the traditional methods of dietary analysis using food tables an unreliable excercise. The best method is by measurement of sodium *excreted* over a 24-hour period. This approach relies on the assumption that, whatever the intake, individuals are in approximate salt balance on a day-to-day basis and thus that sodium excretion is equal to sodium intake. The method usually involves collecting a 24-hour urine specimen from the subject. Normally, well over 90 per cent of total body sodium loss is via the urine and the figure can be corrected for losses via the skin and in faeces which are small under most circumstances (not if there is severe diarrhoea or heavy sweating). Ideally, a marker substance should be used to ensure that the 24-hour urine specimen is complete; that is, a substance that is consumed by the subject and excreted in the urine in 24 hours, and only when there is complete recovery of the marker is the sample considered to be complete.

In a large sample of British adults, Gregory *et al.* (1990) found a very poor correlation ($r=0.25$) between salt intake as measured by 24-hour urinary sodium excretion and that calculated from the average salt content of foods recorded during a 7-day weighed inventory. There are at least three factors that might contribute to this poor agreement between the two methods:

- the sodium excretion method used just one day, which was at a different time to the 7 days of the weighed inventory (the intake of many nutrients fluctuates widely from day to day)
- no allowance was made for salt added during cooking or at the table in the weighed inventory.
- no marker was used to ensure completeness of the 24-hour urine specimen.

Nevertheless, the lack of agreement between these methods underlines the difficulty of estimating a subject's habitual salt intake in order to correlate this with, for example, blood pressure in epidemiological studies. Both methods have been used as the measure of habitual intake in epidemiological studies. Nutrient intakes fluctuate from day to day and several days' intake needs to be recorded to get a useful estimate of average daily intake. This means that this disagreement between the two methods is in line with what is found with other nutrients. For example, potassium intake in food and 24-hour excretion of potassium were also both measured in this sample of people. In this case there was no discretionary intake. Despite this, the correlation between the two methods for measuring potassium intake was almost as bad as for sodium. This strongly suggests that, even though 24-hour sodium excretion may be an accurate reflection of sodium intake *on that day*, large day-to-day variations may make it a relatively poor predictor of the *habitual* salt intake of an individual. This would make it unlikely that individual salt intake measured in this way would correlate with blood pressure even if habitual salt intake is an important determinant of blood pressure (see Chapter 3).

Average 24-hour sodium excretion should be a much better reflection of the habitual intake of a population or group. Using this method, James *et al.* (1987) concluded that average salt intake in the UK was around 10.7 g/day for men and 8.0 g/day for women. More recently, Hoare *et al.* (2004) reported average daily intakes of 11 g and 8.1 g for men and women, respectively, using the 24-hour excretion method; only 15 per cent of men and 31 per cent of women were below the 6 g/day recommended maximum. James' team found that 75 per cent of cooking salt was not consumed but was discarded with the cooking water, so failure to fully recognise this had previously resulted in too high estimates.

James *et al.* (1987) provided their subjects with pots of table and cooking salt that had been 'labelled' with lithium, so recovery of lithium in the urine enabled the team to estimate what proportion of the total salt excreted was from these sources. By comparing the amount removed from the pot with recovery, they were also able to make their estimate of the proportion of this salt that was not consumed (discarded in cooking water or in uneaten food). They concluded that discretionary salt made up only about 15 per cent of total intake – 9 per cent

from table salt and 6 per cent from cooking salt. They estimated that a further 10 per cent of total intake was from salt naturally present in foods, but that the remaining 75 per cent was derived from salt added by food manufacturers during processing. (The salt contents of some common foods are shown in the key facts box.) Such figures indicate that there is very limited scope for individuals to reduce their salt intake by restricting their discretionary use of salt. If salt intake is to be substantially reduced then either the salt content of manufactured foods must be reduced or the contribution of high-salt manufactured foods to the total diet must be reduced.

Hoare *et al.* (2004) estimated salt intake by 7-day weighed food intake at 8.3 g/day for men and 5.8 g/day for women; this excludes salt added during cooking or at the table, and estimates of total salt intake using urinary sodium excretion give figures of 11 g/day for men and 8.1 g/day for women. These results did not show any reduction compared to those of Gregory *et al.* (1990).

Hoare *et al.* (2004) also present an analysis of the contribution of different foods to the total intake from food, as follows.

- Cereals and cereal products provided over 35 per cent of the salt in food, with white bread alone contributing 14 per cent of the total.
- Meat, meat dishes and meat products provided 26 per cent of the total, with bacon and ham contributing 8 per cent.
- Milk and milk products provided 8 per cent of the total.
- Vegetables and vegetable dishes (excluding potatoes) contributed 7 per cent.
- Fish and fish products contributed 4 per cent.
- Miscellaneous foods which include soups, sauces and relishes contribute 8 per cent.
- All other categories of food provided substantially less than 5 per cent each.

Reduced-salt versions of several salty foods are now widely available in the UK and marketed on their lower salt content (e.g. cured meats and some canned foods). In 2006, the Food Standards Agency published a series of voluntary targets for salt reduction in the form of maximum levels for the salt contents of a wide range of processed foods, including:

- meat-based products like hams, sausages, bacon and pies
- bread, rolls and bread products like crumpets and bagels
- breakfast cereals
- baked beans and canned vegetables
- savoury snack foods
- cheeses, butter and margarine
- bottled sauces and relishes
- cook-in and pasta sauces
- a wide range of ready meals.

In the release document for these targets the FSA highlighted substantial progress by parts of the food industry in reducing the salt content of manufactured foods, such as those listed below:

- substantial reduction by several supermarket chains in reducing the salt content of their own-brand products
- a reduction of a third in the salt content of breakfast cereals since 1998
- a 30 per cent reduction in the salt content of bread, soups and sauces and cheese spreads
- a 10 per cent reduction in sales of household table and cooking salt in the previous year.

Reductions in salt content of foods may not be entirely without problems. Reduced salt content may be perceived to adversely affect the palatability of foods. Changes to the recipes for some traditional products, like bottled sauces, may lead to customer complaints and dissatisfaction. Salt is also used by manufacturers as a preservative and processing aid, so reducing the salt content could have effects other than on palatability. In particular, shelf life may be adversely affected, thus increasing costs and perhaps even the microbiological safety of the food compromised. The FSA acknowledges some of these problems in its comments on the targets it has set. If salt is replaced by alternative preservatives then this increased intake of alternative preservatives may itself be undesirable. In a chapter entitled 'The industrial conspiracy', MacGregor and de Wardener (1999) argue that salt producers and food processors have resisted pressure to reduce the salt content of manufactured foods for commercial reasons rather than out of any necessity to maintain food safety or quality.

Key points

- A normal man's body contains around 250 grams of salt, and sodium is the major cation in extracellular fluid.
- Sodium and chlorine are essential minerals but current salt intakes are 10 times minimum requirements.
- Individuals adapt to low salt intakes and heavy sweating by reducing the sodium concentrations of sweat and urine.
- The UK RNIs for sodium and chlorine are equivalent to about 4 g/day of salt.
- 24-hour sodium excretion is regarded as the best measure of salt intake. There is very poor correlation between salt intake as measured by conventional dietary analysis and 24-hour sodium excretion.
- 24-hour sodium excretion is a good measure of any day's salt intake or the average intake of a population. It is a poor measure of an *individual's* habitual salt intake because of large day-to-day variations.
- More than 75 per cent of UK dietary salt is from manufactured foods and only around 15 per cent is salt added at the table and during home cooking. However, most cooking salt in not consumed but is thrown away with the cooking water.
- Substantial reductions in total salt intake require that either less is used by food processors or that consumption of high-salt processed foods is reduced.
- The salt contents of many processed foods have been reduced and low-salt versions of a number of processed foods are now available.
- Voluntary targets for the maximum salt contents of a very large range of processed foods were set in 2006 by the Food Standards Agency in the UK. Substantial progress had been made prior to this in reducing the salt content of some processed foods, notably bread, breakfast cereals, soups, sauces and cheese spreads.

REVIEW OF EVIDENCE FOR A SALT–HYPERTENSION LINK

Observational evidence

In some populations that have very low salt intakes of around 1 g/day, hypertension is practically unknown and there is no general increase in blood pressure with age as is seen in the UK and USA (e.g. Kalahari bushmen and the Yanomamo indians of Brazil). In Japan and Korea, in contrast, average salt intake may be 2–3 times that seen in the UK and there is a very high incidence of strokes and gastric cancer, which have both been causally linked to high salt intake. The 'low-salt populations' often have diets and lifestyles that are very different from those of affluent societies, so any number of confounding variables could be involved – obvious examples being higher physical activity, lower levels of obesity, lower alcohol and tobacco use and higher potassium intake of those populations with low salt intakes. There are, however, some examples of fit, active populations still leading a fairly traditional lifestyle who nonetheless have high salt intakes and they have blood pressure and hypertension profiles that are more typical of those seen in Western populations. For example, Solomon Islanders who cooked their food in seawater had eight times the incidence of hypertension compared to those living on nearby islands where salt intake was low. Tobian (1979) and MacGregor and de Wardener (1999) both provide interesting summaries of the early work in this area.

The level of salt intake in these low-salt populations is too low to be a realistic goal for those living in affluent countries. However, more extensive cross-population studies, like those of Gliebermann (1973), suggested that there was an apparent linear relationship between the average salt intake of a population and the average blood pressure in middle-aged and elderly people (see Figure 4.1 in Chapter 4). This would mean that even modest reductions in population salt intake could be expected to lead to reduced average blood pressure, reduced incidence of hypertension and thus eventually to reduced morbidity and mortality from those conditions that are precipitated by hypertension. In Gliebermann's paper, the reliability and validity of many of the measures of salt intake were questionable. As in all such cross-cultural studies, there was the recurring problem of confounding variables. Gliebermann's data also included some black populations who are genetically salt sensitive and prone to hypertension, and this could account for some of the most divergent points on her graphs.

In a later cross-population study, Law et al. (1991a) related blood pressure to salt intake from reported data on 24 populations around the world. By the following means they overcame some of the criticisms of Gliebermann's earlier work.

- They restricted their analysis to data in which salt intake was measured by 24-hour sodium excretion.
- They excluded African and other black populations from their study.
- They analysed data from developed and economically underdeveloped countries separately so as to reduce the problem of confounding lifestyle variables.
- Their study included people across a wide age range, enabling them to look at the relationship between salt intake and blood pressure in age groups.

Despite these improvements in methodology the conclusions were similar to those of Gliebermann. They found a highly significant relationship between average blood pressure and population salt intake in both developed and economically underdeveloped populations. The effect of salt intake on blood pressure increased with age and with initial blood pressure level. They derived an equation that they suggested would predict the average change in blood pressure of a group that would result from a specified change in salt intake. The variables in this equation were: the group's age, current salt intake and initial blood pressure. They predicted, for example, that in a developed country like the UK a 60 per cent reduction in salt intake in 60- to 69 year olds with a systolic pressure of 183 mmHg might be expected to lead to a 14 mmHg reduction in systolic pressure.

Studies of migrant populations confirm that much of the international variation in blood pressure and incidence of hypertension-related diseases is due to environmental rather than genetic factors. People of

Japanese origin in the USA, where salt intake is much lower than in Japan, have reduced incidence of strokes as compared to Japanese people living in Japan. Samburu tribesmen in Kenya have a traditional low-salt diet in their villages, but if they join the Kenyan army the high-salt army rations are associated with a rise in their average blood pressure after 2–3 years (Tobian, 1979).

Reduced reliance on salting as a means of modern food preservation has been associated with falling mortality from strokes and gastric cancer in the UK, the USA and most industrialized countries. On an international basis, there is a strong positive correlation between stroke and gastric cancer mortality rates in industrialized countries. This is consistent with there being a common causative factor (i.e. high salt intake) for the two diseases (see Figure 4.2 in Chapter 4). Joossens et al. (1996) reported a strong positive correlation between average salt intake and death rate from stomach cancer in a study of 24 populations from around the world.

The weak point in the evidential link between salt intake and hypertension has traditionally been the lack of association between salt intake and blood pressure in individuals from within the same community. This has been a fairly consistent finding in many within-population studies (Tobian, 1979; Law et al., 1991b) and may be because of the general tendency for the influence of other factors on blood pressure to obscure the relationship with salt intake. The difficulty of reliably measuring habitual salt intake would also be an important factor; many studies have used 24-hour sodium excretion as the measure of habitual salt intake of individuals but it is almost certainly a very poor measure of this.

It has also been argued that this lack of association is because only a relatively small proportion of the population are sensitive to salt. There will be genetic variation in salt sensitivity, but if this variation is so great that effectively only a small subgroup of the population is salt sensitive then this would greatly weaken the case for population intervention to reduce salt intake.

Frost et al. (1991), in a complex re-analysis of 14 published within-population studies of the relationship between salt intake and blood pressure, concluded that the results were consistent with the results predicted from their equation derived from between-population analysis (Law et al., 1991a). They argued that day-to-day variation in an individual's salt intake tends to obscure the true association between sodium intake and blood pressure in within-population studies. This is consistent with the poor correlation between 24-hour sodium excretion and salt content of food in weighed inventories that was discussed earlier in the chapter.

There thus seems to be a large body of evidence stretching back more than 40 years indicating that there is a causal link between increasing habitual salt intake and increasing blood pressure. The Scientific Advisory Committee on Nutrition's report on *Salt and Health* in 2003 concluded that the evidence for an association between salt intake and blood pressure had increased over the previous 10 years and that this effect was consistently found in a variety of different study populations and different ethnic groups (SACN, 2003).

Experimental studies

There have been several intervention trials aimed at reducing salt intake of a population as a means of reducing blood pressure and the incidence of hypertension. The results of trials conducted in Japan and Belgium are consistent with the belief that salt restriction will have beneficial effects on blood pressure but are less than conclusive (MacGregor and de Wardener, 1999). Forte et al. (1989) reported the effects of an intervention trial using two small, rural populations in Portugal. Over a 2-year period the intervention succeeded in reducing average salt intake by at least 25 per cent in the test village while that in the control village did not change. By the end of the study period the average systolic blood pressure in the test village had fallen by 13 mmHg relative to the control village.

Denton et al. (1995) conducted a 2-year controlled study of the effects of salt on the blood pressure of chimpanzees. Salt was added to the normal vegetable and fruit diet of the experimental group and over the first 18 months of the study blood pressure rose substantially in 10 of the 13 animals in the experimental group.

When the salt supplements were withdrawn, the blood pressure of these chimps returned to normal within 20 weeks.

Moderation of salt intake is widely promoted as a preventative measure but it has also long been used as a method of treating hypertension. Before the advent of the antihypertensive drugs, extreme salt restriction was one of the few treatments available for severe hypertension. The Kempner rice and fruit diet aimed to restrict salt intake to 1 gram daily. This diet was effective in some individuals but it was associated with very poor compliance, anorexia and side-effects that greatly limited its practical usefulness. These early therapeutic studies of patients with severe (malignant) hypertension generally suggested that, although extreme salt restriction was effective in some hypertensives, more moderate salt restriction (say 2.5+ g/day) was not effective. The advent of antihypertensive drugs heralded a general loss of interest in this method of treating severe hypertension. There is now, however, renewed interest in the use of moderate salt restriction as a therapy for those people with asymptomatic mild to moderate hypertension where the principal aim is to reduce the long-term risk of hypertension-linked diseases. Drug therapy is effective in reducing hypertension in such subjects, but lifelong consumption of drugs is clearly not an ideal solution and may be associated with a new range of hazards.

A large number of trials of the effectiveness of salt restriction in the treatment of hypertension have been conducted in recent decades; note, for example, the rigorous double-blind, random crossover study of MacGregor et al. (1982) discussed in Chapter 4. Law et al. (1991b) analysed the results of 78 controlled salt-reduction trials. They concluded that in those trials where salt restriction was for 5 weeks or more then the results obtained closely matched those that they had predicted from the cross-population analysis of Law et al. (1991a). Effects of salt restriction were less than predicted when shorter periods of salt restriction were used. They concluded that in 50- to 59 year olds in industrialized countries, a reduction in salt intake of 3 g/day could be expected to lead to an average reduction in systolic blood pressure of 5 mmHg with greater reductions in those who were hypertensive. They argued that such a level of salt reduction would, if universally adopted, lead to major reductions in stroke and heart disease mortality.

A systematic review of the long-term effects (at least 6 months) of intensive advice to reduce dietary salt consumption in normotensives, treated hypertensives and untreated hypertensives was conducted by Hooper et al. (2003). They found that there was a statistically significant but very small reduction in blood pressure when measured between 1 and 5 years after the start of the programme. There was a substantial reduction in the 24-hour sodium excretion, equivalent to a 2 g/day reduction in salt intake, but there was no correlation between the reduction in salt intake and the reduction in blood pressure. A low-salt diet did seem to help maintain lower blood pressure in some hypertensives when they stopped taking their antihypertension medication. They concluded that the type of intensive intervention in these trials was unsuitable for population prevention programmes or primary care, and yet they produced only minimal reductions in blood pressure. They did conclude that this type of intervention could be warranted in hypertensive subjects receiving antihypertensive drugs who might be able to reduce or stop their medication while still maintaining a lower blood pressure.

He and MacGregor (2004) conducted a meta-analysis of 31 controlled salt-reduction trials involving either normotensive subjects or subjects with elevated blood pressure. These trials recorded more than double the daily reduction in sodium excretion reported in the trials reviewed by Hooper et al. (2002) – equivalent to about 4.5 g reduction in daily salt intake. They found larger reductions in blood pressure than reported by Hooper et al., and they did find a significant correlation between the reduction in salt intake and the reduction in blood pressure.

Does reduced salt intake reduce morbidity and mortality?

Observational evidence, evidence from controlled animal experiments and from long-term clinical salt-reduction trials does support the salt–hypertension link and suggests that substantial reductions in population salt intake would reduce average blood pressure and reduce the incidence of hypertension. The weight of evidence also suggests that moderate reduction in dietary salt can help in the management of hypertension. However, there is still no substantial evidence that salt reduction in a clinical trial situation results in reduced morbidity from cardiovascular disease or reduced mortality.

In the meta-analysis of Hooper *et al.* (2002) discussed in the previous subsection, they were unable to evaluate whether there was any effect on mortality because there were only 17 deaths recorded in the trials they reviewed, and these were equally distributed between the control and intervention groups. More recently, Taylor *et al.* (2011) reviewed seven long-term, controlled salt-reduction trials that had used normotensive, hypertensive or mixed subjects. There were a total of 665 deaths recorded in these trials, but they found no evidence that salt reduction had any effect on total mortality or cardiovascular morbidity. In a subgroup with congestive heart failure, mortality was actually higher in the salt-restricted group.

In a recent highly publicized 8-year prospective cohort study of 3600 healthy, normotensive Belgians, Stolarz-Skrzypey *et al.* (2011) found that higher sodium excretion (i.e. higher salt intake) was associated with a higher systolic but not diastolic blood pressure. However, low salt intake was associated with a greater number of cardiovascular deaths; there were 50 deaths in the tertile with the lowest salt intake, 24 in the middle quartile but only 10 in those with highest salt intake. This observational association in just one trial with a fairly young and normotensive population should be viewed with extreme caution at this stage; association may not mean cause and effect.

Data from the Dietary Approaches to Stop Hypertension Trial (Appel *et al.*, 1997) showed that a diet rich in fruits, vegetables and low-fat dairy products, and reduced saturated and total fat coupled with a low-salt diet, was the most effective dietary strategy for reducing hypertension.

Other factors involved in the aetiology of hypertension

Much of the evidence implicating salt in the aetiology of hypertension could also be used to support the proposition that high potassium intake

is *protective* against hypertension. In acute studies of sodium loading in both salt-sensitive rats and in people, high potassium intake seems to ameliorate the effects of high sodium loads. Some correlation between Na:K ratio and blood pressure may be found in within-population studies where no relationship can be shown between blood pressure and sodium intake alone. SACN (2003) concluded that it is difficult to relate blood pressure to specific nutrients because of strong correlations between potassium, calcium, magnesium and fibre intakes. They did find that there was consistent evidence that increased intake of fruits and vegetables did have a positive effect in lowering blood pressure.

There is some epidemiological evidence that low calcium intake may be associated with increased risk of hypertension. People who suffer from osteoporosis also have higher incidence of hypertension, a finding consistent with a common aetiology. Some have used this latter observation to suggest that high salt may cause osteoporosis, while others have argued that low calcium intake might be a factor in hypertension. A recent meta-analysis by Beyer *et al.* (2006) found no evidence that supplements of any combination of potassium, magnesium or calcium had any effect on blood pressure in adults, but only three trials satisfied their inclusion criteria.

Overweight and obesity are generally agreed to lead to increases in blood pressure and weight loss reduces blood pressure in the overweight hypertensive. White *et al.* (1993) reported that blood pressure in English adults rose with increasing body mass index (BMI). Increased physical activity reduces the tendency to gain excessive weight and also contributes directly to a reduction in blood pressure. Excessive alcohol consumption also leads to a rise in blood pressure and increases the risk of stroke even in the absence of hypertension. White *et al.* (1993) found that blood pressure was positively associated with alcohol consumption in male drinkers, but they also found that non-drinkers had higher blood pressures than low and moderate drinkers. SACN (2003) reviewed evidence that had accumulated since 1994 and concluded:

• blood pressure rises with increasing adiposity, and weight reduction in hypertensive patients is associated with a reduction in blood pressure

- alcohol is an independent risk factor associated with hypertension
- increased physical activity and especially aerobic exercise has been associated with reductions in blood pressure.

Box 15.2 has a list of several of the factors associated with an increase in blood pressure and an increased risk of hypertension.

Box 15.2

Factors associated with increased risk of hypertension

- Being black; prevalence is higher among blacks in the USA and UK than in whites (there are almost certainly also large individual variations in susceptibility within races)
- Being overweight
- High alcohol consumption
- Sedentary lifestyle
- High population salt intake
- High dietary fat intake
- Low potassium or calcium intakes?

Conclusions on the hypertension link

An active lifestyle, moderate alcohol consumption and good control of body weight are undoubtedly factors that will lessen the risk of hypertension and the hypertension-linked diseases. Increased intake of fruits and vegetables will have a beneficial effect on blood pressure. Fruits and vegetables increase potassium intake and lower the Na:K ratio in the diet; processing of foods generally involves an increase in this ratio by some loss of K and addition of salt; this is one favoured mechanism by which fruits and vegetables may exert their effects on blood pressure.

There is compelling evidence of some causal link between dietary salt intake and hypertension. The argument tends to be about how significant and widespread the benefits of salt restriction would be. Would salt intake moderation lead to a general fall in average population blood pressure, or would effects be limited to a relatively small proportion of salt-sensitive people? Moderate salt restriction will almost certainly be of some value to some salt-sensitive people, and the general consensus is that it would have wider benefits. Salt restriction may also be useful in the treatment of mild-to-moderate hypertension either as an alternative to drug use or as an adjunctive therapy. Processed foods contain most of the salt in Western diets and so any substantial reduction in salt intake requires either less reliance on these high-salt foods or reduced use of salt by food manufacturers. It is difficult for populations to sustain a reduction in salt intake in the current environment because of the predominance of processed food as our main source of salt.

Key points

- Cross-population studies show that average blood pressure of adult populations is highly correlated to average salt intakes. This correlation remains strong even when developed and developing countries are analysed separately.
- When migration is accompanied by changes in salt intake, measured changes in blood pressure or stroke mortality are consistent with salt intake being a cause of hypertension.
- Falls in salt consumption over the last century have been associated with reductions in stroke mortality.
- Internationally, death rates from stroke and gastric cancer are highly correlated and this suggests a common aetiology. An international correlation between average salt intake and gastric cancer mortality has also been reported.
- In general, there is no correlation between salt intake and blood pressure in individuals from the same population. This is not unexpected because the usual measure of salt intake, 24-hour sodium excretion, is a poor measure of habitual salt intake and other dietary and lifestyle factors affect blood pressure.
- Limited evidence from population interventions is consistent with the salt–hypertension hypothesis.
- When salt was added to the fruit and vegetable diets of chimpanzees, their blood pressure rose →

relative to control animals and fell when the supplemental salt was withdrawn.

- Several clinical trials suggest that sustained moderate reductions in salt intake reduce the blood pressures of people with mild-to-moderate hypertension.

- Very severe salt restriction was the first partly effective therapy for severe hypertension, although it fell into disuse with the advent of effective antihypertensive drugs.

- Evidence from recent meta-analyses of long-term salt-reduction trials suggests that reductions in salt consumption of 4.5 g/day but not 2 g/day lead to useful reductions in blood pressure in normotensive and hypertensive people.

- Moderate salt reduction in hypertensive patients can maintain reductions in blood pressure when their medication is stopped.

- There is as yet no evidence that long-term moderate salt reduction leads to reduced mortality or reduced frequency of adverse cardiovascular events.

- One widely publicized cohort study found that mortality rose in healthy Belgian adults with decreasing measured salt consumption.

- Other factors associated with increased risk of hypertension are listed in Box 15.2, and attention to these will contribute to a reduction in hypertension prevalence.

- A diet high in fruits, vegetables and low-fat dairy products, coupled with lower fat, saturated fat and salt intakes, is the most effective dietary strategy for reducing hypertension.

- Substantial reductions in salt consumption towards the target of 6 g/day will almost certainly help to reduce average population blood pressure and thus the prevalence of hypertension.

PART FOUR

VARIATION IN NUTRITIONAL REQUIREMENTS AND PRIORITIES

16 Nutrition and the human lifecycle   435

17 Nutrition as treatment   484

18 Some other groups and situations   507

16

NUTRITION AND THE HUMAN LIFECYCLE

Introduction	435	Infancy	449
Nutritional aspects of pregnancy	437	Childhood and adolescence	462
Lactation	448	The elderly	469

INTRODUCTION

When I show my students Table 16.1 and ask for their comments, they almost invariably consider it a very bad diet because it is so far removed from the dietary guidelines for adults discussed in Chapter 5. Many of them doubt whether anyone could actually be eating such a diet because it is also very different from the average intakes recorded in dietary surveys and household budget surveys.

Table 16.1 An unbelievably bad diet?

	% energy
Fat	53
Saturated fat	23
Carbohydrate	39
Sugars	39
Starch	0
Protein	8
Fibre (g)	0

Table 16.1 in fact shows the approximate composition of mature human milk, the ideal food for babies. This extreme example illustrates the general point that nutritional needs and priorities are likely to change during the human lifecycle; in this case it shows that what is nutritionally ideal for newborns is far from ideal for fully grown adults. One would also, for example, expect the relative nutritional needs of an active rapidly growing

adolescent to be markedly different from those of an elderly housebound person, or even of a sedentary middle-aged person. Such differences mean that the dietary reference values (DRVs) vary with age, sex and reproductive status, and they also mean that there should be differences in the priority and nature of the general dietary guidelines offered for different lifecycle groups. This chapter focuses on their differing requirements and nutritional priorities.

Overt deficiency diseases are uncommon in industrialized countries but that is no guarantee that many people are not more subtly affected by suboptimal nutrition. Thus evidence is presented in Chapters 13–15 that many adults have intakes of essential vitamins and minerals that are considered inadequate or have biochemical indications of poor nutrient status even where average intakes of the nutrient are considered satisfactory; in a few cases even average intakes were less than ideal. Those people who are subject to particular nutritional stresses, such as pregnancy, lactation or rapid growth, are likely to be the most sensitive to any marginal deficiencies or suboptimal intakes of nutrients.

If essential nutrient requirements vary during the human lifecycle, this could suggest that certain groups, especially rapidly growing children, might need diets that are richer in essential nutrients (more nutrient-dense) than the general diet suitable for adults. Children have higher relative requirements for several essential nutrients (i.e. they need more per kilogram of body weight than adults), but on the same relative basis they also need more energy (i.e. need to eat more food). This is well illustrated in Chapter 11 where it is noted that young children not only require between 1.5 and 2 times as much protein per kilogram as adults, they also need to consume three times as many calories or three times as much food. This means that any diet with a sufficient concentration of protein to meet adult needs should also comfortably provide for the needs of growing children provided they eat enough to satisfy their energy needs. This principle applies more widely; even though the relative vitamin and mineral needs of a growing child may be higher than those of adults, this may be wholly or partly offset by the increased relative energy (food) requirement of the child.

Table 16.2 shows some selected *reference nutrient intakes* (RNIs) expressed as a percentage of the standard adult (19–50 years) value for the same sex, and it also shows the *estimated average requirements* (EARs) for energy expressed in the same way. Several age groups of children and other lifecycle groups have been selected to illustrate the general principle. The energy values in the table are a general indication of the relative food intakes of the various groups. For example, if the energy value is shown as 50 per cent then this suggests that this group should consume around 50 per cent of the energy of adults and a value of 125 per cent that they are expected to consume about 25 per cent more than the standard adult (19–50 years) of the same sex. Assuming that the same basic diet is consumed, this also means that those with a 50 per cent value in the energy box should also consume 50 per cent of the amount of nutrients consumed by adults of the same sex, and those with a 125 per cent value for energy should consume 25 per cent more nutrients than standard adults. This logic would indicate that only where the value for the nutrient RNI in Table 16.2 is significantly greater than that for the energy EAR will this group need a diet that is richer in this nutrient (more nutrient-dense) than that required by standard adults.

There are in fact relatively few examples in the table where the RNI percentage is significantly higher than the energy EAR; the adolescent requirement for calcium and several of the values for lactating women are examples where it is substantially higher. In most cases, though, diets that contain enough essential nutrients for standard adults will probably also be adequate for most other lifecycle groups. Often the increased relative requirement for energy in children wholly or partly cancels out any relative increase in nutrient needs. This principle justifies the traditional cultural practice of fully weaned children sharing in family meals with their parents and other adults; any 'real' extra needs can easily be met by drinking extra milk or additional nutritious snacks. This traditional family meal is now, of course, not always the norm as children often graze on self-selected foods or eat preprepared foods at times different from their parents; often these are high-energy low-nutrient foods like confectionary, cakes, biscuits, savoury snacks and sugary drinks.

Table 16.2 Selected reference nutrient intakes (RNIs) (estimated average requirements for energy) for various UK age groups, expressed as a percentage of the appropriate adult (19–50 years) value

	Pregnancy	Lactation	Girls 1–3 years	Girls 4–6 years	Girls 11–14 years	Boys 15–18 years	Men 75+ years
Energy	100*	127	60	80	95	108	82
Protein	113	124	32	44	92	99	96
Vitamin A	117	158	67	83	100	100	100
Riboflavin	127	145	55	73	100	100	100
Folic acid	Supplements	130	35	50	100	100	100
Vitamin C	125	175	75	75	88	100	100
Calcium	100	179	50	64	114	143	100
Iron	100	100	47	41	100	130	100

*1st two trimesters (110% last trimester)

NUTRITIONAL ASPECTS OF PREGNANCY

Pregnancy overview

Effects of malnutrition in pregnancy

Healthy well-fed women have the best chance of having healthy babies and of lactating successfully after the birth. This was graphically illustrated by studies of the effects of the Dutch Hunger Winter of 1944–5. In October 1944, the Nazi occupiers imposed a punitive embargo on food transport in Holland which led to widespread starvation especially in the urban areas and especially among the less affluent members of society. This famine was not relieved until Holland was liberated in May 1945. It is estimated that 40 000 pregnant women in Holland were subjected to a period of starvation during this winter and the effects of this are summarized below (Diamond, 1999).

- During the winter of 1944–5, the rates of conception fell to around a third of their normal level. Starvation and low body weight markedly reduce fertility in women (as well as in men).

- Women who were starved during the last trimester of their pregnancy, when most fetal growth occurs, had babies that were on average over 10 per cent lighter than those born before the famine (even before the famine food supplies were low).

- Babies born 3 months after the famine ended were of normal weight.

- However, babies exposed to famine in the first trimester of pregnancy had double the rate of stillbirth and were twice as likely to have a neural tube defect like spina bifida.

- Babies who were exposed to famine in the second and third trimesters had much higher mortality in the first few months of life and mortality rates did not normalize until they were a year old.

- The famine babies who survived into adulthood seemed to be of normal weight and intelligence.

- One interesting observation was that girls who were exposed to intrauterine starvation in the first and second trimesters had underweight babies when they became adults, despite being of normal birth weight themselves.

The scale of increased nutritional needs in pregnancy

One would expect pregnancy to be a time of significantly increased nutritional needs for the mother – the expression 'eating for two' has been widely used to sum up this expectation. As it is a time of physiological stress, the health and well-being of many pregnant women and their babies might be adversely affected by suboptimal nutrition despite the low frequency of overt malnutrition within the population. Morning sickness affects over half of women in the early part of pregnancy and this could compound with other stresses to deplete nutrient stores.

Cross-species comparisons show that human babies are much smaller than would be predicted from the size of the mother and that gestation is also longer than would be predicted. Thus the nutritional burden of pregnancy is likely to be less in women than in other, non-primate species. The small size and relatively slow postnatal growth of human babies mean that similar arguments apply to lactation. This difference in the relative burdens of pregnancy and lactation in different species is illustrated in Table 16.3. An extreme comparison is between a female

Table 16.3 Species variations in the relative burdens of pregnancy and lactation

Species	Maternal weight (kg)	Litter weight (% of maternal)	Gestation (days)	Days to double birth weight
Mouse	0.025	40	21	5
Rat	0.200	25	21	6
Guinea-pig	0.560	68	67	14
Rabbit	1.175	19	28	6
Cat	2.75	16	64	7
Woman	56	6	280	120–180

Data source: Webb (1992b).

mouse and a woman. The mouse produces a litter that represents around 40 per cent of her pre-pregnant weight in 21 days of gestation. She then provides enough nutrients in her milk to enable this litter to double its birth weight within 5 days. A woman produces a baby that represents 6 per cent of her body weight after 9 months of pregnancy and a breastfed baby might then take 4–6 months to double its birth weight. Extrapolating or predicting the extra nutritional needs of pregnant or lactating women from studies with small laboratory animals may be misleading and tend to greatly exaggerate the extra needs of these women.

Behavioural and physiological adaptations to pregnancy and the utilization of maternal nutrient stores also tend to minimize the extra nutritional needs of pregnant women. These extra nutritional needs may thus turn out to be small in comparison to the needs of non-pregnant women. 'Eating for two' implies a much greater increase in need than is indicated by measurements of the actual increase in intakes that occur in pregnant women and those indicated by current dietary reference values for pregnant women.

Reference nutrient intake and dietary allowance for pregnancy

Table 16.4 summarizes current UK and US recommendations on the extra nutritional needs of pregnant women. This table highlights some differences between the UK and US dietary standards, although these are not as great as noted in previous editions of this book. The American increments are often higher than those in the UK, examples being those for iron, zinc and niacin. As

noted in Chapter 3, baseline adult values also tend to be higher in the USA. This means that, for all nutrients, the absolute American RDA for pregnancy equals or exceeds the corresponding UK value. In the UK there is no RNI for non-pregnant women but an RNI of 10 μg/day for pregnant women, whereas in the USA there is an RDA of 15 μg/day for both pregnant and non-pregnant women.

Table 16.4 Daily extra increments for pregnancy (values in parentheses are percentages of the value for other women)*

Nutrient	UK RNI[1]	US RDA
Energy (kcal)	200 (10)[2]	340–450[3] (14–19)
(MJ)	0.8	1.43–1.90
Protein (g)	6 (13)	25 (50)[4]
Vitamin A (μg)	100 (17)	70 (10)
Vitamin D (μg)	10[5]	0 (0)
Thiamin (mg)	0.1 (13)[2]	0.3 (27)
Riboflavin (mg)	0.3 (27)	0.3 (27)
Niacin (mg)	0	4 (29)
Folic acid (μg)	(supplements)	200 (50)
Vitamin B$_{12}$ (μg)	0	0.2 (8)
Vitamin C (mg)	10 (25)	10 (13)
Calcium (mg)	0	0 (0)
Iron (mg)	0	9 (50)
Zinc (mg)	0	(38)

*Data sources: COMA (1991), NAS (2004).
[1] EAR for energy.
[2] Last trimester only.
[3] Last two trimesters.
[4] Last two trimesters only.
[5] No RNI for non-pregnant women.

As noted earlier when discussing Table 16.2, where the percentage increase in the requirement for a nutrient (compared to non-pregnant women) exceeds the percentage increase in the energy value, this implies the need for increased nutrient density or supplementation. In most cases the extra increments for vitamins suggested by the British standards are relatively modest and there are no increases for the minerals. Often the average intakes of relatively affluent British women will comfortably exceed the pregnancy RNI for many nutrients prior to pregnancy – and so, in practice, avoid the need for dietary change. For example, average intakes of vitamin C in British women are more than double the RNI and so the 10 per cent increase in the RNI during pregnancy looks small in relation to this. Average intakes of all vitamins in British women in 2000 were in excess of the RNI (Hoare *et al.*, 2004), although average vitamin A intakes of younger women were only 80 per cent of the RNI. (Note that even where the RNI is apparently satisfactory there may still be substantial numbers of women, particularly young ones, with frankly unsatisfactory intakes.)

Some values, such as the American RDA for iron and the British and American RNI/RDA for vitamin D, require the use of supplements to be realistically achievable without adequate sunlight exposure. Many well-nourished women take supplements during pregnancy, the assumption being that even if they do no good then neither will they do any harm. Apart from folic acid, which is briefly discussed later in this chapter and more fully discussed in Chapter 14, there is little evidence that such supplements do any good when taken by well-nourished women in affluent countries. On the contrary, there is clear evidence that high levels of retinol are teratogenic and that concentrated protein supplements reduce birth weight. There is also some evidence that routine iron supplements can increase the risk of low birth weight and prematurity when given to women who do not need them. Fetal malformations in zinc-deficient animals are also more frequent when calcium supplements are given than when both minerals are deficient, which suggests that supplements of one nutrient can adversely affect the absorption and metabolism of others (these studies are reviewed by Mathews, 1996). A controlled trial of large supplements of anti-oxidant vitamin supplements in women at high risk of pre-eclampsia found that they did not reduce pre-eclampsia but may have reduced birth weight, and the onset of pre-eclampsia was slightly earlier in the supplemented group; if these supplements had any effect at all they were negative (Poston *et al.*, 2006)

Pregnancy outcomes

There is a strong association between infant mortality rate and birth weight. Newborns who weigh less than 2.5 kg are classified as low-birth-weight (LBW) babies and they have higher mortality and morbidity rates. Thus, birth weight of babies is a useful, quantitative measure of pregnancy outcome. Anything that restricts fetal growth is liable to be detrimental to the chances of the baby's survival and subsequent well-being. Many of the risk factors for having a LBW baby are listed in Box 16.1. When birth weight is plotted against mortality then there is a U-shaped curve. As babies get heavier then initially mortality risk drops until an optimum birth weight is reached which is slightly higher than average birth weight of around 3.5 kg. As birth weight rises above this optimum so mortality risk starts to increase again (Symonds and Clarke, 1996). Many LBW babies are born prematurely and gestational diabetes can be a cause of high birth weight.

Box 16.1

Risk factors for having a baby with low birth weight

- Low social class of the mother
- Mother under age 18 years or over 35 years
- Previous delivery of a low-birth-weight baby
- Maternal drug or alcohol abuse
- Cigarette smoking
- Mother underweight at the time of conception
- Low weight gain in pregnancy
- Dieting or restricted energy intake during pregnancy
- Poor quality of diet during pregnancy
- Excessive exercise or work during pregnancy

The ideal outcome to pregnancy is not only a healthy baby but also a healthy mother who is nutritionally well prepared to lactate. The preparedness of the mother to begin lactation and the general well-being of the mother after parturition are not as readily quantifiable as birth weight but can be important determinants of successful reproduction. In poorer countries the presence or absence of a healthy lactating mother may be a key determinant of the baby's chance of survival.

Maternal weight gain during pregnancy may be one quantifiable measure of the mother's preparedness for lactation. In rats, there is a 50 per cent increase in maternal fat storage during pregnancy and this fat is rapidly depleted during the subsequent lactation. The fat store is a physiological adaptation to enable the female rat to provide enough milk for her large and rapidly growing litter. The increases in maternal fat typically seen in human pregnancy can also be assumed to be physiological. In women in industrialized countries, who have access to an essentially unlimited food supply, this store of energy for lactation may not be critical. It may be much more important to women who are subsisting on a marginal diet and who may have limited opportunity to boost intake to meet the extra needs of lactation.

Estimating the extra nutritional needs of pregnancy

For those nutrients that accumulate during pregnancy, either in the mother's stores or in the products of conception, it is possible to use factorial calculations (see Chapter 3) to predict the likely extra requirements for these nutrients during pregnancy. However, it should be remembered that these are only theoretical predictions and while they may provide a useful basis for discussion, they may not truly indicate extra dietary needs because of behavioural and physiological adaptations to pregnancy.

There has, over the years, been considerable discussion about how any extra nutritional requirements of pregnant women are distributed throughout the pregnancy. At the end of the first trimester the fetus weighs around 5 grams, and around 500 grams at the end of the second trimester. This compares with an average birth weight of 3.5 kg. Thus fetal growth accelerates throughout the gestation, with most of the fetal weight gain concentrated in the final trimester.

Should any extra nutritional allowances be concentrated in the last trimester when fetal growth rate is highest? Several adaptive mechanisms ensure that the burden is distributed more evenly throughout the pregnancy. In the first dietary standards published in 1943, the increases in RDAs in pregnancy were generally higher than current US values, but the increases in 1943 were all confined to the second half of pregnancy whereas most current increases are for the whole of the pregnancy.

Before conception

Maybe as few as 50 per cent of pregnancies are planned, but women who are planning to become pregnant can take steps to improve the chance of a successful outcome. Obesity at the time of conception is a significant risk factor for *pre-eclampsia* or pregnancy-induced hypertension and is linked to increased risk of a number of fetal abnormalities. Ideally, women intending to become pregnant should try to ensure that their body mass index (BMI) is within the range 20–25 kg/m^2 prior to conception. Women seeking pre-conception advice can be counselled to normalize their weight. Menstruation ceases and fertility is reduced in women who are underweight, so only 10 per cent of women with a BMI of less than 18 kg/m^2 are fertile. Underweight women who do manage to conceive have an increased risk of having a baby with low birth weight; in general, the risk decreases with increasing pre-conceptual BMI of the mother. Some other steps that should be taken if a pregnancy is planned are listed below.

- Folic acid supplements should be taken prior to conception (discussed later in this chapter and in more depth in Chapter 14).
- Vegan women should take vitamin B$_{12}$ supplements.
- Iron status should be checked and if necessary any anaemia treated.
- Alcohol intake should be minimized or preferably eliminated.
- A nutrient-rich diet should be selected.
- Extra care should be taken in the management of conditions such as diabetes and phenylketonuria (PKU) because poor management of these can have adverse effects on the fetus.

Key points

- Malnutrition reduces fertility and the chances of conception.
- Malnutrition in late pregnancy reduces birth weight and increases infant mortality.
- Malnutrition in early pregnancy increases stillbirths, fetal abnormalities and infant mortality even though birth weight is normal.
- Girls born to mothers malnourished in early pregnancy have smaller babies when they themselves become mothers.
- The extra nutritional needs of pregnant women are modest and much less than the expression 'eating for two' implies.
- Behavioural changes, physiological adaptations and utilization of maternal reserves all tend to minimize extra requirements in pregnancy and the impact of suboptimal intakes on the fetus.
- The nutritional burden of human pregnancy is much less than that in non-primate species.
- American allowances for pregnancy tend to be higher than those in the UK.
- Large increases in nutrient intakes may be difficult to achieve if there is only minimal increase in total food intake in pregnancy. They may only be realistic if supplements are used.
- For several nutrients, the average habitual intakes of non-pregnant women exceed the UK RNI for pregnant women.
- Apart from folic acid, there is little evidence that nutrient supplements are beneficial in pregnancy unless a woman is undernourished.
- Overdoses of some nutrients, especially retinol, are harmful during pregnancy.
- Low-birth-weight babies (under 2.5 kg) have higher postnatal mortality and morbidity, and some of the risk factors are listed in Box 16.1.
- Too high a birth weight increases obstetric complications and also increases mortality risk.
- A successful pregnancy should produce a healthy normal-weight baby and a healthy mother who is well prepared for lactation.
- Several mechanisms may serve to distribute the nutritional burden of pregnancy more evenly than the concentration of fetal growth in the last trimester might imply.

→

Key points *continued*

- Obesity at conception is associated with higher risk of pre-eclampsia and fetal abnormalities.
- Women who are underweight are less likely to conceive, have a higher risk of miscarriage, and are at higher risk of having a low-birth-weight baby if they do go to term.
- Women planning a pregnancy should be encouraged to normalize their body weight, take folic acid supplements and generally to make sure that they enter pregnancy with good nutritional status.

Energy aspects of pregnancy

A typical British woman gains around 12.5 kg in weight during a typical pregnancy. This weight gain is made up of around 3.5–4 kg of extra maternal fat and around 6 kg as the increased weight of the uterus and contents; the remainder is due to increased body fluids. The total theoretical energy cost of this weight gain, i.e. the increase in basal metabolic rate (BMR) and the energy costs of moving a heavier body in a typical pregnancy, has been estimated at 70–80 000 kcal (c300 MJ). In undernourished women in developing countries, total weight gain during pregnancy may be only half of this value, with no net increase in maternal fat stores. Immediately prior to the Dutch Hunger Winter discussed earlier (see p. 437), average intakes of pregnant women in Holland were estimated at around 1500 kcal/day (6.3 MJ/day). These women maintained the average birth weights of their babies during this period but lost weight themselves.

The theoretical energy cost of the average British pregnancy with 3.5 kg of maternal fat gain works out at just under 300 kcal (1.3 MJ) per day. If this theoretical energy cost is distributed throughout the pregnancy in proportion to the rate of fetal growth, this would amount to an extra energy cost of over 750 kcal/day (3.1 MJ/day) in the last trimester. Most of the gain in maternal fat occurs in the middle of the pregnancy and this fat store represents not only a reserve for lactation but also a potential reserve for the last trimester if intake is inadequate during this period of rapid fetal growth.

The current UK estimated average requirement (EAR) for pregnant women is only 200 kcal (0.8 MJ) above that for non-pregnant women and is for the last trimester only (see Table 16.4). The UK panel on dietary reference values (COMA, 1991) did suggest that women who are underweight at the start of pregnancy or who remain active during the pregnancy may need more than suggested by this EAR. According to COMA, several studies have suggested that pregnant women in the UK tend to eat more than non-pregnant women only in the last few weeks of pregnancy and then less than 100 kcal/day (0.4 MJ/day). These and similar findings in other industrialized countries suggest that the spontaneous increases in energy intake during pregnancy are very small in previously well-nourished women. As energy balance is physiologically regulated this strongly implies that the extra energy needs of pregnant women are also very small. Clearly, many women in industrialized countries markedly reduce their activity levels during pregnancy and so save much of the anticipated energy costs of the pregnancy. Studies on marginally nourished pregnant women, using the doubly labelled water method of measuring long-term energy expenditure, further suggest that physiological energy-sparing mechanisms operate during pregnancy (Prentice, 1989). Lack of maternal fat storage during pregnancy and energy-sparing physiological mechanisms may all but eliminate any theoretical energy costs of pregnancy in developing countries.

In the 1989 version of its recommended dietary allowances, the US panel recommended an extra energy increment for pregnancy of 300 kcal/day (1.25 MJ/day) for the second and third trimesters only. These figures have since been revised by the Institute of Medicine who recommended an increase of 340 kcal/day (1.43 MJ) for the second trimester rising to an extra 452 kcal/day (1.9 MJ) in the third trimester. These new values have been set by using estimates of the rate of energy deposition during pregnancy plus an estimate for the increase in total energy expenditure of 8 kcal/day for every week of gestation that was obtained using the doubly labelled water method.

The best practical guide to the adequacy of energy intake during pregnancy is the maternal weight gain. The US National Academy of Sciences has published guideline values for recommended weight gain that depend on the pre-pregnant weight:

- underweight at conception – 12.5–18 kg gain
- normal weight – 11.5–16 kg gain
- overweight – 7–11.5 kg gain
- obese – at least 6 kg gain.

Any reduced energy supply to the fetus during pregnancy is likely to restrict fetal growth and thus increase the risk of a low birth weight. There is strong evidence linking maternal weight gain during pregnancy with birth weight of the baby. Low weight gain is associated with increased risk of low birth weight and perinatal mortality. Excessive weight gain is associated with prolonged labour, birth injury, higher rates of death and complications in the neonatal period and increased risk of maternal obesity. In a survey of 10 000 births in the USA (summarized in Morgan, 1988), the chance of having a low-birth-weight baby was inversely related to maternal weight gain in pregnancy:

- 15 per cent of women who gained less than 7 kg had LBW babies
- 8 per cent with 7–12 kg weight gain
- 4 per cent with 12–16 kg weight gain
- 3 per cent with more than 16 kg weight gain.

Restricting maternal weight gain by dieting during pregnancy may increase the risk of having a low-birth-weight baby. In animal studies, even food restriction of obese mothers during pregnancy reduced fetal weight. This suggests the need for extreme caution in the use of an energy-restricted diet even if a woman is overweight at the start of her pregnancy. Weight reduction should not be attempted during pregnancy but diet should be moderated to achieve a desirable level of weight gain.

Glucose that has been transferred from maternal blood in the placenta is the primary energy source of the fetus. The concentration of glucose in the fetal blood is always lower than that in the maternal blood, so transfer of glucose is by facilitated diffusion down a concentration gradient. Therefore, if the maternal blood glucose concentration is low, this can limit the availability of glucose to the fetus. Active transfer of nutrients from maternal blood makes it less likely that supplies of other nutrients, like amino acids, to the fetus will be restricted. Starvation or heavy exercise during pregnancy may restrict fetal growth by reducing glucose concentration in the placental blood. Fetal nutrient supply depends not only on nutrient concentration in maternal blood but also on placental blood flow; therefore anything that reduces placental blood flow may also restrict fetal growth and nutrient supply. One effect of smoking may be to reduce placental blood flow and thus retard the supply of nutrients to the fetus. Purely anatomical factors, such as the precise site of implantation and development of the placenta, may affect fetal blood flow and may account for some unexplained incidence of LBW babies. Uncontrolled gestational diabetes can increase the supply of glucose to the fetus and cause babies to be born too heavy.

Poverty is associated with low birth weight. Average weights of babies born in developing countries are lower than in industrialized countries and the proportion of LBW babies is also much higher in many developing countries. These differences are not removed by correcting for differences in maternal stature. Even in industrialized countries, social class and economic status affect birth weight. Leon (1991) found a progressive increase in the percentage of LBW babies and increased postnatal mortality with decrease in the socioeconomic status of the mother. Evidence from a number of studies indicates that nutritional factors are a likely explanation for some of these differences. Women from a poor community in the UK who had a LBW baby had lower average energy intakes than those who had babies of ideal weight. During the Dutch Hunger Winter at the end of the Second World War, the average birth weight of babies was reduced by over 300 g. Studies in Guatemala have shown that women who were marginally nourished, with typical unsupplemented intakes of 1600 kcal/day (6.7 MJ/day), had significantly heavier babies and fewer LBW babies when they were given food supplements prior to conception and throughout the pregnancy. A similar study in Taiwan, with women whose unsupplemented intake was higher, typically 2000 kcal/day (8.4 MJ/day), showed no significant effect on average birth weight (both studies reviewed in Naismith, 1980). This is backed up by what was noted earlier about the Dutch Hunger Winter – that when calorie intake was restricted to around 1500 kcal/day prior to the food

blockade, fetal weight was maintained at the expense of maternal weight, but when maternal food intake dropped further in the last trimester then birth weight dropped. In the Gambia there are significant differences in average birth weight between the hungry season and the harvest season. This difference can be eliminated by the use of energy-protein supplements and the perinatal mortality is also reduced.

Dietary intervention studies generally suggest that, at very low baseline levels of intake, energy supplements do favourably affect birth weight and reduce incidence of LBW babies. However, this favourable effect on birth weight is not seen at slightly higher baseline levels despite the use of very substantial supplements. A lack of measurable effect of supplements on birth weight in the less undernourished women does not necessarily mean that supplementation had no beneficial effects because the supplements may have increased maternal fat stores and made mothers better prepared to lactate. In a review of such intervention trials, Morgan (1988) concluded that the supplements probably had a beneficial effect despite their disappointing effect on birth weight, because of increased maternal weight gain and improved lactation.

Key points

- British women gain an average 12.5 kg in pregnancy and this represents a theoretical energy cost of 70–80 000 kcal (300 MJ) or 300 kcal (1.3 MJ) per day.
- In the UK, the energy standard is increased by 200 kcal (0.8 MJ) per day but only for the last trimester.
- In the USA, the energy standard increases by 340 kcal/day (1.43 MJ) in the second trimester and by 452 kcal/day (1.9 MJ) in the third trimester.
- Estimates of energy expenditure in pregnancy by the doubly labelled water method suggest that it increases by an average of 8 kcal/day for each week of gestation.
- Spontaneous increases in food intake by well-nourished women may rise by only 100 kcal (0.4 MJ) per day in the last few weeks of pregnancy.   →

- Reduced activity and perhaps energy-sparing physiological changes may account for the difference between the theoretical energy costs of pregnancy and the low apparent increases in intake.

- In undernourished women, lack of maternal fat gain and energy-sparing mechanisms may eliminate even the theoretical energy cost of pregnancy.

- Low weight gain during pregnancy and being underweight at conception both reduce birth weights.

- Attempts at weight reduction should be avoided during pregnancy unless medically advised and supervised.

- Being overweight at conception increases the risk of pre-eclampsia.

- Being underweight reduces fertility, increases the risk of miscarriage and increases the risk of a LBW baby in women who do go to term.

- Glucose transfer across the placenta is passive and fetal blood glucose concentration is lower than maternal. Low maternal blood glucose or low fetal blood flow will restrict glucose supply to the fetus and so limit its growth.

- Poverty and low social class are both associated with reduced birth size and increased postnatal mortality of babies.

- Malnourished women have smaller babies, more LBW babies and higher postnatal mortality.

- Energy supplements increase birth weight and reduce LBW in women with very low baseline intakes.

- In marginally undernourished women, supplements do not usually have a measurable effect on birth weight but they probably increase maternal weight gain and fitness to lactate.

Protein in pregnancy

The current UK RNI for protein is increased by 6 g/day throughout pregnancy. The American RDA is increased by 25 g/day which is a 50 per cent increase and represents a considerable increase on the 1989 RDA of an extra 10 g/day. If the UK RNI is expressed as a percentage of the EAR for energy, then in the first two trimesters (when the energy EAR is unaltered) it represents a rise from 9.3 to 10.7 per cent of energy as protein. Average adult intakes of protein in the UK are 1.5 times the RNI and protein represents around 17.5 per cent of total energy intake, so protein seems unlikely to be a limiting nutrient for pregnant women in the UK – or indeed in other industrialized countries where low protein intake is likely to occur only as a secondary consequence of low total food intake. In dietary intervention studies, protein-rich supplements appeared to offer no additional benefits over and above their energy value. Even in marginally nourished women, it is energy rather than protein that seems to be the limiting factor. Amino acids are actively transported across the placenta, so adequate levels can be maintained in the fetal blood even when levels in the maternal blood are low. Some studies even suggest that concentrated protein supplements may depress birth weight (Mathews, 1996).

Factorial calculations suggest a total 'protein cost' of about 925 grams for a typical pregnancy. Theoretical calculations of protein accretion rates during the four quarters of pregnancy suggest rates of 0.6, 1.8, 4.8 and 6.1 g/day, respectively (NRC, 1989a). Naismith (1980) provided direct evidence that, in the rat, extra protein is laid down in maternal muscle in early pregnancy and that this is released in late pregnancy when the demands from the growing fetuses are highest. He argued that some observations in women are consistent with these observations in the rat and may serve to distribute the extra protein need more evenly throughout the pregnancy. Measurements of nitrogen balance in pregnant women show that a small and fairly constant positive balance occurs throughout the pregnancy. Excretion of the amino acid 3-methyl histidine is taken as an indicator of muscle protein breakdown and it increases in the second half of human pregnancy.

Habitual consumption of protein in industrialized countries is almost always in excess of requirements and thus, in practice, it is unlikely that protein supply will be limiting during pregnancy. Pregnant women do not usually need to take specific steps to increase their protein intake despite their increased

RNI/RDA. Even in developing countries, energy is more likely than protein to be the limiting factor in pregnancy.

Minerals in pregnancy

The current RNIs for minerals in the UK indicate no routine extra increment for any mineral in pregnancy. High priority has historically been given to increased mineral intakes during pregnancy, and in the USA the RDAs for most minerals are increased during pregnancy (see examples in Table 16.4). The major exception is calcium where, although there is no increase in RDA for pregnancy, the RDA of 1000 mg/day for adult women is 43 per cent higher than the UK RNI of 700 mg/day which also applies to both pregnant and non-pregnant women. Data discussed in Chapter 13 suggest that the average mineral intakes of British women were below the RNI in several cases and that the mineral intakes of many British women were unsatisfactory. Some examples from Chapter 13 are listed here:

- 25 per cent of women and 42 per cent of younger women had unsatisfactory iron intakes; 11 per cent showed biochemical evidence of iron depletion and 8 per cent were anaemic

- 5 per cent of women and 8 per cent of younger women had unsatisfactory intakes of calcium
- for all of the minerals, substantial numbers of women recorded unsatisfactory intakes with higher rates in the youngest age group.

As the American RDAs for pregnancy are all higher than the corresponding British values (often substantially so), this must mean that many women in both the UK and the USA have mineral intakes that are well below those considered desirable by the American Institute of Medicine.

Calcium

Around 30 grams of calcium accumulate in the fetal skeleton during pregnancy. This represents just over 100 mg/day when spread throughout the gestation. If one assumes that only a fraction of ingested calcium is retained (say 25–35 per cent), this factorial approach suggests an increase of around 400 mg in the RDA for calcium in pregnancy; this is actually what was recommended in the 1989 version of the American RDA (although the value for non-pregnant women was lower than current values). The 'calcium cost' of pregnancy represents only about 2–3 per cent of the calcium in the maternal skeleton, and there is clear evidence that the efficiency of calcium absorption in the gut increases during pregnancy. The UK panel on DRVs has concluded that, in most women, the extra calcium cost of the pregnancy can be met by utilization of maternal stores and by improved efficiency of absorption (COMA, 1991). In certain cases (e.g. adolescent pregnancy), it suggests that some extra increment of calcium might be advisable, and in the USA the RDA for adolescent girls (14–18 years) is 1300 mg/day whether they are pregnant or not.

Iron

During pregnancy the plasma volume increases by around 1.5 litres and the red cell mass by 200–250 mL. This means that during a normal pregnancy the large increase in plasma volume causes a fall in haematocrit and blood haemoglobin concentration, despite an increase in the number of circulating red cells and the amount of circulating haemoglobin. This physiological fall in haemoglobin concentration in pregnancy was historically interpreted as iron-deficiency anaemia and iron supplements have traditionally been given to pregnant women. The American RDAs clearly suggest that universal iron supplementation in pregnancy should continue. Iron supplements often cause adverse gastro-intestinal symptoms and it is likely that many of them are not actually taken.

The net iron cost of pregnancy, allowing for the savings due to cessation of menstruation, has been estimated at between 500 and 1000 mg, which represents 2–4 mg/day throughout the pregnancy (Sadler in 1994 suggested a figure of 680 mg). The UK panel on DRVs suggested that, in most women, the iron requirements for pregnancy can be met by the following adaptations:

• utilization of maternal iron stores
• a considerable increase in the efficiency of iron absorption during pregnancy – the intestinal absorption of iron may rise from a normal 10 per cent to over 50 per cent in the last trimester
• the cessation of menstruation.

In the UK there is considered to be no need for routine iron supplementation during pregnancy, although targeted supplementation (e.g. to women whose iron status is poor when they enter pregnancy) may be necessary. The need for, and benefits of, iron supplements in pregnancy are still a matter of scientific debate. The American and UK panels have thus come up with very different practical 'recommendations' using essentially the same body of factual knowledge.

Mathews (1996) drew the following conclusions from a review of the literature.

• Iron-deficiency anaemia is associated with increased risk of low birth weight and prematurity.
• High haemoglobin and haematocrit levels are associated with similar increased risks, although this may not be a simple cause-and-effect relationship.
• Randomized controlled trials have shown no benefit for routine (i.e. to all women) iron supplements in pregnancy.

Screening and targeted supplementation are feasible options for industrialized countries. In developing countries where iron-deficiency anaemia is very prevalent and often severe, routine supplementation may be the only practical option.

> ### Key points
>
> • In the UK, no routine increases in mineral RNI are considered necessary during pregnancy, although they may be necessary for some individuals or groups.
> • It must be borne in mind, however, that evidence discussed in Chapter 13 suggests that many women, especially younger ones, have intakes of minerals that are below the lower reference nutrient intake (LRNI).
> • In the USA, there are substantial increases in many mineral RDA during pregnancy. In all cases the American RDA is higher, often substantially higher, than the UK RNI.
> • In the UK, it is assumed that the mineral costs of pregnancy can be met by physiological adaptation, increased efficiency of absorption, and utilization of maternal mineral reserves.

Folic acid, folate and neural tube defects

For this edition of the book, the bulk of the discussion of this topic has been moved to Chapter 14 because it has implications for people other than pregnant women. In over 50 countries, flour or other food is now fortified with folic acid and so everyone in the population is exposed to this 'artificial' form of folate. There has been longstanding advice from several expert groups that UK flour should also be fortified, although at the time of writing in 2012 this has not been implemented. Nevertheless, the recommendation first made in 1992 that all women planning to become pregnant should take supplements of folic acid has been widened to advice that all sexually active fertile women should take these supplements (400 μg/day for most women).

There is clear evidence that, under clinical trial conditions, folic acid supplements greatly reduce the incidence of *neural tube defects*. Advice aimed at encouraging women to take supplements prior to becoming pregnant has been given since 1992, but this advice has generally not been effective in reducing the incidence of neural tube defects in countries where it has been used. Food fortification, in contrast, has had an immediate effect in reducing the incidence of these birth defects in countries where it has been implemented, including the USA, Canada and Chile.

Fortification is thus clearly effective in preventing many neural tube defects and probably other congenital defects, but several hundred thousand people are exposed to the extra folic acid for every affected pregnancy prevented. The safety and efficacy of folic acid in preventing birth defects, and the possible wider benefits of folic acid fortification, are discussed at length in Chapter 14.

Other vitamins in pregnancy

The increases in vitamin RNIs and RDAs in the UK and the USA have been summarized in Table 16.4.

The table shows that the UK RNI for vitamin A is increased by 100 μg in pregnancy. The extra increment in the USA is only 70 μg, but the baseline value for American women is the same as that for pregnancy in the UK, at 700 μg. The average intake of vitamin A of younger British women in 2000 was well below the RNI, and 9 per cent of women had unsatisfactory intakes rising to 19 per cent in the younger women (see Chapter 13). This suggests that many women take in less vitamin A than is considered desirable during pregnancy. It is, however, the possible consequences of excessive doses of retinol in pregnancy rather than potential inadequacy that is the current focus of concern about vitamin A in pregnancy in the UK. Very high intakes of retinol during pregnancy are *teratogenic*, so they increase the risk of birth defects. Women in the UK are currently advised *not* to take supplements containing vitamin A during pregnancy, and are advised also to avoid eating liver or products containing liver (e.g. pâté) because of the high levels of retinol in animal livers (COMA, 1991). American women are advised not to take supplements that contain more than the RDA of any vitamin (except folic acid).

It was assumed by the UK panel on dietary reference values that most of the adult population obtain their vitamin D principally from endogenous production in the skin via the action of sunlight on 7-dehydrocholesterol, so there is no published RNI for these groups. Pregnant women are one of the groups where the panel felt that endogenous production could not be relied on and therefore an RNI was given (see Table 16.4). This RNI for vitamin D is over three times average UK intakes, so supplements are necessary to achieve it; in the USA

the same higher RDA of 15 μg/day is given for all women whether pregnant or not.

Increases in the RNIs and RDAs for most other vitamins and average intakes of most of these vitamins in British women are well in excess of even the raised RNI for pregnancy, even though relatively large numbers of individual women may have unsatisfactory intakes or biochemical evidence of poor status; see Chapter 13 for details.

Vitamin B_{12} interacts with folic acid in methyl transfer reactions and poor vitamin B_{12} status is a risk factor for a neural tube defect. The RNI remains unaltered in pregnancy and the American RDA rises only very slightly. For omnivorous women, and even for lacto-vegetarians, there is probably little need to consider B_{12}; however, vegan women will not have a natural dietary source of this vitamin and so should take supplements or fortified foods to ensure their adequacy, because only newly absorbed vitamin B_{12} is readily transported across the placenta.

Key points

- There is some increase in the dietary standards for several vitamins during pregnancy – see Table 16.4.
- Retinol is teratogenic, so pregnant women should avoid concentrated retinol supplements and in the UK are advised to avoid all liver, liver products, cod liver oil and any vitamin supplements that contain retinol unless advised otherwise by their physician.
- The RNI for vitamin D in pregnancy can only realistically be achieved by taking supplements, although for other adults it is assumed that they can manufacture enough if adequately exposed to sunlight.
- Vegan women should take supplements of vitamin B_{12} or eat foods fortified with this vitamin.

Alcohol and pregnancy

Fetal alcohol syndrome (FAS) is a recognizable clinical entity that is caused by heavy drinking during pregnancy. Babies with this syndrome have the following characteristics:

- they are small
- they have characteristic facial abnormalities
- they are often mentally retarded
- they are immunodeficient
- they show slow postnatal growth.

This syndrome starts to occur with habitual alcohol intakes in excess of 50 g/day (four glasses of wine) and the frequency increases as alcohol intake rises. The alcohol probably exerts a direct toxic effect on the fetus and may also increase the risk of oxygen or glucose deficit to the fetus.

Moderate amounts of alcohol in pregnancy (habitual intakes of 10–50 g/day) may increase the risk of low birth weight. It may be prudent to advise women to limit their alcohol consumption during pregnancy to the occasional small amount, while the Royal College of Obstetricians and Gynaecologists advises that they should avoid alcohol altogether. Alcohol binges should be avoided during pregnancy.

Heavy drinking prior to conception not only reduces fertility but also affects fetal growth even if drinking stops after conception. The fetus is also most vulnerable to the harmful effects of alcohol in the early stages of pregnancy. Taken together, such observations suggest that moderation of alcohol consumption should ideally begin prior to conception.

Key points

- Heavy drinking during pregnancy has serious adverse effects on the fetus. This is fetal alcohol syndrome.
- The effects of moderate and low alcohol intakes during pregnancy are less clear. Ideally, women should avoid alcohol during pregnancy *and* when planning to become pregnant.

LACTATION

Lactation is nutritionally far more demanding for the mother than pregnancy. A woman will daily be producing up to 800 mL of milk containing as much as 9 g of protein and 700 kcal (2.9 MJ) of energy, as well as all the other nutrients necessary to sustain the growing infant. The extra increments for lactation in the US and UK dietary standards are summarized in Table 16.5.

Table 16.5 Extra increments for selected nutrients for lactation in the UK and USA dietary standards (values in parentheses are percentages of the value for other women)*

Nutrient	UK RNI[1]	US RDA
Energy (kcal)	520 (27)[2]	330 (14)
(MJ)	2.18	1.38
Protein (g)	11 (24)	25 (54)
Vitamin A (µg)	350 (58)	500 (63)
Vitamin D (µg)	10[3]	0
Thiamin (mg)	0.2 (25)	0.3 (27)
Riboflavin (mg)	0.5 (45)	0.5 (45)
Niacin (mg)	2 (15)	3 (21)
Folate (µg)	60 (30)	100 (25)
Vitamin C (mg)	30 (75)	45 (60)
Calcium (mg)	550 (79)	0
Iron (mg)	0	0
Zinc (mg)	6 (86)	4 (50)

*Data sources: COMA (1991), NAS (2004).
[1] EAR for energy.
[2] Average for first 3 months.
[3] No RNI for non-pregnant/lactating women.

The amounts by which the British EARs for energy exceed those of other women during the first 3 months of lactation are:

- month 1–450 kcal/day (1.9 MJ)
- month 2–530 kcal/day (2.2 MJ)
- month 3–570 kcal/day (2.4 MJ).

After that, the EAR depends on whether the breastfeeding is the primary source of nourishment for the baby or whether the baby is receiving substantial amounts of supplementary feeds. The American RDA for lactating women is increased by a set 500 kcal/day (2.1 MJ).

The UK EARs have been estimated by measuring the energy content of milk production and assuming an efficiency of 80 per cent for the conversion of food energy to milk energy. The contribution from the maternal fat stores laid down during pregnancy has been taken as 120 kcal/day (0.5 MJ). These increases in the EARs for energy during lactation are said by COMA (1991) to closely match the extra intakes observed in lactating women in affluent societies.

The RNI for protein is increased by 11 g/day throughout lactation of up to 6 months' duration. When this is expressed as a proportion of the EAR for energy, it does not rise significantly above that for other women (i.e. 9.3 per cent of energy). As in pregnancy, it seems unlikely that protein will be a limiting nutrient in lactation because habitual intakes are usually well in excess of this.

The RNIs for eight vitamins and six minerals are also increased during lactation, reflecting the panel's judgement of the extra needs of women at various stages. Some of these increases are substantial proportions of the standard RNIs for adult women, and the increases in the American RDAs are generally even bigger (see Table 16.5).

Moderate weight loss of around 0.5 kg per week does not affect milk output, and changes in the proportions of fat, carbohydrate and protein in the maternal diet do not affect milk composition. The fatty acid profile of milk is affected by the fatty acid profile of the maternal diet. The concentrations of the major minerals in milk are not affected by maternal intake; maternal stores are depleted if intake is inadequate. Maternal intake and the size of maternal stores affect milk content of selenium, iodine and the vitamins. During periods of low maternal intake, milk vitamin content is initially maintained at the expense of maternal stores.

Key points

- Lactation is nutritionally demanding and this is reflected in substantial increases in the dietary standards for energy and many nutrients (detailed in Table 16.5).
- Successful lactation is compatible with moderate weight loss.
- The macronutrient and major mineral content of the maternal diet has little effect on milk composition.
- The fatty acid profile of milk reflects that of the maternal diet.
- Maternal intake and stores of the vitamins and trace elements do affect milk composition.

INFANCY

Breastfeeding versus bottle feeding

The assumption of most biologists would be that, through the process of natural selection, evolution will have produced, in breast milk, a food very close to the optimum for human babies. Only in a few circumstances such as those listed below will breast milk not be the preferred food for a baby:

- babies with an inborn error of metabolism, which leaves them unable to tolerate lactose or some amino acid in milk protein
- babies born to women infected with agents like the HIV virus that may be transmissible in the milk
- babies of mothers taking drugs or radioactive isotopes that may be transmitted in the milk.
- if the mother has herpes simplex infection of the breast.

A detailed list of contraindications to breastfeeding is given in Gartner *et al.* (2005).

The UK Department of Health has confirmed that it believes breast milk is the best form of nutrition for babies. It recommends that babies should be exclusively breastfed for the first 6 months of life and that solid food should then be introduced, but babies should continue to receive breast milk or formula after the first 6 months along with other foods. These recommendations, which are listed in Bolling *et al.* (2007), are consistent with World Health Organization recommendations.

Key points

- With few exceptions, breastfeeding is the best way of feeding newborn babies.
- It is recommended that babies should be exclusively breastfed for 6 months and that babies should continue to receive some breast milk or formula after this 6-month period.
- It is recommended that solid food should be introduced for the first time at 6 months of age.

Prevalence of breastfeeding

In the 1960s, the majority of babies born in the UK would not have been breastfed after leaving hospital. Perhaps only a quarter of babies born in the USA and parts of western Europe in the 1960s would have been breastfed for any significant time after delivery. Since then there has been a marked increase in breastfeeding led by women in the upper socioeconomic groups, the same groups that led the earlier trend away from breastfeeding.

Table 16.6 shows the estimated prevalences of breastfeeding in babies in England and Wales between 1975 and 2005. At the end of that period more than three-quarters of women made some initial attempt to breastfeed their babies, and preliminary data for 2010 suggest that the trend seen in Table 16.6 has been maintained so that the figure had risen to exceed 80 per cent. Only 49 per cent of babies were still being breastfed 6 weeks after delivery and, by 4 months, this had dropped to just over a third of all babies. These figures represent major increases over the figures for 1975 and since 1990 there has been a significant trend for increasing proportions of babies being breastfed at any time between birth and 9 months of age. The substantial increase shown between 1975 and 1980 has been maintained and built on in the last 20 years.

The figures in Table 16.6 understate the use of bottle feeds because data collected in the 2005 survey (Bolling *et al.*, 2007) indicate that many women were using a mix of breast milk and other feeds. Table 16.7 compares the percentage of women who were using some breastfeeding (plus some other nutrition) with those who were exclusively breastfeeding at sample time intervals after birth. Even in the immediate postnatal period, a significant proportion of women (around 10 per cent) were using a mix of breastfeeding plus some alternative feeds, and the gap between the proportions who were using exclusively and partial breastfeeding widened sharply with time. By 4 months after delivery, only 7 per cent of women were using breastfeeding exclusively, and almost none by 6 months.

Most of the statistical data used in this discussion of infant feeding practices are for England and Wales or for the UK as a whole, but this is intended to illustrate principles, patterns and trends that are likely to be common to several industrialized countries. The prevalence of breastfeeding in Scotland and Northern Ireland is below that in England and Wales. In 2005, 71 per cent of Scottish babies were initially breastfed and 44 per cent were still being breastfed at 6 weeks (corresponding figures for NI are 62 and 32 per cent, respectively). These Scottish and NI figures do represent significant positive shifts since 1995.

In *Healthy People 2000* (DHHS, 1992), the goal was for 75 per cent of US mothers to be breastfeeding in the immediate postpartum period by the year 2000 and for 50 per cent to continue to breastfeed for 5–6 months, and these goals have remained essentially unchanged in the updated *Healthy People 2010*. Assumed baseline figures in the USA for 1988 were that 64 per cent of women made some attempt to breastfeed while still in hospital, that just 54 per cent of mothers were breastfeeding on discharge, and 21 per cent were breastfeeding at 5–6 months. Only 32 per cent of low-income US mothers breastfed their babies at time of discharge, and fewer than 10 per cent were still breastfeeding at 5–6 months. American data for 2005–6 indicate that 77

Table 16.6 Prevalence (%) of breastfeeding in England and Wales*

Age	Year						
	1975	**1980**	**1985**	**1990**	**1995**	**2000**	**2005**
Birth	51	67	65	64	68	71	78
1 week	42	58	57	54	58	57	65
2 weeks	35	54	53	51	54	54	61
6 weeks	24	42	40	39	44	43	49
4 months	13	27	26	25	28	29	35
6 months	9	23	22	21	22	22	26

*Data for England and Wales used to facilitate historical comparisons. Data sources: DHSS (1988) and Bolling *et al.* (2007).

Table 16.7 Comparison of the prevalence of partial (receiving some nutrition other than breast milk) and exclusive breastfeeding by UK mothers at different times after birth*

Age	Partial breastfeeding (some additional nutrition) (%)	Exclusive breastfeeding (%)
Birth	76	65
2 weeks	60	38
6 weeks	48	21
4 months	34	7
6 months	25	<1

* Data source: Bolling *et al.* (2007).

per cent of mothers breastfed initially and thus for the first time the original target for 2000 set in 1992 had been realized; around a third of women were still breastfeeding at 6 months. The initial rates for the USA are similar to those in the UK but the proportion of women who are still breastfeeding at 6 months is rather higher than those recorded in the UK in 2005 (see Table 16.6).

Much higher breastfeeding rates have been reported for Canada, the Netherlands, Scandinavia, New Zealand and parts of Australia. In Sweden in 1973, only 20 per cent of babies were being breastfed at 2 months, but by 1993 this had risen to 85 per cent – which shows what can be achieved by effective promotion and facilitation measures (Wharton, 1998). According to Laurent (1993), 99 per cent of Norwegian mothers breastfeed their babies at birth and 90 per cent were still at least partially breastfeeding at 3–4 months.

UNICEF (2012) gives detailed information on the rates and duration of breastfeeding in many of the less industrialized countries. Overall, it estimates that, at 5 months, about 40 per cent of children in developing countries were being exclusively breastfed and just under 60 per cent of babies aged 6–9 months continued to receive some breast milk while also being given other foods. Estimated rates of breastfeeding vary widely from country to country. Listed below are selected examples of rates of exclusive breastfeeding at 4 months:

- Sierra Leone – 11 per cent
- Kenya – 18 per cent
- Nigeria – 22 per cent

- Turkey – 28 per cent
- Cuba – 42 per cent
- Ethiopia – 57 per cent
- India – 58 per cent
- Ghana – 65 per cent
- North Korea – 67 per cent
- Peru – 67 per cent
- China – 77 per cent
- Chile – 85 per cent.

Key points

- Around 80 per cent of UK women start to breastfeed their babies but a third of these cease doing so within the first 6 weeks.
- Prevalence of breastfeeding in the UK rose substantially between 1975 and 1980 and has also increased significantly in the last 20 years.
- By 6 weeks of age, many breastfed UK babies have received additional feeds and only around 20 per cent are being wholly breastfed.
- There is wide international variation in the prevalence of breastfeeding. Rates in Scandinavia are among the highest in the industrialized world – the proportion of Swedish babies being breastfed at 2 months more than quadrupled in a 20-year period (1973–93).
- Around 40 per cent of babies in developing countries are exclusively breastfed for the first 5 months of life. At between 6 and 9 months, around 60 per cent continue to receive some breast milk along with other foods.
- Examples of rates of exclusive breastfeeding in some less industrialized countries are given and a comprehensive list can be found in UNICEF (2012).

Factors influencing choice of infant feeding method

Table 16.8 shows the percentage of babies being breastfed at three ages according to selected characteristics of the mother. Although only selected examples are shown, the data are representative of the full data sets; for example, there is a progressive increase in prevalence of breastfeeding at all infant ages as the age of the mother increases.

Table **16.8** Prevalence (%) of breastfeeding at various ages according to social class, education level, ethnicity, age and parity of the mother*

Maternal categorization	Birth (%)	6 weeks (%)	4 months (%)
Socioeconomic grouping			
Professional and managerial	88	65	47
Routine and manual	66	32	21
Age of finishing full-time education			
16 years or less	61	27	17
Over 18 years	90	68	51
Maternal age			
Under 20 years	52	14	8
25–29 years	76	47	32
35+ years	85	62	48
Ethnicity			
White	75	46	32
(British) Asian	93	66	47
Black (British)	97	87	72
Mixed	82	66	47
Parity			
1st baby	80	47	32
Later baby	73	49	36

*Selected data from Bolling *et al.* (2007).

Choice of infant feeding method is very strongly dependent on social class in the UK. In 2005, 88 per cent of UK women in the highest occupation category attempted to breastfeed their babies and 65 per cent were still breastfeeding at 6 weeks. The corresponding figures for women in the lowest occupation category were 66 per cent and 21 per cent, respectively. Women with higher levels of education are also much more likely to breastfeed their children in the UK, and 68 per cent of those in the highest education category were still breastfeeding at 6 weeks compared to just 27 per cent in the lowest educational category.

There are substantial differences in the prevalence of breastfeeding in different ethnic groups in the UK. White women are the least likely to start breastfeeding and the least likely to continue at all ages up to 6 months.

There are small differences between the feeding choices of first-time mothers and mothers on the second or later birth. A first-time mother is more likely to try to breastfeed but slightly less likely to be breastfeeding at 6 weeks or 4 months after birth. Some of these differences may well be attributable to other characteristics of the first time sample, such as the mother's age. The mother's choice of feeding method for her first baby is a major influence on feeding of subsequent children. Figures below show the percentage of women who start breastfeeding their new baby classified according to their experience of feeding their previous baby:

- never breastfed before – 33 per cent start
- had breastfed for less than 6 weeks – 79 per cent started again
- had breastfed for 6 weeks or more – 98 per cent started again.

So, mothers who had breastfed their first baby usually breastfeed subsequent children whereas women who had bottle-fed the first baby usually did not. Women with previous experience of successful breastfeeding also were less likely to stop early. For UK women in 2005 who had solely bottle-fed their first baby, only 33 per cent changed to breastfeeding for their next baby, but this was a substantial increase on the 18 per cent recorded in 1995.

Many factors will have compounded to decrease the prevalence of breastfeeding, but the availability of a cheap, simple and 'modern' alternative was clearly an essential prerequisite. There may even have been a temptation to think that science had improved on nature if bottle-fed babies grew faster than breastfed babies. Some other factors that have probably contributed to the decline in breastfeeding are considered below.

- Breastfeeding may be inconvenient in the lifestyle of many women, especially those who wish to resume their career soon after birth or those whose income is considered to be a vital part of the family budget. Statutory paid maternity leave should have decreased this influence in more recent years in the UK. According to Foster *et al.* (1997), a third of UK women who stopped breastfeeding at between

3 and 4 months in 1995 gave returning to work as their reason, but this reason was given by only 8 per cent of those stopping before 4 months in 2005 (Table 16.9). Only a third of women in this survey were on paid maternity leave when their babies were 6 weeks old.

Table 16.9 Reasons UK women give for early cessation of breastfeeding*

Reason for stopping	First week (%)	During 2nd week (%)	At 6 weeks to 4 months (%)
Lack of milk	25	42	48
Failure of baby to suckle/rejected breast	35	24	13
Painful breasts/nipples	24	30	9
Did not like breastfeeding	8	5	1
Too time-consuming/tiring	10	17	19
Mother was ill	8	10	8
Return to work/college	1	–	8

*Data source: Bolling et al. (2007).

- Breastfeeding prevents fathers and others sharing the burden of feeding, especially night feeds in the early weeks after birth.
- There are undoubtedly some women (and men) who find the whole idea of breastfeeding distasteful. There is a strong taboo in the UK against breastfeeding in public or even among close friends or relatives. This, coupled with the limited but improving provision of facilities for breastfeeding in many public places, can only increase the inconvenience of breastfeeding and restrict the range of activities that women can participate in during lactation.
- The figures in Table 16.6 clearly indicate that many women who initially try to breastfeed give up after a short time. Many women experience discomfort in the early stages of lactation and many women believe that they are unable to produce sufficient milk. Delay in starting suckling (e.g. to allow the woman to rest after delivery) or any prolonged break from suckling is likely to reduce the likelihood of initiating and maintaining lactation.
- Bottle-feeding has been promoted in many developing countries as the modern, sophisticated, 'Western' way of feeding babies – the high-prestige option. Yet, in industrialized countries, breastfeeding is more common among the higher socioeconomic groups and so in these countries it is the high-prestige option.

In a 2005 survey (Bolling et al., 2007), the following reasons were given by UK women as important reasons for choosing to breastfeed their babies:

- 81 per cent because they thought it was best for the baby's health
- 28 per cent because breastfeeding was more convenient
- 19 per cent because it promotes bonding between mother and baby
- 15 per cent because it is cheaper/free
- 14 per cent because it is more natural
- 17 per cent because it is better for the health of the mother
- 11 per cent because the mother loses weight more easily
- 13 per cent because they had breastfed their previous baby (stated by 27 per cent of non-first-time mothers).

To set against this, listed below are the most common reasons given for choosing to bottle-feed:

- 25 per cent because someone else can feed the baby
- 32 per cent because they didn't like the idea of breastfeeding or would be embarrassed
- 58 per cent because of the mother's previous experience for second or later babies.

Note that, in 2005, 32 per cent of mothers who chose to bottle-feed said they did so because they didn't like the idea of breastfeeding, compared with 19 per cent in the 2000 survey. It may be that these are the women who are most resistant to measures to promote breastfeeding; so, as the proportion of women who choose not to breastfeed declines, this will become more prominent as the major barrier to change. Just 3 per cent of women gave returning to work or college as their reason for choosing to bottle-feed.

The earlier discussion of Tables 16.6 and 16.7 noted that, although the proportion of women who start to breastfeed is around 80 per cent, many cease to breastfeed so that only around a third are still doing so at 4 months and only 7 per cent are exclusively breastfeeding. Around 80 per cent of those who stopped within the first 4 months said they would have liked to breastfeed for longer. Table 16.9 shows the reasons women gave for stopping breastfeeding during the first and second weeks and between 6 weeks and 4 months after the birth. Very few women at any stage gave reasons that would be interpreted as considered maternal choices, such as returning to work/college, too time-consuming or tiring, or not liking breastfeeding. At all three stages women's perceptions were that 'problems' beyond their control caused them to stop, examples being lack of milk, failure of the baby to suckle, painful breasts or nipples or maternal illness.

If these perceptions are taken at face value, health promoters should look for reasons why these problems occur and how they can be overcome or prevented. It is possible that in the current climate some women may feel guilty about choosing to stop breastfeeding and give a problem beyond their control as the reason they stopped.

Early feeding experience in the hospital also strongly affects the likelihood of early cessation of breastfeeding. Mothers attempting to breastfeed but whose babies were also given some bottle feeds were more than three times as likely to give up breastfeeding within a fortnight as were women whose babies received no bottle feeds. Delay in initiating breastfeeding is also strongly associated with early cessation. Early cessation occurred in 30 per cent of cases where there was a delay of 12 hours or more in putting the baby to the breast but in only 16 per cent of cases where this occurred immediately after birth; even a delay of 1 hour had a significant effect (Hamlyn *et al.*, 2002). White *et al.* (1992) reported that women were almost twice as likely to continue breastfeeding if feeding on demand rather than at set times was practised in the hospital.

Hamlyn *et al.* (2002) noted that there had been some changes in UK maternity hospital practices between 1990 and 2000, including the following.

- The number of women starting to breastfeed within 1 hour had increased from 63 per cent in 1990 to 72 per cent in 2000.
- The proportion of mothers who had their babies with them continuously in hospital rose from 63 to 79 per cent.
- The proportion of breastfed babies who were given some bottles in hospital dropped from 46 to 31 per cent.
- In 2000, most first-time mothers said they had been given some useful help or advice about breastfeeding.

Many UK women reported that they had experienced problems in finding somewhere to feed their baby in public places, and in fact almost 30 per cent never attempted to feed their baby outside the home. In 2000, over a third of bottle-feeding mothers had never attempted to feed their baby outside the home, compared with just 8 per cent of those who breastfed – although the breastfeeding mothers were more likely to have encountered problems with feeding outside the home (Hamlyn *et al.*, 2002).

Key points

- Breastfeeding in the UK decreases in prevalence with decreasing social class and with decreasing educational attainment of the mother.
- Breastfeeding rates increase with the age of the mother.
- White women are less likely to breastfeed than other major ethnic groups in the UK.
- Women chose to breastfeed because it is good for the baby and for them, because it promotes bonding between mother and baby, and/or because it is convenient, natural and cheap.
- Women chose to bottle-feed because someone else can help with feeding or because they do not like the idea of breastfeeding or are embarrassed by it.
- The feeding method used for second and subsequent births is very influenced by the mother's experience with her first baby.
- Women often give up breastfeeding prematurely because of difficulties with successfully and comfortably feeding the baby.

→

The benefits of breastfeeding

It was noted earlier that both the UK Department of Health and the WHO have concluded that breast milk is the best nutrition for a baby during the first 6 months of life. Table 16.10 illustrates just how different are human milk, cow milk and infant formula. Cow milk is an ideal food for rapidly growing calves but unless substantially modified is now regarded as an unsuitable food for human babies. This table also demonstrates the scale of changes that are necessary to convert cow milk into a formula that is compositionally similar to human milk. Even though modern 'humanized' formula is closer to human milk than formulations like National Dried Milk that were used until 1976 in the UK, they are nonetheless still quite different from the human milk they are trying to imitate.

Most formulas are based on cow milk. Although soy-based types can be used from birth they are not recommended unless there is a specific reason (e.g. allergy to cow milk protein). It is recommended that babies should not drink unmodified cow milk until they are a year old because it does not have sufficient levels of iron and other nutrients; it can be used to mix and make up other foods. In children up to 2 years old, whole cow milk should be used. Semi-skimmed milk should not be given to under-twos and skimmed milk not be given to under-fives. Goat and sheep milk are not considered suitable for children under 12 months.

Table 16.10 Composition of human milk, cow milk and modern infant formula (per 100 mL as consumed)*

	Human milk	Cow milk	Infant formula	1970s formula[1]
Energy (kcal)	70	67	67	55
(kJ)	293	281	281	231
Protein (g)	1.3	3.5	1.4–1.9	2.5
Carbohydrate (g)	7	4.9	7.2–7.7	5.9
Fat (g)	4.2	3.6	3.3–3.6	2.4
Sodium (mg)	15	52	19–25	40
Calcium (mg)	35	120	51–71	83
Iron (μg)	76	50	670–680	480
Vitamin A (μg)	60	40	80	23
Vitamin C (mg)	3.8	1.5	8	2.4
Vitamin D (μg)	0.01	0.03	1.1–1.2	0.8

*Data sources: Poskitt (1988) and Wharton (1998).
[1] UK National Dried Milk that was withdrawn in 1976.

Cow milk has around three times the protein content of human milk. This means that babies will need to excrete substantial amounts of urea if fed on cow milk, whereas with breastfeeding the bulk of the *nitrogen* is retained for growth. Around 20 per cent of the nitrogen in cow milk and breast milk is non-protein nitrogen (e.g. urea, creatine and free amino acids). Its biological significance is unclear, but this fraction will be absent from infant formula.

The amino acid *taurine* is present in relatively large amounts in human milk and is added to some infant formulas. Taurine is normally made from the amino acid *cysteine*, which in turn can be made from the other sulphur-containing amino acid *methionine*. However, premature babies have a low synthetic capacity and a relatively high requirement for both cysteine and taurine, so they are normally regarded as conditionally essential in premature babies. In breastfed infants, the principal bile acid is *taurocholic acid*, but in infants fed on cow milk it is *glycocholic acid* and this may adversely affect the emulsification and therefore digestion and absorption of milk fat.

The principal proteins in milk are *casein* and *whey*. The casein:whey ratio is much higher in cow milk than human milk. Casein forms hard clots in the stomach and is also relatively low in cysteine (the usual precursor of taurine). Infant formulas vary in the extent to which the casein:whey ratio has been modified to make it closer to that of human milk. Most infant formulas used in the first few months after birth are whey-based because this makes them closer in composition to breast milk and easier for the baby to digest. Use of casein-dominant formulas becomes more prevalent in older infants because it takes longer to digest and is thus said to be more satisfying for hungry babies than a whey-dominant formula, although there is no evidence to support this belief. In a casein-dominant formula the casein:whey ratio is 80:20 (as in cow milk) but in a whey-dominant formula it is closer to the 40:60 ratio in human milk.

Follow-on formulas are produced as an alternative to cow milk for infants who are over 6 months old. They are not intended to be a complete diet but a component of a weaning diet, and at 8–10 months they are used by just over a half of UK mothers. By 8–10 months, just 39 per cent of UK mothers had introduced cow milk to their babies in one way or another and most of them used whole milk. Only 6 per cent of mothers were using cow milk as the main milk at this stage; most were using it to mix with food or as an occasional drink. The statistical data used in this section are mainly taken from Bolling *et al.* (2007) and much more detailed information can be found in that source.

Cow milk fat is poorly digested and absorbed compared to that in breast milk; it is also much lower in essential polyunsaturated fatty acids. Some or all of the butterfat will be replaced by vegetable oils by infant formula manufacturers to give a fatty acid composition closer to that of human milk. Cow milk has only around 1 per cent of energy as *linoleic acid* whereas the figure for human milk is up to 16 per cent, depending on the diet of the mother. The differences in digestibility of cow and breast milk fat may be due to the three factors listed below.

- There are differences in the nature of the fat itself. Palmitic acid is generally not well absorbed by infants, but in human milk most of it is in the 2-position and is absorbed as monoacylglycerol.
- Breast milk contains lipase, which is activated by bile salts. Lingual lipases make a major contribution to fat digestion of bottle-fed and breastfed babies.
- The differences in bile acid secretion mentioned earlier may contribute to the better fat digestion by breastfed babies.

Breast milk is particularly high in lactose and this lactose content may increase calcium absorption and act as a substrate for lactobacilli in the lumen of the gut, thus creating an acid environment that will inhibit the growth of pathogens. Breast milk contains factors that stimulate the growth of *Lactobacillus bifidi* – small amounts of oligosaccharides and nucleotides may be important in this respect. The stools of healthy breastfed babies have a low pH and contain almost exclusively lactobacilli whereas formula-fed babies have a more mixed gut flora. Formula manufacturers increase the carbohydrate content so that it corresponds to that of human milk, and they may or may not use lactose for this purpose. Oligosaccharides of glucose produced by partial hydrolysis of starch are often used.

Cow milk contains much higher concentrations of the major minerals than human milk. The sodium content is over three times higher. This is a high solute load for the immature kidney to deal with and it can precipitate *hypernatraemic dehydration*. The risk of dehydration will be exacerbated by fever, diarrhoea or by making up the formula too concentrated. High sodium content was the single most important reason why, in the UK in 1976, several formulas including National Dried Milk were withdrawn.

The calcium contents of cow milk and breast milk differ by even more than the sodium content, but calcium uptake is homeostatically regulated – calcium absorption from cow milk may be poor despite the high concentration. Unabsorbed fat from cow milk or formula hinders calcium absorption while the presence of lactose increases it.

The vitamin and trace mineral contents of formula are generally set to match or exceed those in human milk. The iron content of formula is higher than in breast milk even though it is normal for breastfed babies to be in negative iron balance for the first few months of their lives. The iron content of breast milk is considered insufficient for older babies (4–6 months). All formulas are fortified with vitamin D.

Table 16.10 shows that formulas are still very different from human milk. Even if manufacturers succeeded in producing a formula that exactly corresponded to breast milk in its nutrient content, there would still be substantial residual benefits to be gained from breastfeeding. In many developing countries, choice of feeding method may greatly affect the chance of survival of the baby. Mortality rates of bottle-fed babies are often much higher than those of breastfed ones (Walker, 1990); sample studies from both developing and developed countries are outlined in the next paragraph. In industrialized countries, deaths from *sudden infant death syndrome* ('cot death') are lower in breastfed babies. A recent meta-analysis of case–control studies found that breastfeeding was associated with a substantially reduced risk of cot death especially in those babies who were exclusively breastfed. Breastfeeding can reduce risk of infection both by preventing exposure to contaminated alternatives and because of the inherent anti-infective properties of breast milk. Although the former may be the dominant benefit in some developing countries, there is evidence that it also reduces gut and respiratory infection rates in industrialized countries and that the latter mechanisms are predominant here (Filteau and Tomkins, 1994).

A WHO-sponsored study in 2000 compared mortality rates for breastfed and bottle-fed babies in three developing countries. It found that, in the first 2 months, mortality rates were six times higher in the bottle-fed babies. This large difference was particularly due to a reduction in deaths from diarrhoea in the breastfed babies, but deaths from acute respiratory infections were also lower; babies who are exclusively breastfed are five times less likely to die from pneumonia than babies who are not breastfed. Although the differences in mortality rates between the breastfed and bottle-fed babies narrowed steadily after the first 2 months, they were still apparent in the second year of life. The protective effect of breastfeeding was highest in those mothers with the lowest level of education.

According to UNICEF (2008), breastfeeding protects babies from diarrhoea and acute respiratory infections, stimulates the immune system, and improves the response to vaccinations; optimal breastfeeding up to 2 years of age has the potential to prevent 1.4 million deaths in young children.

Chen and Rogan (2004) have reported that, in the USA, breastfeeding is also associated with a significant reduction of post-neonatal death. Mortality was just over 20 per cent lower in those babies who had ever been breastfed compared to those who had never been breastfed. While it is not possible to say with certainty that this reduction in mortality in the USA is caused by breastfeeding, these authors did correct for the most obvious confounding variables. In a 2005 policy statement, the American Academy of Pediatrics gave a detailed and referenced summary of the benefits of breastfeeding for babies and their mothers (Gartner *et al.*, 2005).

Some other benefits of breastfeeding are discussed below.

- *Bonding.* Breastfeeding is thought to increase bonding between mother and baby.
- *Anti-infective properties.* Breast milk contains immunoglobulin A, which protects the mucosal surfaces of the digestive tract and upper respiratory tract from pathogens. It also contains immune cells which aid in the immunological protection of the infant gut. The iron-binding protein *lactoferrin* has a bacteriostatic effect. The enzyme *lysozyme* breaks down bacterial cell walls and oligosaccharides, and *nucleotides* promote the growth of lactobacilli. *Colostrum*, the secretion produced in the first few days of lactation, is particularly rich in these anti-infective agents. Colostrum is quite different in its composition from mature human milk. Anti-infective agents in cow milk will probably be destroyed during processing and many are in any case likely to be species-specific. There is some benefit to be gained by even a very short period of breastfeeding because at least then the infant will receive the colostrum.
- *Hygiene.* It is taken for granted in most industrialized countries that an infant formula will be made up with clean boiled water, in sterile bottles, and the final mixture pasteurized by being made up with hot water. The risk of contamination in many other countries is a very serious one. The purity of the water, facilities for sterilization of water and bottles and storage conditions for pre-mixed feeds may all be poor. This means that bottle-fed babies may have greatly increased risk of gastro-intestinal infections. Gastroenteritis is a major cause of death for babies in developing countries – a strong reason why breastfeeding should be particularly encouraged. This is an important

cause of the higher mortality of bottle-fed babies in developing countries.

• *Restoration of maternal pre-pregnant weight.* It is generally assumed that maternal fat laid down during pregnancy serves as a store to help meet the energy demands of lactation. In countries like the UK and USA, where obesity is prevalent, the assumed effect of lactation in reducing this maternal fat after delivery may be an important one. It was noted earlier that 13 per cent of UK women quoted this as a reason for choosing to breastfeed. A Swedish study found that even modest weight gain after a first pregnancy increased the risk of pre-eclampsia, diabetes, stillbirth and caesarean delivery in future pregnancies (Villamor and Cnattingius, 2006).

• *Cost of formula.* In industrialized countries the cost of formula is usually regarded as relatively trivial. Nevertheless, modern infant formulas are high-technology products, so in many developing countries feeding an infant with formula will absorb a very substantial proportion of the total household budget. This may seriously reduce resources available to feed the rest of the family, or it may lead to the baby being fed over-diluted formula as an economy measure and so effectively starving it.

• *Anti-fertility effect.* Although breastfeeding cannot be regarded as a reliable method of contraception, it does greatly reduce fertility. Suckling suppresses the release of pituitary gonadotropins which are necessary for development of ovarian follicles and ovulation. In cultures where suckling occurs for extended periods rather than in discreet 'meals', this effect may be increased. In many developing countries, prolonged breastfeeding will have an important birth-spacing effect and will make a contribution to limiting overall population fertility. Full breastfeeding may be up to 98 per cent effective in preventing pregnancy in the first 6 months after birth; return of fertility will be hastened by use of supplementary formula or solid food during breastfeeding (Picciano and Macdonald, 2006).

• *Reduced risk of breast cancer.* A large case–control study in the UK has suggested that breastfeeding reduces the risk of developing breast cancer in young women (UK National Case Control Study Group, 1993). Breast cancer risk declined both with the duration of breastfeeding undertaken by the woman and with the number of babies that she had breastfed. Several other studies in other countries have reported similar findings and also suggested a possible protective effect against ovarian cancer (Picciano and Macdonald, 2006).

Key points

• Breast milk is very different in composition to either cow milk or even modern infant formulas.

• Most infant formulas are based on cow milk. Although soy-based formulas can be given from birth they are not recommended unless there is a specific reason for using them.

• Unmodified cow milk should not be given to babies under 12 months old, nor should goat or sheep milk.

• Semi-skimmed (2 per cent) milk should not be given before the baby is 2 years old and skimmed milk not before it is 5 years old.

• Exclusive breastfeeding is recommended for the first 6 months of life, although some experts believe the introduction of other foods should begin at 4–6 months. In practice, very few women breastfeed exclusively for 6 months.

• The casein:whey ratio is higher in cow milk, and formulas can either be casein-dominant or whey-dominant like breast milk.

• In infant formulas, some of the highly saturated butterfat of cow milk is replaced by vegetable oil.

• Human milk fat is much better digested and absorbed than that in cow milk.

• Breast milk has more lactose than cow milk. Infant formulas are supplemented with carbohydrate, which may not be lactose.

• Cow milk is high in sodium and some early infant formulas were withdrawn in the UK in 1976 because of their high sodium content.

• Mortality and infection rates of breastfed babies are much lower in developing countries than those of bottle-fed babies. Even in industrialized countries, breastfed babies have lower rates or severity of infection, reduced risk of cot death, and reduced post-neonatal mortality.

→

Weaning

When to wean?

Weaning is the process of transferring an infant from breast milk or infant formula on to solid food. The process begins when the child is first offered food other than breast milk or formula. The process may be very gradual, with other foods forming an increasing proportion of total energy intake over several months until breast or formula is eventually phased out completely. During weaning there is ideally gradual transition from a very high-fat, high-sugar liquid diet to a starchy, moderate-fat, low-sugar and fibre-containing solid diet. The magnitude of the compositional and textural changes involved would seem to indicate the advisability of a gradual transition to allow babies to adapt to them.

In the report *Weaning and the Weaning Diet* (COMA, 1994b) it was recommended that the majority of infants should not be given solid food before the age of 4 months and that a mixed diet should be offered by the age of 6 months. Morgan (1998) suggested that 14 weeks should be the minimum age for weaning, or when the infant's weight reaches 7 kg. Authorities in both the UK and USA as well as the WHO now recommend that exclusive breastfeeding should be continued for the first 6 months of life. It is quite clear from data discussed earlier in this chapter that almost no UK mothers stick to this advice and only 7 per cent are exclusively breastfeeding at 4 months. Even some experts on the US panel disagreed over this 6-month recommendation (Gartner *et al.*, 2005).

This means that the current ideal window for the start of weaning in industrialized countries is probably somewhere between 4 and 6 months; the benefits of longer exclusive breastfeeding will be greater in developing countries. After around 6 months, it is thought that breast milk can no longer supply all of the nutritional needs of the infant and growth is likely to be impaired if the baby receives only breast milk. Breast milk or formula should continue to make a contribution to total food supply for at least some months after weaning has begun.

Earlier introduction of solid foods is considered undesirable because:

- some babies do not properly develop the ability to bite and chew before 3–4 months
- the infant gut is very vulnerable to infection and allergies
- early introduction of energy-dense weaning foods may increase the likelihood of obesity.

Full production of *pancreatic amylase* may not occur in human infants until 6–9 months of age. As milk contains no starch but most weaning foods are starchy, this may be a physiological indicator that a relatively late introduction of starches into the diet is desirable. Introducing starchy solid foods too early may produce symptoms similar to *infectious gastroenteritis* because of poor digestion and absorption resulting from the lack of pancreatic amylase.

In 1975, 18 per cent of British babies had been given some food other than milk in their first month and 97 per cent by the time they were 4 months old; corresponding figures for 1995 were 2 and 91 per cent, respectively (COMA, 1988; Foster *et al.*, 1997). The practice of introducing solid foods to infants very soon after birth has almost ceased in the UK, and in 2005 only 2 per cent of babies had received some solid food at 8 weeks. Table 16.11 shows the percentage of UK babies who had been given some solid foods at different times after birth in 1995, 2000 and 2005. The figures indicate a marked and continuing trend for the later introduction of solid foods in the UK, but half of mothers had introduced solid food before the 17 weeks recommended by COMA (1994b) and many before the 14-week minimum (or 7 kg body weight) suggested by Morgan (1998). Almost all mothers had introduced solid food before the current 6-months recommendation. Introduction of solid food occurs at between 3 and 5 months for around three-quarters of UK babies.

Table 16.11 Percentage of UK babies who have been introduced to solid food at various ages in 1995, 2000 and 2005*

Age of baby	Year		
	1995	2000	2005
6 weeks	7	3	1
8 weeks	13	5	2
3 months	56	24	10
4 months	91	85	51
5 months	n/a	n/a	82
6 months	99	98	98
9 months	100	100	100
Age at first introduction to solids (% of babies)			
Before 13 weeks	10		
At 13–22 weeks	72		
After 22 weeks (5 mo)	18		

*Data sources: Hamlyn *et al.* (2002) and Bolling *et al.* (2007).

The following are some factors associated with early introduction of solid foods.

- *Maternal age.* There was a clear trend for younger mothers to introduce solid foods earlier. For example, only 36 per cent of mothers over 35 years had introduced solid food by 4 months, compared with 74 per cent of teenaged mothers.
- *Socioeconomic group.* There was a marked trend for mothers in the lower socioeconomic grouping to introduce solid food earlier.
- *Ethnicity.* Minority ethnic mothers introduce solid food later than white mothers.
- *Return to work.* Mothers who returned to work before 6 months were slightly more likely to have introduced solid food before 4 months.

The most common reason women gave for the early introduction of solid food was their perception that the baby was not satisfied by their milk feeds (63 per cent). Other mothers stipulated advice from a health professional (35 per cent), experience with a previous baby (32 per cent), or advice from family and friends (14 per cent).

What weaning foods?

In the UK, the first weaning foods for most babies are cereals, rusks or commercial preparations rather than home-prepared foods. At 4–6 months, mothers who gave solids tended to use commercially prepared foods on a daily basis, but by the time their babies were 8–10 months they had become much less reliant on these and were preparing food themselves. The most commonly avoided added ingredients by mothers of 8- to 10-month-old babies were salt (51 per cent), sugar (35 per cent) and food additives (9 per cent); most women avoided salt and sugar because they saw them as not needed, or harmful in some way. The most commonly avoided foods were nuts (48 per cent), eggs (14 per cent), honey (13 per cent) and dairy produce, with concerns about allergies or food poisoning being the most commonly cited reasons. Very few babies (<7 per cent) were given vitamin or mineral supplements.

Priorities for weaning foods

Morgan and her colleagues asked a large sample of British mothers for their views on good infant feeding practices and some of the findings of this survey are summarized in Table 16.12.

Table 16.12 Priorities of a sample of UK mothers for infant feeding*

	Percentage mothers' responses	
	Not important	(Very) important
Wide variety of foods	3	95
Plenty to drink	1	98
Plenty of calories	20	76
Low fat intake	10	88
High fibre intake	15	83

*Adapted from Morgan (1998).

Clearly, most of these women thought that a high-fibre and low-fat diet should be the priority for weaning foods, and a fifth did not think that an energy-rich diet was important for a rapidly growing infant. These maternal priorities are very different from the current consensus of expert nutritional opinion such as those of COMA (1994b) listed below. The numerical values in Table 16.12 represent the views of women sampled over a decade ago and they would almost certainly be very different if a similar survey were conducted now (e.g. only 6 per cent of women said they specifically avoided fat as an ingredient in their baby's food). Nevertheless these views do emphasize the importance of informing pregnant women and new mothers about the different nutritional priorities for young children and the well-publicized advice to adults.

- Provision of adequate dietary energy for growth was the principal determinant of the diets of the under-fives.
- Adult recommendations on reducing fat consumption should not apply to the under-twos and should fully apply from the age of 5 years.
- Diets of the under-twos should not contain fibre-rich foods to the extent that they limit energy content and the absorption of micronutrients.

Poskitt (1998) suggested that weaning foods should be:

- rich in energy, including energy from fat
- rich in vitamins and minerals
- fed frequently
- used initially as a supplement to milk rather than a replacement
- fed in a form that develops the child's feeding skills while still allowing assistance.

One of the main aims of weaning is to raise the energy density of the infant's diet above that for breast milk. The weaning food should have a suitable texture, but be of high enough energy and nutrient density for the baby to meet its nutritional needs without having to consume an excessive volume of food. If very viscous foods are introduced too early in the weaning process then the infant may reject them by spitting them out. A typical weaning food in a developing country, made up to give a suitable viscosity from a starchy cereal or root staple such as cassava or millet flour, might contain only 0.3 kcal/g (1.3 kJ/g). This compares with around 0.7 kcal/g (3 kJ/g) for breast milk and perhaps 1.5 kcal/g (6 kJ/g) for a typical UK weaning diet (Church, 1979). At the lower extreme, the child is incapable of consuming the volume of food required to meet its energy needs. This problem may be exacerbated if the child is fed infrequently, has frequent periods of infection and anorexia, and perhaps by the poor sensory characteristics of the food itself. In industrialized countries, this could be a problem if parents mistakenly apply the recommendations for low-fat, low-sugar and high-starch and high-fibre

diets in adults too rigorously to infants. Some strict vegetarian weaning diets in industrialized countries may also be of insufficient energy density because of their low fat and high starch content.

The lower limit for the energy density of weaning foods should be 0.7 kcal/g (3 kJ/g). Puréed fruits or vegetables are not suitable as weaning foods unless they have their energy density enhanced, for example by the addition of a source of fat. Skimmed and semi-skimmed milk are not suitable for very young children. Bolling *et al.* (2007) found that very few women were giving their babies these low-fat milks in 2005, although 4 per cent of women were using semi-skimmed milk for 9-month-old babies in 2000.

Weaning foods should be clean and not contaminated with infective agents. Poverty, poor hygiene and contaminated food precipitate much malnutrition in developing countries. Even when dietary intakes are judged sufficient to permit normal growth, infection and diarrhoea may be an indirect cause of dietary deficiency. One survey reported that 41 per cent of traditional weaning foods and 50 per cent of drinking water specimens in rural Bangladesh were contaminated with faecal micro-organisms (Walker, 1990). Although substantial progress has been made in improving sanitation and water supplies especially in South Asia since 1990, around 1.3 million children died from diarrhoea in 2008 and 90 per cent of cases of diarrhoea are caused by contaminated water (Black *et al.*, 2010). Millions of children worldwide have little or no access to safe water and proper sanitation.

In affluent countries, like the UK and USA, other aims are also considered important for infant feeds. They should be:

- low in *salt*
- low in *added sugar*
- possibly *gluten-free*.

High-salt foods expose the immature kidney to a high solute load and increase the risk of hypernatraemic dehydration, and maybe increase the later risk of high blood pressure. Sugar is regarded as empty calories and is detrimental to the baby's new teeth. Over-consumption of sugar in infancy may also be creating bad preferences for the future. There is very strong evidence that fluoride is protective against dental caries, so the UK panel on dietary reference values suggested a safe daily fluoride intake for infants of 0.05 mg/kg – around 50 per cent of the amount likely to cause fluorosis. To achieve this safe intake, most UK infants would need supplements and the amount of supplemental fluoride required depends on the fluoride content of the local water supply (see Chapter 15 for details). Swallowing fluoridated toothpaste is one way that many young children receive supplemental fluoride!

While most babies will suffer no harm by early exposure to the wheat protein called gluten, those sensitive to gluten – and thus at risk of coeliac disease (see Chapter 17) – cannot be identified in advance. The incidence of coeliac disease in children has been falling in recent years at the same time as there have been trends towards later introduction of solid foods and towards the use of gluten-free, rice-based weaning cereals.

Key points

- It is generally recommended that weaning should start after the baby is 6 months old. In practice it usually occurs 3–6 months after birth in the UK.
- Babies should be fed frequently during weaning.
- Breast milk is not adequate for babies after 6 months but should continue to contribute to their diet.
- Very early introduction of solid foods is undesirable. Very few babies in the UK are now given solid food in the first few weeks. Half of UK women still introduce solid foods before the baby is 17 weeks old.
- Mothers in the UK usually use some form of commercial weaning food in the early stages.
- Weaning foods should be free from contamination and should be energy- and nutrient-dense. They should not be low in fat or too high in fibre, and they should be low in salt and added sugar.
- In 1995, many British mothers mistakenly believed that weaning foods should be low in fat and high in fibre.
- Puréed fruits and vegetables are unsuitable for weaning unless their energy density has been increased, and very young children should not be given low-fat milk.
- In many developing countries, the traditional starchy weaning foods have such low energy density that they limit energy intake and precipitate malnutrition.

CHILDHOOD AND ADOLESCENCE

Even when fully weaned, children still have nutritional needs and priorities that differ from those of adults. They need enough energy and nutrients to enable them to grow and develop, especially during the intensely anabolic adolescent period. Too heavy an emphasis on a low-fat, low-sugar and high-fibre diet may limit growth. These differing needs have to be reconciled with the need to start good dietary habits early and to prevent the development of obesity. Note that inactivity is now regarded as the key factor in childhood obesity (see Chapter 9).

Table 16.13 shows selected UK RNIs for children in the age categories 1–3 and 4–6 years, expressed in both absolute terms and as an approximate percentage of the value for adults. These values

Table 16.13 Selected dietary reference values (per day) for UK children and their percentage of the corresponding adult values*[1]

Nutrient	1–3 years	% adult[2]	4–6 years	% adult[1]
Boys' energy (kcal)	1230 (5.15 MJ)	48	1715 (7.16 MJ)	67
Girls' energy (kcal)	1165 (4.86 MJ)	60	1545 (6.46 MJ)	86
Protein (g)	14.5	29	19.7	40
Thiamin (mg)	0.5	55	0.7	78
Riboflavin (mg)	0.6	50	0.8	50
Niacin (mg)	8	53	11	73
Folate (µg)	70	35	100	50
Vitamin C (mg)	30	75	30	75
Vitamin A (µg)	400	62	500	77
Vitamin D (µg)[3]	7	–	–	–
Calcium (mg)	350	50	450	64
Iron (mg)	6.9	60	6.1	52
Zinc (mg)	5.0	61	6.5	79

*Data source: COMA (1991).
[1] Note that the body weight of a 1- to 3 year old is c20 per cent that of an adult and that of a 4- to 6 year old is c30 per cent of the adult value.
[2] In most cases this is calculated using the average of the male and female values for 19- to 50 year olds.
[3] For adults and older children there are no reference values as it is synthesized in the skin when exposed to sunlight.

confirm that children require proportionately much more energy than do adults. A 1- to 3-year-old girl weighs perhaps one-fifth of an adult woman but requires three-fifths of the dietary energy of the woman. The values for the other nutrients are generally in line with this proportionately higher energy requirement. In the case of protein, the proportional values are much less than those for energy and so children should be able to manage on a diet with a lower concentration (i.e. percentage of energy) of protein than adults; see the discussion in Chapter 11. A diet that is compositionally suitable for adults should therefore contain adequate amounts of nutrients for young children – provided they eat enough of it to satisfy their energy needs. Of course, children may be more sensitive to the effects of nutrient deficiencies. For example, they may have smaller body stores than adults, or their growth may be impaired.

The rate of growth of children decelerates steadily from birth until puberty. During adolescence there is a very pronounced and sustained growth spurt. Between the ages of 12 and 17 years, boys gain an average 26 cm in height and 26 kg in weight; between the ages of 10 and 15 years, girls gain 23 cm in height and 21 kg in weight. Adolescence is thus an intensely anabolic period and a time when there is inevitably a relatively high demand for energy and nutrients to sustain this rapid growth. In a proportion of adolescents, high levels of physical activity because of participation in games and sports will still further increase needs for energy and perhaps other nutrients. Adolescence is also a time of major psychological changes brought on by the hormonal changes of puberty, and these too may have major effects on children's attitudes to food. Adolescent girls are the most common sufferers from anorexia nervosa. Paradoxically, obesity is also a common nutritional problem of adolescence.

Increasing secretion of sex hormones at puberty produces a major divergence in the body composition of boys and girls. Male sex hormones cause boys to gain more muscle than fat and to adopt a more abdominal distribution of their body fat. Female sex hormones cause girls to gain more fat than muscle and to increase their deposition of fat in the hip and thigh region. This increase in fatness that is a natural part of female adolescence may be an important contributor to the unhealthy preoccupation with body image and dieting experienced by many adolescent girls. Many adolescent girls perceive themselves as 'too fat' when they are not and diet when it is inappropriate. They sometimes adopt unhealthy dietary and other strategies for losing weight, such as fasting, avoidance of meat and other staple foods, and even smoking (e.g. Ryan et al., 1998). Girls need to be better prepared for these physiological changes and be reassured that they are a normal consequence of maturation.

During adolescence, diets that are very low in energy density (e.g. very low in fat and high in fibre) may tend to limit growth. Strict vegetarian diets tend to be bulky and have low energy density; this is indeed often cited as one of their advantages. Vegan children tend to be smaller and lighter than other children (Sanders, 1988). Over-zealous restriction of energy-dense foods by health-conscious middle-class parents may lead to under-nutrition in rapidly growing children (sometimes referred to as 'muesli belt malnutrition').

During the 5-year period of adolescence, boys accumulate an average of around 200 mg/day of calcium in their skeleton with a peak value of about double this average. They also accumulate an average of 0.5 mg/day of iron and 2 g/day of protein. The onset of menstruation represents a further major stress on the iron status of adolescent girls.

Table 16.14 shows some selected DRVs for 11- to 14 year olds and 15- to 18 year olds compared to those for adults. The energy EAR for boys aged 15–18 years is 8 per cent higher than that for adult men despite their smaller size. The calcium RNI is 43 per cent higher for both age groups of boys than that for men and clearly reflects the DRV panel's assumptions of the extra calcium needs required for skeletal growth. This calcium RNI would be difficult to meet without drinking good amounts milk. Similarly, relatively high DRVs for girls compared to women are also shown in this table. Similar trends are also seen in the American RDA; the relative allowance (i.e. allowing for size) is higher in adolescents than in adults. American values for all groups tend to be higher than the corresponding British values. Note particularly that the calcium RDA for both ages of boys and girls is 1300 mg/day (cf. adult value 1000 mg/day); the calcium RDAs for American girls are thus 50 per cent higher than the corresponding UK values.

Table **16.14** Comparison of some UK reference nutrient intakes for adolescent boys and girls with those for adults (figures in parentheses are LRNIs)*

		Age group		
		11–14 years	15–18 years	Adult
Energy EAR (kcal)	Male	2200	2755	2550
	Female	1845	2110	1940
Energy EAR (MJ)	M	9.21	11.51	10.60
	F	7.92	8.83	8.10
Calcium (mg)	M	1000 (480)	1000 (450)	700
	F	800 (450)	800 (480)	700
Iron (mg)	M	11.3 (6.1)	11.3 (6.1)	8.7
	F	14.8 (8.0)	14.8 (8.0)	14.8
Potassium (mg)	M	3100 (1600)	3500 (2000)	3500
	F	3100 (1600)	3500 (2000)	3500
Selenium (mg)	M	45 (25)	70 (40)	75
	F	45 (25)	60 (40)	60
Zinc (mg)	M	9.0 (5.3)	9.5 (5.5)	9.5
	F	9.0 (5.3)	7.0 (4.0)	7.0
Vitamin A (μg)	M	600 (250)	600 (300)	600
	F	600 (250)	600 (250)	600
Riboflavin (mg)	M	1.2 (0.8)	1.3 (0.8)	1.3
	F	1.1 (0.8)	1.1 (0.8)	1.1
Niacin (mg)	M	15 (10)	18 (12)	17
	F	12 (8)	14 (9)	13
Folate (μg)	M	200 (100)	200 (100)	200
	F[1]	200 (100)	200 (100)	200
Vitamin C (mg)	M	35 (9)	40 (10)	40
	F	35 (9)	40 (10)	40

*Data source: COMA (1991).
[1] Women 'at risk' of pregnancy are advised to take 400 μg/day as supplements.
EAR, estimated average requirement.

Table 16.14 also shows the lower RNI for these older children for these nutrients. As discussed in Chapter 13, people with intakes below their LRNI are usually classified as receiving inadequate amounts of that nutrient. In some instances the LRNI is strikingly low, examples being 9–10 mg/day for vitamin C, 250–300 μg/day for vitamin A, 6.1–8 mg/day for iron, 450–480 mg/day for calcium, and 100 μg/day for folate. This makes it particularly disturbing that data presented later in this section will indicate that a substantial number of children have recorded intakes that are below their LRNI for one or more micronutrient.

Data from past UK surveys of children's diets

In a survey of the diets of UK pre-school children (1.5–4.5 years old), Gregory *et al.* (1995) made the following observations.

- Energy intakes of the children were less than the EAR – which was probably because the EARs are set too high.
- The proportion of food energy contributed by the major nutrients was 13 per cent from protein, 51 per cent from carbohydrate and 36 per cent from fat.
- Within the major macronutrient categories, sugars (including milk and fruit sugars) provided 29 per cent of energy, non-milk extrinsic sugars 19 per cent and saturated fat 16 per cent.
- Average intakes of most vitamins and minerals were generally well above the RNI, except for vitamin A, iron and zinc.
- About half of children had intakes of vitamin A that were below the RNI and around 8 per cent below the LRNI.
- A large majority of children had iron intakes below the RNI and a fifth of the very young ones had intakes that were below the LRNI.
- Inadequate iron intakes in many of the sample were confirmed by blood analyses which showed that 10 per cent were anaemic and 20 per cent had less than satisfactory iron stores (serum ferritin <10 μg/L).
- Intakes of vitamin D were under 2 μg/day and this amount is clearly insufficient if children do not get adequate exposure to summer sunlight.

While the macronutrient composition of the diets of UK pre-school children recorded in this survey was close to the guideline values for adults, the levels of added sugars and saturated fat were high. More than half of the added sugar in the diet came from soft drinks and sweets. These are practically devoid of nutrients, lower the overall nutrient density of the diet and are damaging to children's teeth. Milk and milk products provided about 40 per cent of the saturated fat and meat and fish about 15 per cent. Biscuits, cakes, chips and savoury snacks provided 20 per cent of the saturated fat.

The message from this survey is what most parents probably would have guessed. Children's diets would be improved if they consumed fewer sugary drinks, sweets, cakes, biscuits and chips, and ate more fruits, vegetables, lean meat, fish, cereals and boiled potatoes.

COMA (1989b) published a survey conducted in 1983 of the diets of a nationally representative sample of British girls and boys at 10–11 years and 14–15 years. It concluded that the main sources of energy in the diets of British children were bread, chips (French fries), milk, biscuits (cookies), meat products (e.g. sausages, burgers, meat pies), cakes and puddings. These foods together accounted for about half of the total energy intake. Mean recorded energy intakes were within 5 per cent of the EAR for all groups when interpolated from actual recorded body weights.

Fat made up about 38 per cent of total energy intake of these British children, very similar to the adult figure recorded just a few years later by Gregory *et al.* (1990). Three-quarters of all children exceeded the target of 35 per cent of food energy from fat. Surprisingly, meat and meat products contributed less than 15 per cent of the total fat, marginally less than that contributed by chips (French fries) and crisps (potato chips).

Average intakes of all four groups of children exceeded the current RNIs for most of the nutrients surveyed. The two main areas of concern highlighted by this study were:

- average calcium intakes of the older children were about 10 per cent below current RNI (more than 40 per cent of calcium came from milk and cheese)

- iron intakes of the older girls were only 62 per cent of the current RNI and around 60 per cent of girls had iron intakes below the RNI appropriate for the start of menstruation.

The overall impression from this survey of British children was that their diets met most criteria for adequacy, although there are a few areas for concern such as the iron intakes of the adolescent girls. In terms of health education priorities, particularly dietary fats, the diets of children seemed to be, as one might expect, very similar to those of their parents at this time. These general conclusions would probably apply also to most other industrialized countries.

A survey of British children aged 4–18 years was conducted as part of the programme of National Diet and Nutrition Surveys (NDNS) by Gregory *et al.* (2000). Energy intakes recorded in this survey were significantly lower than those recorded 15 years earlier by COMA (1989b), even though the children in the more recent survey were bigger and heavier. This probably reflects the general decline in population activity leading to reduced energy expenditure and higher weight gain despite lower food intake; this is a major factor in the increased levels of overweight and obesity in all age groups. Information collected on activity in those children aged over 7 years indicated that most young people were inactive. Generally, girls were less active than boys and activity tended to fall as children got older. In this survey, 40–50 per cent of the children failed to meet the recommendation that young people should participate in at least moderate activity for an hour each day.

The proportions of energy derived from fat were 35 per cent for boys and 36 per cent for girls, which are close to the recommended value of 35 per cent. This suggests that the proportion of fat in children's diets had dropped in the couple of decades after COMA (1989b) was completed, which is true also of adult diets (see Chapter 12). Saturated fat intakes at around 14.2 per cent of energy were above the recommended 11 per cent. Intakes of non-milk extrinsic sugars were 16.5 per cent of energy compared to the recommended 11 per cent, with fizzy drinks and chocolate confectionery being the main sources of these added sugars.

Although average intakes of most nutrients were above the RNI, a number of problems with the micronutrient intakes were highlighted by the survey, some of which are listed below.

- Average intakes of vitamin A were close to the RNI in younger children but below it in older children. Around 20 per cent of older girls and 12 per cent of older boys had intakes that were below the LRNI.
- A fifth of older girls had inadequate riboflavin intake.
- Biochemical evidence of poor vitamin D status was found in 13 per cent of 11- to 18 year olds, with a higher proportion in winter samples.
- Biochemical evidence of poor nutritional status in some individuals was also found for thiamin, riboflavin, folate and vitamin C.
- There were substantial numbers of children with mineral intakes that were below the LRNI: for zinc in all groups; for potassium, magnesium and calcium in older children; and for iron in older girls.
- Some 50 per cent of older girls had an iron intake below the LRNI. Low serum ferritin levels, indicating low iron stores, were found in 27 per cent of girls and 13 per cent of boys.

It was noted in Chapter 13, when discussing adults' micronutrient intakes, that even where average intakes appear satisfactory there may still be many individuals with unsatisfactory intakes and/or biochemical indications of poor nutrient status. About 20 per cent of the children sampled by Gregory *et al.* (2000) reported that they took a micronutrient supplement. About 10 per cent of girls in the 15- to 18-year age band were vegetarian and about 16 per cent were dieting (comparable figures for boys were, respectively, 1 and 3 per cent). Those children with lower socioeconomic status tended to have lower quality diets as indicated by lower recorded intakes of many nutrients and lower biochemical status for several vitamins and for iron.

Data from the newer rolling NDNS programme

Up to 2001, the NDNS survey programme used large representative samples of people from specific age groupings at intervals of some years between samplings for each age group. In 2006, the new rolling programme of surveys was commissioned in which people of all age groups from 1.5 years upwards are surveyed annually in a combined sample with much smaller numbers in each age group than in previous surveys. Further details of the new methodology are discussed in Chapter 3.

The first data were collected in 2008–9 and a limited amount published by Bates *et al.* (2010). A considerable amount was not published because at this stage the sample sizes were considered too small. Direct comparisons have not been made between this survey and earlier surveys because of the small sample sizes and differences in the collection period (4 days, compared with 7 days in earlier surveys). Detailed comparisons with earlier surveys can be found in Bates *et al.* (2010), although they do warn about not assuming that recorded differences between this and past surveys are 'significant'.

The next three tables presented here show selected data from this survey in which the diets and nutrient intakes of children split into three age bands are compared with those of people aged 16–64 years. Most of the figures in these tables are for the two sexes combined, although female-only data are shown where the two sexes diverge substantially.

- Table 16.15 shows the total energy intakes of the four age groups, the contribution of selected macronutrients to the food energy intake (to minimize the distorting effects of alcohol), and the contribution made by particular foods to total energy intake. Average energy intakes for all groups were significantly below the EAR and this is a common finding in surveys of this type. The diets of children generally had slightly less protein and more carbohydrates than those of adults; in the older age groups the higher carbohydrate intake was due to higher intake of added sugars. Average fat intakes were below the adult target vale of 35 per cent of food energy for the three age groups of children. The saturated fatty acid intake of younger children was higher than that of adults, but this was due to their higher intake of dairy foods, especially whole milk. Its temporary effect on saturated fatty acid intakes is no reason to discourage this relatively high use of milk and dairy foods – and especially whole milk – in younger children. Older children consumed more soft drinks, savoury snacks, chocolate and confectionery than adults and this accounted for about twice the proportion of their energy intake compared to adults.

Table 16.15 Comparison of the macronutrient composition of the diets of children and adults and the contribution of selected food groups to total energy intake (values in parentheses are for females only)*

	Age group (years)			
	1.5–3	**4–10**	**11–18**	**19–64**
Total energy (MJ)	4.79	6.56	8.07 (7.02)	8.19 (6.92)
(kcal)	1136	1558	1917 (1668)	1949 (1645)
Percentage of food energy from:				
Protein	15.4	14.5	14.6	17.6
Fat	34.3	34.5	35.0	35.1
Saturated fatty acids	15.0	13.6	12.9	12.8
Carbohydrate	50.3	51.0	50.3	47.3
NMES	11.2	14.5	15.7	12.5
NSP (g)	8.2	10.8	11.9	14.0
Percentage contribution to total energy intake:				
Cereal products	29	35	33	28
Dairy products	26	15	9	9
Whole milk	11	3	1	1
Meat and products	10	14	17	18
Vegetables and potatoes	8	10	11	12
Potato foods	5	7	9	7
Fruits	6	3	2	3
Soft drinks	2	3	5	2
Savoury snacks	2	3	4	2
Confectionery (incl. chocolate)	3	5	4	2

*Data source: Bates *et al.* (2011).
NMES, non-milk extrinsic sugars; NSP, non-starch polysaccharide.

- Table 16.16 shows that, for both adults and children, average intakes of vitamins were above the RNI; and only for two vitamins in the oldest

children, folate and vitamin A (especially girls), were average intakes within 20 per cent of the RNI. While there is no RNI for vitamin D for any of these age groups, the recorded intakes in all groups were clearly insufficient to meet the needs for this vitamin (>10μg/day) if there is not adequate exposure of the skin to summer sunlight. The average mineral intakes shown in Table 16.16 are much less satisfactory than those for vitamins. In the 11- to 18 year olds, average intakes of iron (especially girls), calcium, magnesium, potassium, selenium, iodine and zinc were all below the RNIs. This low average intake of a number of minerals is also seen in adults, especially in younger women (discussed in Chapter 13). The iron intake of the youngest

Table 16.16 Comparison of vitamin and mineral intakes from food sources of children and adults, expressed as a percentage of the reference nutrient intake (RNI) (values in parentheses are for females only)*

Nutrient	Age (years)			
	1.5–3 (%)	**4–10 (%)**	**11–18 (%)**	**19–64 (%)**
Vitamin A	139	131	112 (103)	163
Thiamin	186	182	170	167
Riboflavin	240	162	127	136
Niacin	244	233	238	263
Vitamin B$_6$	204	183	191	185
Vitamin B$_{12}$	786	431	325	369
Folate	223	157	113	140
Vitamin C	246	275	224	235
Iron	89	115	79 (58)	111 (82)
Calcium	220	115	90	118
Magnesium	180	121	75	93
Potassium	226	141	73	83
Selenium	163	132	76	73
Iodine	215	133	99	122
Zinc	104	95	91	109
Vitamin D	2.0μg	2.0μg	2.3μg	2.9μμg

* Data source: Bates *et al.* (2011).

children was also below the RNI and is consistent with their high intake of cow milk and relatively low intake of meat.

- Table 16.17 shows the percentage of children and adults whose recorded intake of selected micronutrients was below the LRNI (i.e. classified as having inadequate intakes). Significant numbers of the oldest children had inadequate intakes of several vitamins, especially vitamin A and riboflavin, and for all of the minerals listed quite a high proportion had intakes below the LRNI. While the values for the oldest children shown in this table look substantially worse than those for adults, it should be remembered that in earlier surveys (discussed in Chapter 13) the micronutrient intakes of 19- to 24 year old adults tended to be the lowest and this trend was particularly marked in young women.

Table 16.17 Percentage of adults and children whose food intake of selected vitamins and minerals is below the lower reference nutrient intake (LRNI) (figures in parentheses are for females only)*

	Age (years)			
	1.3–3 (%)	4–10 (%)	11–18 (%)	19–64 (%)
Vitamin A	5	3	11	8
Riboflavin	0	0	7	7
Folate	0	0	4	2
Vitamin C	0	0	2	1
Iron	6	1	26 (46)	11 (21)
Calcium	0	1	9	6
Magnesium	0	2	36 (46)	10
Potassium	0	0	22 (30)	15 (21)
Zinc	3	7	13 (15)	6
Selenium	0	1	33 (46)	37
Iodine	0	2	9 (16)	6

*Data source: Bates *et al.* (2010).

Supplement use recorded by Bates *et al.* (2010) was slightly lower in the two youngest age groups and much lower in the oldest children. Just 7 per cent of 11- to 18 year olds used some supplement during the recording period, compared with 24 per cent of adults.

Key points

- Children need enough dietary energy and nutrients to allow them to grow and develop properly.
- Young children need proportionately much more energy than adults and so good energy density is still an important priority.
- Inactivity is a major cause of child obesity.
- Diets that are adequate for adults should be adequate for growing children if they meet their energy requirements.
- Adolescence is an intensely anabolic period and there are substantial increases in body weight, body protein and body calcium content.
- At puberty, boys increase their lean:fat ratio.
- Female sex hormones cause a substantial increase in the body fat content of girls, particularly increases in fat around the hips and thighs. Girls who are unprepared for these pubertal increases in body fat may be encouraged to diet inappropriately and to adopt unhealthy practices to try to lose weight.
- Average energy intakes of British children are generally significantly below their EARs.
- Children generally get less of their energy from protein and more from carbohydrates than adults. In older children the higher carbohydrate content is due to a higher intake of added sugars.
- All groups of children get just under 35 per cent of their food energy from fat. This represents a significant improvement for older children, similar to that seen in adult diets over recent decades.
- The relatively high intake of saturated fatty acids seen in younger children is due to their higher intake of dairy foods and particularly of whole milk.
- The relatively high intake of dairy products and whole milk is a positive factor despite its temporary effect on saturated fatty acid intakes.
- British children should consume fewer sugary drinks, sweets, cakes, biscuits and chips but more fruit/vegetables, lean meat, cereals and potatoes.
- Average intakes of all vitamins for children are above their RNIs.

→

- Substantial numbers of individual children have inadequate intakes of vitamin A (especially those aged 11–18 years) and, in the oldest children, of riboflavin, folate and vitamin C.
- British children need regular exposure to summer sunlight to achieve satisfactory vitamin D status. Past surveys have found biochemical evidence of poor vitamin D status in many British children.
- Average intakes of minerals are at or below the RNIs for all minerals shown in Table 16.16, and the iron intakes of younger children are less than the RNI.
- Past surveys of children have also reported frequent occurrence of depleted iron stores and even anaemia in all age groups of children.
- Although the prevalence of micronutrient inadequacies appears to be higher in 11- to 18 year olds than in adults, previous surveys of adults have found lower micronutrient intakes in the 19–24 year age band, especially in women in this age group.

THE ELDERLY

Demographic and social trends

Much of this section is based on updated material from the first chapter of Webb and Copeman (1996).

Table 16.18 gives an approximate breakdown of the proportion of the population of England and Wales in various age bands. The proportion of elderly people in the populations of industrialized countries rose substantially during the twentieth century and is projected to continue rising. At the start of the new millennium, around 16 per cent of the population of England and Wales were over 65 years and almost 2 per cent were over 85. There are now well over a million people aged over 85 in England and Wales compared with not much more than half a million in 1981. At the start of the twentieth century, life expectancy at birth was around 47 years in both the UK and USA but had

risen to well over 76 years by the end of the century. In 1901, only 4.7 per cent of the population of England and Wales were over 65 years. The increase in life expectancy during the twentieth century has not been confined to the younger age groups.

Table 16.18 Percentage of the population of England and Wales in various age bands from the 2001 census

Age band	Percentage of total[1]
0–14 (children)	18.9
15–44 (young adults)	41.3
45–64 (middle-aged)	23.8
65+ (elderly adults)	16.0
65–74	8.39
75–84	5.64
85–89	1.30
90+	0.65

[1] Total population of 52.0 million.

- Between 1901 and 1991, the life expectancy of a 1 year old rose from 55 to 76 years (38 per cent increase).
- Expectancy for a 60 year old increased from 14 to 19 more years (36 per cent)
- Expectancy for a 75 year old increased from 7.5 to 10.5 more years (40 per cent).

In England and Wales in 2008–10, the life expectancy at birth was 78.5 years for males and 82.5 years for females and at 65 years it was a further 18.2 years for men and 20.8 years for women. Comparison with the figures in Table 16.19 for 2001 shows that life expectancy is still increasing and that there is perhaps a slight narrowing of the difference between men and women.

The ratio of females to males in the elderly population increases progressively with age, so in the over-85s there are three times as many women as men. In 2001, men made up about 48 per cent of 65- to 69 year olds, about 37 per cent of 80- to 84 year olds and just 23 per cent of those over 90 years.

By 2026, the over-65s are expected to represent 19 per cent of the UK population and the over-85s almost 2.5 per cent. In the USA in 1990, about 13 per cent of the population were over 65 and this

Table **16.19** Comparison of estimates of life expectancy, healthy life expectancy and life expectancy without disability in England in 2001, at birth and at age 65 years*

	Males (years)	Females (years)
Life expectancy at birth	76.0	80.7
Life expectancy at 65 years	16.1	19.2
Healthy life expectancy:		
At birth	69.1	72.3
At 65 years	12.5	14.7
Life expectancy without disability:		
At birth	61.7	64.2
At 65 years	8.1	9.1

*Data source: www.data4nr.net/resources/older-people.

proportion is projected to rise to around 22 per cent by 2040.

A third of the over-65s in England and Wales live alone, and this proportion increases markedly with advancing age as a result of the deaths of spouses. In 2001, 70 per cent of men and 63 per cent of women aged 65–69 years were living as a couple, but these figures decreased to 49 and 25 per cent, respectively, in the 80- to 84 year olds, and to 14 and just 7 per cent in those aged over 90 years.

The number of people living in residential homes for the elderly increased from around 150 000 in 1977 to around 374 000 in 2001, and this later figure represents over 0.7 per cent of the total population of England and Wales. The chance of an elderly person living in care accommodation rises steeply with age, and the increase in the number of people living in care accommodation is entirely due to increases in the size of the elderly and very-elderly population. In 2001, the proportions of older people recorded as living in some form of communal establishment were:

- <1 per cent of 65- to 69 year olds
- 3 per cent of 75- to 79 year olds
- 14 per cent of 85- to 89 year olds (9.5 per cent of men)
- 31 per cent of those aged over 90 years (20 per cent of men).

Very elderly women were more likely than men to live in a residential home, which increases still further the female to male ratio of the population in residential homes.

Catering for the dietary and nutritional needs of the elderly is thus a topic that should warrant an increased educational and research priority.

In the previous edition of this book, data from 1992 suggested that many elderly people in the UK spent their last years of life in relative poverty compared to younger adults. Data for 2008–9, summarized from official sources on The Poverty Site (www.poverty.org.uk/64/index.shtml), suggest that the economic position of the elderly population in the UK has since improved relative to other UK adults. About 1.2 million pensioners in the UK have no other income than their state pension and other state benefits; that is, about 18 per cent of single pensioners and 6 per cent of couples. The proportion of pensioners living in households classified as 'low income' (i.e. below 60 per cent of median income after deducting housing costs) has fallen sharply since 2000, and this fall has been particularly marked among single pensioners. In 2000–1, 21 per cent of pensioner couples and 35 per cent of single pensioners were in this low-income category, but by 2008–9 these figures had fallen to 15 and 18 per cent, respectively. Pensioners are now less likely to be in this category than working-age families, especially single-parent families. Pensioners who are over 75 years are more likely to be in the low-income category partly because more of them are now single after the death of a spouse. Relatively few pensioners have very low incomes (i.e. below 40 per cent of median income). Removing housing costs considerably improves the comparative position of pensioners compared to working-age adults because many pensioners own their own houses without a mortgage to repay.

More than half of all the over-65s report being affected by some longstanding health issue, and the proportion rises to around 72 per cent of the over-85s. Bone and joint diseases, including arthritis and rheumatism, are the most common longstanding conditions. Other important causes of longstanding illness include heart diseases, hypertension, respiratory diseases like bronchitis and emphysema, stroke and diabetes. Ageing inevitably leads to increasing rates of mortality, morbidity and disability. Despite this, the majority of elderly people consider themselves to be in good or fairly good general health. In 2001, about 80 per cent of men and women aged over 65 years perceived their own health as good or fairly good, and even in the over-85s only around 34 per cent described their health as 'not good'. This suggests that some level of disability is seen by elderly people as being inevitable and does not stop many of them from perceiving their overall health as good. More than 80 per cent of elderly people still report seeing friends or relatives at least once a week, and even in the over-85s this figure is still around 75 per cent. More than 95 per cent of the over-65s still live either in their own home or with their family.

As average life expectancy starts to approach its inevitable plateau, so improving the quality of life of the elderly population has become an increasing priority for health education in industrialized countries. A major goal in the USA is to 'increase the span of healthy life for Americans'. Similarly, in England the aim is not only to reduce premature deaths and 'add years to life' but also to 'add life to years' by increasing the years that are free from ill-health and minimizing the adverse effects of illness and disability.

Bebbington (1988) calculated 'the expectation of life without disability' from self-reported rates of disability and longstanding illness recorded in the British General Household Survey together with estimates of the numbers of people living in institutions for the 'disabled'. Although total life expectancy in the UK increased over the period 1976 to 1988 (from 70 to 72.4 years in men and from 76.1 to 78.1 in women), the 'expectation of life without disability' remained essentially unchanged. Over this same period the years of illness and disability increased by 2.1 years in men and 2.5 years in women. The main effect of the increases in life expectancy was to increase the number of years spent suffering from illness and disability. A similar study in the USA (Crimmins *et al.*, 1989) concluded that, between 1970 and 1980, increases in life expectancy were largely concentrated in years with a chronic disabling illness. Table 16.19 shows more recent figures for estimates of life expectancy, life expectancy free of disability and healthy life expectancy at birth and at 65 years in English men and women. These figures

show that only about half of the years of life expectancy of 65 year olds are healthy and disability-free years.

A good diet and an active lifestyle would contribute both to increasing total lifespan and to compressing the years of morbidity and disability at the end of the lifespan.

Key points

- Improved life expectancy during the twentieth century caused large increases in the proportion of elderly and very elderly people in the populations of industrialized countries.
- By the year 2001, 16 per cent of British people were aged over 65 years and around 2 per cent over 85 years.
- Not only are more people surviving to 65 years, but elderly people are also living longer.
- Women greatly outnumber men in the older age groups.
- Many elderly people in the UK live alone or in care accommodation and the proportions increase sharply with age.
- The proportion of elderly pensioners classified as 'low income' has decreased sharply in the UK in recent years. They are now less likely to be in this category than families with children, especially single-parent families.
- Few pensioners are classified as having a very low income, indicating that welfare payments to older people seem to be achieving their objective of preventing poverty.
- Many elderly people are affected by some longstanding disease, but this does not prevent most of them perceiving their general health as good or fairly good.
- Some increase in life expectancy in recent decades in the UK and USA has been achieved at the cost of more years spent with an illness or disability. Improving the quality of life in the later years, rather than simply increasing life expectancy, is now being given a higher priority in health promotion.
- A good diet and an active lifestyle should help to improve life expectancy and compress the period of chronic morbidity at the end of life.

The effects of ageing

Ageing is characterized by a gradual decline in the ability of an organism to adapt to environmental stresses and an inability to maintain homeostasis. This results in increasing mortality rates, increased morbidity and higher rates of disability. There is measurable age-related deterioration in the functioning of most systems of the body.

Ageing of the immune system leads to a decline in the efficiency of the immune surveillance and defensive mechanisms, resulting in higher incidences of infection, autoimmune disease and cancer. Shrinking or involution of the thymus gland is one of the most obvious age-related changes in the immune system, and this is coupled with a reduced capacity to produce naive T-lymphocytes which react to a new infective agent. There is also a reduced T-cell response to previously encountered infective agents. There is an age-related decline in function of natural killer (NK) cells which secrete cytokines that kill other cells, and this reduces the response to viruses and to cancer cells. Impaired functioning of B-lymphocytes also occurs in older people and this reduces their ability to produce antibodies, and older people respond less well to vaccination than younger people. There is, however, increased production of auto-antibodies that attack the person's own body, so the prevalence and severity of autoimmune conditions both increase with age. There is dysregulation of inflammatory responses – a reduced ability to mount an acute inflammatory response which plays an important role in wound healing and responses to infection. In contrast to this, older people have higher circulating levels of certain inflammation-provoking cytokines, which makes them more susceptible to conditions where chronic inflammation plays an aetiological role, including atherosclerosis, cancer and osteoporosis. These age-related changes make older people:

- more susceptible to infective agents
- less able to detect and destroy cancer cells
- less able to mount a protective immune response to vaccination
- more likely to suffer adverse effects of autoimmune tissue damage and chronic inflammation.

Malnutrition has similar deleterious effects on the immune system (see Chapter 17). Malnutrition could compound with the effects of ageing in depressing the immune function of elderly, malnourished people.

The absorptive area of the small intestine decreases with age, so it is likely that the absorption of several nutrients decreases. Deterioration is usually earliest and fastest in those systems where there is no replacement of dead cells (e.g. brain, muscle and heart) than in those where continual replacement occurs (e.g. red cells and intestinal epithelium). Generally, complex functions involving coordination are more affected than simple ones; for example, reaction time increases more rapidly than the slowing in nerve conduction velocity.

There is a marked change in body composition with age: the proportions of lean tissue and bone decline and the proportion of fat increases. There is also a loss of height from about 30 years. There is a decline in the basal metabolic rate (BMR), which is probably linked to the decline in lean body mass because, when the BMR is expressed per kilogram of lean body mass, there is no decline with age.

The speed of homeostatic regulation is reduced as people become elderly. Some examples are given below.

- In response to cold stress, old people tend to start shivering later and in response to heat stress they sweat later. Old people are also more susceptible to hypothermia because of their reduced BMR and their reduced levels of physical activity.
- There is slower restoration of acid–base balance if it is disturbed. Elderly people have reduced buffering capacity, a diminished respiratory response to acid–base disturbance. and a reduced ability to eliminate excess acid or base via the kidneys.
- There is a decline in the efficiency of the mechanisms regulating salt and water balance. For example, there is an age-related decline in the acuity of the thirst mechanisms. Rolls and Phillips (1990) found that, immediately after a period of water deprivation, elderly men drank much less than younger men and experienced much less thirst even though their levels of dehydration were similar.

Key points

- All body systems deteriorate during ageing and there are increasing rates of mortality, morbidity and disability.
- There is an age-related decline in certain measures of immune function:
  - involution of the thymus
  - reduced production of naive T-lymphocytes that respond to new infective agents
  - reduced functioning of natural killer (NK) cells which kill virus-infected and cancer cells
  - reduced production of antibodies by B-lymphocytes, which means elderly people have a reduced response to vaccination
  - increased production of auto-antibodies, increasing autoimmune damage to cells and tissues
  - a reduced acute inflammatory response, which adversely affects wound healing and responses to infections
  - higher circulating levels of pro-inflammatory cytokines, which makes elderly people more prone to diseases like cancer and atherosclerosis where chronic inflammation has an aetiological role.
- The proportions of muscle and bone in the adult body decrease with age and the proportion of fat increases.
- The loss of lean tissue in the elderly leads to a fall in basal metabolic rate.
- Ageing is characterized by a reduced speed of homeostatic regulation and a reduced ability to adapt to environmental changes.

Nutritional requirements of the elderly

Energy expenditure (and therefore energy requirement too) falls as people become elderly. The two factors listed below are thought to be responsible for this.

- Levels of physical activity decline. This may be accelerated by retirement and is inevitable in those who are housebound or bedridden.
- Basal metabolic rate decreases. This is due to the decline in lean body mass, which might itself be largely a consequence of muscle wasting due to reduced levels of physical activity.

Table 16.20 shows the UK EARs and the American dietary reference intakes for energy for age categories of men and women. These standards represent quite substantial reductions in the estimated energy requirements – and therefore likely total food intake – of elderly people, particularly men. The UK values for younger adults are set by multiplying the calculated average BMR by a multiple of 1.4 (the *physical activity level*, PAL) whereas that for older adults is set using a PAL multiple of 1.5. This is despite clear evidence that physical activity decreases in the elderly. The rationale for this decision is discussed in Chapter 7. The US standards clearly acknowledge the decline in average energy requirements with age because the standards drop by 10 kcal/day for men and 7 kcal/day for women for each year after the age of 19 years.

Table 16.20 UK and US dietary reference values for energy in older adults

Age (years)	Men		Women	
	kcal	MJ	kcal	MJ
United Kingdom (EAR)				
19–50	2550	10.60	1940	8.10
51–59	2550	10.60	1900	8.00
60–64	2380	9.93	1900	7.99
65–74	2330	9.71	1900	7.96
75+	2100	8.77	1810	7.61
United States[1]				
20	3075	12.78	2396	10.02
40	2857	11.94	2256	9.43
60	2657	11.10	2116	8.84
80	2457	10.27	1976	8.26

[1] Note that the dietary reference intakes are listed for healthy and moderately active Americans and Canadians at 19 years and then 10 kcal/day subtracted for each year for males and 7 kcal/day for females.

Table 16.21 summarizes differences between the dietary standards for elderly people and those for younger adults. For nutrients not listed in the table the values for younger and older adults are the same. Although energy requirements and total food intakes tend to fall in the elderly, Table 16.21 suggests that there is no corresponding decrease in the requirement for most other nutrients.

Table 16.21 UK and US differences between dietary reference values for elderly and younger adults (for other nutrients the values are the same)

Nutrient	United Kingdom RNIs			
	Male (years)		Female (years)	
	19–50	50+	19–50	50+
Protein (g)	55.5	53.3	45.0	46.5
Thiamin (mg)	1.0	0.9	–	–
Niacin (mg)	17	16	13	12
Vitamin D (μg)[1]	0	10	0	10
Iron (mg)	–	–	14.8	8.7

Nutrient	United States RDAs			
	31–50 years	51–70 years	70+ years	
	M/F	M/F	M/F	
Vitamin D (μg)[2]	15/15	15/15	20/20	
Vitamin B_6 (mg)	1.3/1.3	1.7/1.5	1.7/1.5	
Calcium (mg)	1000/1000	1200/1200	1200/1200	
Iron (mg)	8/18	8/8	8/8	
Chromium (μg)	35/25	30/20	30/20	

[1] RNI applies after 65 years.
[2] In the absence of adequate sunlight exposure.

The UK RNIs for the elderly suggest small reductions in the RNI for:

- protein in men – due entirely to differences in the assumed body weight of young and elderly men
- thiamin and niacin – which are set according to the assumed energy expenditure
- a substantial reduction in the female RNI for iron – which reflects the cessation of menstrual blood losses. (The American standards for iron in elderly women are also reduced to the same as those for men.)

In young adults, endogenous production of vitamin D in the skin is the primary source of the vitamin. The UK RNI for vitamin D in older adults shown in Table 16.21 reflects the view that endogenous production can no longer be relied on in elderly people who may be housebound and inadequately exposed to sunlight. In the USA there is also an RDA of 10μg/day set for those aged 51–70 years (none for those aged 30–50) which rises to 15μg/day for the over-70s. Poor vitamin D status is identified in Chapter 15 as a major aetiological factor for osteoporosis in the very elderly.

The US standards also suggest a substantial increase in vitamin B_6 requirement in the elderly and a 200mg/day increase in the calcium requirement which, in younger adults, is already well above the UK RNI. The UK dietary standards for older adults have often been set at the same value as for younger adults because at the time they were set (1991) there was a lack of data on how nutrient requirements change with ageing. It now seems probable that requirements for some nutrients (e.g. calcium and vitamins B_6 and B_{12}) may increase in the elderly and that reduced efficiency of absorption in the gut may affect requirements more generally. The raised American standards for calcium and vitamin B_6 have occurred relatively recently and may reflect this change in attitude.

Thus elderly people are perceived as requiring intakes of most nutrients that are similar to, or higher than, those for other adults but requiring average intakes of energy up to 20 per cent lower than those of other adults.

For many elderly people, the real fall in energy expenditure and food intake may be even greater than the figures in Table 16.20 suggest. COMA

(1992) suggested that for many inactive elderly people who spend only an hour a day on their feet, a multiple of 1.3 times BMR would represent their balance rather than the 1.5 times BMR used to set the EARs in COMA (1991). Of course, if very elderly people are losing weight then they are not even eating enough to maintain energy balance. This increases the risk that energy intakes can be met without fulfilling the requirements for all other nutrients. This risk increases if the nutrient density of the diet is low, perhaps if a substantial proportion of the energy is obtained from nutrient-depleted sources such as fatty or sugary foods or from alcohol. Energy intakes may be so low in many elderly people that it becomes difficult to obtain good intake of the other nutrients without substantial alterations in the nature of the diet. Elderly people, or those responsible for providing meals for the elderly, were advised in COMA (1992) to ensure that their diet is of high nutrient density so that adequate intakes of the other nutrients can be maintained despite a considerable decline in total food intake. They concluded that the general dietary guidelines suggesting limiting non-milk extrinsic sugars to 10 per cent of energy might be especially appropriate for older people to ensure a high nutrient density of their diets. This expert group also suggested that intakes of these sugars in elderly people tended to be at the top end of the UK range, although this is not supported by recent survey data (presented later in Table 16.23).

Key points

- Energy requirements fall in the elderly owing to the combined effects of reduced activity and lower BMR. In elderly immobile people, energy expenditure may be as low as 1.3 times BMR.
- There is no fall in the estimated requirement for most nutrients to compensate for the fall in energy needs and food intake.
- The iron needs of elderly women are reduced substantially because menstruation has ceased.
- Elderly housebound people are unlikely to obtain sufficient vitamin D from their diet and should either take supplements or ensure exposure to summer sunlight.   →

Key points *continued*

- Very low energy requirements mean that the nutrient density of the diet needs to be good.
- The need for some nutrients probably increases in the elderly (e.g. due to reduced absorption) and this is reflected in the recent substantial increase in vitamin B_6 and calcium standards for older people in the USA.

The diets and nutritional status of elderly people

Historical surveys

A survey of 750 elderly people living in the UK in the late 1960s (DHSS, 1972) indicated that only around 3 per cent of the surveyed population were suffering from malnutrition, and that in the great majority of cases malnutrition was associated with some precipitating medical condition. Around half of this population were reassessed in 1972, by which time they were all aged over 70 years (DHSS, 1979). In this second survey the prevalence of malnutrition was found to be around 7 per cent but twice as high as this in the over-80s. Once again, most of the nutritional deficiencies were related to some underlying disease; certain social factors were also identified as being associated with the risk of malnutrition in the elderly, such as being housebound and having a low income. According to this survey, the diets of elderly British people were in their general nature very similar to those of other adults.

The general impression created by the results of these early surveys was that if elderly people have good general health, are reasonably mobile and affluent then they tend to have few specific nutritional problems. However, as people get older they are more likely to suffer from a medical condition that predisposes to a nutritional problem. The elderly are also more likely to be affected by a range of social factors that were associated with higher risk of nutritional inadequacies, such as:

- immobility and being housebound
- social isolation
- recent bereavement and depression
- low income
- living alone

- low social class
- low mental test score.

Finch *et al.* (1998) conducted a dietary and nutritional survey of a representative sample of British over-65s that included both free-living elderly people and those living in care accommodation. Some results from this survey are still used in the following analysis even though the data were collected in the early 1990s. The precise numerical values may have changed, but the data from this large sample of both institutionalized and free-living elderly people may still usefully demonstrate some points (e.g. the higher energy intakes of very elderly people living in residential homes compared to those catering for themselves).

Some data were released in 2011 from the first 2 years of the rolling NDNS programme (Bates *et al.*, 2011), and this contained some dietary information about adults aged 65 years or over. Data from the first release did not include elderly people because the sample size was not large enough, and even this latest release did not contain blood analysis data for the over-65s. Also, adults are separated into just two age bands (19–64 years and ≥65 years) and the data do not include a separate category of elderly people living in care accommodation.

Energy and macronutrients

Table 16.22 shows the average energy intakes recorded for various age groups of men and women living independently and living in care accommodation, from Finch *et al.* (1998), and shows for comparison that recorded about 5 years later in adults aged 19–64 years, from Hoare *et al.* (2004).

For the elderly people who were living independently, energy intakes were significantly lower than those of younger adults and dropped progressively with age in both sexes. The average intakes of those living in care accommodation were significantly higher than those of similar age living independently. In women, the average for those aged 65–84 years and living in care accommodation was actually higher than that for all other categories, including those aged 19–64 years. These latter figures may indicate that perhaps problems with obtaining or preparing food depress the intakes of very elderly free-living people and they might eat more if it were

Table 16.22 Average recorded energy intakes (MJ) for different age groups of British adults*

Age group (years)	Free-living		Institutionalized	
	Men	**Women**	**Men**	**Women**
19–64	9.72	6.87		
65–74	8.21	6.07		
75–84	7.75	5.88		
65–84			7.99	6.77
85+	7.20	5.77	8.22	7.14
More recent limited data from Bates *et al.* (2011)				
19–64 (kcal)	9.24 (2200)	6.88 (1638)		
65+ (kcal)	8.30 (1976)	6.39 (1522)		

*Data for 16–64 years from Hoare *et al.* (2004) and that for older adults from Finch *et al.* (1998).

easily available to them. Table 16.22 also shows recorded energy intakes of adults aged under and over 65 years from the first 2 years of the new rolling NDNS programme (Bates *et al.*, 2011), which confirms the reduced intakes of older adults; men aged over 65 years consume about 225 kcal (*c*1 MJ) per day less than men aged 19–64 years.

Table 16.23 compares the sources of energy for people aged 65 years and over with adults aged 16–64 years, as recorded in Bates *et al.* (2011). In terms of macronutrient composition, the diets of elderly people had higher contributions of fat and saturated fatty acids, and at 36.4 and 14.4 per cent these were substantially above the recommended levels of 35 per cent and 11 per cent, respectively. These differences in dietary fat content are because fat spreads and foods from the milk group contributed more to the energy supply in older adults, with much greater use of butter and whole milk. Elderly people obtained less of their energy from non-milk extrinsic sugars and their average contribution to food energy was close to the recommended 11 per cent of food energy; this is consistent with their reduced consumption of sugars, preserves, confectionery and non-alcoholic drinks. The average contribution of alcoholic drinks in older adults was just over half that of younger adults.

In the extensive survey of the elderly of Finch *et al.* (1998), about two-thirds of the free-living sample

Table 16.23 Comparison of the macronutrient and food sources of energy recorded in samples of British adults*

	Age group (years)	
	16–64 years	65+ years
Percentage contribution to food energy		
Protein	17.5	17.4
Fat	34.8	36.4
Saturated fatty acids	12.8	14.4
Carbohydrate	47.7	46.2
Non-milk extrinsic sugars	12.6	11.1
Percentage contribution to total energy intake		
Cereal foods	29	30
Milk and milk products	9	12
Whole milk	1	2
Fat spreads	3	5
Butter	1	3
Meat, fish, eggs	22	23
Fruits and vegetables (incl. potatoes)	14	15
Sugars, preserves, beverages (not alcohol), savoury snacks	11	9
Alcoholic drinks	7	4

*Data source: Bates et al. (2011).

and just under half of the institutional sample were overweight or obese (BMI <25). About 16 per cent of the institutionalized sample were underweight (BMI >20), as were 3 per cent of the free-living men and 6 per cent of the women. The proportions of those who were overweight and those who were obese declined markedly with age in both sexes in the free-living sample and for women also in the institutionalized sample; for institutionalized men the proportion who were overweight increased between the two age bands (65–84 and ≥85 years) but the proportion who were obese decreased.

Table 16.24 summarizes the latest and limited anthropometric data for older people from the NDNS rolling programme (Bates et al., 2011). More older adults are overweight and obese than their younger counterparts, and 84 per cent of older men and 67 per cent of older women are either overweight or obese. The prevalence of underweight looks lower than that recorded by Finch et al. (1998), although the criterion for being underweight has now been reduced to <18.5 kg/m². The majority of elderly people had high levels of abdominal adiposity and exceeded the threshold values for waist circumference for their sex (see Chapter 3). Bates et al. (2011) do not give values for different age bands in the large over-65s category, nor do they give values for the institutionalized elderly. The implications of being overweight and underweight for elderly people are discussed in the next section.

Table 16.24 Percentages of men and women who are underweight, overweight and obese and have a raised waist-to-hip ratio (WHR) or a raised waist circumference*

	Age group (years)			
	Men		Women	
	16–64	65+	16–64	65+
Underweight	1	–	2	1
Overweight	41	54	30	32
Obese	27	31	26	34
Overweight or obese	68	84	55	67
Raised WHR	35	70	29	63
Raised waist circumference	34	66	42	57

*Data source: Bates et al. (2011).

Average intakes of all vitamins recorded by Bates et al. (2011) for the over-65s were well above the RNI, with the exception of vitamin D (33 per cent of the 10 μg/day RNI). This is consistent with the general finding that British diets overall do not contain enough vitamin D without exposure of the skin to summer sunlight or the use of supplements. In general, average intakes of minerals were a higher proportion of the RNI than in younger adults ,with only magnesium and selenium below the RNI. Average intakes of older women were above the RNI for iron compared to only 79 per cent of the RNI in younger women because the RNI for iron is reduced in post-menopausal women.

Relatively fewer elderly people were found to have intakes of micronutrients that were below the LRNI, and estimates of the percentages below the LRNIs for selected micronutrients from food sources are listed here:

- vitamin C – 1 per cent
- iodine – 1 per cent
- vitamin A – 2 per cent
- riboflavin – 2 per cent
- iron – 2 per cent
- calcium – 2 per cent
- folate – 3 per cent
- zinc – 5 per cent
- potassium – 15 per cent
- selenium – 42 per cent.

Bates *et al.* (2011) also list the values for total intakes including supplements, and only one value is different from those listed above (the value for selenium falls slightly to 41 per cent). This illustrates the point that dietary supplements are taken by those who need them least; and, although they increase average intakes, they make almost no difference to the number of people whose intake is deemed to be inadequate. This is despite the fact that 37 per cent of older adults recorded using some type of dietary supplement compared to 25 per cent of those aged 19–64 years

Back in 1998, Finch and associates reported that relatively few elderly people had intakes of micronutrients that were below the LRNI and their results were similar to those listed above. This earlier report also included statistics on the biochemical status of elderly people for certain micronutrients as determined by *blood analysis*. The numbers of people recorded with poor biochemical status were high in comparison to the small numbers of individuals recording inadequate intakes. This observation adds some weight to the argument that the requirements for some nutrients increase in the elderly, and that perhaps the dietary standards for elderly people may need to be raised over those used for younger adults (as shown by Table 16.21). It is also possible that the biochemical thresholds indicating inadequate nutritional status for some nutrients may be set too high (there is a strong suggestion that this is the case for riboflavin – see Chapter 13). Some of the areas of concern highlighted by Finch *et al.* (1998) are listed below.

- About 10 per cent of the total sample had serum ferritin levels that were indicative of poor iron status, but fewer than 5 per cent had iron intakes that were below the LRNI. Nevertheless, about 10 per cent of the free-living sample, 52 per cent of institutionalized men and 39 per cent of institutionalized women had blood haemoglobin concentrations that were below the WHO standards for anaemia (13 g/dL for men and 12 g/dL for women).
- About 8 per cent of the free-living sample and 37 per cent of those living in institutions had biochemical indications of poor vitamin D status. As in the more recent survey of Bates *et al.* (2011), vitamin D intakes were only around a third of the RNI. Elderly people should either get regular exposure to summer sunlight or take vitamin D supplements.
- About 40 per cent of the total sample had biochemical indications of low riboflavin status although, as noted in Chapter 13, this may reflect the high sensitivity of this test.
- Of the institutionalized sample, 40 per cent had low biochemical status for folate, compared with around 30 per cent of the independent sample. (Only 1 per cent of men and 6 per cent of free-living women had intakes below the LRNI, as did 5 per cent of the total institutionalized sample.)
- Of the institutionalized sample, 40 per cent had low biochemical status for vitamin C, compared with around 14 per cent of the independent sample. (Only 2 per cent of the free-living sample and fewer than 1 per cent of the institutionalized sample had intakes below the LRNI.)
- Low biochemical status for thiamin was found in 10–15 per cent of all groups. (Fewer than 0.5 per cent of the total sample had recorded intakes below the LRNI.)
- Of the people in institutions, 15 per cent of men and 7 per cent of women had biochemical indications of zinc deficiency. This is not dissimilar to the numbers recording inadequate intakes.

This clear mismatch between prevalence of low intakes and prevalence of biochemical insufficiency needs further consideration and explanation, particularly by those setting dietary standards and biochemical thresholds of adequacy.

Key points

- Recorded energy intakes decline in middle-aged and elderly people.

- Only a few per cent of elderly Britons in the 1960s and 1970s were found to be malnourished, but the prevalence did rise with age. A survey conducted in the mid-1990s suggested that about 16 per cent of elderly people living in care accommodation were underweight (although the BMI threshold for underweight was then $20\,kg/m^2$ compared with $18.5\,kg/m^2$ now).

- Nutritional inadequacy in elderly people is often precipitated by some illness or is associated with adverse social circumstances.

- The early surveys suggested that elderly British people who were mobile, in good health and reasonably affluent had few specific nutritional problems and had diets that were in their general character similar to those of other Britons.

- Table 16.23 shows a recent comparison of the dietary energy sources of elderly and other British adults from the NDNS report of Bates et al. (2011).

- Older adults obtained more of their energy from fat and saturated fatty acids than younger adults and were above guideline values for both. They also obtained more of their energy from spreading fats and dairy products, including butter and whole milk.

- Older adults obtained less of their food energy from non-milk extrinsic sugars than younger adults and consumed less alcohol.

- Recorded intakes of micronutrients by Bates et al. (2011) found the following.

  - Average intakes of vitamins were well above the RNI except for vitamin D (33 per cent of RNI).
  - Average intakes of minerals were generally a higher proportion of the RNI than in younger adults, with only magnesium and selenium below the RNI.
  - Only small percentages of elderly people had recorded intakes of less than the LRNI for most micronutrients. Only for selenium (42 per cent), potassium (15 per cent) and zinc (5 per cent) were more than 3 per cent consuming less than the LRNI.

  →

Key points *continued*

  - Although 37 per cent of older adults reported using a dietary supplement, supplement use made no discernible difference to the proportions recording inadequate intakes.

- In a survey conducted in the mid-1990s, the proportion of elderly British people classified as having poor biochemical status for a micronutrient was substantially higher than those recording inadequate dietary intakes for iron, folate, riboflavin, vitamin C and thiamin.

- Substantially higher numbers of elderly people showed biochemical indications of micronutrient inadequacy than would have been expected from the dietary data. This may suggest that:

  - requirements for some nutrients may increase with age and thus higher dietary standards may be needed for the elderly
  - biochemical thresholds for inadequacy may be set too high and exaggerate the apparent prevalence of inadequacy (probably true for riboflavin).

- Many elderly people, especially those living in care accommodation, showed evidence of vitamin D insufficiency. This reinforces the earlier conclusion that elderly people need either regular exposure to summer sunlight or vitamin D supplements.

Diet and disease risk in the elderly

There is an age-related deterioration in the immune system and some specific measurable changes were discussed earlier in this chapter (see p. 472). Coupled with the well-known effects of malnutrition on immune functioning, this could make elderly people with poor nutritional status particularly vulnerable to systemic and wound infections and more susceptible to cancers. Improving the nutritional status of elderly people by the use of dietary supplements might reduce their susceptibility to infection particularly if targeted to those with the poorest nutritional status. Although many elderly people currently take dietary supplements they tend to be those with the best micronutrient intakes from food, so supplement use makes almost no difference to the numbers recording inadequate intakes.

In previous editions of this book, a considerable body of evidence was discussed which suggested that micronutrient supplements could improve the immune function and reduce episodes of infection in elderly people. Most of the results discussed were published by the award-winning Canadian scientist Dr Ranjit Chandra and his group who published dozens of papers in this area. Dickinson (2002) stated a widespread view when she acknowledged Dr Chandra as the 'internationally recognized expert in nutrition and immunity', and she goes on to quote Dr Chandra himself who wrote that studies 'indicate that a causal relationship does exist between under-nutrition and impaired immunity and that this is a correctable abnormality in the majority'. Unfortunately, Dr Chandra has since been accused of fabricating results and making a considerable fortune by selling 'evidence-based' dietary supplements – see Hamblin (2006) and Smith (2005). At least one of Dr Chandra's papers has been withdrawn by a journal's editors and doubts have been raised about the many other papers published by his group. Stephen and Avenell (2006) published a systematic review of controlled trials of the effectiveness of micronutrient supplements for preventing infections. They reported that when results from Dr Chandra's group were excluded then, in the relatively small number of remaining trials, there was no significant difference in the number of episodes of infection in those who were and were not receiving supplements.

Woo *et al.* (1994) reported that nutritional supplements given to elderly people recovering from chest infections were effective in helping them to recover from their illness. Mowe *et al.* (1994) assessed the diets and nutritional status of a large sample of elderly people admitted to hospitals in the Oslo area for an acute cause like a stroke or myocardial infarction. They compared these results with those obtained from a matched sample of well elderly people living within the same area. They concluded that there were several indicators that suggested that the food and nutrient intakes of the hospitalized group had been inferior to those of the well group in the 3 months prior to admission. They raised the possibility that poor food and nutrient intakes might be a contributory factor in the acute illnesses that led to hospitalization.

In the Allied Dunbar National Fitness Survey (1992), ageing was associated with a substantial decline in aerobic fitness, muscle strength and flexibility. Only a relatively minor proportion of this decline seems to be due to age *per se*, much of it representing a form of disuse atrophy. The average aerobic fitness of the top 10 per cent of men aged 65–74 years was higher than the average of the bottom 10 per cent of men aged 25–34 years. The report's authors concluded that 'much functional disability among older people could be reversed or avoided through continued regular exercise as people grow older'. Fiatarone *et al.* (1994) found that resistance training led to significant increases in muscle strength, walking speed, stair climbing power and spontaneous physical activity even in very elderly nursing home residents (mean age 87 years). In this same study a multi-nutrient supplement had no effect on the measured outcomes.

Maintenance of a reasonable level of physical activity would seem to be strongly advisable for the elderly as a complement to sound nutrition in maximizing good health and quality of life. In addition to the general beneficial effects on the cardiovascular system, increased activity will maintain energy expenditure and help to maintain lean body mass. Exercise and improved fitness, strength and flexibility will help elderly people to continue with the everyday activities that are essential to independent living. The general benefits of regular exercise and physical fitness are reviewed in Chapter 17 and these benefits are maintained and perhaps even greater in older people. Nied and Franklin (2002) tabulate an extensive range of benefits of exercise in older adults, including beneficial effects on the cardiovascular system, glycaemic control and diabetes risk, osteoporosis and fracture risk, osteoarthritis symptoms, cancer risk, psychological health and obesity. Regular exercise reduces total mortality and total morbidity in older people.

Overweight and obesity are generally associated with excess morbidity and reduced life expectancy (see Chapter 9). However, this conclusion is less secure in older people. Lehmann (1991), in a review of nutrition in old age, concluded that *underweight* is a more important indicator of increased mortality and morbidity risk than is obesity She suggested that, in the elderly, being moderately overweight is not associated with any excess mortality risk whereas underweight is associated with the following adverse outcomes:

- increased mortality
- increased risk of hip fracture
- increased risk of infections
- increased risk of specific nutrient deficiencies.

An expert working party in the UK (COMA, 1992) recommended that there should be more research on the prognostic significance of BMI in the elderly. It reviewed data from a 10-year cohort study of elderly people (aged 65–74 years) which found that the relationship between mortality and BMI was U-shaped with a tendency for mortality to rise at the extremes of the range (i.e. at very low or very high BMIs). More recent data have supported these earlier indications of an inverse relationship between BMI and mortality in older people as opposed to the positive relationship seen in younger adults and particularly in younger men (see Chapter 9).

Janssen et al. (2005) found that, after controlling for waist circumference, mortality risk decreased by 21 per cent for every standard deviation increase in BMI in a sample of 5200 men and women aged over 65 years. When waist circumference was corrected for BMI, this was associated with higher mortality risk; that is, having a little bit of extra weight is associated with lower mortality but, at any given BMI, high waist circumference was associated with higher mortality. Large stores of abdominal fat seem to have similar negative health associations to those in younger adults, as discussed in Chapter 9.

Al Snih et al. (2007) did a detailed analysis of the relationship between BMI and mortality and disability risk in an ethnically mixed cohort of 12 000 elderly Americans (aged over 65 years) with a 7-year follow-up. They found that lowest mortality rates were in the BMI categories 25–30 and 30–35 kg/m^2 (RR 0.78 and 0.8, respectively) with subjects who were above or below these ranges experiencing higher mortality risk. A similar pattern was seen for disability risk when those with BMI under 18.5 or above 30 kg/m^2 were significantly more likely to suffer disability during the follow-up period.

While studies suggesting a reduced risk of mortality associated with higher BMI in older people are numerous and convincing, that does not mean they demonstrate a reversal of risk with age and that being overweight or obese is directly protective in elderly people. Many groups, including Elia (2001) and Schooling et al. (2007), have suggested reasons why this apparent risk reversal may be artefactual, a selection of which is noted here.

- Many studies have not adequately accounted for confounding factors like smoking, associated with reduced BMI and increased mortality.
- Existing poor health may affect mortality. In an older person with multiple health problems, a high BMI may indicate that the disease process is not yet overwhelming and causing cachexia, whereas a low BMI may indicate overwhelming disease and approaching death.
- It is common for older people to lose weight in the period leading up to their death. The lower BMI categories will contain both people who have always been thin and the previously fat who have lost weight on their trajectory towards death. This may mean that BMI underestimates the detrimental effect of adiposity on mortality risk.

Schooling et al. (2007) conducted a prospective cohort study of 56 000 elderly Chinese residents of Hong Kong, looking at the relationship between BMI and mortality. They found that initial analysis of their data, after adjusting for age, sex, socioeconomic status and lifestyle habits, suggested that higher BMI was associated with reduced mortality in a dose-dependent way. However, the relationship between BMI and mortality varied with cause of death and especially with baseline health status. In those people with poor baseline health there was a strong dose-dependent relationship between higher BMI and lower mortality. However, in those elderly people with good baseline health and who had never smoked there was the same positive relationship between obesity and higher mortality seen in younger adults. They found that being underweight was consistently associated with higher mortality. They concluded that interventions to prevent obesity were justified at all ages including the elderly.

There have been numerous reports suggesting that weight loss in elderly people is associated with increased mortality, although there are also contradictory reports (Elia, 2001). This has prevented consensus recommendation of weight loss for elderly overweight and obese people. However, most of these studies have not distinguished between intended weight loss (for obesity and related conditions) and unintentional weight loss which is likely due to underlying disease and thus likely to predict increased risk of mortality and/or disability. In an expert evidence assessment report for the USDA (www.nel.gov/evidence. cfm?evidence_summary_id=250331) it was concluded that there was moderate evidence that intentional weight loss in elderly overweight and obese subjects reduced risk of mortality and morbidity and reduced levels of diabetes and cardiovascular risk factors. Zamboni *et al.* (2005) also concluded that, although there were relatively few studies on the effects of voluntary weight loss in the elderly, they do suggest that even small amounts of weight loss (5–10 per cent) may be beneficial.

The general dietary guidelines reviewed in Chapter 5 are still regarded as being appropriate for the majority of elderly people. Despite this, the nutritional priorities for older people are different from those of younger adults. Dietary adequacy assumes a greater priority in the face of declining energy intakes. In those elderly people suffering weight loss, loss of taste perception and reduced ability to chew, maintaining high palatability and good food intake may be more important than conforming to current nutritional education guidelines. These guidelines are intended to reduce the long-term risk of degenerative diseases. It seems inevitable that, even if these preventative benefits still occur in the elderly, they are likely to be reduced. The application of several of these guidelines to the elderly is briefly reviewed below.

- The association between increased serum cholesterol concentration and increased risk of coronary heart disease has in the past often been assumed to be less convincing in elderly people than in young and middle-aged adults. According to COMA (1992), more recent data from both the USA and the UK had indicated that the predictive value of a raised serum cholesterol for increased coronary heart disease risk was maintained in later years and thus that the general cholesterol lowering guidelines should also apply to the elderly. Table 16.23 indicates that the proportion of food energy from saturated fat is still well above the target value of 10 per cent. More recent studies do suggest that cholesterol lowering is effective in reducing both fatal and non-fatal heart attacks in older people. For example, Shepherd (2004)

reviews the results of the PROspective Study of Pravastatin in the Elderly at Risk (PROSPER), which showed that this cholesterol-lowering (statin) drug markedly improved blood lipoprotein profiles, reduced CHD deaths and non-fatal heart attacks and strokes. Although this was a drug trial it does confirm that, as with younger people, effective management of high blood lipid levels is effective in reducing heart disease in elderly at-risk people. In a review of the treatment of high blood lipids in the elderly, Pohlel *et al.* (2006) concluded that modern lipid-lowering strategies have been shown to prevent or delay the progression of diseases associated with abnormal blood lipid profiles such as cardiovascular disease and cerebrovascular disease in the elderly.

- Increased intakes of non-starch polysaccharides (fibre) are likely to reduce constipation and beneficially affect existing minor bowel problems such as haemorrhoids. Increased activity and prevention of dehydration would also improve bowel function. Dehydration is common among elderly people because of reduced acuity of the thirst mechanism, reduced ability to concentrate urine, and physical problems with getting drinks (or even voluntary suppression of fluid intake because of fears of incontinence or difficulties in using the toilet). Dehydration is also a cause of confusion in the elderly. Elderly people are advised to drink the equivalent of 6–8 glasses of water a day, and those charged with care of the elderly should make sure that immobile patients are regularly offered palatable drinks.
- Hypertension is very prevalent in the elderly population and only just over a third of the over-65s are classified as normotensive and untreated; all the rest are taking anti-hypertensive drugs and/or have high blood pressure (Bates *et al.*, 2011). COMA (1992) concluded that an average intake of 6 g/day of salt was a reasonable target for elderly people as well as other adults.
- COMA (1992) recommended that the targets for non-milk extrinsic sugars for elderly people should be the same as for the rest of the population. Moderating the intake of added sugar should help to ensure a high nutrient density of the diet. The majority of elderly people now still have some natural teeth, so the effects of sugars on the teeth and gums are not irrelevant.

The average intakes of non-extrinsic milk sugars of elderly people do actually comply with the recommended 11 per cent of food energy (Bates *et al.*, 2011).

- Like the rest of the population, elderly people are advised to eat more fruits and vegetables (five portions a day). This should increase intake of many vitamins, anti-oxidants, non-starch polysaccharide and some minerals including potassium. Just over a third of elderly people do actually reach this five portions per day target, which is slightly more than for younger adults (Bates *et al.*, 2011).

Key points

- Immune function deteriorates with age and is also depressed by malnutrition.
- Several papers have suggested that nutrient supplements can improve immune function and reduce infections in the elderly. However, many of these papers have come from a research group headed by a scientist accused of fabricating data. Meta-analysis of controlled trials excluding those conducted by this group do not show any significant benefit of these supplements.
- Aerobic fitness, strength and flexibility all decline sharply with age in the UK, largely because of decreased activity rather than as an inevitable consequence of ageing.
- Resistance training can increase strength and performance even in people in their 80s and 90s.
- Increased activity and fitness in elderly people would increase life expectancy and improve the quality of life in the later years, and so enable more elderly people to remain independent for longer.
- Being underweight is an important indicator of mortality risk in the elderly.
- Overweight and moderately obese elderly and very elderly people tend to have reduced mortality and disability risk. This apparent reversal of the risks of high BMI in older adults is probably an artefact caused by:
  - failure of many studies to adequately consider confounding variables like smoking and baseline health status

Key points *continued*

  - the lower BMI categories containing both always-lean people and people who have lost weight due to ill-health.
- One very large cohort study found a high dose-dependent association between high BMI and reduced mortality but when they considered only people with good baseline health status and lifelong non-smokers, they found the same positive association between BMI and high mortality seen in younger adults.
- Weight loss is associated with increased mortality in older people, but this includes unintentional weight loss due to ill-health.
- Intentional weight loss probably reduces mortality, morbidity and risk factors for diabetes and cardiovascular disease in the elderly.
- Prevention and treatment of obesity are still beneficial in the elderly despite the association between high BMI and mortality in older people.
- A high waist circumference remains a positive indicator of mortality risk in the elderly, confirming the negative health implications of large abdominal fat stores in the elderly.
- Maintaining dietary adequacy becomes an increasingly important goal as people become elderly and very elderly.
- The dietary guidelines for other adults are still generally appropriate for elderly people provided that they do not compromise dietary adequacy, i.e. lower intakes of fat, saturated fat, added sugar and salt but more non-starch polysaccharide, starch and fruits and vegetables.
- Studies with statins confirm that effective management of hyperlipidaemia yields considerable benefits even in old age.
- Dehydration is common in the elderly. It causes confusion and constipation. The equivalent of 6–8 glasses of water a day is recommended for elderly people.
- Good intakes of non-starch polysaccharide, increased activity and ample fluid intakes should all contribute to improved bowel functioning in the elderly.

17

NUTRITION AS TREATMENT

Diet as a complete therapy	484	Malnutrition in hospital patients	496
Diet as a specific component of therapy	488		

DIET AS A COMPLETE THERAPY

Overview and general principles

There are a small number of diseases or conditions where dietary change can be an effective and complete therapy, where the patient is intolerant of a specific nutrient or component of food. *Food intolerance* has been defined as:

a reproducible, unpleasant (i.e. adverse) reaction to a specific food or ingredient, which is not psychologically based.

Where there is 'evidence of an abnormal immunological reaction to the food' then this is termed a *food allergy* (Mitchell, 1988).

The therapeutic principles in cases of food intolerance are very simple.

- *To identify the nutrient or foodstuff to which the patient is intolerant.* In practice, it may prove difficult to pinpoint the food or foods causing the symptoms, or even to establish with certainty that the symptoms are really due to food intolerance.
- *To devise a dietary regimen that provides a healthful and acceptable diet while either keeping intakes of the problem nutrient within tolerable limits or completely excluding the offending foodstuff.* This may be difficult if the offending food is a staple and an ingredient of many foods or dishes (e.g. flour, egg or milk). It may also be difficult if a person is intolerant to excessive amounts of an essential nutrient found in many foods, such as an essential amino acid like phenylalanine.

These problems will be illustrated in this chapter by *coeliac disease* and *phenylketonuria* (PKU) as examples of the dietary management of food intolerances.

In addition to diseases where exclusion is the primary dietetic aim, there are a few diseases that are not of primary dietary origin but can be alleviated by nutrient supplements. *Pernicious anaemia* is probably the best known example, in which autoimmune destruction of the parietal cells of the stomach results in a failure of vitamin B_{12} absorption. Most of the symptoms of this potentially fatal disease can be alleviated by regular injections of B_{12}. *Hartnup disease* is a rare but fatal inherited disorder with symptoms that resemble those of pellagra (niacin deficiency). The symptoms of this disease result from a failure to absorb the amino acid tryptophan (the precursor of niacin) which leads to niacin deficiency. The condition responds to niacin treatment which reduces the dermatitis and neurological consequences of pellagra. If plenty of protein is given, tryptophan may be absorbed in di- and tripeptides.

L-carnitine is an important cellular metabolite that does not qualify as an essential nutrient because it is normally synthesized in the body from the amino acid lysine. There are several relatively rare hereditary disorders that respond to therapy with pharmacological doses of L-carnitine. Examples include a defect in the enzyme that normally transfers carnitine across the plasma membrane, and some disorders of fatty acid metabolism. There is a short discussion of L-carnitine in Chapter 13 under the heading of conditionally essential nutrients.

Food allergy: immediate hypersensitivity reactions

Most food allergies are immediate hypersensitivity reactions that are mediated by a class of antibodies or immunoglobulins known as *immunoglubulin E* (IgE). Symptoms begin within a few minutes of ingesting the food. The symptoms vary from case to case but can include one or more of the following:

- gastro-intestinal symptoms like abdominal pain, diarrhoea and vomiting
- eczema or urticaria (hives)
- asthmatic symptoms and laryngeal swelling
- allergic rhinitis (runny nose) and itchy, watering eyes.

In rare cases the symptoms may be severe enough to be life-threatening – including anaphylactic shock, which is widespread blood vessel dilation resulting in a fall in blood pressure and circulatory collapse.

Exposure to the allergen, which is usually a food protein (e.g. in cow milk, eggs, peanuts, tree nuts or shellfish), results in production of IgE antibodies which bind to and sensitize tissue mast cells and their circulating form, the basophils. Once a person is sensitized, during subsequent exposures the allergen binds to the antibodies on the mast cells causing them to release histamine and other chemical mediators which bring about the allergic symptoms.

Many people believe that they or their children are allergic to particular foods, but many of these client diagnoses are inaccurate or involve too many foods. People may not respond to the food to which they believe they are allergic if they do not know that they have eaten it, and conversely may respond to something they are told contains the suspected allergen even if it does not. A first step towards a firm diagnosis is for the patient to keep a *food diary* to record everything eaten and drunk and to record the severity of any allergic symptoms or the occurrence of allergic episodes. This should give an indication of likely allergens. For chronic symptoms like dermatitis, the suspected food can be withdrawn to see whether this leads to gradual easing of symptoms which – provided they are not too severe – can be provoked again by reintroduction of the food.

Again provided the symptoms are not too severe, the most reliable way of establishing an allergy to a particular food is to use a *blind challenge* – a double-blind, placebo-controlled food challenge analogous to a double-blind clinical trial. Neither the patient nor the clinician knows which is the real and placebo challenge until after the trial is completed. If a patient responds to the placebo that would suggest a psychological component.

Skin prick tests are now used widely to identify causes of food allergy. Small amounts of potential allergens are injected into the skin and the extent of any inflammatory skin reaction is then used to assess sensitivity. A positive skin test does not automatically mean that a person will have an allergic reaction to that substance when it is given by mouth, although a negative response means that the substance is an unlikely cause of allergic symptoms. Skin prick tests are useful in confirming a suspected allergy and in deciding which foods might need to be considered in challenge tests. The *radio-allergosorbent test* (RAST) is a more expensive alternative, which assesses the amount of specific IgE present in a patient's blood. The patient's serum is reacted with allergen which is adsorbed on to a solid paper matrix and the specific IgE in the serum will compete with added radioactive IgE for binding to this antigen. The more specific IgE there is in the patient's blood, the less radioactivity will remain on the paper.

Food allergies seem to affect up to 4 per cent of the population, with shellfish being the most common sensitivity in adults. Rates of food allergies are higher in young children, perhaps double that for the population as a whole, but many of them grow out of these allergies and are able to tolerate the food later in childhood. The most common sensitivity in young children is to eggs, followed by cow milk and peanuts.

The main treatment is dietary avoidance of the offending substance, although drugs like antihistamines can alleviate the symptoms of the allergy.

Key points

- Most food allergies are mediated by IgE antibodies and are immediate hypersensitivities where symptoms appear within minutes of exposure.
- A double-blind, placebo-controlled food challenge is the most reliable method of diagnosis unless the severity of the symptoms prevents its use.
- Skin prick tests can be useful in identifying or confirming suspected allergies.
- The presence of specific IgE antibodies to suspected allergens in a patient's blood can be measured using the in-vitro RAST.
- Perhaps up to 4 per cent of the population have IgE-mediated immediate hypersensitivities to food, with perhaps double this frequency in young children who may grow out of their allergies.
- Shellfish is the most common sensitivity in adults. Egg, cow milk and peanuts are the most common in young children.

Coeliac disease: delayed-type hypersensitivity

Coeliac disease (gluten-induced enteropathy) results from a hypersensitivity or allergy to the gliadin component of the wheat protein gluten, and similar proteins that are found in barley, rye and some other less well-known cereals. Pure oats do not cause symptoms in most people with coeliac disease unless they have been contaminated with wheat; this is despite the presence of a protein called avenin which is similar to gluten. The disease is sometimes termed *gluten-sensitive enteropathy*.

The disease is classified as a food allergy because it involves an 'abnormal immunological response to food', but it differs from a classical allergy such as hay fever and does not involve production of IgE antibodies. It is an example of the other type of food allergy in which symptoms do not develop until some hours after the ingestion of the offending food and may not reach their peak until 48 hours or more after ingestion. This is known as *delayed-type hypersensitivity* (DTH).

Exposure to the allergen leads to sensitization of T-cell lymphocytes. After sensitization, re-exposure to the antigen causes the sensitized T-cells to release inflammatory mediators and cause a localized inflammatory response. Patients with coeliac disease are also more likely to suffer from other autoimmune diseases like type 1 diabetes, thyroiditis, pernicious anaemia and the chronic skin condition dermatitis herpetiformis; the symptoms of this latter condition respond to a gluten-free diet.

In people with untreated coeliac disease, the villi of the small intestine atrophy and there is excessive secretion of mucus. Diagnosis is confirmed by a biopsy of the jejunal mucosa using an endoscope. These changes in the small intestine result in severe malabsorption of fat and other nutrients, leading to fatty diarrhoea, distended abdomen, weight loss or growth failure. There will be other symptoms that are the result of nutrient deficiencies, such as anaemia, rickets/osteomalacia and bleeding due to vitamin K deficiency. In the long term, there may be cancerous changes in the intestine induced by continued exposure to gluten-type proteins, leading to small bowel lymphoma. Some patients diagnosed with this condition can tolerate some dietary gluten without overt symptoms but this may increase their later risk of small bowel lymphoma.

The aim of dietary management in coeliac disease is to avoid all gluten-containing foods as well as foods that contain the similar rye and barley proteins. Achievement of this goal is complicated because bread and cereals are not only staple dietary items but flour is also an ingredient of many prepared foods. Gluten-free flour, bread, pasta and some other basic foods are available on prescription in the UK, and gluten-free cakes and biscuits (cookies) are commercially available. Many food manufacturers use a 'crossed grain' symbol to indicate that a particular product is free of gluten. The charitable organization Coeliac UK has a website (www.coeliac.org.uk) that gives guidance to both patients and healthcare professionals about the dietary management of coeliac disease. This website gives a list of gluten-free foods that are available on prescription and also produces an updatable *Food and Drink Directory* that is available in downloadable and paper format and contains a list of many thousands of foods that are safe for patients to eat.

The symptoms of coeliac disease may present in early childhood, but in most cases it starts in adulthood in people who have not displayed symptoms earlier. It appears to be more common in women and the peak incidence has been said to occur at between 35 and 44 years. It has been suggested that increased use of rice-based weaning foods – and thus delayed exposure to wheat – has caused a delay in the onset of the disease with more adult and fewer childhood presentations. There is strong evidence that there is an inherited disposition to this condition as its occurrence in the first-degree relatives of existing sufferers is up to 100 times greater than in the general population. Certain human leucocyte antigens (HLAs) are found in most sufferers of coeliac disease. Its frequency varies around the world, with a high prevalence in some European countries (e.g. 1:300 in Ireland), but it is rare in Chinese, Japanese and Africans. Details of the pathology and other scientific aspects of this condition can be found in Connon (2006).

> **Key points**
>
> - Coeliac disease is an example of *delayed-type* hypersensitivity where symptoms appear some hours after ingestion of the food. Sensitized T-cells release inflammatory mediators when exposed to the antigen and cause local inflammation.
> - Coeliac disease is a hypersensitivity to components of the wheat protein gluten and similar proteins in barley and rye.
> - Gluten causes atrophy of the villi in the small intestine, which leads to diarrhoea, malabsorption, and a variety of abdominal symptoms.
>
> →

> **Key points** *continued*
>
> - If untreated, the condition leads to growth failure, weight loss and a range of nutritional deficiencies. It may eventually result in cancerous changes in the small bowel.
> - The treatment is to exclude from the diet the wheat, barley and rye that contain the gluten-like proteins. Dietary compliance is made difficult by the widespread use of wheat flour in manufactured foods.
> - Rice, maize and uncontaminated pure oats do not contain gluten, and a range of gluten-free wheat products are available, some of them on prescription in the UK.
> - A *Food and Drink Directory* produced by the charity Coeliac UK identifies thousands of foods that can safely be eaten.

Phenylketonuria

Phenylketonuria (PKU) is an inherited disease which affects around 1 in 10 000 babies in the UK. Since the 1960s, all babies born in the UK have been tested for this condition within the first 2 weeks of life. The blood phenylalanine concentration is measured using the Guthrie test. Classical PKU is caused by a genetic defect in the enzyme *phenylalanine hydroxylase* that converts the essential amino acid phenylalanine to tyrosine.

Normally, excess phenylalanine, either from the diet or from endogenous protein breakdown, is metabolized via its conversion to tyrosine. In normal adults, 90 per cent of the phenylalanine consumed is converted to tyrosine and only about 10 per cent is used for protein synthesis. In PKU this route is blocked, so excess phenylalanine and unusual metabolites of phenylalanine accumulate in the blood where they seriously impair mental development. In PKU, tyrosine becomes an essential amino acid and some of the symptoms of PKU are probably associated with tyrosine deficiency. The mental development of untreated children is severely retarded and they are prone to epilepsy but they grow normally and have a normal life expectancy.

The objective of dietary management in PKU is to restrict phenylalanine intake so that mental development is not impaired, while providing enough of this essential amino acid and all other nutrients to allow growth and physical development. In particular, adequate amounts of tyrosine must be provided.

These objectives cannot be achieved with normal foods because all foods with good amounts of protein and tyrosine also contain high levels of phenylalanine. The tolerance to phenylalanine depends on the precise nature of the biochemical lesion and varies from child to child. The amount of phenylalanine the child can consume while keeping his or her blood level within the acceptable range for age is first determined. The phenylalanine allowance defined in this way is then taken in the form of normal foods, usually milk, cereals and potatoes. Meat, fish, eggs, cheese and pulses will be totally excluded, and only sugars, fats, fruits and non-leguminous vegetables can be eaten relatively freely – and even for these there will be some restrictions.

The resultant diet is, by design, very low in protein and tyrosine and is unlikely to provide adequate amounts of energy. Children are therefore given medical supplements that provide amino acids, energy and other nutrients such as vitamin B_{12} that are likely to be deficient. Infant formulas that are low in phenylalanine are available prior to weaning.

The prognosis for children with PKU depends on how strictly the dietary regimen is followed, but even in a family where control is poor the child should still be educable. Prior to the 1960s, and the introduction of universal screening, the mental development of most PKU children would have been very severely impaired (the average IQ of untreated PKU patients is about 50), and many would have spent much of their life in an institution for the mentally handicapped. Children whose blood phenylalanine levels have been well controlled have normal IQs at 9 years old (Elsas and Acosta, 2006). Current consensus suggests that some dietary regulation needs to be maintained throughout life.

Neurological changes occur in adults with PKU when their blood phenylalanine concentration is allowed to rise, but these symptoms can be reversed by reintroduction of a low-phenylalanine diet. Special care needs to be taken over the diet of

women intending to become pregnant because the developing fetus is vulnerable to high phenylalanine levels. Babies born to mothers with uncontrolled PKU often have congenital defects that are incompatible with life, and those that do survive fail to grow and develop normally. The dietary management of PKU and other inborn errors of metabolism has been reviewed by Elsas and Acosta (2006).

Key points

- PKU is caused by an inherited defect in the enzyme phenylalanine hydroxylase. This leads to accumulation of phenylalanine and its metabolites which impair brain development and tyrosine becomes an essential nutrient.
- Management involves severe dietary restrictions and extensive use of medicinal dietary supplements.
- If phenylalanine levels are tightly controlled then children can develop with normal IQs.
- Pregnant women with PKU must control their phenylalanine levels to permit normal fetal development.

DIET AS A SPECIFIC COMPONENT OF THERAPY

There are a number of conditions where diet does not give complete relief from symptoms nor is it the sole treatment, but where there is an apparently sound theoretical and empirical basis for a specific role for a particular dietary regimen in its management. Three examples are considered briefly here.

Diabetes mellitus

Classification and aetiology

Diet has long been regarded as a key element of the treatment of diabetes. Diabetes mellitus results from insufficient production of the pancreatic hormone insulin. In the severe *type 1 diabetes*, which usually develops during childhood, there is destruction of the insulin-producing cells in the pancreas and this results in an almost total failure of insulin supply. It is envisaged that some environmental factor like a viral infection triggers the autoimmune destruction of the cells in the pancreas that produce insulin, the β-cells in the islets of Langerhans. This type of diabetes accounts for around 10–15 per cent of all cases of diabetes. Type 1 diabetes is always treated by a combination of diet and insulin injections. Patients cannot survive long without insulin therapy and before insulin therapy was available they usually died within a few weeks of diagnosis.

In the much more common and milder *type 2 diabetes* there is no primary failure of insulin supply or any obvious β-cell pathology. The primary defect is reduced target tissue sensitivity to insulin, and this results in compensatory increases in insulin production. In genetically susceptible people, there is an inadequate compensatory increase in insulin production resulting in a progressive shortfall of insulin and gradually increasing symptoms of diabetes. In Chapter 9 it is noted that high insulin production caused by insulin resistance leads to increases in several cardiovascular disease risk factors and to increased risk of heart disease even in the absence of overt diabetes. This insulin resistance is referred to as the *metabolic syndrome* or *syndrome X* and many of these individuals will go on to become diabetic. Insulin sensitivity decreases as body fat content increases and excessive weight gain is the most important trigger for the onset of type 2 diabetes in those who are genetically susceptible to it.

Excessive weight gain is particularly detrimental if it is associated with a high waist circumference, because adipose tissue within the abdominal cavity has less sensitivity to insulin than that stored subcutaneously. A high-fat, low-fibre diet and inactivity are other important lifestyle characteristics that decrease insulin sensitivity and predispose to this type of diabetes.

Type 2 diabetes is usually treated either by diet alone or by a combination of diet and oral hypoglycaemic drugs. Insulin injections may be used to improve the management, particularly in those who have had the condition for some time. Around 5 per cent of the UK population aged over 65 years are diagnosed diabetics but there may be an equal number who are undiagnosed and untreated but still at risk of the long-term complications of

diabetes. The risk of this form of diabetes increases with age, so the number of diabetics will continue to increase as the numbers of very elderly people in the population continue to grow and as the prevalence of obesity continues to rise. Until recently, type 2 diabetes was almost exclusively confined to the over-40s, but cases now occur with increasing regularity in younger adults and even in children because of the increased prevalence of obesity in younger people.

Diagnosis

The normal fasting blood glucose concentration of a healthy young adult is 4–5 mmol/L and this will rise to just over 7 mmol/L in the period after a carbohydrate meal and return to the fasting level an hour or so after absorption is complete. All diabetics have an elevated blood glucose concentration and this is the basis for diagnosis. Traditionally, diagnosis was confirmed by a glucose tolerance test; the fasting subject was giving a 75 g oral load of glucose and blood glucose concentration monitored over the subsequent 2 hours. This is less often used nowadays and diagnosis is often made on the basis of clinical symptoms and a simple elevated blood glucose measurement. The following criteria are indicative of diabetes:

- clinical symptoms plus a casual plasma glucose concentration of ≥11.1 mmol/L
- a fasting (8-hour) plasma glucose concentration of >7.0 mmol/L or a whole-blood concentration of 6.1 mmol/L
- a 2-hour plasma glucose concentration of ≥11.1 mmol/L during an oral glucose tolerance test.

A single measurement of hyperglycaemia without clinical symptoms of diabetes would need a repeat test to confirm the diagnosis. Those with a fasting plasma glucose concentration of 6.1–7.0 mmol/L would be classified as having impaired glucose tolerance, and half of these will become overtly diabetic within 10 years.

Symptoms and long-term complications

As a consequence of their high blood glucose concentration, diabetics of both types excrete glucose in their urine. This is because glucose is freely filtered in the renal tubule, and as blood glucose rises so the amount filtered exceeds the capacity of the reabsorption system in the proximal part of the renal tubule and the excess spills into the urine. This glucose in the urine acts as an osmotic diuretic and causes increased water loss, increased thirst and propensity to dehydration. The blood glucose concentration in an untreated diabetic may reach 10 times the normal fasting value and hundreds of grams of glucose may be lost in the urine each day. In untreated type 1 diabetes there are other severe and even life-threatening symptoms:

• rapid weight loss (weight loss also occurs in type 2 and so tends to obscure the strength of the association between obesity and diabetes)
• very high blood glucose concentration and severe dehydration
• excessive production and excretion of ketone bodies leading to acidosis, electrolyte imbalance and eventually to coma and death.

The symptoms of the disease suggest that the diabetic is intolerant of carbohydrate, so severe restriction of dietary carbohydrate and almost total exclusion of dietary sugar were the rule for diabetic diets for most of the twentieth century. Prior to 1975 most diabetic diets would have contained no more than 40 per cent of the calories as carbohydrate and often much less than this. These low-carbohydrate diets were inevitably high in fat. According to Leeds (1979), when insulin treatment was first used in the 1920s, diabetic diets typically contained less than 10 per cent of calories as carbohydrate and more than 70 per cent as fat. Diabetics in Western countries have traditionally suffered much higher mortality from cardiovascular diseases than do non-diabetics. This is *not* an inevitable consequence of diabetes because Japanese and black East African diabetics have been relatively free of cardiovascular disease, unlike either Japanese American or black American diabetics (Keen and Thomas, 1988). Insulin resistance and hyperinsulinaemia lead to detrimental changes in blood lipoprotein profiles (see metabolic syndrome in Chapter 9), and a high-fat diet is an accepted risk factor for cardiovascular diseases; and so the very high-fat diet that was in the past prescribed for diabetics almost certainly increased their propensity to cardiovascular disease still further.

Diabetics also suffer from a range of conditions that are attributed to degenerative changes in their microvasculature (i.e. capillaries). These changes in the microvasculature are responsible for the *diabetic retinopathy* that causes many diabetics to go blind, and for the high levels of renal disease (*diabetic nephropathy*) seen in diabetics. Persistent hyperglycaemia also leads to cataract and degeneration of peripheral sensory nerves (*peripheral neuropathy*). Changes in capillaries also lead to poor oxygenation of peripheral tissues and this, together with the peripheral neuropathy, leads to chronic ulceration in the extremities and to enhanced risk of *gangrene* in the toes and feet.

Changes in the capillaries are thought to stem from a chemical change in the proteins of the basement membrane of capillary cells that results from their continued exposure to high glucose levels; the proteins react abnormally with glucose and become glycosylated. Glycosylation probably also plays a role in the development of *cataract* and the degeneration of peripheral nerves seen in older diabetics. Glycosylation of low-density lipoproteins (LDLs) may increase their atherogenicity. The proportion of glycosylated haemoglobin is used as an indicator of average blood glucose concentration over the previous 2–3 months. In a healthy person, glycosylated haemoglobin is less than 6 per cent of the total but it can rise to over 25 per cent in some diabetics.

Principles of management

The historical aim of diabetic therapy was to alleviate the immediate symptoms of the disease, which are at best unpleasant and incapacitating and at worst acutely life-threatening. Therapies that are effective in this limited aim for almost all diabetics have been available for many years. Despite this, the life expectancy of diabetics remains considerably less than that of others, and diabetics have continued to suffer a high-level disability in their later years for the reasons discussed in the previous section. A major additional objective of modern diabetic therapy is to increase life expectancy and to reduce long-term morbidity. From the previous discussion the two major considerations below seem to be important in this respect:

- the hyperlipidaemia that is associated with diabetes (and high-fat diets) and the consequent increase in risk of atherosclerosis
- the persistent hyperglycaemia of diabetes.

Modern management seeks to reduce these longer term complications by:

- achieving and maintaining a more normal body weight
- minimizing hyperlipidaemia and hyperglycaemia.

The modern diabetic diet is thus almost the complete opposite of that recommended prior to 1970. It is a low-fat diet that is high in complex carbohydrate and fibre. More than half of the energy should come from carbohydrate, with the emphasis on unrefined foods high in complex carbohydrate and fibre. It has moderate levels of fat and saturated fat, ideally less than 35 per cent of energy as fat and less than 10 per cent as saturated fat. The very strict avoidance of sugar has been relaxed provided it is a component of a meal. The general avoidance of isolated sugary foods except for hypoglycaemic emergency is still recommended. A diet considered ideal for diabetics with type 2 diabetes is very similar to that recommended for the population as a whole.

The matching of carbohydrate to insulin dose in type 1 diabetes is a specialist topic beyond the scope of this text, but the overall dietary strategy is as outlined here. Note that overdose of insulin causes blood glucose level to fall below normal (*hypoglycaemia*) and this fall in blood glucose can lead to a variety of symptoms ranging from confusion and disorientation through to coma and even death. Hypoglycaemia is treated by consuming a sugary snack or by infusion of glucose if the patient is unconscious. It occurs, for example, if the patient misses or unduly delays a meal or takes too much insulin.

Obesity is a major risk factor for type 2 diabetes, and normalization of body weight and regulation of caloric intake to match expenditure improve the symptoms of type 2 diabetes. Much of the success of traditional low-carbohydrate diabetic diets may

have been due to their regulation of energy intake rather than carbohydrate restriction *per se*. Provided the person is in energy balance then the proportions of energy that come from fat and carbohydrate do not really affect short-term diabetic control. A raised carbohydrate intake increases peripheral sensitivity to insulin and thus does not increase the need for insulin. This adaptation cannot occur in the absence of insulin, so carbohydrate does have adverse effects in untreated severe diabetes – thus explaining the past assumption that carbohydrate was inevitably bad for diabetics.

The well-documented effects of fibre in improving glucose tolerance are discussed in Chapter 10. An increase in the proportion of energy from carbohydrate, together with an increase in dietary fibre, has a generally favourable effect on blood glucose control in both type 1 and type 2 diabetes. The moderate levels of fat and saturated fat in diabetic diets would be expected to reduce blood lipid levels, especially LDL cholesterol, and contribute to a reduction in atherosclerosis.

The Diabetes Control and Complications Trial (DCCT, 1993) provided the first direct evidence that type 1 diabetics who achieved good long-term glycaemic control had reduced risk of nephropathy, retinopathy and neuropathy compared to those with poor glycaemic control. Data from the UK Prospective Diabetic Study (UKPDS) also suggested that better glycaemic control considerably reduced the macrovascular and microvascular complications of type 2 diabetes (Stratton *et al.*, 2000). This group used mean concentration of glycosylated haemoglobin as the indicator of glycaemic control in over 4000 type 2 diabetics in the UK. It found that there was a highly significant and progressive improvement in all measured outcomes with each 1 per cent reduction in glycosylated haemoglobin. Reduced diabetes-related mortality, incidence of heart attacks, amputations, retinal degeneration and cataract were all found in those with better glycaemic control (as indicated by lower glycosylated haemoglobin concentration), and the best outcomes were seen in those patients whose glycosylated haemoglobin levels were within the normal range for non-diabetics.

There have since been several randomized controlled trials and meta-analyses that have tried to assess the overall benefits of intensive versus conventional glycaemic control on the complications of both types of diabetes. Mattila and Boer (2010) summed up the findings of existing trials and meta-analyses with the following conclusions.

- Intensive glucose control has substantial beneficial effects on the microvascular complications of both types of diabetes (i.e. retinopathy, nephropathy and neuropathy).
- There was some reduction in non-fatal myocardial infarction with intensive glucose control, especially in type 2 diabetes.
- There was no reduction in strokes, cardiovascular deaths or all-cause mortality with intensive glycaemic control in either type of diabetes.
- There was more than double the risk of serious hypoglycaemia in those given intensive glycaemic control.

Jenkins and Wolever (1981) coined the term *glycaemic index* (GI) to describe in a quantitative way the rise in blood glucose that different carbohydrate foods produce. It is the rise in blood glucose induced by 50 grams of carbohydrate present in a test food expressed as a percentage of that induced by the same amount of a standard carbohydrate source (discussed further in Chapter 9). For example, bread and corn flakes have high glycaemic index, porridge oats and All-Bran have moderate values, and pulses have low values. It is generally accepted that foods with low glycaemic index would be beneficial for glycaemic control in diabetes management. Thomas *et al.* (2007) did a meta-analysis of 11 controlled trials (400 patients) of at least 4 weeks' duration which compared diets with low and high glycaemic indices in the management of both types of diabetes. They found that there were significantly lower levels of glycated haemoglobin and fewer hypoglycaemic episodes in patients on the diets with low glycaemic index. On the basis of these narrow and short-term outcome measures, they concluded that a low-GI diet can improve glycaemic control in diabetics without increasing hypoglycaemic episodes.

Table 17.1 shows examples of the glycaemic indices of several foods compared to that of white bread.

Table 17.1 Glycaemic indices of sample foods*

Food	Glycaemic index (GI)[1]
White bread	100
Wholemeal bread	100
Sugar	83
Milk[2]	c45
Spaghetti (boiled)	67
Corn flakes	121
Shredded wheat	97
All-Bran	74
Porridge	88
Baked beans	70
Frozen peas	85
Dried lentils	38
Butter beans	46
Red kidney beans (dried)	43
White rice (boiled 10–25 min)	81
Parboiled rice (boiled 15 min)	54
Boiled new potatoes	80
Apple	62
Orange	59
Orange juice	71
Honey	126
Potato crisps	77

*Data source: Shils *et al.* (2006).
[1] The glycaemic response to 50 grams of carbohydrate in the test food is compared to that of 50 grams of white bread (designated GI 100).
[2] Values for whole or skimmed milk are very similar.

Key points

- Diabetes mellitus is caused by insulin deficiency.
- In type 1 diabetes, there is β-cell destruction in genetically susceptible children which results in an absolute insulin deficiency.
- In type 2 diabetes, the primary change is reduced sensitivity to insulin which precipitates a relative insulin deficiency.
- Type 2 diabetes is triggered in genetically susceptible people by excessive weight gain (particularly increased abdominal fat), a high-fat and low-fibre diet, and inactivity.

→

Key points *continued*

- The acute symptoms of type 2 diabetes are relatively mild whereas those of type 1 are acutely life-threatening and insulin therapy is an absolute requirement.

- More than 85 per cent of diagnosed diabetics have type 2. Many more remain undiagnosed and the numbers are rising with the growth in the elderly population and the increasing prevalence of obesity.

- Cases of type 2 diabetes are now starting to occur in obese young adults and even children.

- Both types of diabetes lead to hyperglycaemia, glucose in the urine, increased urine flow and increased thirst.

- Diagnosis of diabetes is by detection of hyperglycaemia, with various threshold values used depending on whether a random sample, a fasting sample or one obtained after glucose challenge is used.

- In untreated type 1 diabetes, there is rapid weight loss, severe dehydration and ketoacidosis which will eventually result in coma and death.

- Diabetics are particularly prone to heart disease, strokes, renal failure, blindness, peripheral nerve degeneration and gangrene.

- Diet is a key part of the treatment of both types of diabetes.
  - Good control of body weight, blood lipids and blood glucose is important for reducing the long-term complications.
  - Obesity reduces insulin sensitivity.
  - High blood lipids increase atherosclerosis and are considered largely responsible for the macrovascular complications of diabetes, atherosclerosis, heart disease and strokes.

- Hyperglycaemia induces the excessive glycosylation of proteins which is responsible for many of the long-term complications, especially the microvascular conditions (nephropathy, retinopathy and neuropathy).

- Modern diabetic diets are low in fat and saturated fat but high in fibre and complex carbohydrate.
  - High-carbohydrate diets improve glycaemic control because they increase insulin sensitivity.

→

Key points *continued*

  - Dietary fibre slows carbohydrate digestion and absorption and so improves glycaemic control.
  - Low saturated fat intake reduces atherosclerosis.

- Intensive glycaemic control has been shown to reduce the microvascular complications associated with both type 1 and type 2 diabetes and to reduce non-fatal heart attacks.

- The consensus of studies suggests that intensive glycaemic control does not significantly reduce cardiovascular or total mortality but does increase the number of hypoglycaemic episodes.

- The blood concentration of glycosylated haemoglobin is used as a measure of glycaemic control.

- The glycaemic index is a measure of the rise in blood glucose produced by individual carbohydrate foods. Increased use of low-GI diets leads to better glycaemic control in short-term studies with both types of diabetics.

Cystic fibrosis

Cystic fibrosis (CF) is an inherited disease caused by an autosomal recessive gene and it affects around 1 in 2400 live births in the UK. It is the most common genetic disease in northern Europeans and about 1 in 25 people carry the CF gene. According to Dodge *et al.* (1997), in 1992 there were 6500 people with this condition living in the UK and two-thirds of these were aged under 16 years. Increasing life expectancy (births were then outnumbering deaths by around 160 per year) was steadily increasing its prevalence. Since 2003, all newborns in Scotland have been screened for the disease. Screening for the CF gene is offered to potential parents in the USA; if both parents carry the gene, then prenatal screening of the baby is available with the option of terminating affected pregnancies. Many people with CF now survive into middle age, and early detection and treatment improve the long-term prognosis.

The genetic lesion results in the production of a sticky mucus which blocks pancreatic ducts and small airways in the lungs. In the pancreas, this blockage leads to formation of cysts and progressive fibrosis and loss of function as these cysts are repaired. Similar changes occur in the lungs; there are repeated chest infections and progressive fibrotic damage to the lungs. In the past, affected children would have been unlikely to survive into adulthood but improved therapy is steadily increasing their life expectancy. The increasing prevalence is evidence of increased survival of affected patients into adulthood.

Regular physiotherapy to clear the lungs of the thick secretions and the availability of antibiotics to treat lung infections have been key factors in the improved survival and quality of life of sufferers. Lung transplant may further extend the life expectancy. Improved dietetic management has also been an important factor in improving the prognosis for CF patients. The fibrosis of the pancreas leads to a failure to produce pancreatic juice, so there is poor digestion and absorption of fat and protein and poor absorption of fat-soluble vitamins. Untreated CF patients are at high risk of general malnutrition, fat-soluble vitamin deficiencies and perhaps even essential fatty acid deficiencies. Evidence of vitamin A deficiency has in the past been found in untreated CF patients, and in some cases xerophthalmia (due to vitamin A deficiency) was the presenting symptom. There is often anorexia, especially associated with infection, and there is often also increased energy expenditure which compound to increase the risks of malnutrition.

The principal dietetic objective in this condition is to maintain nutritional adequacy. Dietetic management should prevent the wasting, the deficiency diseases and the fatty diarrhoea of untreated CF. Nutritional status is strongly associated with pulmonary function and survival in cystic fibrosis patients (Munck, 2010). Malnourished patients are more prone to respiratory infections, whereas well-nourished patients suffer fewer episodes of pneumonia. Experience of other sick and injured patients suggests that weak, malnourished people have an impaired ability to cough and expectorate.

The strategies employed to meet this objective of maintaining dietary adequacy are summarized below.

- Pancreatic supplements containing the missing digestive enzymes are given with food. These are now in the form of coated microspheres that are protected from destruction in the stomach but disintegrate in the small intestine (duodenum).
- Patients are prescribed a diet that is high in energy and protein and, with the more effective pancreatic supplements, this need not now be low in fat.
- Vitamin supplements (particularly fat-soluble vitamins) are given.
- Dietary supplements or artificial feeding are given when the person is unable to take adequate food by mouth.

Munck (2010) has reviewed the role of diet and maintaining nutritional status in the management of cystic fibrosis.

Key points

- Cystic fibrosis is an inherited condition that results in progressive fibrotic damage to the lungs and pancreas.
- A combination of effective physiotherapy, antibiotic treatment of lung infections and improved dietary management allows many CF patients to survive into middle age.
- Failure of pancreatic secretion leads to malabsorption of fat, protein and fat-soluble vitamins.
- Anorexia and malabsorption reduce energy and nutrient supply and raised energy expenditure increases energy requirements.
- The aim of dietary management is to prevent the wasting and deficiency diseases that CF can precipitate.
- Improved nutrition slows pulmonary deterioration and maintains muscle strength and the ability to cough and expectorate.
- Oral supplements of pancreatic enzymes ensure proper digestion of food and enable patients to eat a normal diet.
- Vitamin supplements are a precautionary measure.
- Supplements or artificial feeding should be used during bouts of infection and anorexia.

Chronic renal failure

The weight of the kidney and the number of functional units (nephrons) both decline with age. There is also an age-related decline in measures of renal function such as glomerular filtration rate (GFR). In large numbers of elderly people, renal function declines to the point where the chronic renal failure (CRF) becomes symptomatic. Incidence of CRF is five times higher in the over-60s than in those aged 20–49 years and 10 times higher in the over-80s.

As the kidney fails, there is reduced excretion of the urea produced by breakdown of excess dietary protein (or body protein in wasting subjects). Levels of creatinine and urea in the blood rise and increased blood urea (*uraemia*) produces unpleasant symptoms such as headache, drowsiness, nausea, vomiting, anorexia, itching and spontaneous bruising. As the condition progresses the patient will eventually lapse into a coma and die unless he or she receives either dialysis or a kidney transplant. A diet that minimizes urea production would be expected to reduce the symptoms of uraemia, and low-protein diets have long been used in the symptomatic treatment of CRF.

There has been a longstanding debate about whether a low-protein diet (*c*40 g/day, about half normal intake) is not only palliative but whether it actually slows the pathological degeneration of the kidney. If this were the case then it would extend the period in which conservative management could be used before either dialysis or transplantation became essential. It has even been argued that chronic over-consumption of protein in early adult life may be a contributory factor in the aetiology (e.g. Rudman, 1988). It has also been suggested that very low-protein diets (*c*20 g/day) should be used in patients with chronic renal failure.

Many of the early studies that claimed a benefit for low-protein diets were small, improperly controlled or short term. Even if very restrictive diets have some effect, this may be outweighed by effects they have on the patient's quality of life and general nutritional status. Locatelli *et al.* (1991) reported only marginal benefits from a low-protein diet and a controlled but 'normal' protein diet on the progression of CRF in a large sample of Italian patients with renal disease. They concluded that any extra benefits of the low-protein diet did not justify the restrictions imposed on the patients. A large and long-term American cohort study suggested that moderate protein restriction slowed the progression of CRF in patients with moderate renal insufficiency. More severe restriction of protein intake in those with more advanced renal failure did not appear to offer any additional benefits as compared to moderate restriction (Klahr *et al.*, 1994).

More recently, Levy *et al.* (2006) compared the effect of a moderately restricted protein diet with an unrestricted diet on the progression of kidney disease in a cohort of almost 600 patients with non-diabetic kidney disease. The intervention period was 2–3 years and the total follow-up time was 12 years, but the results were inconclusive. A group from this same laboratory compared the effects of a very low-protein diet with that of a moderately reduced protein diet (Menon *et al.*, 2009). The very low-protein diet had no effect on the progression to kidney failure but it did appear to significantly increase the risk of death during the follow-up period.

Most low-protein diets for chronic renal disease aim to restrict protein intake to around 40 grams per day (and phosphorus intake to around 600 mg/day) and to give a high proportion of this protein in the form of high-quality animal protein. The typical protein intake of a UK man is 84 g/day. Intakes of lower quality cereal proteins with their attendant relatively high nitrogen losses are restricted, and the diet also aims to be high in energy in order to prevent the breakdown of endogenous protein as an energy source. The overall aim is a high-energy, low-protein intake with protein of high quality. A range of high-energy but protein-reduced foods such as protein-reduced flour, bread, pasta and crackers are available not only as direct sources of low-protein calories but also to act as vehicles to carry fats and sugars; examples are butter and jam (jelly). High-energy, low-protein supplements may also be used. In the past, dietary restriction was often initiated in asymptomatic patients based on biochemical evidence of mild insufficiency, but there was little evidence to support use of this early intervention.

The available evidence does not justify the use of severe protein restriction. Moderate protein restriction can be justified if it produces symptomatic benefits, but there is no consistent evidence that it delays renal deterioration or reduces overall mortality.

Key points

- Renal function declines with age. In many (usually elderly) people, chronic renal failure becomes symptomatic owing to high blood urea concentrations.

- Blood levels of urea and creatinine increase as the capacity of the kidney to excrete them declines.

- Low-protein diets reduce production of urea and give symptomatic relief in CRF.

- Maintenance of good nutrient and energy intakes is necessary as wasting will increase urea production from endogenous protein breakdown.

- There is no consistent evidence that moderate restriction of protein to around half normal intake slows the deterioration in renal function.

- Severe protein restriction may actually increase mortality rate in renal patients.

MALNUTRITION IN HOSPITAL PATIENTS

Overview

Every careful observer of the sick will agree in this, that thousands of patients are annually starved in the midst of plenty, from want of attention to the ways which alone make it possible for them to take food.

Florence Nightingale, Notes on Nursing (1859)

Many people with severe illness are at risk from an unrecognised complication – malnutrition. ... Doctors and nurses frequently fail to recognise undernourishment because they are not trained to look for it.

King's Fund Centre report, A Positive Approach to Nutrition as Treatment (1992)

Malnutrition is both a cause and consequence of disease; it predisposes to and delays recovery from illness. ... the problem often goes unrecognised and untreated ... Yet there is no consistent or coherent framework in place to deal with this problem.

British Association for Parenteral and Enteral Nutrition, press release (2003)

Those three quotations span almost a century and a half, but all three suggest a high prevalence of malnutrition among hospital patients that is partly the result of inadequate care. Despite much research and writing about this problem since 1980, the conclusions of the 2003 quote are strikingly similar to those of Florence Nightingale in 1859.

Several examples of conditions where diet is a specific part of the therapy have been discussed earlier in the chapter. In such patients there is likely to be careful monitoring of their intakes and early recognition of nutritional problems. However, good nutrition is not unimportant for all long-stay hospital patients; rather, it is a vital, if non-specific, complement to their medical or surgical treatments. Unfortunately, general medical and nursing staff are likely to be less vigilant in monitoring the food intakes and nutritional status of the general hospital population.

Historically, nutrition has been given low priority in medical and nursing education. Many doctors and nurses are neither trained to recognize signs of inadequate nutrition nor educated about the key importance of good nutrition in facilitating recovery. The key to improving the nutritional status of hospital or community patients is heightened awareness among all medical staff of the importance of sound nutrition to prognosis and their increased vigilance in recognizing indications of poor or deteriorating nutritional status. A specialist nutrition team can only personally supervise the nutritional care of a small number of patients. This team must rely on other medical and nursing staff to identify nutritionally 'at-risk' patients and refer them quickly to the team. The general nutritional care of those patients not specifically at risk is also dependent on non-nutrition specialists.

Budgetary pressures may encourage hospital managers to economise on the 'hotel' component of hospital costs and to concentrate resources on the direct medical aspects of care. However, pruning the catering budget is likely to be a false economy if it leads to deterioration in the nutritional status of patients. Any deterioration in nutritional status will lead to higher complication rates, longer hospital stays and increased costs in spite of maintained or even improved surgical, medical and nursing care. In the report of an expert working party, it was estimated that the potential financial savings in the UK from a nationwide introduction of nutritional support for undernourished patients amounted to the equivalent of over £400 million at 2011 prices (KFC, 1992). In a major report for the British Association of Parenteral and Enteral Nutrition (BAPEN), Elia *et al.* (2003) estimated that the healthcare cost of malnutrition, specifically under-nutrition, in the UK in 2003 was around £7.3 billion, and this was revised up to £13 billion by Elia *et al.* (2009). Compared to well-nourished people, malnourished patients had more GP visits, more hospital admissions, a longer hospital stay and more admissions to care homes. Of this total of £7.3 billion in 2003, more than half was for the treatment of malnourished patients in hospital. This total represents about 10 per cent of the total health budget, so even modest fractional savings would have a significant impact on resources within the health system.

Key points

- Malnutrition is still prevalent among hospital patients more than 150 years after Florence Nightingale first highlighted this problem.
- Nutrition has traditionally been inadequately covered in medical and nursing education. Hospital staff are neither trained to monitor nutritional status nor sufficiently aware of its importance to successful treatment.
- Improving the nutritional support for hospital patients could generate considerable financial savings.
- Under-nutrition and its consequences may well cost the healthcare system more than those associated with obesity.

Prevalence of hospital malnutrition

Two papers published in the 1970s are widely credited with focusing attention on the problem of hospital malnutrition. Bistrian *et al.* (1974) in

the USA and Hill *et al.* (1977) in the UK reported that up to 50 per cent of surgical patients in some hospitals showed indications of malnutrition, both general protein energy malnutrition and vitamin deficiencies. Since these landmark publications there have been reports of high prevalence of suboptimal nutrition in children's wards, medical and geriatric wards and in hospitals in other countries. For example, almost one in six children admitted to a Birmingham (UK) hospital were stunted or severely wasted – at least a quarter of children admitted with chronic respiratory, cardiac and digestive problems were short for their age; see KFC (1992) and Powell-Tuck (1997) for further examples and references. More recently, Elia *et al.* (2003) have estimated that up to 60 per cent of patients in hospitals are clinically malnourished.

Consequences of hospital malnutrition

Following a general review of the relationship between nutritional status and outcome in hospital patients, an expert committee in the UK concluded that malnutrition is associated with increased duration of stay, increased hospital charges, increased requirements for home healthcare after hospital discharge, increased rates of complications and increased mortality. Some of the specific consequences of under-nutrition in hospital patients are summarized in Box 17.1.

Box 17.1

Some consequences of under-nutrition in hospital patients

- Higher rates of wound infection because of slow healing and reduced immunocompetence
- Increased risk of general infections, particularly respiratory infections and pneumonia
- Muscle weakness – which means that patients take longer to re-mobilize, and weakness of the respiratory muscles will impair the ability to cough and expectorate and predispose to respiratory infections
- Increased risk of pressure sores because of wasting and immobility

→

Box 17.1 *continued*

- Increased risk of thromboembolism because of immobility
- Malnutrition reduces the digestive functions of the gut and probably also increases its permeability to bacteria and their toxins
- Increased liability to heart failure because of wasting and reduced function of cardiac muscle
- Apathy, depression and self neglect

Wasting of muscles and fat is one of the most obvious outward signs of starvation, but there is also wasting of vital internal organs including the heart and intestines. In the classical starvation studies of Keys *et al.* (1950), chronic under-nutrition in healthy subjects was also found to cause apathy and depression. This would clearly hinder the recovery of malnourished hospital patients.

It is a general observation that, in famine areas, malnutrition is associated with high rates of infectious diseases, with increased severity and duration of illness and ultimately with higher mortality. Providing medicines and medical personnel has limited impact if the underlying problem of malnutrition is not addressed.

There are numerous demonstrable changes in the functioning of the immune system as a consequence of protein-energy malnutrition. An illustrative, but by no means exhaustive, list of some of the best documented effects is given below (reviewed by Scrimshaw and Sangiovanni, 1997).

- There is atrophy of the thymus gland, lymph nodes, tonsils and spleen in malnourished children.
- There is reduced production of T-lymphocytes and various T-cell subsets, including natural killer cells which kill cancers cells and virus-infected cells.
- Cell-mediated immune function is profoundly depressed by protein-energy malnutrition. Delayed-type cutaneous hypersensitivity responses to injected antigens are markedly depressed even in moderate nutritional deficiency, and these responses are a measure of cell-mediated immune responses. The best

known of these reactions is the Mantoux reaction in which individuals immune to the organism that causes tuberculosis respond to a cutaneous tuberculin injection with an inflammatory reaction some hours after the injection.

- Secretion of immunoglobulin A (IgA), the antibody fraction that protects epithelial surfaces such as those in the gut and respiratory tract, is markedly depressed. This would make malnourished patients more prone to respiratory, gut and genito-urinary infections.
- Circulating antibody responses (IgG) are relatively unaffected in protein-energy malnutrition.
- White cells kill bacteria after they have ingested them by generating an oxidative pulse of superoxide radicals. Their capacity to kill ingested bacteria in this way is reduced in malnutrition.
- Changes in the skin and mucous membranes of the gut, respiratory tract and genito-urinary tract reduce their efficiency as barriers to infection. Malnutrition leads to defects in their integrity, reduced mucus secretion and decreased ciliary activity. Decreased gastric acid secretion may also increase the risk of gastro-intestinal infections.

There is also a vast literature detailing the effects of specific micronutrient deficiencies on immune function. Two examples are noted here.

- Zinc has an important role. In experimental zinc deficiency there are multiple adverse effects on both the humoral and cell-mediated arms of the immune system.
- Vitamin A deficiency reduces cell-mediated and humoral immunity and greatly increases the incidence and severity of infections. It also affects the integrity of epithelial tissue, making it less effective as a barrier to infection.

Scrimshaw and Sangiovanni (1997) write about a synergism of nutrition, infection and immunity – infections have adverse effects on nutritional status, and almost any severe nutrient deficiency will impair resistance to infection and have measurable adverse effects on measures of immune function.

Note that trauma and ageing also have deleterious effects on immune function. This means that, for example, the immune systems of poorly nourished elderly patients undergoing major and traumatic surgery will be triply depressed. Minimizing surgical trauma with modern techniques should lessen the immunosuppressive effect of surgery.

Key points

- Malnutrition of hospital patients increases their duration of stay, their risk of complications, their requirements for medical care after discharge and their mortality risk.
- Malnutrition decreases immune function and predisposes hospital patients to infections.
- In general malnutrition, the cell-mediated immune response is reduced, there is reduced secretion of IgA, and white cells have a reduced capacity to generate an oxidative pulse to kill ingested bacteria.
- The ability of skin and epithelial tissues to act as non-specific barriers to infection is impaired by malnutrition.
- Several micronutrient deficiencies adversely affect the immune system, particularly zinc and vitamin A.
- Ageing and trauma also have adverse effects on immune function. An elderly malnourished patient undergoing traumatic surgery experiences a triple depression of immune function.
- Some specific consequences of malnutrition for hospital patients are summarized in Box 17.1.

Causes of hospital malnutrition

Hospital malnutrition is not solely or even primarily a consequence of things that happen in the hospital environment. Up to 40 per cent of patients are already malnourished when they are admitted. For example, McWhirter and Pennington (1994) surveyed the nutritional status of 100 consecutive admissions to each of five areas of a major Scottish acute teaching hospital; they found that about 40 per cent of patients were malnourished at admission.

A study by Mowe et al. (1994) suggested that, at least in the elderly, malnutrition might have been one factor in precipitating the illnesses that necessitated admission. They made a nutritional assessment of a large sample of elderly patients admitted to an Oslo hospital because of an acute illness (e.g. stroke, myocardial infarction, pneumonia). They also assessed the nutritional status of a matched sample of older people living within the hospital catchment area. Between 50 and 60 per cent of patients were undernourished at the time of admission, and the nutritional status of the hospital group was much worse than that of the home group. Using several measures of nutritional status, they found that 86 per cent of the home subjects showed no sign of malnutrition compared to only 43 per cent of the hospital group. They found that poor food intake in the month prior to admission was much more common in the hospital group than the home group. They suggested that reduced nutrient intakes and deteriorating nutritional status in the period prior to admission could have raised the risk of hospitalization. Recall that in the third quotation at the start of this section, this expert group stated that 'malnutrition is both a cause and a consequence of disease'.

Although many patients are already malnourished when they reach hospital, there is a tendency for any under-nutrition to worsen during their stay (Powell-Tuck, 1997). In their survey of 500 Scottish hospital admissions, McWhirter and Pennington (1994) reported that two-thirds of patients lost weight during their stay, and this loss was greatest in patients identified as most malnourished on admission. Very few patients were given any nutritional support, but those who were then showed a substantial mean weight gain. Those selected for nutritional support obviously tended to be the most severely malnourished on admission. The deterioration in nutritional status that often accompanies hospitalization can usually be avoided with appropriate care. Fewer than half of the malnourished patients in this survey had any nutritional information documented in their notes. The authors concluded that 'malnutrition remains a largely unrecognized problem in hospital and highlights the need for education on clinical nutrition'. In their earlier study, Hill et al. (1977) also found that only 20 per cent of patients' notes contained any reference to their nutritional status, and then only a brief note such as 'looks wasted'. Only around 15 per cent of the patients they surveyed had been weighed at any stage during their hospital stay.

Depressed intake is usually the main cause of nutritional inadequacy during illness or after injury.

Several of the factors that can depress food intake in the sick and injured are noted below.

- *Physical difficulty in eating.* Reasons can be unconsciousness, facial injury, difficulty in swallowing, oral or throat infection, lack of teeth, arthritis, and diseases affecting coordination and motor functions.
- *Anorexia induced by disease or treatment.* Severe anorexia is a frequent consequence of malignant disease, but anorexia is a symptom also of most serious illnesses and a side-effect of many treatments. It is likely in anyone experiencing pain, fever or nausea.
- *Anorexia resulting from a psychological response to illness, hospitalization or diagnosis.* Starvation itself may lead to depression and apathy and may thus reduce the will to eat in order to assist recovery.
- *Unacceptability of hospital food.* This is most obvious in patients offered food that is not acceptable on religious or cultural grounds. Equally, low-prestige, unfamiliar and just plain unappetizing food may severely depress intake in people whose appetite may already be impaired.
- *Lack of availability of food.* Patients may be starved prior to surgery or for diagnostic purposes, and they may be absent from their ward at meal times. This may help to depress overall nutrient intakes.

In general, the more specific and more obvious these influences are the more likely they are to be addressed. It will be obvious that particular measures are needed to ensure that someone with a broken jaw can eat, but a patient who lacks teeth and has a sore mouth and throat is more likely to be overlooked. More allowance is likely to be made for a Jewish patient known to require kosher food than for a patient who simply finds hospital food strange and unappetizing. Some service provision factors that may help to depress the food intake of hospital patients are listed in Box 17.2.

A recent survey of over 2200 patients in 97 English hospitals highlighted and quantified several of these problems that tend to depress food intake in hospital patients (CPPIH, 2006). This survey reported that:

- 40 per cent of patients had their hospital food supplemented by their visitors

---

Box 17.2

Service provision factors that may depress energy and nutrient intakes in hospital patients

- Meals may be bunched together during the working day, with long enforced fasts from early evening to morning.
- Prolonged holding of food prior to serving leads to deterioration of both nutritional quality and palatability.
- Inherently unappetizing food and limited choice.
- Failure to allow choice (e.g. patients may initially be given meals selected by the previous occupant of the bed).
- Providing patients with portions of food that are insufficient for their needs, perhaps because staff underestimate the needs of bedridden patients.
- Plate wastage not monitored or recorded by staff and so very low intakes are not recognized early.
- Inadequate amount of time allowed for slow feeders to finish their meals.
- Lack of staff help for those who need help with eating. Staff shortages may mean that by the time help is provided, the food is cold and unappetizing.

- 37 per cent left their meal because it smelt, looked or tasted unappetizing
- 26 per cent didn't receive the help they needed in feeding themselves
- 22 per cent of meals were served at the incorrect temperature
- 18 per cent of patients didn't get their choice of meal.

In addition to the myriad factors that tend to depress intakes, the factors listed below may also increase the nutrient requirements of many sick and injured patients.

- *Increased nutrient losses.* Reasons can be loss of blood, the protein lost in the exudate from burned surfaces, loss of glucose and ketones in the urine of diabetics, and protein in the urine of patients with renal disease.
- *Malabsorption of nutrients.* Reasons can be disease of the alimentary tract or simply age-related

deterioration in the efficiency of absorption. Malnutrition itself produces adverse changes in gut function with reduced efficiency of digestion and reduced absorption of several nutrients.

- *Increased nutrient turnover.* Illness and injury lead to hypermetabolism, the metabolic response to injury.

In a classical series of studies that began in the 1930s, Cuthbertson demonstrated that in patients with traumatic injury the initial period of shock after injury was followed by a period of hypermetabolism. He used the term 'ebb' to describe the period of depressed metabolism or shock in the first 12–24 hours after injury, and the term 'flow' to describe the state of hypermetabolism that occurs once the initial period of shock is over. The flow phase is characterized by increased resting metabolism and oxygen consumption and an increased urinary loss of nitrogen associated with increased muscle protein breakdown, increased gluconeogenesis and increased fat breakdown and fatty acid oxidation. Cuthbertson found that the magnitude of this flow response was greater the more severe the injury and the better nourished the patient. Long bone fractures may increase the resting metabolic rate by 15–25 per cent and extensive burn injuries can double the metabolic rate. In severe trauma, sepsis or advanced disease, nutritional support can only partly ameliorate the severe depletion of body fat and protein reserves that this hypermetabolic state produces (Cuthbertson, 1980).

Following a traumatic injury, Cuthbertson found that the flow response generally reached its peak 4–8 days after injury and that the overall loss of body protein could exceed 7 per cent of total body protein within the first 10 days. The increased metabolism was a consequence of the increased rate of body protein turnover and the use of body protein as an energy-yielding substrate. Cuthbertson regarded this *catabolic response* as an adaptive mechanism to provide a source of energy when incapacitated by injury (traumatic or infective) and a means of supplying amino acids for the synthesis of new tissue and for the functioning of the immune system. The aim of nutritional management during this phase is to supply sufficient energy and protein to prevent or minimize use of endogenous protein and energy reserves and to maintain an adequate intake of essential micronutrients. Some nutrients, in particular the amino acid glutamine, may become conditionally essential during this phase, and there is likely to be increased turnover of other micronutrients, especially zinc and vitamin A.

This catabolic response is partly mediated through hormonal responses to the stress of injury or illness. Levels of cortisol and catecholamine hormones from adrenal glands rise in the flow phase, but induced hormonal changes in healthy subjects are not able to reproduce the magnitude of protein catabolism seen in severe injury. Levels of inflammatory mediators known as *cytokines* are elevated during the hypermetabolic phase, and several of these have clearly identified metabolic effects that contribute to the multiple metabolic changes seen during the metabolic response to injury.

A patient who is well nourished and able to mount a bigger flow response is enabled to recover more quickly. This would suggest that improving nutritional status prior to planned major surgery should facilitate the recovery process – although studies designed to test this hypothesis have produced variable results (KFC, 1992).

In a recent review of the current literature, Hebbar and Harte (2007) confirmed that poor preoperative nutritional status was associated with delayed wound healing, increased susceptibility to infections and respiratory problems, prolonged hospital stay, and higher mortality. However, they found little evidence that the routine use of preoperative nutrition interventions, whether parenteral or enteral, had any measurable effect on *overall mortality* – although they did appear to reduce postoperative complications in severely malnourished patients. They concluded that there was no justification for delaying surgery to improve nutritional status except for those patients who were severely malnourished.

Key points

- The high prevalence of hospital malnutrition is largely explained by the high prevalence of malnutrition among new admissions.
- In some cases, malnutrition might be a contributory factor to the illness that has necessitated hospitalization.

→

Key points *continued*

- Many patients lose weight during their hospital stay and any under-nutrition at the time of admission tends to worsen.
- Much of the deterioration in nutritional status could be avoided if there were effective nutritional support, but there is inadequate monitoring and recording of nutritional status in many hospitals.
- Weight loss is due to depressed food intake and sometimes to increased requirements. Intake of hospital patients is depressed for many reasons, including:
  - eating difficulties
  - anorexia due to illness treatment or anxiety
  - unacceptability of hospital food
  - enforced periods of fasting.
- Some more specific service provision factors are listed in Box 17.2.
- Nutritional requirements may be increased if there are increased nutrient losses in urine or from the site of injury or if absorption of nutrients is impaired.
- Major trauma, sepsis and serious illness induce a hypermetabolic state in which there is increased metabolic rate and protein catabolism leading to rapid wasting of muscle and adipose tissue.

Improving the nutritional care of hospital patients

Aims of dietetic management of general hospital patients

The two main aims of dietetic care of hospital patients are noted below.

- Steps should be taken to assess and monitor the nutritional status of all patients and, where necessary, take measures to correct nutritional inadequacy. Where feasible, the nutritional status of poorly nourished patients should be improved prior to planned surgery, but unless the patient is severely malnourished this would not justify delaying the surgery.
- After injury or surgery, or during illness, the inputs of energy, protein and other essential and conditionally essential nutrients should be

sufficient to maintain body reserves or even to increase them in undernourished patients. In grossly hypercatabolic patients it may be possible to only partly compensate for losses caused by this hypercatabolism.

The basal energy requirements of a patient can be estimated from his or her body weight, as described in Chapter 3. The following additional allowances can then be added to this basal figure to estimate the patient's total requirements.

- Add an amount to allow for the hypermetabolism of illness and injury, which will depend on the exact nature of the condition. It might range from an extra 5–25 per cent in postoperative patients, those with long bone fractures or mild-to-moderate infections, up to as much as an extra 90 per cent in patients with extensive burns.
- Add an amount to allow for the mobility of the patient, ranging from +20 per cent in the immobile, +30 per cent in the bed-bound but mobile, to +40 per cent in those able to move around the ward.
- Add an increment to allow replenishment of stores if the patient is already depleted.

Protein allowances will also need to be increased in line with the extent of the calculated hypermetabolism.

Aids to meeting nutritional needs

The simplest and cheapest way of satisfying the nutritional requirements of sick and injured people is to encourage and facilitate the consumption of appetizing and nutritious food and drinks. In some patients, additional support measures may be needed.

- *Nutritional supplements.* Concentrated energy and nutrient sources are usually consumed in liquid form and are readily digested and absorbed.
- *Enteral feeding.* Nutrients are introduced directly into the stomach or small intestine through a tube that has been inserted through the nose and into the stomach or intestine via the oesophagus. Tubes may be introduced directly into the gut by surgical means, particularly if there is likely to be an extended period of enteral feeding.

- *Parenteral feeding.* The patient may be supplied with nutrients intravenously, either as a supplement to the oral route or as the sole means of nutrition – total parenteral nutrition (TPN). In TPN the nutrients must be infused via an indwelling catheter into a large vein. In some cases (e.g. of extreme damage to the gut) patients may be fed for years by TPN. A major factor that has enabled patients to be maintained indefinitely with TPN was the development of a means of safely infusing a source of fat intravenously.

When supplementary feeding is being given via the gut either as nutritional supplements or enteral feeds, it is important that they really do increase total nutritional intake and that they do not suppress voluntary intake and thus simply replace what the patient would voluntarily consume. Systematic reviews and meta-analysis of the use of oral nutritional supplements indicate that they do increase total energy and nutrient intakes in a variety of types of patient, that they have little depressing effect on voluntary food intake, and that, in post-surgical patients, they may even increase appetite and voluntary food intake. Experimental studies with healthy subjects suggest that quite substantial supplementary enteral feeds when given by slow continuous infusion have almost no appetite-suppressing effect and substantially increase total energy intake. Clinical trials also report that enteral feeding in this way does increase total nutritional intake in patients when used as a supplement to normal oral feeding. If the supplement is given as a bolus or 'meal' then it does depress voluntary food intake. The reader is referred to reviews by Stratton (2005) and Stratton *et al.* (2008).

When a patient is being fed totally by the parenteral route because normal intake is contraindicated (e.g. by severe intestinal disease), then ideally the parenteral feed should not only supply the needs for energy and essential nutrients but also satisfy the person's hunger and reduce the desire to eat normal food. However, even though the parenteral nutrition supplies all nutritional needs and maintains the person's body weight within the normal range, three-quarters of these patients report that they still feel hungry and almost half report that they are distressed by this. Many report specific food desires. The presence of hunger

in people being maintained on long-term parenteral nutrition is clearly a very unpleasant consequence of their therapy, akin to intractable pain experienced by many other people with chronic conditions.

Ideally a specialist nutrition team should supervise these artificial feeding methods. TPN, in particular, requires specialist management and is usually used only where the oral route is ruled out, such as in patients who have had a large part of the intestine removed or have severe inflammatory disease of the intestine. Infection of the intravenous lines can be a major problem in TPN but with skilled specialist management can be largely eliminated.

The King's Fund Centre (KFC, 1992) estimated that over 1000 patients were receiving enteral nutrition at home and 100–150 parenteral nutrition. A comparison of these figures with those given in Stratton (2005) demonstrates that there was a very steep rise in the home use of these artificial feeding regimes in the following decade. At the end of 2003 it was estimated that 25 000 patients in the UK were using enteral feeding at home, and 600 patients per year were using parenteral feeding at home.

Use of oral supplements costs just a few pounds per week while the cost of artificial feeding rises steeply the more sophisticated the method. Enteral feeding is many times more expensive than oral supplements, and total parenteral nutrition many times more expensive than enteral feeding. It is therefore important that patients receive a level of intervention that is appropriate for their needs. Figure 17.1 shows a scheme that could be used to select the appropriate level of nutritional support for a given patient.

Measures that could improve the nutritional status of hospital patients

- Improve nutrition education for doctors and nurses and heighten awareness of the importance of adequate nutrition for patient recovery. Staff must be aware of the effect of illness and injury on nutritional needs and must be able to carry out simple nutritional monitoring and to interpret the results.
- Include a nutritional assessment as part of the standard admissions procedure. This might

Is the patient malnourished? —No→ No action

Yes ↓

Can the patient tolerate enough —Yes→ Normal food
ordinary food to meet needs?

No ↓

Would oral supplements help? —Yes→ Oral supplements

No ↓

Is the gut functioning sufficiently —Yes→ Enteral feeding
for enteral feeding?

No ↓

Parenteral feeding?

Figure 17.1 Scheme for deciding on the appropriate level of nutritional support for a patient. Based on a scheme in RCN (1993).

include information about appetite, recent weight changes, oral and dental health, social characteristics and physical indicators of nutritional status such as BMI or arm circumference. Many hospitals do now include such information in their admission forms and have developed simple scoring schemes to screen for those people who are nutritionally 'at risk'. In Scotland, all patients entering hospital are nutritionally screened. In 2003, the Malnutrition Universal Screening Tool was launched to be used to simply and quickly assess nutritional status in hospitals, the community or in other care accommodation and is simple enough to be used by any care workers (Elia *et al.*, 2003). This is briefly discussed later in the chapter.

• Regularly monitor a patient's food intake and weight or any other simple anthropometric indicator. This would facilitate early identification of depressed food intake and deteriorating nutritional status.

• Provide appetizing, acceptable and nutritious food that reaches patients in good condition, and ensure they receive the correct level of assistance with feeding. Ways of minimizing the adverse impact of the service provision factors listed in Box 17.2 should be sought and proper provision should be made for patients with special cultural

needs. There should be formal procedures to record absences from the ward at meal times and active measures to provide food for patients who are absent for meals and after a period of enforced fasting. Despite several well-publicised initiatives since the late 1990s, a recent large survey of English hospitals still found very high levels of patient dissatisfaction with the hospital food and high levels of wastage (CPPIH, 2006).

• Rapidly refer a patient with poor or deteriorating nutritional status to a nutrition specialist. The patient can then be given the appropriate level of support by a specialist team. Several of the authors who have reported a high prevalence of malnutrition in hospitals have also noted that very few of the malnourished patients had received any nutritional support; see, for example, Hill *et al.* (1977) and McWhirter and Pennington (1994).

Outcomes of supplementation

In many acute conditions, nutritional support can substantially reduce mortality. A number of controlled studies on the effects of supplementary feeding in hospital patients have been conducted. Reduced complication rates, decreased length of hospital stay and reduced mortality rates are general findings from such studies (KFC, 1992; Powell-Tuck, 1997; Pennington, 1997). Larsson *et al.* (1990) carried out a randomized study of the effects of energy supplements using 500 patients admitted to a long-stay geriatric ward of a Swedish hospital. The supplements reduced the deterioration in nutritional status following admission and reduced the mortality rate. Two studies on the effects of supplementation in patients with hip fractures suggest that oral or enteral supplements improve both the nutritional status of the patients and measures of outcome. Supplementation was associated with reduced hospital stay, more rapid mobilization, reduced rates of complications and lower mortality (Delmi *et al.*, 1990; Bastow *et al.*, 1983). In more recent reviews (Stratton, 2005; Stratton *et al.*, 2008) it was reported that several systematic reviews had indicated that, compared with those receiving routine care, patients receiving oral supplements or tube feeding had significantly lower mortality, significantly lower rates of complications like wound infections and pneumonia, greater respiratory and skeletal muscle strength, improved wound healing and other physical and psychological benefits.

The Malnutrition Universal Screening Tool

The 'MUST' is a screening tool for malnutrition that is said to be simple enough for use by any care workers and suitable for use in almost any setting – in hospitals, care homes, doctors' surgeries and outpatient clinics and in other community settings. It was developed by Elia *et al.* (2003) for the British Association for Parenteral and Enteral Nutrition (BAPEN). The basic protocol and explanatory notes can be downloaded and printed from www.bapen. org.uk/must_tool.html. It involves a five-step process (Box 17.3).

Box 17.3

The Malnutrition Universal Screening Tool (MUST)

Step 1: Measure height and weight and calculate the BMI
- <18.5 kg/m² – score 2
- 18.5–20 – score 1
- >over 20 – score 0
- >30 score 0 (but classify as obese)

Step 2: Record amount of unplanned weight loss in last 3–6 months
- <5% – score 0
- 5–10% – score 1
- >10% – score 2

Box 17.3 *continued*

Step 3: If patient is acutely ill and it is likely that there has been no nutritional intake for more than 5 days
- score 2

Step 4: Add scores from steps 1, 2 and 3
- total score 0 – **low risk**
- total score 1 – **medium risk**
- total score ≥2 – **high risk**

Step 5: Management guidelines
- **Low risk**. Give routine care with regular repeat screening.
- **Medium risk**. Monitor intake for 3 days – if improved or adequate then there is little clinical concern. If intake is poor or not improved there should be clinical concern. Follow local management policy. Continue to monitor regularly.
- **High risk**. Treat by reference to a nutrition specialist or team, improve and increase intake and monitor and review treatment plan regularly.

Alternatives for patients when the required measurements cannot be obtained
- If height cannot be measured, then either (a reliable) self reported height can be used or knee height, demispan or ulna length can be used and tables are given for estimating height from these measures.
- If neither height nor weight can be measured, mid upper arm circumference (MUAC) can be used and guideline values are given.
- Subjective evaluations can be used as an alternative to an objective BMI measure/estimate.
- Subjective indicators of recent weight loss can be used where numerical values/estimates cannot be made (e.g. loose-fitting clothes or jewellery, or a history of low food intake or feeding problems).

Key points

- The nutritional status of all patients should be routinely monitored and all appropriate measures taken to minimize any deterioration in nutritional status.
- The MUST screening tool developed for BAPEN is simple to use and suitable for almost any clinical or community setting, including hospital patients. It is a five-step process whereby height, weight, BMI, recent weight loss and recent clinical condition are used to produce a score which classifies patients as at low, medium or high risk (see Box 17.3).

Key points *continued*

- Where necessary, special nutritional supplements can be given orally or patients can be fed by an enteral tube or parenterally (intravenously).

- Feeding costs increase steeply with increasing sophistication of nutritional support, so the minimum effective level of support should be used (see Figure 17.1).

- Controlled trials and systematic reviews have shown that nutritional support can lead to significant patient benefits, including:

  - lower mortality
  - reduced complications like local infections and pneumonia
  - improved muscle strength, including respiratory muscles
  - improved healing
  - faster re-mobilization
  - psychological benefits.

- Some measures that could improve the nutritional status of hospital patients are:

  - improved nutrition education for medical and nursing staff
  - nutritional screening of patients at admission and regular monitoring during hospitalization
  - improvements in catering and the delivery of food to patients
  - rapid referral of patients identified by screening as 'at risk' to a nutrition specialist or team.

18

SOME OTHER GROUPS AND SITUATIONS

Vegetarianism	507	Nutrition and physical activity	519
Racial minorities	513		

VEGETARIANISM

Overview

A strict vegetarian, or *vegan*, avoids consuming any animal products – meat, fish, eggs, dairy produce and perhaps even honey. Others are less strict in their avoidance and, although they do not eat meat, they may eat dairy produce, eggs or fish or any combination of these three. The prefixes *lacto*, *ovo* and *pesco* are used alone or in combination to describe these degrees of vegetarianism; so, for example, one who avoids meat and fish but eats eggs and dairy produce is an ovolactovegetarian.

Johnston and Sabate (2006) have written a wide-ranging and extensively referenced review of health aspects of vegetarianism, and most of the uncited references for statements made in this section can be found in that review.

An American survey conducted in 1994 suggested that about 7 per cent of Americans called themselves vegetarians. Only around 4 per cent of self-styled vegetarians are vegans and many of them occasionally ate meat and many more ate poultry or fish. The term 'vegetarian' clearly has a variety of different meanings to different consumers. People who consume little meat and poultry but are not strictly vegetarian are sometimes referred to as semi- or demi-vegetarians. Detailed analysis of the questionnaires from this 1994 survey suggested that only about 1 per cent of Americans actually refrained from eating any meat, fish or poultry at that time. These survey results highlight the difficulties of making accurate estimates of the extent of vegetarianism. A similar poll conducted in 2000 concluded that 2.5 per cent of the US population could then be classified as vegetarian using this criterion.

The Vegetarian Society in the UK (www.vegsoc. org) produces updated factsheets that give useful statistical information about vegetarianism and sales of meat-free foods (and meat/fish) gleaned from government and independent sources.

Estimates of the prevalence of vegetarianism in the UK vary between 3 and 5 per cent, with many more people saying they are partly vegetarian (i.e. avoiding some types of meat and fish). Much less than 1 per cent of UK adults are vegans. About twice as many women as men are vegetarians, and the peak prevalence is in younger women (under 35 years). It is less common in people aged over 65 years. Vegetarianism is much more common among people with high incomes than those in the lowest income category. The market for meat-free foods has been growing in the UK from £548 million in 2001 to £739 million in 2008, and about £170 million of this latter figure was for foods using meat substitutes like Quorn.

The major reasons cited for adopting vegetarianism in the USA and UK are identified below:

- health reasons – the vegetarian lifestyle may reduce the risk of several chronic diseases, and there have been several major alarms about the safety of animal foods such as the BSE crisis in the late 1990s in the UK

- ecological and environmental reasons (in Chapter 2 it was noted that it requires between 3 and 10 kilograms of grain to produce 1 kilogram of meat)
- animal welfare and cruelty concerns
- not liking the taste of meat.

Several major religions restrict or discourage the consumption of meat, including Buddhism, Hinduism and Seventh Day Adventism. In the UK, many members of the large south Asian community are lactovegetarians and these people probably represent the biggest group of vegetarians in the UK. Religious considerations and lack of meat availability mean that many people in developing countries eat little or no meat.

Nutritionists have traditionally been concerned about the adequacy implications of vegetarian and particularly vegan diets. From an adequacy viewpoint, any major restriction of the categories from which food may be selected cannot be regarded as ideal. The greater the degree of restriction the greater are the chances of the diet being inadequate, and also of any toxicants in food being consumed in hazardous amounts. Paradoxically, most recent interest has been shown in vegetarian diets as a possible means to increasing wellness. There have been numerous reports of low incidence of chronic disease among vegetarian groups. This change has been reflected in the focus of scientific research about vegetarianism. Between 1966 and 1975, 48 per cent of scientific papers about vegetarianism were concerned with their nutritional adequacy and only 24 per cent about their possible role in disease prevention or treatment; but between 1986 and 1995 these figures were almost reversed at 24 and 40 per cent, respectively. Indeed, the possible health benefits are now frequently cited as the reason for adopting vegetarianism in the UK and USA.

A recurring theme of the dietary guidance offered in this book has been to encourage diversity of food choice. The avoidance of whole groups of foods runs contrary to that theme and is therefore regarded by the author as suboptimal. Paradoxically, another recurring theme has been to encourage adults in industrialized countries to reduce their consumption of meat and other animal foods and to increase their consumption of cereals, fruits and vegetables – effectively to move towards a more vegetable-based diet.

It is clear that a thoughtfully constructed vegetarian or even vegan diet is compatible with nutritional adequacy and may well be more diverse and adequate than the current diets of many omnivores. When people decide for cultural, religious, ethical or ecological reasons to adopt some degree of vegetarianism then the role of the nutrition educator should be to facilitate the healthful implementation of that personal choice. Nutritionists should only try to discourage practices that are irrevocably dysfunctional.

Key points

- Only a small proportion of vegetarians are vegans who avoid all animal products.
- Most vegetarians consume milk and dairy produce (lactovegetarian); many consume eggs (ovo) and/or fish (pesco).
- Some people classify themselves as vegetarian despite eating some poultry or meat, and they could be termed demi-vegetarian.
- Several major religions encourage vegetarianism but many affluent Western vegetarians choose to be vegetarian for health, ecological or ethical reasons or simply because they claim not to like the taste of meat.
- Vegetarianism restricts dietary choice and so theoretically increases the risks of dietary inadequacy.
- Most dietary guidelines in Western countries imply that a move towards a more vegetable-based diet would have health benefits.
- Most, but not all, vegetarian groups in Western countries have lower rates of chronic disease and lower mortality than omnivores.
- The potential health benefit of partial or complete vegetarianism is now the predominant theme of research, rather than its potential to cause dietary inadequacies.

Adequacy of vegetarian diets

Animal-derived foods are the only, or the major, sources of some nutrients in typical UK and USA diets. The possibility that supplies of such nutrients might be inadequate in vegetarian or vegan diets needs to be considered and, where necessary, remedial measures identified that are consistent with maintaining the chosen diet. The degree to which less strict vegetarians are threatened by these potential inadequacies will depend on the extent of individual restrictions. Many vegetarians make liberal use of dairy produce and in some cases also of eggs and fish, so most of the theoretical deficiencies of totally vegetable-based diets will not apply to them.

Vegan diets theoretically contain no natural vitamin B_{12}, vitamin D or retinol. They are also likely to contain less total energy, protein, calcium, zinc, riboflavin and available iron. Several studies do indeed suggest that intakes of vitamin B_{12}, vitamin D, retinol, calcium and zinc are lower in vegetarians.

Vegan and probably other vegetarian diets are likely to be less energy-dense than omnivorous diets because they have less fat and more starch and fibre. Total energy intakes are, as a consequence, also likely to be lower than those of omnivores. Indeed, the reduced energy density of vegetarian diets is perceived as one of the major advantages of such a diet for affluent adult populations where overweight and obesity are common. There is a general consensus that Caucasian vegans have lower energy intakes than omnivores and are lighter and have a lower proportion of body fat. Most studies also suggest that other vegetarians are lighter than omnivores and are less likely to be overweight or obese, although the difference is smaller than that between vegans and omnivores. As discussed later, this does not necessarily mean that meat avoidance *per se* will prevent excessive weight gain or be an effective strategy for weight loss in those who are already overweight or obese.

A less positive view of the low energy density of vegetarian diets is usually taken when children are the consumers. A diet that has too low an energy density could impair their growth. Studies in the USA, Holland and the UK have found that younger vegan children tend to be lighter and smaller in stature than omnivorous children. The differences are generally small and the growth patterns and growth curves of vegan children are usually within normal limits and they tend to catch up this growth

later in childhood (by the age of 10 years). In a sample of British vegan children, Sanders (1988) found that energy intakes were below the then recommended dietary allowances (RDAs) and that fat intakes were, on average, low but very variable (ranging from 16 to 39 per cent of calories). Sanders concluded that low fat intake and the low energy density were probably the major determinants of the low energy intakes. In turn, the low energy intakes were probably responsible for the anthropometric differences between vegan and omnivore children rather than any differences in dietary quality. American Seventh Day Adventist children who are ovolactovegetarians grow similarly to other children and have no greater evidence of nutritional deficiencies.

Vegan diets are likely to be lower in protein than omnivorous or lactovegetarian diets. Individual plant proteins are also generally of lower quality than individual animal proteins. Thus one of the traditional concerns of vegetarians has been about the protein adequacy of their diets. The priority attached to protein deficiency as a likely cause of human malnutrition has declined very sharply in recent decades (see Chapter 11). Mutual supplementation also means that the overall protein quality of a good mixed-vegetable meal or diet may not be substantially different from an omnivorous one. This means that, according to current estimates of requirements, vegetarian and even vegan diets are likely to be more than adequate both in terms of their overall protein content and in their ability to supply the essential amino acids.

Vitamin D (cholecalciferol) is naturally present only in foods of animal origin (see Chapter 15). Vitamin D is added to soya milk, many infant foods and several breakfast cereals and to margarine and other spreading fats in the UK. Milk in the USA is also often supplemented with vitamin D. Average intakes of vitamin D in the UK are generally well below estimated requirements, but even intakes of British vegans do not differ substantially from those of omnivores provided they eat vitamin D-supplemented foods. Endogenous production (via the action of sunlight on the skin) rather than dietary intake is regarded as the principal source of vitamin D for most adults and children. Endogenous production should therefore ensure adequacy of vitamin D status in strict vegetarians even if they avoid supplemented foods. In some lifecycle groups, endogenous production cannot be relied on as a source of vitamin D, so supplements of vitamin D may be necessary. In such groups and in anyone who has limited exposure to summer sunlight, the case for supplements is even stronger if they are vegan, especially if they avoid supplemented foods.

Retinol (vitamin A) is present only in animal foods, but ample supplies of carotene in fruits and vegetables will make the total vitamin A content of many affluent vegetarian diets higher than those of typical omnivorous diets.

In strictly vegetarian diets there is no apparent vitamin B_{12}. Symptoms of megaloblastic anaemia and the neurological manifestations of vitamin B_{12} might thus be expected to be prevalent among vegans. However, the human requirement for vitamin B_{12} is extremely small (the UK reference nutrient intake, RNI, is 1.5 µg/day) and stores of the vitamin in the liver are large and could amount to several years' supply in an omnivore. In the UK, meat substitutes are usually supplemented with B_{12} and many vegans take B_{12} supplements. Even in the absence of such alternative dietary sources, cases of clinical B_{12} deficiency among Caucasian vegans are rare. There are indirect sources of B_{12} even for those who consume no animal products or supplemented foods, such as:

- from micro-organisms and moulds contaminating plant foods
- from insects or insect remains consumed with plant foods
- absorption of vitamin produced endogenously by gut bacteria, although most of this is produced below the point of absorption in the ileum and is excreted in faeces
- from fermented foods or yeast extracts
- from faecal contamination of foods like seaweed.

A combination of the large stores, extremely low requirement and incidental consumption from the sources listed above means that the practical hazard of B_{12} deficiency is less than might be expected even for vegans who take no active measures to ensure the adequacy of their B_{12} supply. Even though overt vitamin B_{12} deficiency is rare even in strict vegans, their serum concentrations are generally lower than those of omnivores, and other less strict vegetarians have intermediate values. Vegans who do not take effective supplements may well have suboptimal status for the vitamin even though they may not show the usual overt symptoms. High intakes of folic acid in vegans tend to mask the haematological consequences of B_{12} deficiency, so if symptoms do occur it is the neurological symptoms that may be manifested. The low incidence of B_{12} deficiency in some developing countries where a largely vegan diet is the norm may be because of higher levels of contamination of food and water with bacteria. It is now clear that in some products marketed and used as B_{12} supplements by vegans, the vitamin is present in an inactive form. The blue-green algae *Spirulina*, for example, contains an analogue of vitamin B_{12} which is detected by the microbiological assays used to measure vitamin B_{12} but it is not biologically active (Watanabe, 1999). Some of these analogues may actually worsen the effects of B_{12} deficiency by interfering with metabolism or absorption of the active form.

Dairy produce and eggs are major sources of riboflavin in UK and US diets, so intakes of riboflavin are likely to be low in vegan, although not lactovegetarian, diets. Carlson *et al.* (1985) found average intakes of riboflavin in vegans of only 75 per cent of the then RDA compared with 140 per cent of the RDA in ovolactovegetarians. There is no evidence of overt riboflavin deficiency among strict vegetarians in affluent countries although it is generally one of the more prevalent micronutrient deficiencies. Plant sources of riboflavin are leafy vegetables, nuts and pulses.

Milk and dairy produce, including soya milk, are major sources of dietary calcium. Strict vegetarians who avoid these foods are likely to have lower calcium intakes than omnivores. High fibre and phytate intakes might also be expected to hinder the absorption of calcium from the gut. However, vegans apparently adapt to low calcium intakes and have reduced faecal losses of calcium. Low prevalence of osteoporosis has frequently been reported in vegetarian groups, like Seventh Day Adventists. Very few studies have looked specifically at vegans and this has been highlighted as a possible area of concern; note that leanness is also a risk factor for osteoporosis and vegans are often leaner than other groups. In general, many largely vegetarian populations in developing countries have very low calcium intakes by American and British standards but also have very low rates of osteoporosis (see Chapter 15).

Haem iron is the most readily absorbed form of dietary iron. Hazel and Southgate (1985) found that between 12 and 25 per cent of the iron in meat and fish was absorbed compared with 2–7 per cent from a variety of vegetable sources. Rice and spinach were at the bottom of the vegetable range and soy at the top. The higher fibre and phytate content of vegetarian diets would also tend to reduce non-haem iron absorption, although high levels of vitamin C in vegetarian diets are an important promoter of inorganic iron absorption. Several groups have reported lower iron stores in lactovegetarians, although there is little evidence of increased clinical anaemia. Some studies have reported lower haemoglobin levels in lactovegetarian children and adults despite their having higher iron intakes than omnivores. This would suggest that poor iron absorption may be a particular problem with some vegetarian diets. NDNS surveys of both British adults and children over the last 15 years have highlighted both low iron intakes and poor biochemical iron status as particular problems for girls and young women generally. For example, Gregory *et al.* (2000) found that 27 per cent of girls had low serum ferritin levels and Hoare *et al.* (2004) found that this was also true of 16 per cent of young women; Bates *et al.* (2011) reported that 46 per cent of girls aged 11–18 years had iron intakes below the lower reference nutrient intake (LRNI). One might expect that, given the increased theoretical risks, iron deficiency in vegetarian women and girls would be even higher. Thane *et al.* (2003) (using the data of Gregory *et al.*, 2000) reported that adolescent girls who were vegetarians had significantly poorer iron status than meat eaters, and they suggested that increased consumption of enhancers of non-haem iron, such as fruit and fruit juice, was a possible way of reducing this problem.

Over 40 per cent of the zinc in omnivore diets comes from meat and fish and a further 20 per cent comes from dairy foods. The overall zinc intake of vegetarians is similar to that of omnivores but it is less well absorbed. Many British adolescents (around 14 per cent) have recorded zinc intakes that are below the LRNI, as do many younger women. There is as yet, however, no persuasive evidence of greater prevalence of unsatisfactory zinc status among vegetarians.

Key points

- The risk of dietary inadequacy in vegetarians is partly dependent on the level of dietary restriction.
- Well-planned vegetarian diets are more varied and have higher levels of adequacy than the diets of many omnivores.
- Vegetarian diets are likely to be less energy-dense than omnivorous diets, and Caucasian vegetarians tend to be lighter and leaner than omnivores.
- A vegan diet can restrict the growth of children although the effect is usually small and temporary.
- Vegan diets reduce growth rates in children because they are low in fat and of low energy density rather than because of protein or other nutrient deficiency.
- If energy intakes are adequate then most diets, even vegan diets, should have ample supplies of protein and essential amino acids.
- If plenty of coloured fruits and green vegetables are consumed then vegetarian diets should have ample vitamin A in the form of carotenoids even though retinol is only found in animal foods.
- Plant foods theoretically contain no vitamin B_{12}.
- Overt vitamin B_{12} deficiency is rarely seen in even in vegans although there may be suboptimal status in some who do not take supplements. The vitamin B_{12} in some algal supplements, like *Spirulina*, is not biologically active and may even interfere with normal B_{12} metabolism.
- Dietary deficiency of B_{12} is uncommon because:
  - requirements are extremely small
  - omnivores have stores sufficient for several years
  - many vegetarians take supplements or eat supplemented foods
  - many plant foods contain some B_{12} as a contaminant (e.g. from microbes).

Key points *continued*

- Vitamin D is not naturally present in vegetable foods although some are supplemented. For most people, the principal source of vitamin D is endogenous synthesis in the skin when it is exposed to summer sunlight. Vegetarians, especially those who do not eat supplemented foods, are even more reliant than omnivores on sunlight as their primary source of vitamin D.

- Vegetarian diets lack haem iron which is the most readily available form of dietary iron. The iron in vegetarian diets is likely to be less well absorbed than in omnivorous diets, and several surveys suggest that vegetarians have lower body iron stores than omnivores.

- Vitamin C is an important promoter of non-haem iron absorption.

- Animal foods are important dietary sources of riboflavin, calcium and zinc, but there is no persuasive evidence of a specific problem of inadequate status for these nutrients in vegetarians or vegans.

Vegetarian diets and nutritional guidelines

A vegetarian diet has been reported, by a variety of authors and using a variety of vegetarian groups, to be associated with:

- lower body weight and reduced prevalence of obesity
- lower blood pressure
- lower prevalence of osteoporosis (not specifically reported in vegans)
- reduced risk of coronary heart disease
- reduced risk of developing type 2 diabetes
- reduced incidence of certain cancers, particularly bowel cancer
- lower all-cause mortality.

It is very difficult to determine to what extent these associations are wholly or partly due to lack of meat consumption *per se*. Caucasian vegetarians in the UK tend not to be from the lower social groups; many of them adopt vegetarianism for health reasons and thus they are likely to pay particular attention to the healthiness of their diet and their lifestyle in general. Those who are

vegetarian for cultural or religious reasons also tend to adopt other practices that are considered healthful, such as avoidance of alcohol and tobacco. American Seventh Day Adventists are a frequently studied group because many are vegetarians. They do indeed have lower rates of the diseases listed above, but they also tend to avoid alcohol and tobacco and are perhaps different in many other lifestyle characteristics to Americans in general. Several studies have compared the health of meat-eating and non-meat-eating Seventh Day Adventists and these have found that the vegetarians have increased life expectancy, lower rates of coronary heart disease and bowel cancer and a reduced risk of diabetes. A study is currently under way with 125 000 American and Canadian Adventists – the Adventist Health Study-2 which is centred on Loma Linda University in California, an Adventist university. Details of this study and its findings may be found at www.llu.edu/llu/health/about.html, and the website has links to academic publications arising from it. This large sample is made up of 48 per cent non-vegetarians and the rest with varying degrees of vegetarianism, including 8 per cent who are vegans. The following are some of the findings of this study.

- There is a progressive increase in body weight as one goes from vegan to omnivore; the closer to a strict vegetarian, the lower the body weight.
- Levels of plasma cholesterol, blood pressure and the incidence of type 2 diabetes and metabolic syndrome also all increase as one gets further from a strict vegetarian diet.
- The findings for fracture risk were less clear-cut, although Adventists did have lower rates of several fractures than non-Adventists, including hip fractures.

As already discussed in Chapters 4 and 10, the European Prospective Investigation into Cancer and Nutrition (EPIC) found strong support for the hypothesis that consumption of red and processed meat increases the risk of colorectal cancer while dietary fibre and fish consumption decrease the risk.

Compared to the UK population in general, Caucasian vegetarians in the UK would probably tend to:

- be more health conscious
- drink less alcohol
- make less use of tobacco
- take more exercise
- be lighter and less likely to be overweight or obese
- be less likely to come from the lower manual social classes
- be more likely to be female.

Compared to omnivores, the diets of vegetarians, and vegans in particular, tend to be lower in fat, saturated fat, cholesterol and alcohol but higher in fruits and vegetables and their associated anti-oxidants and phytochemicals, and also be higher in complex carbohydrates, fibre and polyunsaturated fatty acids.

To assume that any differences in mortality or morbidity patterns of vegetarians are largely due to the avoidance of meat or animal foods *per se* is probably premature. Non-dietary risk factors may be very different in vegetarian and non-vegetarian groups. There are also numerous compositional differences between the diets of vegetarians and omnivores. Some of these are almost inevitable, but a thoughtfully constructed omnivorous diet could match even a good vegan diet in many respects.

The key question is not whether vegetarians are healthier than omnivores, but rather how the health records of vegetarians compare with omnivores of similar racial, religious and social backgrounds who have similar smoking, drinking and activity patterns and who take equal care in the selection and preparation of a healthy diet. The point of this discussion is to suggest, to those reluctantly contemplating vegetarianism on health grounds alone, that giving up meat or 'red meat' may well *by itself* be ineffective but that adopting some of the lifestyle and dietary practices characteristic of vegetarians will almost certainly be beneficial. This point is even more important for nutrition educators seeking to influence the behaviour of others.

The discussion in the next section on the health of British Asians makes the point that vegetarianism and good health statistics are not invariably linked. Thorogood (1995) has reviewed earlier epidemiological studies of the relationship between vegetarianism and chronic disease.

Key points

- Affluent Western vegetarians tend to:
  - be leaner than omnivores
  - have reduced levels of several risk factors and lower prevalence of several chronic diseases
  - have reduced all-cause mortality.
- There are numerous social, lifestyle and dietary differences between affluent vegetarians and the rest of the population that may contribute to the observed health differences between them.
- Studies with Seventh Day Adventists suggest that those of them who avoid meat have higher life expectancy, reduced rates of bowel cancer, heart disease and diabetes. The ongoing Adventist Health Study-2 has found a progressive increase in body weight, blood cholesterol, blood pressure and prevalence of type 2 diabetes and metabolic syndrome as the diet becomes less vegetarian.
- Adopting a more vegetarian diet and lifestyle should produce more health benefits than simple meat avoidance.

RACIAL MINORITIES

Overview

Williams and Qureshi (1988) and Bush *et al.* (1997) have reviewed nutritional aspects of the dietary practices of racial minorities in the UK. Davey Smith *et al.* (2000) have published a detailed review of the variations in disease incidence and causes of mortality in different minority ethnic groups within the UK.

Several topics and issues discussed in Chapter 2 are also of relevance when considering the nutrition of racial minorities:

- the effects of migration on dietary habits and nutrition
- economic influences on food choices
- cultural and religious factors that influence food selection and dietary practices.

Those offering dietary or other health education advice to people from a different cultural background need to carefully identify the particular needs and priorities of the target group and the reasons for them. This should enable them to determine what advice is appropriate from the scientific viewpoint. However, before they attempt to translate these scientific goals into practical advice and recommendations they need to assure themselves that they are aware of and understand the cultural and social determinants of the group's practices. Only by doing this can they ensure that their advice is compatible with the beliefs and normal practices of the group.

There is a general tendency for the health of racial minority groups living in industrialized countries to be inferior to that of the majority population. Indeed, one of the health promotion goals set for the USA in 1992 was to 'reduce the health disparity among Americans' (DHHS, 1992). If improved nutrition is credited with being a major factor in the improving health and longevity of the majority population, then one would have to assume that some of this disparity is due to nutritional improvements lagging behind in minority groups. Racial minorities often tend to be economically and socially disadvantaged compared with the majority population, and this is almost certainly an important factor in some of these ethnic disparities in health. One of the most striking inequalities in health of Americans is that between low-income groups and all other groups (DHHS, 1992); and when the mortality statistics of black Americans were adjusted for socioeconomic factors the differences between whites and blacks largely disappeared. Socioeconomic disadvantage has also been highlighted as a major barrier to sound nutritional health in ethnic minorities in the UK (Bush *et al.*, 1997).

Health and nutrition of particular minority groups

The health record of Native Americans is particularly poor, with two nutrition-related risk factors, alcohol abuse and obesity, clearly identified as important. Death rates from accident, homicide, suicide and cirrhosis of the liver are all much higher in Native Americans than in other Americans and are all associated with alcohol abuse. Rates of diabetes are also very high among Native Americans,

with more than 20 per cent of the members of many tribes affected by the disease; diabetes and the metabolic syndrome are acknowledged as major determinants of coronary heart disease risk (see Chapter 9). The increasing rates of diabetes in Native Americans have paralleled increasing rates of obesity; the proportion of overweight adults varies between one-third and three-quarters depending on the tribe. In Chapter 8 it was noted that Pima Indians living in Mexico have much lower rates of obesity and diabetes than those living in the USA; adults in the USA were on average 25 kg heavier than those living in Mexico. Clearly nutritional factors, including alcohol abuse, are major determinants of the poor health statistics of this minority group (DHHS, 1992).

In 1987, black Americans had a life expectancy of 69.4 years, compared with 75 years for the American population as a whole, and this gap widened during the first half of the 1990s. Mortality rates for heart disease are considerably higher for black Americans than white Americans. The poverty rate among blacks was also three times that of whites; and when heart disease rates of blacks and whites were compared within income levels, the black rates were actually lower than those for whites. A good proportion of the poor health record of some American racial groups seems to result from their generally lower socioeconomic status.

In the UK, the two largest racial minority groups are African Caribbeans and South Asians. The former originated from the British colonies in the West Indies and large-scale immigration of this group started in the 1950s. British Asians are a racially and culturally mixed group and most of the immigration has occurred since 1960. They originate from the countries of Southern Asia (India, Pakistan, Bangladesh and Sri Lanka) or from the Asian communities of East Africa. In their review, Bush *et al.* (1997) also identified the Irish as a large minority ethnic group with particular evidence of nutrition-related health disadvantages, including low stature, high rates of coronary heart disease (CHD), cancer and high overall mortality which persists among those who are British-born. They identified poverty and solitary living as barriers to nutritional health in older Irish people living in the UK, especially Irish men. In future editions it may be necessary to consider the nutritional health of the very large numbers who have recently migrated to the UK from the eastern European countries that are relatively new members of the European Union.

Many British Asians are in three major religious groups – Hindus, Sikhs and Muslims. Rates of vegetarianism are high. Hindus are usually lactovegetarians and they do not usually eat Western cheese. Sikhs do not eat beef, rarely eat pork, and many are lactovegetarian. Muslims should not eat pork or consume alcohol and any meat or animal fat should have come from animals slaughtered and prepared according to Islamic ritual.

The potential health problems of vegetarianism, discussed earlier in the chapter, would thus apply to many within these groups. For example, Robertson *et al.* (1982) suggested that (at that time) nutritional deficiencies of folic acid and vitamin B_{12} were virtually confined to the Asian population in the UK. They suggested that the practice of boiling milk with tea leaves when making tea destroys much of the B_{12} present in the milk and strict Hindus would have no other apparent source of B_{12} in their lactovegetarian diet. They also suggested that prolonged gentle heating of finely cut-up foods also destroys much of the folic acid initially present in some Asian diets.

Biochemical indications of poor vitamin D status are common in all groups of the UK, especially when samples are taken during the winter months. British diets do not provide enough vitamin D to meet estimated physiological needs without regular exposure to summer sunlight. Levels of deficiency are much higher in British Asians than in the white population. For example, in a survey conducted in Birmingham, Shaw and Pal (2002) found that 85 per cent of the Asians had plasma 25-hydroxycholecalciferol levels below 20 nmol/L compared with just 3.3 per cent of non-Asians. Mini epidemics of rickets and osteomalacia occurred in the 1960s and 1970s among Asian children and women in the UK. For example, a 5-year-old Asian child living in Glasgow between 1968 and 1978 had a 3.5 per cent chance of being admitted to hospital with rickets before the age of 16 years whereas the equivalent risk for a white child was negligible (Robertson *et al.*, 1982). Vitamin D deficiency has also been reported as common among pregnant Asian women in the UK, which has serious implications for the health of the baby. Fortification of chapatti flour was advocated at the time as likely to be the most effective preventative measure (e.g. Pietrek *et al.*, 1976) but the problem had largely disappeared by the mid-1990s without fortification (Shaw and Pal, 2002).

Several factors such as those listed below probably contribute to this high prevalence of vitamin D deficiency among British Asians.

- There is avoidance of those few foods that contain good amounts of vitamin D, such as fatty fish, liver, fortified margarine and infant foods and eggs.
- There is a cultural tendency not to expose the skin to sunlight. This, perhaps coupled with pigmentation of the skin, would be expected to reduce endogenous vitamin D synthesis.
- There are high levels of fibre and phytate in chapattis (a traditional unleavened bread). This might impair calcium absorption and perhaps also prevent enterohepatic recycling of vitamin D (Robertson *et al.*, 1982).
- There is prolonged breastfeeding by mothers with poor vitamin D status (Shaw and Pal, 2002).

Robertson *et al.* (1982) suggested that the initial mini epidemic problem was particularly associated with new immigrants and diminished in those who were well established because of acculturation and partial adoption of a Western diet. Bush *et al.* (1997) recognized rickets/osteomalacia as an area where intervention was needed in South Asians, and Shaw and Pal (2002) document a more recent resurgence of rickets among British Asian children and young women. At least one local health authority in the UK with a large South Asian community (Bradford) was so concerned about rickets and poor vitamin D status among its children that, in 2006, it offered free supplements for young children. Zipitis *et al.* (2006), in a study in Burnley (England), found that clinical rickets was re-emerging as a problem in Asian children in the town. Although the number of clinical cases was small, almost all of them had occurred in the second half of the 10-year study, suggesting a rising trend. If these results are typical of British Asian children, they point to a significant and growing problem and, of course, clinical cases of rickets are likely to represent 'the tip of the iceberg' with many more children having poor vitamin D status and impaired functioning. This group recommended that health authorities should provide supplements of vitamin D for Asian children for at least the first 2 years of life.

The prominence of the different causes of mortality also varies quite considerably between different ethnic groups in the UK. The incidence of hypertension and strokes is high in the African Caribbean population of the UK. It is also high among black Americans, with stroke mortality among the men almost twice that in the total male population. Africans and African Caribbeans may have an ethnic predisposition to hypertension owing to a hypersensitivity to salt (Law *et al.*, 1991a).

The rates of coronary heart disease among the Asian groups in the UK are higher than in the white population, despite the high prevalence of vegetarianism among British Asians. Age-standardized mortality is around 50 per cent higher for Asians in England and Wales than for the general population, and mortality in those aged under 40 years is up to three times higher. A similar trend has been reported for Asians living in other industrialized areas, and heart disease generally starts about a decade earlier in South Asian countries than elsewhere (Joshi *et al.*, 2007). This problem was first highlighted in the UK by McKeigue *et al.* (1985) who compared the dietary and other risk factors for coronary heart disease among Asians and non-Asians living in London. They confirmed that rates of CHD were much higher among the Asians and that the excess morbidity and mortality were common to the three major religious groups despite considerable differences in dietary and lifestyle characteristics between the three. They found that the diets and lifestyles of Asians differed from their white neighbours in the following ways.

- The Asians had lower intakes of saturated fat and cholesterol and had lower serum cholesterol concentrations. (Note that a recent study of UK children found that this historically lower LDL cholesterol level in black and Asian British children had been lost, with serious implications for their future heart disease risk (Donin *et al.*, 2010).)
- The Asians smoked fewer cigarettes and drank less alcohol.

- Vegetarianism was much more common among the Asians.
- The Asians had had lower rates of bowel cancer than the white population even though high rates of bowel cancer and coronary heart disease tend to go together in populations.

McKeigue *et al.* (1991) reported high levels of insulin resistance among British Asians, and the prevalence of diabetes was more than four times higher than in the population as a whole. They also reported very high incidence of central obesity in this Asian population. Vegetarianism among the Asian population does not seem to protect against overweight and obesity as it usually does for Caucasian vegetarians. McKeigue and associates suggested that this insulin resistance was associated with high caloric intake and inactivity. They therefore proposed that these Asian groups are adapted to life in environments where high levels of physical activity and frugal use of food resources have been traditionally required. When these groups migrate to countries where levels of physical activity are low and caloric intakes high, this leads to insulin resistance, central obesity and other associated metabolic disturbances (see metabolic syndrome in Chapter 9), including maturity-onset diabetes. This in turn predisposes them to CHD.

A more recent major report on heart disease in South Asians (DH/BHF, 2004) confirmed that the increased risk applies to all of the major ethnic and religious groups encompassed by the broad term South Asian. A high genetic susceptibility to insulin resistance and diabetes is triggered by inactivity and abdominal obesity leading to low plasma HDL levels, increased plasma triglycerides, hypertension, and hyperglycaemia (the metabolic syndrome) or frank diabetes, which in turn leads to increased risk of CHD. In a prospective cohort study in south London, Forouhi *et al.* (2006) compared conventional cardiovascular risk factors and those associated with insulin resistance in middle-aged Asian and European men living in north London. They confirmed the very high heart disease mortality in Asian men and the high prevalence of diabetes; but from a multivariate analysis they concluded that conventional risk factors, insulin resistance and the metabolic syndrome criteria could not fully explain the high heart disease mortality in Asian men.

Unmeasured risk factors and probably genetic factors contributed to this risk.

Most authors who write about this topic assume that South Asians in Britain are less active than the rest of the population and that this contributes to their increased levels of obesity, diabetes and heart disease. In a systematic review of the literature, Fischbacher *et al.* (2004) found evidence of substantially lower levels of activity among all South Asian groups in the UK. Although there were methodological flaws with the 17 studies they reviewed (12 adult studies and five with children), they did nevertheless confirm the general assumption of high levels of inactivity contributing towards their diabetes and heart disease risk. In a more recent study using an objective measure of physical activity in a large (2000+) ethnically mixed sample of 9- and 10-year-old English children, Owen *et al.* (2009) found that South Asian children had lower activity levels than either white European or black African Caribbean children.

Dietary comparison of ethnic groups in Britain

Table 18.1 shows a very selective comparison of the purchases and expenditure of British families classified as white, Asian or black; examples of substantial differences between these groupings

have been selectively included in this table. Note that 95 per cent of the participants were classified as white and there were some differences in average family composition and age structure between the ethnic groups. Compared to the majority white category, the Asia families purchased:

- slightly less milk and cream and much less cheese
- much less meat and meat products
- more fats and oils
- fewer potatoes
- less confectionery
- much less alcohol.

The Asian grouping also spent much less per head on both household food and eating out than the white majority despite having a higher average gross household income.

Compared to the white majority, the black grouping purchased:

- much less milk and cream and much less cheese
- slightly less meat and meat products
- slightly more fats and oils
- fewer potatoes, confectionery and alcohol.

The black grouping also spent much less per head than the white majority on both household food and eating out, and they also had a much lower gross weekly household income.

Table 18.1 Selective comparison of the weekly food purchases and expenditure of British families where the household reference person (HRP) is classified as white, Asian or black British*

Household purchases (grams or mL) per person	Asian	Black	White
Milk and cream	1948	1319	2031
Cheese	48	44	117
All meat and products	605	919	1073
Fats and oils	275	203	182
Potatoes	460	485	875
Confectionery	70	61	135
All alcohol (home and outside)	337	507	1496
Average gross weekly household income	£640	£424	£565
Weekly expenditure per person (excluding alcohol)			
All household food and drink	1423p	1520p	2149p
All eating out	478p	429p	765p

*Data source: DEFRA (2006).

Some of these differences are very predictable in the light of cultural differences, such as:

- the low meat purchasing of Asians because the grouping includes a large number of vegetarians
- the high potato consumption of the white grouping, which reflects the greater importance of potatoes as a staple in the traditional British diet compared to the other groups
- the low alcohol consumption of the Asian grouping because it contains many Muslims who should not drink.

Table 18.2 shows selected comparisons between these groups of nutrient intakes estimated from the recorded food purchases. In general, the estimated micronutrient intakes of the Asian and black groupings are less than that of the white majority. In several cases the average intakes of micronutrients fall below the RNI in one or both of the non-white groups (e.g. for calcium in the black grouping and for iron, zinc and vitamin A in both the black and Asian groupings). The low calcium intakes are in line with the low milk and cheese purchases of the two non-white groupings, and the iron and zinc are in line with the lower meat intakes of the non-white groupings. When macronutrients are expressed as a percentage of food energy (excluding alcohol), then the white grouping has the highest total fat intake, highest added-sugar intake and the lowest carbohydrate intake. The saturated-fat intake of the white grouping is much higher than the other two (reflecting the higher use of meat, cheese and milk and cream by the white group). The Asian grouping has a much higher intake of starch than the white grouping. These differences in macronutrient content between the Asian and white groupings are, as noted earlier, superficially at odds with the high rates of coronary heart disease and high obesity rates recorded in British Asians.

Key points

- The health statistics of racial minorities are often worse than those of the majority population.
- Native Americans are much more likely to be obese and to develop the metabolic syndrome and type 2 diabetes than other Americans. Obesity and alcohol-related problems are major contributors to the generally poor health record of Native Americans.

Table 18.2 Selective comparison of nutrient intakes in British families where the household reference person (HRP) is classified as white, Asian or black British*

Nutrient intake as % RNI[1]	Asian	Black	White
Total energy (% EAR including alcohol)	93	85	98
Calcium	109	89	130
Iron	84	87	106
Zinc	86	89	104
Folate	113	120	139
Vitamin A	90	88	127
Macronutrient as % food energy (excluding alcohol)			
Fat	36.3	35.9	37.8
Saturated fatty acids	11.9	11.7	15.0
Carbohydrate	51.9	50.7	48.0
Non-milk extrinsic sugars	12.7	15.6	15.7
Starch and intrinsic sugars	39.2	35.2	32.3

*Data source: DEFRA (2006).
[1] Nutrient intakes have been estimated from food purchases.

- Black Americans have shorter life expectancy and higher heart disease mortality than white Americans. The relatively poor health statistics of black Americans can be largely attributed to their relative poverty, and this probably applies to other minority groups in industrialized countries.
- African Caribbeans and South Asians are the largest racial minority groups in the UK.
- The potential problems of a lactovegetarian diet are relevant to many British Asians who are lactovegetarian for religious reasons.
- Poor vitamin D status is prevalent among British Asians, and rickets is starting to recur owing to the combined effects of low dietary availability and low endogenous synthesis because of inadequate exposure of the skin to sunlight.
- People of African and Caribbean origin have high prevalence of hypertension and more strokes because they are genetically sensitive to the hypertensive effects of salt.
- Coronary heart disease is very prevalent among British Asians, even among those who are lactovegetarian, and even though they generally have lower exposure to several established risk factors than the white population.
- People in South Asian countries develop heart disease up to a decade earlier than people in other countries.
- High rates of inactivity and abdominal obesity leading to insulin resistance among British Asians probably account for their susceptibility to coronary heart disease.
- Despite some methodological issues, there is a substantial body of evidence which suggests that all South Asian groups are more inactive than the rest of the UK population. Asian children in the UK are less active than white or black African Caribbean children when an objective measure of activity is used.
- Insulin resistance and abdominal obesity of British Asians lead to frank diabetes or the metabolic syndrome, which in turn predisposes them to premature heart disease.
- Rates of type 2 diabetes are around five times higher in British Asians than in the rest of the population.

→

- Dietary comparisons between white, Asian and black groupings of British families suggest substantial differences in the food purchasing and expenditure of these three groupings. Table 18.1 has some examples.
  - Asian and black families purchase much less alcohol than white British families.
  - Asian and black families' food purchases contain fewer essential micronutrients per person than those of white families. In several cases the estimated average intakes of the non-white groups are well below the RNI.
  - Compared to white families, the purchases of Asian families contain less fat, much less saturated fat, more carbohydrate and much more starch (similar but slightly lower trends are seen in the black families).
- These dietary comparisons between British Asians and white Britons are superficially inconsistent with the high rates of obesity and heart disease recorded in British Asians.

NUTRITION AND PHYSICAL ACTIVITY

Fitness

It does not require scientific measurement to convince most of us that regular exercise leads to an increased level of physical fitness. Any normally sedentary person who undertakes a programme of regular vigorous exercise will soon notice that he or she can perform everyday activities – like garden and household chores, climbing stairs, walking uphill or running for a bus – with much less breathlessness and pounding of the heart than previously. Simple personal monitoring would show a reduction in resting heart rate and smaller increases in pulse rate in response to an exercise load.

Scientific appraisal of the benefits of physical activity on long-term health or the effects of different training schedules on fitness requires a precise definition of fitness and an objective method of measuring it. This allows changes in fitness levels to be monitored during training and allows the fitness levels of different individuals or populations to be compared.

The scientific criterion normally used to define fitness is the *aerobic capacity* or the rate of oxygen uptake of the subject when exercising maximally – the VO_{2max}. This VO_{2max} is a measure of the functional capacity of the cardiopulmonary system to deliver oxygen to the body muscles and other tissues. Direct measurement of oxygen uptake in maximally exercising subjects is feasible but it requires relatively sophisticated laboratory equipment and trained personnel. It also requires subjects to perform sustained exercise to the limit of their capacity, which might be undesirable and sometimes dangerous in untrained people. The heart rate measured at several submaximal exercise levels is therefore often used to derive a measure of aerobic capacity.

In one widely used test, the subject cycles on a static bicycle ergometer at defined work loads. The external work performed by the subject is calculated from the speed of cycling and the resistance applied to the bicycle flywheel. In the steady state, heart rate is assumed to equate with oxygen uptake. Three graded levels of work are performed and the steady-state heart rate is measured at each. The calculated work rate is then plotted against the heart rate on a graph and the best straight line drawn through the three points (Figure 18.1). By extending this straight line, the graph can be used in either of the following ways:

- to predict the work rate for the subject at the predicted maximum heart rate (220 minus the age in years) – the *maximum physical work capacity*, PWC_{max}
- to predict the work rate at a defined heart rate – for example, the *physical work capacity at 170 beats per minute*, the PWC_{170}.

The rate of 170 beats per minute is approximately 85 per cent of the maximum heart rate in young adults and using this value involves less extrapolation than predicting the maximum heart rate. In older subjects, a lower defined heart rate would be used. Similar tests are available that involve walking or running on a treadmill rather than the use of a static bicycle.

Conditioning of the cardiopulmonary system to produce measurable improvements in aerobic capacity requires that the system be significantly exerted for sustained periods. A nominal three sessions each week in which heart rate is raised to 60–70 per cent of maximum for at least 20 minutes duration has been suggested.

Regular exercise not only produces measurable increases in aerobic capacity but also produces other rapid and readily demonstrable benefits in the short term, such as those listed below.

- Training increases muscle strength.
- Training increases endurance – the maximum duration that one is able to sustain a particular activity. Both the endurance of individual trained muscle groups and the endurance of the cardiopulmonary system are increased.
- Training improves or maintains joint mobility or flexibility, so the range of movements that subjects are able to safely and comfortably perform is increased.
- Training increases (or at least maintains) muscle mass. During bouts of sustainable activity like aerobics, jogging or walking, the supply of oxygen to the muscles is sufficient for the muscle to produce energy by the normal aerobic (oxygen-requiring) processes – hence 'aerobic exercise'. The most effective exercises for increasing muscle mass are high-intensity, short-duration activities where the effort involved is

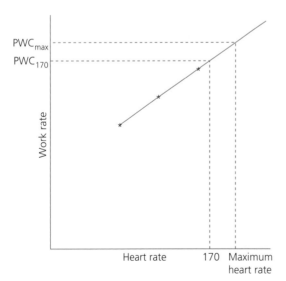

Figure 18.1 Work load plotted against heart rate. The straight line through the three measured points can be used to predict the PWC_{170} or the PWC_{max}.

close to the maximum; examples are lifting a heavy weight, pushing against a resistance, press-ups, jumping, climbing stairs or sprinting. Such exercises are so intense that the oxygen supply to the muscle is insufficient to produce all the energy needed for the intense activity, so the muscle temporarily 'tops up' the energy supply by switching to energy-producing processes that are anaerobic (not requiring oxygen) – hence 'anaerobic exercise'.

• Training leads to measurable increases in psychological well-being, including less depression.

Several of these latter benefits of exercise accrue at intensities and durations of activity that are considerably below those necessary to produce measurable changes in aerobic capacity. These latter effects of increased strength, endurance and flexibility may be of even greater importance to some subjects (e.g the elderly) than increases in aerobic fitness. As noted in Chapter 16, much of the loss of physical capacity and functional disability associated with ageing is not a result of the ageing process *per se* but is largely the result of inactivity. Even in extreme old age, resistance training resulted in measurable increases in strength and functional ability (Fiatarone *et al.*, 1994). These findings back up the conclusions in the Allied Dunbar Health Survey (1992), which showed that there was a dramatic decline in aerobic fitness, strength and flexibility with age. However, the authors concluded that much of this decline was not an inevitable consequence of ageing but a form of disuse atrophy which could be greatly reduced by regular exercise; the aerobic fitness of the top 10 per cent of men in the 65- to 74-year-old category was higher than the bottom 10 per cent in the 25- to 64 year olds.

There is also a substantial body of evidence suggesting that participation in regular physical activity produces psychological benefits. It improves the general sense of well-being and self-confidence, improves the ability to cope with stress, and may even reduce the frequency and severity of personality disorders. Some of these psychological benefits may well be a consequence of the physiological conditioning (Fentem, 1992; Bowen *et al.*, 2006). As the result of an extensive meta-analysis of previously published studies, Fedewa

and Ahn (2011) claimed that physical activity, especially aerobic exercise, improved children's academic performance.

It is now recognized that setting activity targets for the general population based on the 20 minutes of vigorous exercise (60–70 per cent of maximum heart rate) is probably unrealistic. In both the UK and USA, encouraging moderate physical activity is seen as a more realistic health promotion goal and offers the prospect of greater health benefits for the population as a whole (see Table 18.3 for a quantitative grading of activity levels). The Chief Medical Officer in the UK has recommended that adults should aim for at least 30 minutes of moderate activity on at least five occasions each week, and that this 30 minutes can be accumulated in up to three shorter activity sessions of at least 10 minutes duration.

In *The Health of the Nation* (DH, 1992a), the stated intention of the British government was 'to develop detailed strategies to increase physical activity' in the light of the activity and fitness levels found in the Allied Dunbar National Fitness Survey. In the follow-up document *Saving Lives: Our Healthier Nation*, the benefits of increased physical activity were mentioned several times and there was general encouragement to increase levels of physical activity and fitness.

Healthy People 2010 in the USA (DHHS, 2000) set a number of specific targets for increasing physical activity by 2010, including:

• reduce to 20 per cent the proportion of adults engaging in no leisure-time physical activity
• 30 per cent of adults should be engaging in 30 minutes of daily moderate activity
• 30 per cent of adults should engage in 20 minutes of vigorous physical activity on at least three occasions each week
• increase the number of adults who engage in physical activities that enhance and maintain flexibility, muscle strength and endurance.

Current levels of physical activity and fitness

The average levels of physical activity of the populations of the wealthy industrialized countries have, by general agreement, declined in recent decades. Car ownership, workplace automation and labour-saving aids in the home and garden have drastically reduced the amount of obligatory physical exertion that most people are now required to undertake. Any increases in voluntary leisure-time activities have not been enough to offset this reduction in obligatory activity. The average Briton now watches twice as much television as in the 1960s, and many people spend more time watching television than they do at work or school. Between 1975 and 1995 the average distance walked by British adults fell by about 20 per cent.

The increased levels of overweight and obesity in the UK and USA in recent decades have occurred despite a substantial decline in average energy intakes and this gives indirect evidence of the scale of this reduction in activity (discussed in Chapter 9). Energy expenditure (i.e. activity) has been declining faster than the decline in energy intake.

There are estimates of activity levels of the US population in *Healthy People 2010* (DHHS, 2000) such as those listed below.

- Forty per cent of adults in the USA engaged in no leisure-time physical activity (i.e. no activity that substantially increased the rate of energy expenditure). Rates of inactivity were higher in black and Hispanic Americans and rates decreased substantially with increasing educational attainment and increased steadily with advancing age. Similar racial, educational and age trends were seen in the other measures of activity listed below.

- Only 15 per cent of adults engaged in 30 minutes of moderate activity on five or more days each week, rising to 31 per cent if the criterion is reduced to 20 minutes of moderate activity on three or more days per week.

- Twenty-three per cent of adults engaged in sufficient vigorous physical activity to improve cardiorespiratory fitness.

Table 18.3 gives a summary of activity levels determined by interview in a health survey of English adults (Sproston and Primatesta, 2004). Only just over a third of the men and a quarter of the women reported engaging in the recommended five 30-min periods of moderate activity each week. Well over a third of adults recorded no 30-min periods of moderate activity each week, rising to more than half of those aged 65–74 years. As with the American data discussed earlier, activity levels declined markedly with increasing age and people with higher educational qualifications were more active.

Table 18.3 Variation by age and sex in the percentage of English adults who reported engaging in different periods of 30 minutes of at least moderate level activity[1]

Weekly occasions	Age in years					Total
	16–24	25–44	45–64	65–74	75+	
5 or more						
Male	53	43	35	17	8	37
Female	30	29	27	13	3	24
1–4 sessions						
Male	29	36	30	32	20	31
Female	39	44	35	31	14	36
None						
Male	18	22	35	52	72	32
Female	31	27	38	56	82	40

[1] **Vigorous activity** is that where the energy expenditure is at least 7.5 kcal (30 kJ)/min. **Moderate activity** is 5–7.5 kcal (20–30 kJ)/min. **Light activity** is 2–5 kcal (8–20 kJ)/min. **Inactive** is below 2 kcal (8 kJ)/min. *Moderate activities* are walking a mile at brisk or fast pace; heavy gardening work such as digging or cutting large areas of grass by hand; heavy DIY work such as knocking down walls or breaking up concrete; heavy housework such as walking with heavy loads of shopping or scrubbing/polishing floors by hand. *Vigorous activities* are running or jogging; playing squash; several other sporting activities if it caused the subject to breathe heavily or sweat a lot such as aerobics, tennis, weight training or swimming.

Using a representative sample of English adults and children, Craig et al. (2009) recorded not just self-reported activity but also an objective measure of activity using a movement indicator (accelerometer) and estimates of physical fitness (VO_{2max}) using a step test. According to self-reported activity, 39 per cent of men and 29 per cent of women achieved government recommended activity levels. An average of 31 min/day of moderate or vigorous activity (MVPA) was recorded for men using the accelerometer measurements (24 min/day for women). However, most of this activity was in short bursts and only about a third of it was sustained for at least 10 minutes in line with government recommendations. Using the accelerometer data, just 6 per cent of men and 4 per cent of women met the government targets and most of those who met the targets by self-reporting did not meet them when this more objective measure was used. Almost all adults were fit enough to walk at 3 mile/h on the flat, but 32 per cent of men and 60 per cent of women were not fit enough to walk at that speed up a 5 per cent incline without severe or maximal exertion (almost exactly the same as recorded in the Allied Dunbar National Fitness Survey in 1992). On all measures, activity and fitness declined with increasing age, and 68 per cent of men and 88 per cent of women aged 55–75 years would only be able to walk at 3 mile/h up a 5 per cent in line with severe or maximal exertion. Men were generally more active, fitter and spent less time in sedentary activities than women.

The Allied Dunbar survey also found very low levels of reported physical activity and low levels of aerobic fitness among a representative sample of 4000 English adults. Some of the data are not directly comparable to those in Craig et al. (2009), but the proportions of men and women who would be unable to sustain walking up a 5 per cent gradient at 3 mile/h were almost identical to those of Craig's team. According to this earlier survey, many elderly women do not have enough strength in their legs to rise from a chair without using their arms, and many elderly and even middle-aged people do not have enough shoulder flexibility to allow them to wash their own hair in comfort.

There is also convincing evidence that activity levels of children in the UK have decreased sharply in recent decades. Durnin (1992) has suggested that average energy intakes of teenagers were up to a third higher in the 1930s than in the early 1990s. Several other studies have also found a reduction in recorded energy intakes of various age groups of children in recent decades. Over these same decades British children have got taller and fatter and this must indicate a decrease in their energy expenditure via physical activity. It was argued in Chapter 9 that the rising prevalence of childhood obesity is primarily a result of declining activity rather than dietary changes per se. There was a 20 per cent decrease in walking among British children in the 10 years up to 1995 and a 25 per cent decrease in the amount of cycling. Between 1975 and 1995, the annual distance walked by 11- to 15 year olds dropped a third from 248 miles to 199 miles. In the NDNS survey of British schoolchildren (Gregory et al., 2000) it was reported that children were taller and heavier than in a similar study conducted in the early 1980s but had lower energy intakes. This clearly points to a decline in energy expenditure (i.e. activity) over this period.

The official UK recommendation for children is that they have an hour each day in at least moderate exertion. According to self-reported activity, about 32 per cent of boys and 24 per cent of girls met this target, the proportion meeting this target declining with age in girls (Craig et al., 2009). Based on objective (accelerometer) measurements, 33 per cent of boys and 21 per cent of girls met the government target, with 47 per cent of boys and 61 per cent of girls in the lowest (light) activity category. Comparison of self and objective activity measurements suggested that self-reporting underestimated activity in young children but, as in adults, overestimated it in older children. Girls are generally less active than boys.

In Healthy People 2010 (DHHS, 2000), evidence was also presented of the assumed levels of activity of American children in 2000, with targets set for 2010. Some of these are summarized below:

- to increase from 27 to 35 per cent the proportion of adolescents who participate in at least five weekly sessions of 30 minutes of at least moderate activity
- to increase from 65 to 85 per cent the proportion of adolescents who engage in three weekly

sessions of activity vigorous enough to promote cardiorespiratory fitness

- to increase the proportion of schools that require daily physical education for students and to increase the proportion of children who participate in them
- to increase from 57 to 75 per cent the proportion of adolescents who watch television for fewer than 2 hours on school days.

Key points

- Scientific assessment of fitness uses some measure of aerobic capacity like the maximum oxygen uptake (VO_{2max}).
- Aerobic capacity is usually extrapolated from pulse rates measured at submaximal exercise loads.
- Measurable increases in VO_{2max} require regular and significant exertion for sustained periods, nominally three weekly sessions of 20 minutes duration when heart intake is raised to 60–70 per cent of maximum.
- Official UK recommendations are that adults should have at least five 30-minute periods of moderate activity per week, and this can be made up of no more than three shorter periods of at least 10 minutes.
- It is recommended that children should have an hour each day of at least moderate activity.
- Training also maintains muscle mass, increases strength, endurance and flexibility and produces beneficial psychological effects. These other benefits of exercise are discernible at lower intensities than that required to produce increases in VO_{2max}.
- The overall activity levels of affluent populations have decreased substantially in recent decades.
- Increasing mechanization has greatly reduced occupational energy expenditure and the energy required to perform the tasks of everyday living.
- The Allied Dunbar National Fitness Survey and the Health Survey for England have confirmed the extreme inactivity and low levels of aerobic fitness, flexibility and strength of many British adults and children. People are much less active than they were even a few decades ago.

Long-term health benefits of physical activity

In the short term, increased physical activity improves aerobic capacity, endurance, strength, flexibility and various aspects of psychological well-being. Over a period of weeks or months it also leads to changes in appearance and body composition – increased lean to fat ratio and improved muscle tone. It is inevitable that low levels of physical activity will lead to reduced energy requirements and predispose people to becoming overweight and obese. In the longer term, regular exercise contributes to reduced morbidity and mortality from several of the diseases of industrialization and therefore increases both life expectancy and years of healthy life. Some of the health benefits of regular exercise and increased fitness are summarized in Box 18.1.

Box 18.1

Demonstrable benefits of regular exercise and increased physical fitness

- Increased activity and fitness are associated with increased bone density in children and younger adults (e.g. Pocock et al., 1986), and reduced levels of osteoporotic fracture in elderly people (e.g. Wickham et al., 1989). Controlled trials show a significant beneficial effect of exercise on bone density (Howe et al., 2011). Further discussion in Chapter 14.
- Increased physical activity (Paffenbarger et al., 1986) and high level of aerobic fitness (Blair et al., 1989; Koba et al., 2011) are associated with reduced all-cause mortality in men and women. These benefits are detectable even in the elderly and may even become more pronounced with age.
- Although most early studies of the benefits of exercise were conducted in men, it is clear that the same dose-dependent benefits on all-cause mortality are also seen in women (Oguma et al., 2002).
- Middle-aged male civil servants who participated in vigorous leisure-time activities had reduced risk of coronary heart disease compared with those who did not (Morris et al., 1980).

→

Box 18.1 *continued*

- Men with active jobs have fewer heart attacks than those in similar but less active jobs (Leon, 1985).
- There are psychological benefits resulting from increased physical activity (Fentem, 1992; Bowen *et al.*, 2006). These may be direct effects of the physical activity, or indirect effects caused by the improved physical capabilities and conditioning that increased activity brings with it.
- Exercise maintains the ability to perform the activities of daily living as people become elderly and so maintains the morale, self-esteem and quality of life of older people (Bennet and Morgan, 1992).
- Increased activity leads to increased energy expenditure, both directly and as a result of the associated higher lean body (muscle) mass (particularly important in the elderly).
- Exercise increases the anti-atherogenic HDL cholesterol concentration in blood (Macnair, 1994; Koba, 2011).
- Those who are physically fit seem to be protected against the consequences of being overweight or even mildly obese (Lee *et al.*, 1998). Discussed in Chapter 9.
- Regular moderate exercise reduced the frequency of colds in post-menopausal women in a study lasting for 1 year (Chubak *et al.*, 2006).

Regular, sustained and moderate (aerobic) activity should aid in the long-term control of body weight. Craig *et al.* (2009) found a clear relationship between BMI and meeting the UK targets for activity levels. For example, 46 per cent of men and 36 per cent of women with BMI under $25\,kg/m^2$ met the activity recommendation compared with 32 per cent of men and 19 per cent of women with a BMI above $30\,kg/m^2$. Regular physical activity is more likely to be effective as a preventative measure rather than as a relatively short-term measure to cure established obesity. An exercise programme is nonetheless an important adjunct to dietary management of obesity. It increases the chances that any short-term weight losses will be sustained in the longer term. See Chapter 9 for a discussion of the role of inactivity in causing obesity and the role of exercise in its treatment.

Exercise increases and maintains bone density and therefore protects against osteoporosis. For example, Pocock *et al.* (1986) found physical fitness to be a major determinant of bone density in two regions frequently associated with osteoporotic fracture: the neck of the femur and the lumbar spine. Howe *et al.* (2011), in a meta-analysis of 43 controlled trials, found that exercise had a small but significant positive effect on bone density in post-menopausal women. Other examples of studies that indicate positive benefits of weight-bearing exercise and physical fitness on bone health can be found in Chapter 15. Note, however, that extremes of physical exercise in women that are accompanied by very low body weight and amenorrhoea almost certainly accelerate bone loss and predispose to osteoporosis (see Chapter 15).

Regular physical activity is protective against cardiovascular disease. This may be a direct effect (e.g. by strengthening heart muscle) or an indirect consequence of its effects on other risk factors. Physical activity reduces the tendency to overweight, insulin resistance and maturity-onset diabetes, it lowers blood pressure, and has beneficial effects on blood lipid profiles (e.g. Blair *et al.*, 1989). As far back as 1980, Morris *et al.* found that middle-aged people who participated in vigorous leisure-time activity had lower rates of both fatal and non-fatal coronary heart disease than those who did not. This was based on an 8.5-year cohort study of 18 000 middle-aged male British civil servants. This apparent protective effect of exercise was maintained in all age groups and in subgroups classified according to smoking behaviour and family history of CHD, and even in those with existing hypertension and subclinical angina. They concluded that vigorous exercise has 'a protective effect in the ageing heart against ischaemia and its consequences'. In a meta-analysis by Williams (2001), there was a marked drop in cardiovascular disease events at higher levels of physical fitness and a reducing risk associated with increasing activity levels.

Several studies have looked at the comparative mortality of different occupational groups with differing levels of work-related activity (Leon, 1985). Studies in California, North Dakota, Georgia and Iowa have all found lower levels of heart disease among farm workers than other inhabitants of these regions (Pomrehn *et al.*, 1982). Less smoking and higher levels of activity were identified as differences between farmers and non-farmers in these studies. Pomrehn and associates found that farmers in Iowa had lower all-cause mortality and mortality from heart disease than non-farmers. They also found that the farmers in Iowa at that time were significantly less likely to smoke, were more active, were fitter and drank less alcohol. The farmers in their sample also had significantly higher total serum cholesterol levels. They attributed the reduced total and heart disease mortality of farmers to higher physical activity and much less use of alcohol and tobacco than non-farmers.

In a 16-year cohort study of 17 000 Harvard graduates, ranging in age from 35 to 74 years, Paffenbarger *et al.* (1986) found that reported exercise level was strongly and inversely related to total mortality. They used reported levels of walking, stair climbing and sports play to calculate a relative activity index. The relative risk of death of those with an index of around 3500 kcal (14 MJ) per week was around half that of those with an index of less than 500 kcal (2 MJ) per week. They found that mortality rates among the physically active were lower with or without consideration of other confounding factors, such as hypertension, cigarette smoking, body weight or weight gain since leaving college, or early parental death.

In an 8-year cohort study of over 13 000 men and women, Blair *et al.* (1989) found a strong inverse correlation in both sexes between measured fitness level and relative risk of death from all causes. The apparent protective effect of fitness was not affected by correcting for likely confounding variables. In Chapter 9 there is a discussion of the data of Blair and his colleagues (Lee *et al.*, 1998) which suggests that people who are overweight or mildly obese but have high levels of aerobic fitness do not have excess mortality compared with those who have similar fitness but are lean. Aerobic fitness seems to offset the usual health risks associated with being overweight or obese.

Phillips *et al.* (2010) found that even self-reported fitness was a good predictor of mortality in the subsequent 16 years in a cohort of people aged 59 years. Koba *et al.* (2011) report that prospective cohort studies in Japan indicate that increased physical fitness and greater activity are of benefit in reducing all-cause and cardiovascular mortality.

They also report that aerobic training increases HDL levels in Japanese subjects.

Most expert reports dealing with strategies for reducing chronic disease and improving long-term health emphasize the importance of increased physical activity and often highlight its role in maintaining normal body weight. See, for example; COMA (1994a, 1998) and WHO (2011).

Diet as a means of improving physical performance

Body weight, athletic performance and energy intake

Athletes in training expend considerably more energy than the average person for whom the dietary reference values are intended. Their total energy expenditure during training and competition may be well over twice their basal metabolic rate (BMR) as compared to the 1.4 or 1.5 times BMR assumed when DRVs are set. During the 10 days of the Tour de France cycle race, athletes may expend up to 5.5 times their BMR (Wilson, 1994). One would also therefore expect that the energy and nutrient intakes of those in training would be considerably higher than those of the average person. Even though requirements for some nutrients may be increased by heavy exercise, one would not expect athletes to have dietary inadequacy.

In some events, where performance is judged on aesthetic appeal (e.g. gymnastics, ice skating and dancing), thinness may be seen to increase the chance of a favourable verdict by judges. In some sports (e.g. middle- and long-distance running, jumping and cycling), being light may improve performance. In some sports, competitors are divided up into weight categories and competitors of both sexes may starve themselves to make the lower weight or even dehydrate themselves. These pressures may cause some athletes to consume much less than one would expect. Many female athletes, in particular, have much lower energy intakes than might be expected from their activity levels. According to Wilson (1994), average recorded intakes of female runners in several studies were only about 100 kcal (420 kJ) per day higher than those recorded in non-athletes. This means that, unless their diets are nutrient-dense, even small increases in nutrient requirements due to exercise may become significant in athletes with such unexpectedly low energy intakes.

Many female athletes have such low body weights that they cease to menstruate and have low levels of circulating sex hormones. This may adversely affect their bone health. It may make them more prone to stress fractures and increase their risk of developing osteoporosis in later life. Several studies have suggested that there is high prevalence of eating disorders among female athletes competing in events where low body weight might be considered advantageous (Wilson, 1994). The *female athlete triad* is a condition in which there are no menstrual periods, disordered eating and osteoporosis brought on by inadequate energy intake.

Energy and nutrient requirements

Adequate intakes of dietary energy and of micronutrients are prerequisites for maximum athletic performance. There is, however, no convincing evidence that any particular vitamin or mineral supplements boost performance in already well-nourished individuals. There may be small increases in the requirements for some water-soluble vitamins such as vitamin C, thiamin, niacin and riboflavin in those undertaking vigorous training schedules. Nevertheless a well-balanced diet should contain sufficient of these vitamins, especially as total food intake will be higher during training. Some vitamins are toxic in excess (e.g. vitamins A and D) and excesses of some others may actually impair performance (e.g. niacin).

In their updated joint position statement, the American Dietetic Association, the American College of Sports Medicine and Dieticians of Canada stated that athletes who obtain adequate energy from a variety of sources will get adequate amounts of vitamins and minerals from their food. Supplements may, however, be required by athletes who restrict their energy intake, use severe weight-loss practices, restrict whole food groups, or consume a high-carbohydrate diet with low micronutrient density (Rodriguez *et al.*, 2009).

Iron status has frequently been reported to be low and iron requirements to be increased in athletes, particularly endurance athletes. The situation with regard to iron is complicated by the fact that endurance training produces a haemodilution effect similar to that in pregnancy. Training increases plasma volume and total circulating red cell mass, but the relatively larger increase in plasma volume causes blood haemoglobin concentration to fall. True anaemia (low circulating haemoglobin) and iron deficiency (low amounts of iron stored as ferritin) in athletes are usually due to low dietary intake. This would be particularly likely in athletes, often female, who restrict their energy intake to keep their body weight low. Exercise may increase iron losses and it may impair the increase in iron absorption that normally occurs when iron stores are low. Training may thus slightly increase iron requirements, so poor iron intakes during training may precipitate iron deficiency or even anaemia in some athletes, especially female ones. Anaemia would certainly impair athletic performance particularly in endurance events. Indeed, artificially boosting blood haemoglobin levels by blood transfusion or injection of the hormone erythropoietin has been used as an unfair way of trying to boost performance.

The protein requirements and optimal protein intakes of athletes and body-builders have been the subject of hundreds of studies stretching back over several decades. While a detailed analysis of these studies is beyond the scope of this book, a few general conclusions are listed below.

- Prolonged heavy exercise does increase protein losses slightly as amino acids start to be used as substrates.
- Habitual protein intakes are almost always well in excess of requirements.
- If athletes consume sufficient energy and carbohydrate then any specific measures to boost protein intakes are unnecessary even in ultra-endurance events.
- The large protein supplements taken by many athletes are almost certainly ineffective either in increasing muscle mass or in boosting athletic performance.
- As was noted in Chapter 11, excess protein intakes have been speculatively suggested to have adverse long-term consequences, such as increased risk of chronic renal failure.

Contrary to the conclusions of several other expert groups, Rodriguez *et al.* (2009) conclude in their position statement that protein requirements are higher in very active people and suggest that protein intakes should be raised to 1.6–1.7 g/kg body weight in resistance athletes and to 1.2–1.4 g/kg in endurance athletes. These quantities of protein can be obtained from normal food in athletes who are eating enough to meet their raised energy requirements.

Substrate utilization during exercise and its implications

In explosive events like short sprints, jumping or throwing, the energy supply of the muscle during the event is mainly from creatine phosphate plus a contribution from the anaerobic metabolism of glycogen. Creatine phosphate is the muscle's short-term energy reserve and it can be used to convert adenosine diphosphate (ADP) to adenosine triphosphate (ATP) by transfer of a phosphate moiety:

$$\text{creatine P} + \text{ADP} \rightarrow \text{ATP} + \text{creatine}$$

Creatine is present in the diet in meat and fish and can be synthesized in sufficient quantities for normal circumstances from other amino acids even if a vegetarian diet is eaten. Some athletes do take supplements of creatine which do elevate the stores of creatine in muscles. In a meta-analysis, Branca (2003) found that creatine supplements produced a measurable increase in performance on some very short-term (up to 30 s) laboratory-based exercise tasks but did not appear to be effective in improving running or swimming performance.

In the longer sprints and other events when there is more sustained and very intense activity, energy supply comes from creatine phosphate, anaerobic metabolism of glycogen plus a contribution from the aerobic metabolism of glycogen. The build-up of lactate from the anaerobic metabolism of glycogen will produce fatigue and limit performance.

In endurance events, the aerobic metabolism of glucose plus a contribution from the metabolism of fat are the major sources of energy. In any endurance event or competitive sport (or even a long training session for a more explosive event), the depletion of muscle glycogen is a factor that potentially limits sustained high performance. One would expect glycogen stores in liver and muscle to be depleted after 1.5–2 hours of vigorous exercise, and depletion of muscle glycogen leads to fatigue – the so-called 'wall' that affects marathon runners. Training for

endurance events increases muscle glycogen stores and also increases the aerobic capacity of muscles, enabling them to use fatty acids more effectively. The contribution made by fatty acids to the total energy supply of the muscle increases as the duration of the exercise increases. Once glycogen reserves have been used up then running speed is limited by the speed at which fatty acids can be metabolized aerobically.

Maximizing the glycogen stores in muscle and liver is now seen as a key element in the preparation for competition in endurance sports (i.e. longer than 1 hour of sustained heavy exercise). In some endurance sports it may also be possible to take in extra carbohydrate during the event. In experimental studies, the maximum duration for which heavy exercise (75 per cent of VO_{2max}) can be sustained is directly proportional to the glycogen content of the muscle at the start. Exhaustion occurs when the muscle glycogen reserves are completely depleted. High carbohydrate diets (70 per cent of energy) during training increase the muscle glycogen content and so increase the maximum duration for which heavy exercise can be sustained. In their position statement, Rodriguez *et al.* (2009) suggested that, in diets for athletes, fat should provide 20–35 per cent of the energy (i.e. 75–80 per cent from protein and carbohydrate) but that less than 20 per cent of energy from fat offered no health or performance benefits. This moderate level of fat should provide adequate amounts of essential fatty acids and fat-soluble vitamins and help provide adequate energy for weight maintenance. Many endurance athletes manipulate their diets and exercise schedules prior to competition in an attempt to increase their body glycogen stores – carbohydrate loading. This extra carbohydrate also increases muscle water content which may not be advantageous for those in explosive events where the size of muscle glycogen stores is not critical.

There are several theories as to the best way to increase muscle glycogen stores. One regimen that is not associated with any obvious side-effects is for the athlete to eat a normal high-carbohydrate diet during heavy training up to a week before the event. Then in the week before competition, a mixed diet (50 per cent carbohydrate) is eaten for the first 3 days followed by a very high-carbohydrate diet (75 per cent carbohydrate) during the rest of the week. Training intensity is wound down in the second half of the week with a complete rest on the day before the competition. A high-carbohydrate diet should be continued during the week following competition to replenish carbohydrate stores. Carbohydrate taken in the first hour or two following the completion of the event seems to be most effective in replenishing muscle glycogen stores.

The need to prevent dehydration

A marathon runner competing in a warm environment may expect to lose up to 6 litres of sweat during the run and, even in a more temperate climate, sweat losses will often be in the range 3–4 litres. Prolonged exercise, particularly in a hot environment, can lead to dehydration which produces fatigue and reduces work capacity. Profuse sweating and an inability to dissipate excess body heat in a warm, humid environment may lead to a combination of dehydration and hyperthermia (heat stroke) which can have serious, even fatal, consequences. Ideally marathon runners should

drink 0.5 L of fluid 15–30 minutes before competition and then take small, regular drinks (say every 3 miles), although competitive rules may prevent drink stops in the early part of the race. Ideally the athlete should take in enough water to replace what is lost rather than simply drink enough to satisfy thirst. These principles apply not just to marathon runners but also to anyone participating in events that involve long periods of heavy exertion and sweating, including tennis players, long-distance cyclists and soccer players.

Rodriguez et al. (2009) recommend that athletes should be well hydrated before starting to exercise and should drink enough during and/or after exercise to balance fluid losses. They suggest that the consumption of sports drinks containing carbohydrates and electrolytes during exercise will help to maintain blood glucose, maintain fuel supplies to the muscles and prevent dehydration and sodium depletion.

The following referenced reviews about nutrition for exercise and sport may be useful for further reading: Powers and Howley (1990), Williams (2006) and Rodriguez et al. (2009).

Key points

- Athletes in training expend much more energy than the average person for whom DRVs are intended.
- Low body weight and consequent amenorrhoea are common among female athletes who restrict their energy intake to enhance performance or because judges favour lean competitors.
- Amenorrhoea reduces bone density in female athletes and could possibly make them more susceptible to stress fractures and to osteoporosis in later life.
- Requirements for some nutrients may be increased slightly by prolonged training.
- A balanced diet should provide sufficient nutrients even during training unless total energy intake is severely restricted.
- There is no convincing evidence that micronutrient supplements improve performance in those who are not deficient, but large excesses of some nutrients can be toxic or hinder performance.

- The iron stores of some female athletes are low and this is largely due to poor iron intake.
- Endurance training produces a haemodilution effect, which may exaggerate the apparent prevalence of iron-deficiency anaemia among athletes.
- Prolonged heavy exercise may increase protein requirements slightly, but habitual intakes are almost always well in excess of even these increased requirements.
- The ACSM/ADA/DC position statement (Rodriguez et al., 2009) did recommend protein intakes that were above the normal DRVs, but these amounts can still be obtained from normal food.
- There is no evidence that the large protein supplements taken by many athletes either increase performance or increase muscle mass.
- In explosive events, creatine phosphate is the principal source of muscle energy.

Key points *continued*

- Creatine is present in meat and fish and can be made from amino acids. Nevertheless, creatine supplements can increase creatine stores in muscle.

- In endurance events, depletion of muscle glycogen limits performance and so maximizing glycogen stores prior to competition is an important goal for endurance athletes.

- A high-carbohydrate diet increases muscle glycogen stores.

- Manipulating diet and training schedules during the week before competition can significantly increase glycogen stores – carbohydrate loading.

- Enormous amounts of fluid can be lost from the body during sustained heavy work or exercise. Dehydration produces fatigue, reduces work performance and can lead to potentially fatal heat stroke.

- Maintaining hydration during prolonged heavy exercise enhances performance, but thirst is an insensitive indicator of dehydration in these circumstances.

- Sports drinks consumed during exercise can help maintain glucose supplies and prevent dehydration and sodium depletion.

PART FIVE

THE SAFETY AND QUALITY OF FOOD

19   The safety and quality of food   533

THE SAFETY AND QUALITY OF FOOD

19

Aims of the chapter	533	Bovine spongiform encephalopathy	554
Consumer protection	533	Food processing	560
Food poisoning and the microbiological		The chemical safety of food	564
safety of food	540	Functional foods	573

AIMS OF THE CHAPTER

This chapter provides an overview of factors that influence the safety and quality of food in industrialized countries and of the legal framework that is designed to try to ensure food safety and quality. The major aims of this chapter are:

- to give readers enough understanding of the sources of potential hazard in their food to enable them to take practical measures to improve the safety and quality of their own food
- to help readers to make a realistic evaluation of the real hazards posed by potential threats to food safety (i.e. to identify priorities for improved food safety)
- to give readers a realistic appraisal of the likely benefits of regularly consuming the major categories of functional foods and superfoods which are heavily marketed on their supposed health benefits.

CONSUMER PROTECTION

Food law

The web pages on UK and European food law prepared by Dr David Jukes of Reading University are recommended for anyone seeking further information on this topic (www.reading.ac.uk/

foodlaw). A discussion of US food legislation can be found in Tompson *et al.* (1991), and Fisher *et al.* (2006) is a more recent source for information on legal regulation of food and supplement labelling in the USA.

Food law has traditionally had three major aims.

- *To protect the health of consumers.* To ensure that food offered for human consumption is safe and fit for people to eat.
- *To prevent the consumer from being cheated.* Food laws try to ensure that verbal descriptions, labels and advertisements for food describe it honestly and that manufacturers and retailers cannot dishonestly pass off some substitute or inferior variant as the desired product.
- *To ensure fair competition between traders.* To prevent unscrupulous traders from gaining a competitive advantage by dishonestly passing off inferior and cheaper products as more expensive ones or by making dishonest claims about the merits of their product.

A further aim could be added for some current legislation governing the labelling of foods.

- *To facilitate healthy consumer choices.* To give consumers enough information about the nutritional content of foods to allow them to make informed food choices that increase their compliance with nutrition education guidelines and also warn them of the presence of ingredients they may wish or need to avoid.

In the UK, the first comprehensive food legislation was passed in the middle of the nineteenth century and there have been regular revisions and additions to this legislation ever since. The *Food Safety Act 1990* is the latest version. The first food legislation was introduced in an attempt to combat widespread adulteration and misrepresentation of foods designed to cheat the consumer but also on occasion resulting in a product that was directly injurious to health. The sweetening of cider with sugar of lead (lead acetate) and addition of red lead to cayenne pepper are examples of practices with serious health repercussions. The watering of milk (often with dirty water), addition of alum and bone ash to flour, dilution of pepper with brick dust and the bulking out of tea with floor sweepings are all examples of practices designed to cheat the consumer. The sale of meat from diseased animals slaughtered in knacker's yards and the passing off of horseflesh as beef also occurred.

Below are some of the main provisions of the Food Safety Act that illustrate a formal legal framework designed to achieve the aims listed above.

- It is illegal to add anything to food, take any constituent away, subject it to any treatment or process, or use any ingredient that would render the food injurious to health.
- It is forbidden to sell food not complying with food safety regulations. Food does not comply with food safety regulations if:
  - it has been rendered injurious to health by any of the above
  - it is unfit for human consumption (e.g. food that contains high levels of food-poisoning bacteria)
  - it is contaminated, for instance by dirt, insect bodies, metal or glass fragments.
- It is illegal to sell any food not of the nature, substance or quality demanded by the purchaser. Customers are given a legal right to expect to be given what they ask for and to expect certain minimum standards for any food product.
- It is an offence to describe, label or advertise a food in a way that is calculated to mislead as to its nature, substance or quality. This is an additional

requirement on top of any specific food labelling requirements.

The Food Safety Act also empowers government ministers to issue, with parliamentary approval, specific regulations to ensure food safety – for example, setting maximum permitted levels of contaminants. There are many such specific regulations or *statutory instruments*. For a successful prosecution under this Act, it is not necessary to prove intent on the part of the manufacturer or retailer. The main defence against prosecution is for the defendant to show that they took all reasonable precautions and 'exercised due diligence' in trying to prevent the defect in the food.

Over the past few decades there have been a series of highly publicised alarms in the UK about the safety of food, most notably the BSE crisis discussed later in the chapter. This undermined public confidence in the safety of British food and in the ability of the old Ministry of Agriculture, Fisheries and Food (MAFF) to balance the interests of farmers and food producers against those of consumers when dealing with food safety issues. As a consequence of these concerns, the *Food Standards Agency* (FSA) was established and began operating as an independent UK government department in 2000. This agency is charged with ensuring public health and consumer interests in relation to food. The agency is expected to consult widely, assess scientific information impartially, and give advice to ministers on legislation and controls that should ensure and improve food safety. The agency is expected to take into account the costs and consequences of any proposed actions so that they are proportionate to the risks involved. MAFF has also been replaced by a new *Department of Food, Environment and Rural Affairs* (DEFRA).

Enforcement of food legislation in the UK is primarily the responsibility of Trading Standards Officers (TSOs) and Environmental Health Officers (EHOs) employed by local authorities. The EHOs are mainly concerned with issues relating to food hygiene and the microbiological safety of food; they are involved in investigating food poisoning outbreaks. The TSOs are primarily concerned with food labelling, advertising and the chemical safety of food. These officials do not just police the food safety laws but also give guidance and advice to local businesses relating to food safety issues.

The *Codex Alimentarius Commission* is an international body that was set up by the United Nations in 1962 to try to establish international food standards. Over 160 countries are members of this commission. Membership of the commission does not oblige members to accept the international standards and most industrialized countries have retained their own national standards. This means that so far the commission has been a useful forum for international debate of food standards and safety issues, but the direct impact of its standards has been very limited.

Key points

- Food law exists to protect consumers' health and to try to ensure high standards of honesty and responsibility in food manufacturing and retailing.
- The UK Food Safety Act 1990 makes it illegal to:
  - do anything to food that would make it harmful to health
  - sell food that is unfit to eat or does not comply with food safety regulations
  - dishonestly describe a food
  - sell food that is of unacceptable quality.
- UK ministers are also empowered by the 1990 Act to make specific food regulations subject to approval by Parliament.
- An offence can be committed under the 1990 Act even if there is no intent, unless the defendant took all reasonable measures and care to try to avoid the defect in the food or its description.
- An independent Food Standards Agency has been set up whose brief is to ensure public health in relation to food.
- Enforcement of food safety legislation in the UK is usually the responsibility of local government.
- The Codex Alimentarius Commission is an international body that sets international food standards.

Food labelling

Labelling in the UK

A guide to all aspects of regulations covering food labelling in the UK may be found within the website mentioned at the start of the chapter that has been developed by Dr David Jukes at the University of Reading. Information relating specifically to food labelling may be found at www.reading.ac.uk/foodlaw/label/index.htm.

Most packaged foods in the UK must contain the following information on the label:

- the name and address of the manufacturer or packer of the food
- the name of the food
- a list of ingredients
- an indication of its minimum durability
- an indication of any special storage conditions or conditions of use that are required (refrigerate, eat within 3 days of opening, etc.).

Most foods must be marked with a 'lot' number so that they can be identified and withdrawn from sale if there is a problem that requires this.

If a food is perishable and likely to become microbiologically unsafe after a relatively short storage period, then it carries a 'use by' date and it is illegal to offer for sale any food that is past this date. Such foods usually need to be stored in a refrigerator or chill cabinet, and these foods should not be eaten after their use-by date; examples are cooked meats, ready meals, sandwiches and meat pies. Other foods that are unlikely to become hazardous on storage are labelled with a 'best before' date. Although unlikely to represent a hazard after that date, their eating quality may be impaired; examples are biscuits (cookies), cakes, bread and chocolate. Foods may be legally offered for sale after their best-before date provided they have not become unfit for human consumption. A few foods are exempt from having to provide a best-before date, examples being wines and spirits, fresh fruits and vegetables (unless they have been cut up or peeled) and solid sugar.

In the UK and the European Union, the ingredients of packaged foods must be listed in order of their prominence, by weight, in the final product. All additives must be listed and their functions given. Certain foods are exempt from the requirement to carry a list of ingredients, examples being fresh fruits and vegetables, cheese, butter, alcoholic drinks and any food composed of a single ingredient.

In the UK, most packaged foods now also carry nutritional information on their label.

Manufacturers voluntarily choose to include this, but such nutrition labelling is compulsory if the manufacturer makes any *nutritional claim* for the product, such as 'low fat' or 'high fibre'. The minimum nutritional information the food must then carry is the energy, protein, carbohydrate and fat contents per 100 grams, together with the amount of any nutrient for which a claim is made.

The Food Standards Agency has developed a new system for labelling foods that is intended to help consumers make healthier food choices. It is based on the red, amber and green colours of traffic lights. The FSA would like this 'traffic light system' to be used on a range of processed foods, including ready meals, pizzas, sandwiches, breakfast cereals, sausages, burgers, pies, and food products with breadcrumb coatings. Many of the major British retailers and food manufacturers have started to use this system, although each has adopted its own slightly different style of presentation. The system is intended to give information about four nutrients that we have been advised to consume less of, namely fat, saturated fat, sugar and salt (it is also sometimes used to indicate energy content). The red, amber and green lights on the label indicate the amounts of these four nutrients per 100 grams of the food (Figure 19.1):

- red = high
- amber = medium
- green = low.

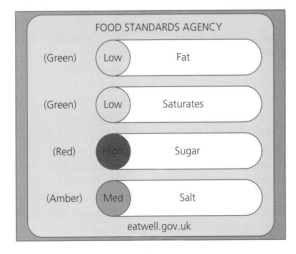

Figure 19.1 Traffic light food labelling system recommended by the Food Standards Agency in the UK.

This means that when comparing alternative versions of similar products consumers can see at a glance which is the healthier choice with respect to these four nutrients. Consumers are advised by the FSA that foods with a red light should be eaten occasionally or as a treat but that generally we should eat less of these. A green light means that the food is low in the nutrient and so the more green lights the healthier the choice. Amber-light foods have moderate amounts of the nutrient and so are a reasonable choice most of the time, although consumers might wish to choose some foods with a green light for that nutrient on some occasions. When assessing overall food choices, consumers are advised to choose more green lights and not too many red lights.

Details of this traffic light system with illustrated examples can be found at www.eatwell.gov.uk/foodlabels/trafficlights.

Some major retailers have actively chosen not to implement this system partly because of fears that red lights on a food may make consumers resist buying the food at all. An alternative system based on *guideline daily amounts* (GDAs) has been developed and is favoured by some retailers (some include both the traffic light and the GDA system on their labels).

Guideline daily amounts are the approximate amounts of a nutrient that should be consumed each day in a healthy diet. They have been developed for men, women, adults and children for calories, fat, saturated fat, carbohydrate, total sugars, protein, fibre, salt and sodium. These GDAs are calculated by using the approximate estimated average requirements (EARs) of energy for the group in question and the dietary reference values (DRVs) for macronutrients and fibre. There are separate GDAs for different age and sex groups of children and a generalized set of GDAs for children aged 5–10 years. The decision about which GDA to include on any given food label will depend on space available and on the likely consumers of the food. This system is much more complex than the traffic light system recommended by the FSA and is essentially very similar to that used on US food labels as outlined below.

Further details of the GDA system, including tables of numerical values, can be found at www.

igd.com/index.asp?id=1&fid=5&sid=42&tid=62. Some retailers use a combination of the traffic light system and guideline daily amounts

Labels in the USA

American food labelling regulations underwent a major revision in the Nutrition Labelling and Education Act of 1990 (NLEA). This very formal and detailed set of regulations covers 4000 pages. A short review is offered here to readers from outside the USA as an illustration of the complexity involved when statutory regulation of full nutritional labelling of food is attempted.

The stated aim of the legislation was to produce a simple, understandable label that clears up confusion and helps consumers to make healthy choices, and also:

> to encourage product innovation, so that companies are more interested in tinkering with the food in the package, not the word on the label.

> *DA Kessler, FDA Commissioner (1991)*

Ironically, one of the original purposes of US food law was to stop producers 'tinkering with the food in the package'! This brief summary of these regulations illustrates the complexity of trying to frame food labelling rules that cover every eventuality. They have tried to ensure that all labels contain all the useful information, in a clear, comprehensible and truly informative form, and free from misleading information and claims. Shortly after these regulations were introduced in 1992, it was suggested in the influential journal *Nature* (vol. 360, p. 499) that the resulting labels were 'all but incomprehensible' and 'leaving the consumer in need of a mainframe computer to translate it all into practical terms'.

Listed below is a sample of the important provisions introduced in the NLEA.

- *Range of foods.* Nutrition labelling is mandatory on almost all packaged foods. Food stores are also asked to display nutrition information on the most frequently consumed raw fruits, vegetables, fish, meat and poultry.
- *List of ingredients.* A full list of ingredients is required on all packaged foods, even those made according to the standard recipes set by the FDA such as mayonnaise, macaroni and bread. The

ingredients must be listed in descending order of weight in food, and a number of additional specific requirements are listed (e.g. all colours must be listed by name, caseinate (used in non-dairy coffee whitener) must be identified as being from milk, and the source of any protein hydrolysate must be indicated (e.g. hydrolysed milk protein)). One purpose of these specific rules is to assist people with food allergies.

- *Serving sizes.* These have to be stated and for many products the serving size is laid down so as to properly reflect what an adult actually eats. For example, the 'reference amount customarily consumed' for a soft drink is 8 ounces (c250 g). There are detailed regulations about what happens if packages contain less than two statutory servings; for example, if the carton contains less than 200 g per 200 mL then the whole package should be treated as one serving. This measure has been introduced to prevent producers misleading consumers as to, for example, the fat, sugar or energy content of their product by using unrealistically small portion sizes.
- *Nutritional information.* The label must contain the amounts of the following per serving: calories; calories from fat; total fat; saturated fat; cholesterol; sodium; total carbohydrate; complex carbohydrate; dietary fibre; sugars; protein; vitamins A and C; calcium; and iron. Other nutritional information that can be voluntarily listed (e.g. B vitamins) is also specified. The label must not only give the amount of the nutrient in absolute terms but must also put it into the context of an average ideal diet. So, for example, if a serving contains 13 g of fat this is equivalent to 20 per cent of the total fat in the ideal 2000 kcal diet. Not only the content of the label but also its format is laid down, and a nutrition information panel from a sample label is shown in Figure 19.2.
- *Descriptive terms.* Several of the descriptive terms that are frequently used on food labels are formally defined and the food must comply with those statutory definitions – for example, *free* as in 'fat free' and 'sugar free', *low* as in 'low calorie' and 'low sodium', and *less* as in 'less fat'. Other descriptive terms are *light, lite, reduced* and *high*. Low-fat versions of products like butter, sour

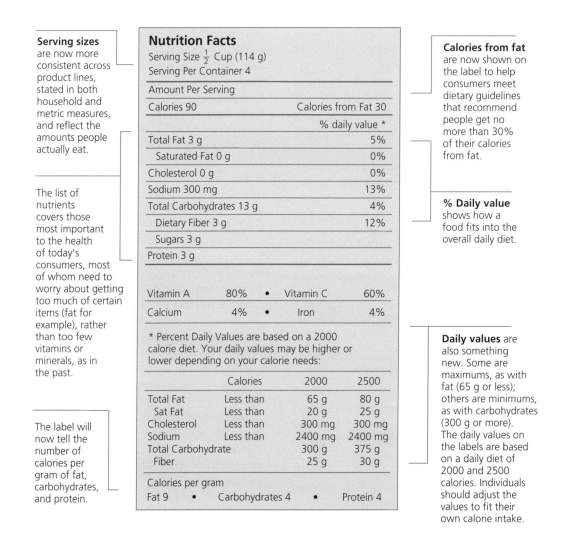

Serving sizes are now more consistent across product lines, stated in both household and metric measures, and reflect the amounts people actually eat.

The list of nutrients covers those most important to the health of today's consumers, most of whom need to worry about getting too much of certain items (fat for example), rather than too few vitamins or minerals, as in the past.

The label will now tell the number of calories per gram of fat, carbohydrates, and protein.

Calories from fat are now shown on the label to help consumers meet dietary guidelines that recommend people get no more than 30% of their calories from fat.

% Daily value shows how a food fits into the overall daily diet.

Daily values are also something new. Some are maximums, as with fat (65 g or less); others are minimums, as with carbohydrates (300 g or more). The daily values on the labels are based on a daily diet of 2000 and 2500 calories. Individuals should adjust the values to fit their own calorie intake.

Nutrition Facts

Serving Size $\frac{1}{2}$ Cup (114 g)

Serving Per Container 4

Amount Per Serving	
Calories 90	Calories from Fat 30
	% daily value *
Total Fat 3 g	5%
Saturated Fat 0 g	0%
Cholesterol 0 g	0%
Sodium 300 mg	13%
Total Carbohydrates 13 g	4%
Dietary Fiber 3 g	12%
Sugars 3 g	
Protein 3 g	

Vitamin A	80%	•	Vitamin C	60%
Calcium	4%	•	Iron	4%

* Percent Daily Values are based on a 2000 calorie diet. Your daily values may be higher or lower depending on your calorie needs:

	Calories	2000	2500
Total Fat	Less than	65 g	80 g
Sat Fat	Less than	20 g	25 g
Cholesterol	Less than	300 mg	300 mg
Sodium	Less than	2400 mg	2400 mg
Total Carbohydrate		300 g	375 g
Fiber		25 g	30 g

Calories per gram

Fat 9   •   Carbohydrates 4   •   Protein 4

Figure 19.2 Typical nutrition information panel from a food label in the USA.

cream and cheese need no longer be called 'imitation' or 'substitute' but may be called simply 'low fat', provided they comply with certain specified criteria. This is aimed at improving the image of low-fat foods.

- *Health claims.* Some relationships between nutrients and disease are regarded as well enough established to be allowed to be used in health claims on food labels. These currently include:
  - calcium and osteoporosis
  - sodium and hypertension
  - saturated fat and cholesterol and coronary heart disease (CHD)
  - fat and cancer
  - folic acid and neural tube defects
  - fibre-containing food and cancer
  - fruits and vegetables and cancer
  - foods that contain fibre (especially soluble) and CHD
  - soy protein and coronary heart disease
  - phytosterols and phytostanols and CHD (discussed at the end of this chapter).

Only foods that meet the compositional criteria specified for each claim can carry the claim, and the suggested wordings for such claims are also laid down. See the next subsection for an overview of health claims.

When these regulations were first introduced in 1992, the US Food and Drug Administration (FDA) estimated the cost of the labelling changes at $1.4–2.3 billion (c£1–1.5 billion) over 20 years. They assumed that these costs would be more than compensated for by the improvements in the diet that they facilitate and the resultant reduction in healthcare costs! More detailed information on American food labelling regulations may be found in Fisher *et al.* (2006).

An overview of health claims

As supplements and functional foods are legally classified as food, the regulations that apply to food also apply to these. In the UK it is not permitted to make claims that a food has tonic properties or that it can prevent or cure a disease. General health claims like 'may help to maintain healthy joints' have historically been permitted, but this is now changing because of the application of *EU Regulation 1924/2006* on nutrition and health claims made on foods.

The situation in the USA is similar to that in the UK up to 2006, although the health claims listed in the previous subsection are additionally allowed in the USA. In order to prevent a legal challenge to health claims restriction being an unconstitutional restriction on freedom of speech, the FDA further allows a number of 'qualified health claims' that do not meet the criterion of significant scientific agreement (SSA), and these may be printed on foods or supplements along with a suitable qualifying disclaimer, such as 'the evidence supporting the claim is not conclusive'. See Fisher *et al.* (2006) for more information.

The general principles of the EU regulations on food and health claims are that claims should not:

- be false, ambiguous or misleading
- give rise to doubt about the safety and/or the nutritional adequacy of other foods
- encourage or condone excess consumption of a food
- state, suggest or imply that a balanced and varied diet cannot provide appropriate quantities of nutrients in general
- refer to changes in bodily functions which could give rise to or exploit fear in the consumer, either textually or through pictorial, graphic or symbolic representations.

It is also a requirement of these regulations that eventually all nutrition and health claims will need to be substantiated by scientific evidence published in scientific journals. The *European Food Safety Authority* is currently engaged in a long and time-consuming effort to sift through and accept or reject many hundreds of claims submitted by food producers that they wish to make for their products. This process is briefly described in Chapter 13 along with examples of judgements made on the first 900 submitted claims. A very high proportion of these claims have not been accepted, and many of those that have relate to relatively uncontroversial claims about the effects of vitamins and minerals, dietary fibre and the effects of different fatty acids on blood cholesterol. Once a claim has been rejected the company will be under notice to stop using that claim on its labels and advertising within a specified time.

Key points

- In the UK, most packaged foods must have on their label the food's name, ingredients, shelf life, storage requirements, batch number and the name and address of the packer.

- A use-by date on a food in the UK indicates that the food is likely to become microbiologically unsafe after that date. A best-before date indicates that a UK food's quality may have deteriorated after that date but it is unlikely to have become unsafe.

- Most British foods carry some nutritional information on the label and they must do so if they make any nutritional claim for the product.

- If nutritional information is used on a British label then it must include the energy and macronutrient content per 100 grams and the amount of any nutrient for which a claim is made.

- The Food Standards Agency has devised a traffic lights system of nutritional labelling which is designed to indicate whether a food is high, moderate or low in fat, saturated fat, sugar and salt. Many UK retailers and manufacturers have adopted the FSA's traffic light system, although each has used its own design.

→

Key points *continued*

- Some retailers have opted to use a more complex system of nutritional labelling based on guideline daily amounts (GDAs) which is similar to the American system.

- There are now very detailed and complex regulations controlling food labelling in the USA. Almost all packaged foods must have a label which must:
  - contain a full list of ingredients
  - use prescribed serving sizes for nutritional information
  - give detailed nutritional information according to prescribed rules
  - only use descriptive terms like 'high' or 'low' if the food meets certain prescribed criteria
  - only make permitted health claims, and then only if the food meets the prescribed criteria.

- In the UK, neither food packaging (including dietary supplements and functional foods) nor food advertisements can make claims that they cure or prevent disease.

- EU Regulation 1924/2006 is now the basis for legal regulation of nutrition and health claims for foods in the UK and other EU countries. The general principles of this legislation are summarized in the text. One main aim of this EU regulation is that only health and nutrition claims substantiated by published scientific evidence will be permitted.

- The European Food Safety Authority is in the process of sifting though and assessing many hundreds of such claims submitted by food producers. Only a small minority of claims so far assessed have been approved.

FOOD POISONING AND THE MICROBIOLOGICAL SAFETY OF FOOD

There cannot be many readers of this book who have never experienced a bout of microbial food poisoning. The number of officially recorded and verified cases in England and Wales rose throughout the 1980s and 1990s from under 15 000 in 1982 to more than 100 000 by the end of the 1990s. Between 2000 and 2005 the number of cases fell to around 80 000, but since then the number has drifted up a bit, largely owing to increased cases of *Campylobacter* infection.

Food poisoning is rarely serious enough to cause death but it can be fatal in the very young, very old and those people whose immune system is suppressed by drugs or disease. Between 100 and 200 people die each year in the UK as a consequence of food poisoning. To put this into perspective, in the 1940s, prior to the introduction of general pasteurization of milk, 1500 people died in the UK each year from bovine tuberculosis contracted from drinking contaminated milk. Bovine tuberculosis has now been all but eradicated in the UK.

The number of officially recorded and verified cases of food poisoning will, almost inevitably, represent only the 'tip of the iceberg' because only a minority of sufferers will even consult a physician. Reported cases have been variously estimated as representing between 1 and 10 per cent of all cases. The Health Protection Agency estimated that in 2000 there may have been as many as 1.3 million cases of food-borne disease in England and Wales, of whom around 370 000 consulted a doctor; and yet in that year only 87 000 cases of food poisoning were notified and a figure of 5.5 million cases of food-borne illness has been suggested (i.e. that as many as one person in 10 experiences a food-borne illness each year). Even though recorded cases represent only a small and indeterminate fraction of actual cases, it seems probable that real cases will change in line with the number of recorded ones. It is also likely that infections that produce a relatively mild or relatively short-lasting illness will probably be under-represented in the recorded data. The relatively high incidence in children may again be because parents are more likely to consult a doctor about a serious stomach upset in a child.

Key points

- Recorded cases of food poisoning rose sharply during the 1980s and 1990s in England and Wales but dropped by around 20 per cent between 2000 and 2005. They have drifted up a little since then, largely driven by increased cases of *Campylobacter* infection.

- Recorded food poisoning cases only represent a small fraction of total cases of food-borne disease, with perhaps as many as 1 in 10 of the population being affected each year.

→

Key points *continued*

- Food poisoning is seldom fatal. Most of the 100–200 annual deaths in the UK are in vulnerable groups like the elderly, infants and those with impaired immune function.

Causes of food-borne diseases

The causative organisms

Textbooks of food microbiology usually list more than 10 organisms or groups of organisms as significant causes of food poisoning. In classical food poisoning, large numbers of organisms generally need to grow in the food to cause illness and this normally presents as *acute gastro-enteritis*. There are a number of other food-borne or water-borne diseases (e.g. typhoid, cholera, and infections with *Campylobacter* and *Shigella* species) which usually require relatively few organisms to cause illness, and in these cases there is usually no need for the organism to grow in food as there is in classical food poisoning. Several organisms that are now important causes of food-borne illness require only a few organisms to cause illness, including *Campylobacter jejuni* which is the most common cause of food poisoning in the UK, and *Escherichia coli* O157 which can cause renal failure and death especially in children and the elderly. This has important implications for safe food handling as contamination of a food with a small number of organisms is enough to cause illness if the food is not subsequently heat treated; proper storage will not remove this risk.

The relative importance of the various organisms in causing food poisoning varies in different countries and communities and depends on the diet and food practices of the population. For example, food poisoning caused by the organism *Vibrio parahaemolyticus* is associated with consumption of undercooked fish and shellfish. In Japan, where consumption of raw fish (sushi) is widespread, food poisoning due to this organism is the most common cause of food poisoning. It is, however, a relatively uncommon causative agent in the UK and USA where sushi bars and Japanese restaurants are frequently the source of infection.

The assumed importance of the various causative organisms has changed markedly over the last 30 years in the UK. Roberts (1982) analysed over a thousand outbreaks of food poisoning that occurred in England and Wales and she found that four organisms or groups of organisms accounted for almost all the outbreaks: the Salmonellae, *Clostridium perfringens*, *Staphylococcus aureus* and *Bacillus cereus*. Similar findings were reported in the USA (Bryan, 1978).

During the 1980s the incidence of food poisoning in the UK caused by *Salmonella* increased dramatically, mainly owing to increases in infection with *S. enteriditis* from poultry and eggs. During the early 1980s it was the most common recorded cause of food poisoning, but it is now second to *Campylobacter jejuni* which was only recognized as a general cause of food poisoning in the late 1970s when techniques for its isolation and identification became available. It is difficult to grow on standard laboratory media and does not usually multiply in food. The *Campylobacter* are now the organisms most frequently causing acute bacterial gastro-enteritis in the UK and account for the majority of all recorded cases. *Campylobacter* were not mentioned in the Roberts report of 1982. It requires only a few of these organisms to cause illness and it can be spread from person to person, and in this respect it is more like the other group of food-borne diseases such as typhoid and cholera. *C. perfringens*, *B. cereus* and *S. aureus* now each represent such a small proportion of cases that they are not recorded by the Food Standards Agency.

Listeriosis was also not mentioned in the earlier report of Roberts (1982), neither is it mentioned in textbooks of food microbiology published well into the 1980s. It has, however, been a cause of great public concern in the UK and USA in more recent years, with the demonstration of the causative agent (*Listeria monocytogenes*) in many supermarket chilled foods. It has been of particular concern because it may cause miscarriage, birth defects and death of newborn infants if pregnant women are infected.

Escherichia coli O157 is another food poisoning organism that has attracted much media and public attention in more recent years. This bacterium was associated with an outbreak of food poisoning in Scotland in 1996 that affected hundreds of people and killed 20 elderly people. This is one of a group of bacteria that produces a verocytotoxin that damages cells in the gut and the endothelium of blood vessels. These verocytotoxin-producing *E. coli* (VTEC) emerged as a cause of food poisoning only in the early 1980s but are now responsible for around a thousand cases of food poisoning each year. Cases have attracted a lot of attention because the organism often causes haemorrhagic diarrhoea and a small proportion of those affected develop renal complications and even acute renal failure (haemolytic uraemic syndrome, HUS), which can be fatal. It has significant mortality especially in children and the elderly. A large outbreak of food poisoning caused by a novel VTEC bacterium (*E. coli* O104) was centred on Germany in the summer of 2011. It was caused by eating raw sprouted seeds imported from Egypt, although initially it was wrongly associated with cucumbers from Spain and caused considerable economic damage to Spanish fruit and vegetable producers. This outbreak caused around 4000 cases of food poisoning in Germany and other countries, with around 45 recorded deaths from renal failure and haemorrhagic diarrhoea.

Viruses can also cause food poisoning, and the *norovirus* is probably the most common cause of acute gastro-enteritis in the UK. It is commonly referred to as the winter vomiting bug. It probably affects up to a million people each year, although lab-confirmed cases are only a small fraction of this total (*c*15 500 in 2010). It causes symptoms of diarrhoea and vomiting that last for 2–3 days. It is very contagious and can be spread from person to person or through food which has been handled by someone carrying the virus. Outbreaks are very common in places where people are confined together, including hospitals, nursing homes, schools and cruise ships.

How bacteria make us ill

Food poisoning organisms produce their ill-effects in one of the three ways listed below.

- Some organisms cause illness by colonizing the gut when they are ingested; examples are *Salmonella*, *Campylobacter* and *V. parahaemolyticus*. They produce an infection.
- Some organisms produce a toxin when they grow in the food, and it is the ingestion of this toxin that is responsible for the illness associated with the organism; examples are *S. aureus*, *B. cereus*

and *Clostridium botulinum*. The illness is caused by chemical intoxication.
- Some organisms like C. *perfringens*, *E. coli* O157 and the other VTEC infect the gut and produce a toxin after ingestion that is responsible for the food poisoning symptoms.

Food-borne viruses like the norovirus account for many mild cases of gastro-enteritis. Some of the major food poisoning organisms and their characteristics are listed in Table 19.1.

Circumstances that lead to food-borne illness

For food-borne disease to arise, the food must have been contaminated with the causative organism at some stage prior to ingestion. There are many possible means by which the food can be contaminated with micro-organisms and some examples are listed below.

- The organism might be widespread in the soil, water, dust or air.
- The organism might be present in the animal carcass at slaughter or transferred from contaminated carcasses during processing.
- Eggs and meat can become contaminated with animal faeces.
- Fish and shellfish can become contaminated by sewage in seawater – particularly important in filter-feeding molluscs like mussels.
- Fruits and vegetables can become contaminated by being washed in or watered with dirty water.
- The food handler can be a source of contamination.
- Insects, like flies, may serve as mechanical vectors for contamination.
- Food may be cross-contaminated from contact with another food – particularly important if cooked food that is to undergo no further heat treatment is contaminated by raw meat or poultry.
- Contamination can occur in the kitchen from work surfaces or dishcloths.

With some of the now most important food-borne bacteria, illness can result from the consumption of small numbers of organisms (say 10–10 000) and thus contamination of any food with these organisms may in itself be sufficient to cause illness. Such an organism is said to have a *low infective dose* and in these cases infection can result

Table 19.1 Some characteristics of important food poisoning bacteria

Bacteria	Effect of 75°C	Incubation	Infective dose	Mode of pathology	Likely source	Other points
Campylobacter	Killed	2–10 days	Low	Infection	Meat, poultry	
Salmonella	Killed	12–48 hours	High	Infection	Meat, poultry, eggs	
C. perfringens	Spores resist	8–12 hours	High	Toxin in food	Meat, poultry	
E. coli O157	Killed	1–14 days	Low	Toxin in gut	Cattle	Can be lethal
S. aureus	Killed	2–6 hours	High	Toxin in food	Food handler	Heat-resistant toxin
B. cereus	Spores resist	1–16 hours	High	Toxin in food	Rice	
C. botulinum	Spores resist	18–36 hours	High	Lethal toxin in food	Improperly canned or bottled food	Rare, often fatal; anaerobic
L. monocytogenes	Killed	2 days–7 weeks	Low in pregnancy and vulnerable groups	Infection	Chilled foods, pâté, soft cheese	Grows at 3°C, tolerates salt and sugar
V. parahaemolyticus	Killed	2–48 hours	High	Infection	Fish, shellfish	

from drinking contaminated water or, in some cases, spread from person to person or from animals to people (e.g. in children's petting farms). Of the major food poisoning bacteria, both *Campylobacter* and *E. coli* O157 also have a low infective dose. Simple contamination of the food is enough to cause food poisoning in such cases if the food is not subjected to further heat treatment. Norovirus is highly contagious and can be spread from person to person as well as from contaminated food.

Foreign travel and gastro-enteritis (travellers' diarrhoea) seem to be very frequently associated. Some of these cases may be due to a wide variety of food poisoning organisms, including those listed earlier, but a high proportion are probably due to strains of *E. coli* to which the traveller has not acquired any immunity. Cook (1998) has suggested that up to 80 per cent of cases of acute diarrhoea among travellers may be due to strains of *E. coli* that are much less virulent than the potentially fatal infection of *E. coli* O157. Faecal contamination of drinking water, bathing water or perhaps contamination of water used to irrigate fruits or vegetables are the likely sources of the organisms.

The lack of immunity means that foreigners may have a much lower infective dose than the indigenous population and so foreigners become ill but the local population is untouched. Low infective doses from water, ice in drinks, or raw fruit and salad vegetables washed in contaminated water may be a source of infection. Those on short visits to foreign countries, especially where the water supply may be suspect, would be well advised to consume only drinks made with boiled or purified water, to avoid ice in drinks, to peel or wash in purified water any fruits or vegetables that are to be eaten raw.

Many of the 'traditional' food poisoning organisms (including *Salmonella*) need to be ingested in higher numbers (often in excess of 100 000) to cause illness in a healthy adult. These organisms are said to have a *high infective dose* and they do not usually cause illness as a result of the consumption of contaminated water because of dilution and because water does not have the nutrients to support bacterial proliferation. Similarly, with some organisms that cause illness by producing a toxin in the food, a large bacterial population needs to have accumulated before sufficient toxin is produced to cause illness. For food poisoning to occur in healthy adults, not only must food be contaminated with these organisms but the following conditions also usually need to be met.

- The food must support growth of the bacteria (and allow production of toxin if relevant).
- The food must at some stage have been stored under conditions that permit the bacteria to grow (or produce toxin).

Note that even within a group of healthy young adults there will be variation in the susceptibility to any particular infective organism. In highly vulnerable groups, infective doses are likely to be at least an order of magnitude smaller. Babies are vulnerable because their immune systems are not fully developed, and the functioning of the immune system also declines in the elderly. Others who are at increased risk of food poisoning are those people whose immune systems have been compromised by illness, starvation, immunosuppressive drugs or radiotherapy. Not only is the infective dose lower in such vulnerable groups, but the severity of the illness is likely to be greater, perhaps even life-threatening, and the speed of recovery slower. Most food poisoning deaths occur in these vulnerable groups.

Key points

- At least 10 groups of bacteria are important potential causes of bacterial food poisoning.
- Classical food poisoning bacteria require large numbers to be present in the food to produce illness. They have a high infective dose.
- Some of the organisms most commonly producing food-borne illness do so even when only a few are present in the food. They have a low infective dose.
- A group's diet and dietary practices determine the relative importance of different food poisoning bacteria.
- In the early 1980s, *Salmonella*, followed by *C. perfringens*, *S. aureus* and *B. cereus*, accounted for almost all recorded outbreaks of food poisoning.
- In recent years, *Campylobacter* has risen from being unrecognized as a cause of food poisoning to being the most recorded common cause in the UK.

→

Key points *continued*

- Other organisms that have attracted particular attention in recent years are:
  - *S. enteriditis* – because it became the most common cause of *Salmonella* food poisoning and its presence in British poultry and eggs was very widespread
  - *L. monocytogenes* – because it is present in may chilled foods and it can cause miscarriage, birth defects and stillbirth if consumed by pregnant women
  - *E. coli* O157 – because it may lead to acute and potentially fatal renal complications in children and elderly people
  - norovirus or winter vomiting bug – produces up to a million yearly cases of short-lived gastro-enteritis and spreads from person to person.
- Food poisoning bacteria produce illness by infecting the gut or by producing a toxin either in the food or in the gut after ingestion.
- Initial contamination of food with the organism is a prerequisite for all food-borne diseases and is sufficient to cause some food-borne illnesses (*Campylobacter*, *E. coli* O157 and norovirus) if the food is not subject to further cooking or heating.
- If organisms have a high infective dose then the bacteria must have multiplied in the food prior to ingestion, so the food and storage conditions must have been suitable for bacterial growth.
- Travellers' diarrhoea is often caused by strains of *E. coli* to which the traveller is more susceptible than is the local population. Contaminated water may be directly or indirectly responsible for many cases of travellers' diarrhoea.

Principles of safe food preparation

Safe preparation of food involves measures and practices that attempt to do some or all of the following:

- minimize the chances of contamination of food with bacteria
- kill any contaminating bacteria, perhaps by heat or irradiation
- ensure that food is stored under conditions that prevent bacterial proliferation.

Some bacteria produce changes in the flavour, appearance and smell of the food that reduce its palatability; that is, they cause spoilage. The growth of spoilage organisms serves as a warning that the food is stale or has been the subject of poor handling procedures, inadequate processing or poor storage conditions. Food poisoning organisms, on the other hand, can grow in a food without producing changes in palatability. Thus, the absence of spoilage is no guarantee that the food is safe to eat – otherwise food poisoning would be a much rarer occurrence!

Requirements for bacterial growth

Many bacteria must actively grow in food before they are numerous enough or have produced enough toxin to cause illness in healthy people. In order to grow in food, bacteria need the following conditions to be met (these factors will also affect the growth of spoilage bacteria).

- *Nutrients.* Many foods are ideal culture media for the growth of micro-organisms. The same nutrients that people obtain from them can also be used to support bacterial growth. One reason why meat, meat products, eggs, seafood and milk products are so often the causes of food poisoning and spoil quickly is because they are nutrient-rich and generally support bacterial growth.
- *A suitable temperature.* Bacterial growth slows at low temperature and growth of most pathogens ceases at temperatures of less than 5°C. At the temperatures maintained in domestic freezers (–18°C), all bacterial growth will be arrested even though organisms can survive extended periods at such freezing temperatures. Growth of food poisoning or spoilage organisms will also not occur at temperatures of over 60°C and most will be slowly killed. At temperatures of over 73°C, non-spore-forming bacteria will be very rapidly killed, although those capable of forming spores may survive considerable periods even at boiling point. Note also that, for example, *S. aureus* produces a heat-stable toxin and so foods heavily contaminated with this organism remain capable of causing food poisoning even if heat treatment or irradiation kills all of the bacteria.
- *Moisture.* Bacteria require moisture for growth. Drying has been a traditional method of extending the storage life of many foods. High

concentrations of salt and sugar preserve foods by increasing the osmotic pressure in them and thus make the water unavailable to bacteria – they reduce the water activity of the food. Moulds generally tolerate much lower water activities than bacteria and grow, for example, on the surface of bread, cheese and jam (jelly).
- *A favourable chemical environment.* A number of chemical agents (preservatives), by a variety of means, inhibit bacterial growth. They create a chemical environment unfavourable to bacterial growth. Many pathogenic and spoilage organisms grow only within a relatively narrow pH range, so they will not, for example, grow in a very acid environment. Acidifying foods with acetic acid (pickling with vinegar) is one traditional preservation method. Fermentation of food using acid-producing bacteria (e.g. the *Lactobacilli*) has also been traditionally used to preserve and flavour foods such as yoghurt, cheese and sauerkraut.
- *Time.* The contaminated food needs to be kept under conditions that favour bacterial growth for long enough to allow the bacteria to multiply to the point where they represent a potentially infective dose. Note that under favourable conditions, bacteria may double their numbers in less than 20 minutes and so a thousand organisms could become a million in 3 hours.
- *Oxygen.* Food poisoning organisms do not require oxygen for growth although it may hasten the growth. *C. botulinum* is an anaerobe that is killed by oxygen.

Some specific causes of food poisoning outbreaks

Roberts (1982) identified the factors that most often contributed to outbreaks of food poisoning in England and Wales. Such analyses give a useful indication of practices that are likely to increase the risk of food poisoning and so indicate some of the practical measures that can be taken to reduce risk. Roberts' analysis would not have included cases of infection with the bacteria that have relatively recently attracted attention and have a low infective dose, such as *Campylobacter* and *E. coli* O157. A more recent analysis of specific factors causing outbreaks of food-borne disease by Gormley *et al.*

(2011) has highlighted similar contributory factors to those listed by Roberts. The results of Roberts are still qualitatively relevant although, because of changes in the frequency of the causative organisms, the quantitative significance of these factors will have changed. Some of the factors contributing to the cause of food-borne disease outbreaks are listed in Box 19.1.

Box 19.1

Some factors that are contributory causes of food-borne disease outbreaks

- Cross-contamination (e.g. hands, utensils, surfaces contaminated by raw food then used for ready-to-eat foods)
- Inadequate heat treatment (e.g. undercooking, inadequate thawing, consumption of raw food)
- Inappropriate food storage (e.g. preparation of food in advance of needs, storage at room temperature, improper warm holding, inadequate cooling, use of leftovers)
- Infected food handler
- Contaminated processed food

A high proportion of recorded outbreaks of food-borne illness are linked to institutions like restaurants, canteens, schools, hospitals, hotels and clubs because there is more likely to be epidemiological data relating to these. Outbreaks of food poisoning that originate from home-prepared food will usually generate far fewer individual cases than outbreaks associated with commercial and institutional catering:

Situations where food is prepared in quantity for a large number of people are most likely to give rise to most food poisoning.

Hobbs and Roberts (1993)

For example, a flaw in the pasteurization process of a major US dairy resulted in over 16000 confirmed cases and around 200000 suspected cases of food poisoning in Illinois in 1985 (Todd, 1991).

Poultry, meat and other animal products are the most commonly implicated food vehicles for outbreaks. In 2011, the Health Protection Agency in the UK identified undercooked chicken or duck liver as the source of 13 out of 14 *Campylobacter* outbreaks that occurred at catering venues. *Campylobacter* organisms are high in most raw chicken, and they are present throughout the liver, not just the surface as in poultry meat (so if the liver is cooked just until pink then many bacteria will survive to cause infection). Eggs, as well as poultry, are a source of the organism causing the most common type of *Salmonella* poisoning (*S. enteritidis*). The magnitude of this problem was such that a series of reduction measures were introduced such as mass vaccination of egg-producing flocks.

Certain foods, such as those listed below, are associated with a low risk of food poisoning:

- dry foods like bread and biscuits or dried foods – the low water activity prevents bacterial growth
- high-sugar or salted foods like jam – because of the low water activity
- fats and fatty foods like vegetable oil – they lack nutrients and provide an unfavourable environment for bacterial growth
- commercially canned foods – because they have been subjected to vigorous heat treatment and maintained in airtight containers
- pasteurized foods like milk – because they have been subjected to heat treatment designed to kill likely pathogens
- highly acid foods like pickles.

Vegetables generally do not support bacterial growth. They can, however, be a source of contamination for other foods, for instance if used in prepared salads containing meat, eggs or mayonnaise. Fruits and vegetables contaminated by dirty water may be a direct source of infection if the infecting organism has a low infective dose. Note the *E. coli* (VTEC) outbreak centred on Germany in 2011 caused by eating raw contaminated sprouted seeds.

Canned or pasteurized foods cannot be assumed to be safe if they may have been contaminated after opening or, in the case of dried foods, after rehydration.

All the foregoing information may be particularly useful if one is obliged to select food in places where food hygiene seems less than satisfactory.

Key points

- Spoilage organisms adversely affect the taste, smell and appearance of food but food poisoning organisms generally do not.
- Safe handling and preparation of food require that the risks of contamination and bacterial proliferation be minimized and/or that the killing of bacteria during preparation be maximized.
- In order to grow, bacteria require nutrients, moisture, warmth, time and a suitable pH.
- Safe storage of food involves depriving likely pathogens and spoilage bacteria of one or more of their requirements for growth.
- Box 19.1 lists some of the factors most often contributing to outbreaks of food poisoning.
- Institutional and commercial catering is responsible for most large outbreaks of food poisoning.
- Meat, poultry and eggs are the sources of most food poisoning outbreaks in the UK.
- Undercooked chicken and duck livers pose a serious risk of *Campylobacter* infection.
- Some foods are seldom associated with food poisoning:
  - foods with low water activity (dry, salted or high-sugar foods)
  - fats and oils
  - newly opened canned or pasteurized foods
  - pickled foods
  - fruits and vegetables – unless they act as vehicles for contaminated water.

Practical guidelines to avoid food poisoning

Minimize the risks of bacterial contamination of food

Some specific steps for reducing the risk of food contamination are listed in Box 19.2. Much of the meat, poultry and eggs that we purchase must be assumed to be already contaminated when they are purchased. It will require improvements in farming and slaughtering practices to reduce the initial contamination of these foods. For example, there

has been a sharp fall in the number of infections with *S. enteriditis* in the UK following the introduction of stringent new safety measures for egg production and handling, including a massive hen vaccination programme.

Box 19.2

Tips for reducing the risk of food poisoning

Reduce the bacterial contamination of food

- Buy food that is fresh and from suppliers who store and prepare it hygienically.
- Keep food covered and protected from insect contamination.
- Wash hands thoroughly before preparing food and after using the toilet or blowing your nose.
- Cover any infected lesions on hands.
- Ensure that all utensils and surfaces that come into contact with food are clean.
- Ensure that any cloth used to clean utensils and surfaces or to dry dishes is clean and changed regularly.
- Avoid any contact between raw food (especially meat) and cooked food.
- Don't store raw meat in a position in the refrigerator where drips can fall onto other foods that will not be heat-treated before being eaten.
- Wash utensils, hands and surfaces in contact with raw food before they are used with cooked food.

Maximize killing of bacteria during processing

- Cook meat, poultry and eggs thoroughly so that all parts of the food reach a minimum of 75°C.
- Defrost frozen meat and poultry thoroughly before cooking.
- Reheat food thoroughly so that all parts of it reach 75°C.

Minimize the time food is kept in conditions that allow bacteria to grow

- Prepare food as close to the time of consumption as is practical (prolonged holding of food also leads to loss of nutrients).
- When food is prepared well in advance of preparation, it should be protected from contamination and should not be stored at room temperature.

→

Box 19.2 *continued*

- Discard foods that are past their use-by dates or show evidence of spoilage (e.g. 'off' flavours and smells or discolouration).
- Food that is kept hot should be kept at 65°C or above.
- Food that is kept cool should be kept below 5°C.
- When food is cooked for storage it should be cooled quickly.
- Leftovers or other prepared foods that are stored in a refrigerator should be covered and used promptly.
- Store eggs in a refrigerator and use them within 3 weeks of purchase.

Most of the tips for reducing bacterial contamination in Box 19.2 are common-sense measures that require little amplification or explanation, but carelessness can cause us to overlook them even though they seem obvious when written down. Most people would require no prompting to avoid a butcher who kept his meat in a warm place where flies could crawl over it, or to avoid buying food that is obviously spoiled or past its use-by date. Lax hygiene can allow the cook's hands to become a source of faecal organisms or of *S. aureus* which is frequently present in skin lesions and in the nasal passages of many people. It is vital to avoid cross-contamination of ready-to-eat foods with raw foods like meat which are usually contaminated with bacteria. The bacteria in the raw food will probably be killed during cooking, but not so the bacteria in the ready-to-eat food where there is no further heat treatment to eliminate them. There are very strict food hygiene regulations that are intended to ensure that raw and cooked meats are separated in supermarkets and butchers' shops, and staff should be trained to avoid cross-contaminating cooked meats.

Maximize the killing of bacteria during home preparation of food

Some tips are included in Box 19.2. Even though many raw foods may be contaminated when bought, if they are thoroughly cooked then almost all of them should be made safe. Most of the common organisms causing food-borne illness are killed rapidly at temperatures above 73°C. Meat that is eaten 'rare' will not have undergone sufficient heat treatment to kill all bacteria and represents a hazard if contaminated prior to cooking; poultry should always be well cooked. Note that this is especially important for hamburgers and other minced meat. With a joint or slice of meat, most of the contaminating bacteria will be on the outside and these will be killed even if the centre of the meat is pink and underdone. However, when meat is minced, the bacteria are spread throughout the meat so that the centre of a hamburger contains as many bacteria as the outside (this is also true of poultry liver).

Raw eggs (e.g. in homemade mayonnaise) and undercooked eggs represent a potential hazard especially to the elderly, the sick and the very young.

Minimize the time food is stored under conditions that permit bacterial multiplication

Some tips are included in Box 19.2. The time between food preparation and consumption should be as short as practically reasonable. Where food is prepared well in advance of serving it should be protected from contamination and should not be stored at room temperature. Buffets, where prepared food may be left uncovered at room temperature for some hours before consumption, are particularly hazardous.

Most bacteria grow only at between 5°C and 65°C and are slowly killed at temperatures above that. This means that food kept hot should be kept above 65°C and any food that is to be reheated should be thoroughly reheated so that all parts of it reach 75°C, the temperature at which non-spore-forming bacteria are rapidly killed. Food that is to be kept cool should be kept below 5°C because most food poisoning and spoilage bacteria will not grow below that. Food that has been cooked but is to be stored cool should be cooled rapidly so that it spends the minimum time within the growth range of bacteria. Leftovers or other prepared foods that are stored in a refrigerator should be covered and used promptly; care should be taken to ensure that they do not come into contact with raw food, especially flesh foods.

The principal aim here has been to encourage greater care and awareness in the home preparation of food. To effect reductions in the rates of food poisoning produced outside the home, there needs to be improved training of catering workers and regulatory changes that lead to improvements to commercial and institutional catering practices. Food hygiene laws and regulations are complex, often extremely detailed, and vary from nation to nation (recent attempts to harmonize food hygiene laws within the EU have highlighted this).

Food hygiene legislation is a specialist topic beyond the scope of this book, but in principle food hygiene laws represent attempts by governments to enshrine the safety principles and practices outlined for home food preparation into a formal legal framework so as to ensure that they are carried through into mass catering situations.

A note about treatment of food-borne disease

Most cases of food poisoning go unrecorded because the symptoms are not severe enough or prolonged enough to prompt people to consult their doctor. The best way of treating simple food poisoning is to maintain the patient's fluid and electrolyte levels with oral rehydration fluids containing glucose and salts. In severe cases, intravenous infusion of fluid may be necessary. In simple food poisoning, antibiotics are not used because they do not affect the course of the disease and their use may simply encourage the development of antibiotic resistance in bacteria. As a general rule, self-medication with preparations that stop diarrhoea by inhibiting gut motility should not be used, especially in children, because they increase retention of the bacteria and increase exposure to toxins. These antimotility agents may, for example, increase the risk of renal damage in cases of infection with *E. coli* O157. They may be helpful in relatively mild cases of travellers' diarrhoea.

Key points

- Many practical measures that will reduce the risk of food poisoning are listed in Box 19.2.
- It should be assumed that meat, poultry, eggs and raw milk are likely to be contaminated when purchased.

→

Key points *continued*

- Heat will kill bacteria, but some heat-resistant spores may survive boiling and some bacterial toxins may be heat-resistant and remain in food even when all the bacteria have been killed.
- Most cases of food poisoning can be treated by simple supportive measures aimed at body fluid balance.
- Antibiotics do not generally affect the course of a bout of food poisoning.
- Compounds that stop diarrhoea by inhibiting gut motility may prolong the infection.

Pinpointing the cause of a food poisoning outbreak

Identifying the cause of food poisoning outbreaks should highlight high-risk practices and thus may be useful for improving food handling. If a single event (e.g. serving a contaminated dish at a buffet) is the cause of an outbreak then a time distribution of cases like that shown in Figure 19.3 would be expected. Each food poisoning organism has a characteristic average incubation period from time of ingestion to the onset of symptoms. Incubation times in individuals will vary around this average; a few people develop symptoms early, most

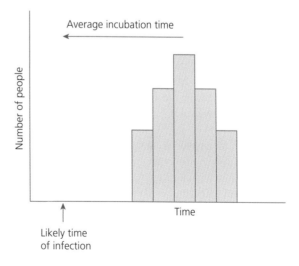

Figure 19.3 Theoretical time course of first experiencing food poisoning symptoms after infection.

towards the middle of the range and a few towards the end of the range. The variation in the speed of onset of symptoms is influenced by all sorts of factors, such as:

- the dose of organism or toxin consumed
- the amount of other food consumed and thus the dilution and speed of passage through the gut
- individual susceptibility.

The organism causing the illness can be identified from the clinical picture and/or laboratory samples and then, knowing the incubation period, the approximate time at which all the victims were exposed to the organism and the meal at which the organisms were consumed pinpointed. Sampling of leftovers or circumstantial evidence can then identify the responsible food and, it is hoped, the unsafe practice that led to the outbreak.

Board (1983) gave an illustrative case history of an outbreak of food poisoning among the passengers and crew of a charter flight. More than half of the passengers developed food poisoning, a few at the end of the flight and large numbers at the airport within 2 hours of landing. The clinical picture (the symptoms, the rapid onset and short duration) indicated that the illness was probably due to ingestion of toxin from *S. aureus*. The time distribution of cases indicated that the breakfast served on the plane 90 minutes before landing was the likely source of the illness and samples of uneaten breakfasts confirmed the presence of this organism in ham omelette. The food had been contaminated by infected sores on the hands of one of the cooks at the catering company that had supplied the breakfasts to the airline. A long time (3 days) had elapsed between the initial preparation of the food and its eventual serving, and the food had not been kept cool for much of that time.

If no food samples are available for analysis then the responsible food can often be implicated by calculation of attack rates. All of those participating in the meal identified as the point of infection are asked to complete a questionnaire about which foods they consumed and whether they became ill. The attack rate is the percentage of people becoming ill. For each food, the percentage of those who became ill is calculated for those who did and those who did not consume that food (i.e. the

food-specific attack rates). A statistically significant higher attack rate for those consuming a particular food compared with those not consuming it indicates that it was the likely source of the infection. In the example in Table 19.2, eating food A significantly increased the attack rate while eating B significantly reduced it. Food B appears protective because A and B were alternative choices on the menu, so people who ate B did not eat A. It would thus seem almost certain that food A was the source of the infection.

Table 19.2 Food-specific attack rates for people present at a social function identified as the point of infection for an outbreak of food poisoning*

Food	Ate			Did not eat		
	Ill	Not ill	Attack rate (%)	Ill	Not ill	Attack rate (%)
A	30	131	19	0	51	0[1]
B	0	27	0	30	154	16[1]
C	8	49	14	21	125	14
D	21	95	18	9	84	10
E	8	69	10	22	107	17
F	13	60	18	17	121	12

*After Hobbs and Roberts (1993).
[1] Statistically significant difference between the attack rates of those who did and did not consume that particular food.

The time distribution of people reporting symptoms of food poisoning may not follow the bell-shaped model shown in Figure 19.3. For example, there may be multiple peaks or the number of new cases may tend to plateau rather than fall away. Such distributions would indicate either person-to-person spread or a continuing source of infection – for example, a processing fault, an infected food handler, continuing use of a contaminated ingredient, or continued sale of a contaminated processed food. If the incubation period of the causative organism is known, a questionnaire should establish what all the victims were doing (and eating) within the window of time when infection is predicted to have occurred. It should then be possible to identify a common factor, such as that all victims ate a particular processed food, ate at a particular place or ate a processed food bought from a particular source during the period when they were likely to have become infected.

Key points

- Food poisoning bacteria each produce a characteristic set of symptoms and have characteristic incubation times.
- Incubation times will vary between individuals depending on dose consumed, its dilution with other food and drink and the susceptibility of the person.
- If the time distribution of cases in an outbreak is 'normal' as in Figure 19.3, this indicates a single point of infection and one can predict when this occurred from the average incubation period of the organism.
- One can identify which specific food was responsible because there will be a higher 'attack rate' among those who ate this food than among those who did not.
- If there is a continuing source of infection or person-to-person spread, the time distribution of cases will show multiple peaks or a tendency to plateau rather than the single peak in Figure 19.3.
- Even with a continuing source of infection, it should still be possible to identify a factor common to all victims during the window of time when they were likely to have been infected.

Review of some common food poisoning organisms and food-borne illnesses

Campylobacter

Campylobacter was only recognized as a general source of food-borne disease in 1977. The organisms do not grow in food at room temperature and do not grow readily on normal laboratory media. This means that suitable methods needed to be developed for their identification. From being almost totally ignored as a cause of food poisoning 30 years ago, this organism is now the most common cause of acute bacterial gastro-enteritis in the UK with around 50 thousand lab-confirmed cases recognized each year.

The illness has a relatively long incubation period (2–10 days) and it produces a quite severe and prolonged illness. It initially produces flu-like symptoms and abdominal pain which last for 1–2 days, and that is followed by profuse, sometimes bloody, diarrhoea lasting for 1–3 days. It may take a week or more for complete recovery. The organism may contaminate water, unpasteurized milk, meat and poultry and it may reside in the intestines of domestic animals. The organism has a low infective dose and thus is potentially transmissible through water, through the hands of children playing with or near domestic or farm animals, or even from person to person. Undercooked poultry is the most common cause. Poultry or meat that has been inadequately cooked on garden barbecues has been blamed for many cases in the UK. The organism has a high optimum growth temperature but is killed rapidly at 75°C.

Salmonella

Many different types of the *Salmonella* group are responsible not only for common food poisoning but also for the more serious food- and water-borne illnesses typhoid and paratyphoid. The common food poisoning organisms usually need in excess of 100 000 bacteria to represent an infective dose. These organisms produce diarrhoea, stomach pain, vomiting and fever about 12–48 hours after ingestion and the illness lasts for between 1 and 7 days. Intensive farming methods and slaughtering practices mean that raw meat, poultry, eggs and raw milk should be regarded as potentially contaminated. These organisms grow at temperatures between 6°C and 46°C. They are relatively sensitive to heat and are killed slowly at 60°C and very rapidly at 75°C. They are not tolerant of very acidic conditions (pH <4.5).

Meat and especially poultry have long been regarded as foods with a high potential to cause *Salmonella* poisoning, but in recent years the contamination of eggs with *S. enteriditis* has been a major cause for concern in the UK. Many thousands of hens were slaughtered in an apparently unsuccessful attempt to eradicate these organisms from the laying flock. Incidence of *S. enteriditis* infection has fallen sharply in the UK in the last few years because of changes in egg production and handling and a mass vaccination programme for hens.

Eggs have a number of natural barriers that tend to reduce the risk of bacterial entry, but they are sold in millions, so even if only a very small proportion are contaminated this can represent, in absolute terms, a large number of potentially infected meals. Eggs also have a number of systems that inhibit bacterial growth (bacteriostatic systems) by making nutrients unavailable to the bacteria. The likelihood of a single fresh egg containing an infective dose for a healthy adult is thus low. However, if eggs are stored at room temperature and kept for long periods then a small number of original contaminating bacteria can multiply to the point where they represent an infective dose. Eggs should be stored in a refrigerator and they should not be kept for more than 3 weeks. Fresh and well-cooked eggs should represent no hazard at all. Any potential hazard from eggs is increased very significantly if uncooked egg is added to other foods (e.g. mayonnaise or cheesecake) and then the mixture stored under conditions that allow bacterial proliferation, such as at room temperature.

Clostridium perfringens

This organism has a high infective dose of between a hundred and a thousand million organisms. Illness is due to a toxin produced by bacteria within the gut. The disease has an incubation period of 8–12 hours and lasts for up to 24 hours. The symptoms are diarrhoea and abdominal pain but not usually either vomiting or fever. The organism grows at temperatures of up to 53°C and the spores need temperatures of 100°C to kill them. Food poisoning from this organism is usually associated with meat and poultry consumption and the organism is of widespread distribution in the gut of animals and people and also in soil and dust. When food is inadequately cooked, these organisms may continue to grow during the initial heating of the food and some will survive at high temperatures by forming spores. Surviving spores may start to grow as the food cools and during storage of the cooked food. The organism grows very rapidly at temperature towards the top end of its tolerable range.

Escherichia coli O157 and the VTEC bacteria

Media and public awareness of E. coli O157 was increased sharply in the UK by an outbreak of food poisoning in Lanarkshire, Scotland, in November 1996 that affected around 500 people and caused the deaths of 20 elderly people. Interviews with the initial cases established that all of them had eaten cooked meat products from a single butcher or had attended a lunch at which a steak pie supplied by this butcher had been served. More recently an outbreak centred on Germany in 2011 of a novel VTEC E. coli caused 40 000 cases and 45 deaths; this was linked to eating raw contaminated sprouted seeds.

Cattle are almost always the source of infection with E. coli O157. Undercooked beef – and more especially beef products like burgers, raw milk and cheese made from unpasteurized milk – are some potentially infective foods. The organism has a low infective dose and so cases have occurred due to contact with farm animals (e.g. children visiting farms), contamination of drinking water and even person-to-person spread.

Escherichia coli O157 is one of a group of bacteria that produce toxins that have potentially fatal effects, the verocytotoxin-producing E. coli (VTEC). These toxins damage gut cells and cells in the vascular endothelium. The onset time is typically 3–4 days after exposure but can range from 1 to 14 days. The symptoms are abdominal cramps, vomiting and diarrhoea, but a proportion of sufferers will go on to develop more serious complications including haemorrhagic diarrhoea and kidney failure that can be fatal in some children and elderly people. It is one of the major causes of acute renal failure in children.

Staphylococcus aureus

The illness caused by this organism is due to a toxin present in food where this organism has grown. In excess of 5 million bacteria are usually regarded as necessary to produce enough toxin to evoke illness. The symptoms are vomiting, diarrhoea, abdominal pain but no fever. Symptoms are rapid in onset (2–6 hours) and of short duration (6–24 hours). The organism is heat sensitive: it grows within the range 8–46°C and is killed at 60°C, but the toxin, once formed in food, is very heat stable and will not be eliminated by further heat treatment or irradiation of the food.

Food handlers are an important source of contamination. Many people carry the organism in their nasal passages and this can lead to contamination of hands and thence food; infected lesions on the hands may contain this organism. The organism needs foods rich in protein to produce toxin, but it is comparatively tolerant of high salt and sugar concentrations as found, for example, in ham and custard. *S. aureus* does not compete well with other bacteria present in raw food but, if essentially sterile, cooked food is then contaminated by the handler then, without any competition, the organism is able to grow even in foods with relatively high salt or sugar contents.

Bacillus cereus

This organism is commonly found in soil and thus on vegetables. It grows in starchy foods and, in the UK and USA, poisoning due to this organism is usually associated with consumption of rice. The organism produces heat-resistant spores which may survive cooking of rice. If the cooked rice, containing viable spores, is stored at temperatures that permit growth of the organism (7–49°C) then an infective dose will accumulate. Boiling rice in bulk and then storing it at room temperature prior to flash frying (e.g. in Chinese restaurants) is a common scenario for food poisoning due to this organism. The resultant illness is acute in onset (1–16 hours) and of short duration (6–24 hours) and it is caused by toxins produced by the organism in food. An infective dose is in excess of 100000 organisms in the food. The symptoms depend on the particular toxin involved but may include diarrhoea, abdominal pain, nausea or vomiting.

Clostridium botulinum

This organism grows under anaerobic conditions in low-acid foods. Canned or bottled meats, fish or vegetables (but not acidic fruit) are potential sources of illness. The organism is killed by oxygen, so storage of these foods in airtight containers allows growth. The organism may also occasionally grow deep within non-canned flesh foods or meat products. Commercial canning processes involve a heat treatment that is specifically designed to ensure that all of the heat-stable spores of this organism are killed – the so-called botulinum cook. Cured meats and meat products contain nitrate, nitrite and salt which are effective in preventing growth of this organism and the addition of these preservatives is legally required in the UK for meat products like sausages. Home canning or bottling of vegetables results in significant numbers of cases of botulism in the USA each year because the heat treatment is insufficient to kill the spores. The very rare cases in the UK have usually been traced to occasional rogue cans of imported meat or fish (after heat treatment, contaminated water might be sucked into the cooling can through a damaged seam). The most recent UK outbreak in 1989 was traced to a can of nut purée that was subsequently used to flavour yoghurt. Honey can contain spores of the organisms and these can survive in the intestines of infants and produce toxin, but only eight cases of infant botulism were recorded in the UK in the 30 years up to 2007. In the USA and now in the UK, it is recommended that honey should not be given to children under 1 year old. Three cases within a year prompted the Health Protection Agency to re-emphasize this advice in May 2010.

The organism produces an extremely potent toxin within the food. This toxin is destroyed by heat, so danger foods are those eaten unheated (e.g. canned salmon or corned beef) or those that are only warmed. The toxin, although a protein, is absorbed from the gut and affects the nervous system, blocking the release of the important nerve transmitter acetylcholine. A dry mouth, blurred vision and gradual paralysis are the symptoms, and death will occur due to paralysis of the respiratory muscles. With rapid treatment, including artificial ventilation, about 75 per cent of those affected survive. In victims who survive, complete recovery may take weeks or months. The incubation period is normally 18–36 hours.

This organism is included in this review even though it rarely produces illness in the UK, because the symptoms are frequently fatal and because the imperative to avoid contamination of food with this organism has had a great influence on food processing practices.

Listeria monocytogenes

Chilling has been a traditional method of storing food because it reduces both microbial growth and the rate of chemical deterioration. An enormous range of chilled foods are available in supermarkets. Such foods are susceptible to the development of infective doses of pathogenic bacteria that continue to grow slowly at low temperatures. Small variations in temperature within the low range (0–8°C) can have marked effects on the rate at which these low-temperature organisms grow. Strict temperature control is therefore of great importance in ensuring safe storage of chilled foods. For foods that are to be eaten without further cooking, or just rewarming, current UK legislation requires that they be stored below 5°C (e.g. cook–chill ready meals, sandwiches, cured meat and fish).

Listeria monocytogenes is one of these low-temperature organisms and it has attracted much media attention and public concern in the UK and USA in recent years. It will grow slowly at temperatures as low as 3°C and it will tolerate a salt concentration of 10 per cent and a pH down to 5.2. Soft cheeses and pâté, which have a relatively long shelf life, are considered to be at particular risk from this organism. Its presence has been reported in many cook–chill ready meals and it is likely to survive mild reheating in a microwave oven.

The organism causes a disease known as listeriosis in vulnerable groups like the elderly, infants, pregnant women and the immunodeficient, although it does not usually cause illness in healthy people. Symptoms range from those resembling mild flu to severe septicaemia and occasionally meningitis. If infection with this organism occurs during pregnancy then abortion, fetal abnormality or neonatal death may result. In the UK, pregnant women are currently advised to avoid those foods that are liable to harbour *Listeria* (e.g. pâté and soft cheese made with unpasteurized milk) and to thoroughly reheat cook–chill foods. Increased use of chilling led to an increase in recorded cases of listeriosis from around 25 a year in the early 1970s to around 300 a year by 1988. In 1988 there were 26 deaths of newborn babies, 52 total deaths and 11 abortions caused by listeriosis. There have been around 200 lab-confirmed cases per year in England and Wales during the period 2000–10.

The rise in the prominence of listeriosis with increased use of food chilling is a good illustration of how changing eating habits and processing methods can lead to changes in the prominence of different types of food poisoning organisms.

BOVINE SPONGIFORM ENCEPHALOPATHY

Historical introduction

In 1994, when the first edition of this book appeared, there was no evidence that bovine spongiform encephalopathy (BSE) would directly affect human beings. It is now clear that the human form of this disease, *variant Creutzfeldt–Jakob disease* (vCJD), *has* affected people. There were 176 deaths up to January 2012, and most of these people acquired the disease by eating contaminated beef products (a very small number may have acquired it through blood transfusions).

When I prepared the second edition of this book in 2001 it was estimated, in a government-sponsored enquiry into the disease, that between a few hundred and 135 000 people in the UK would eventually die as a result of this food-borne disease. In the intervening years it has become clear that many of the wildest predictions about the likely scale of this human epidemic were much too pessimistic; there were suggestions that 'hospices would be overflowing with terminally ill disease sufferers'. In January 2012 there were no known live cases of vCJD. This means that, even allowing for a small number of infections from blood transfusions or surgical transmission, the total number of deaths from the vCJD will probably remain below 200 in total. Perhaps, in the next edition of this book, BSE will be reduced to a brief historical footnote.

There is a wealth of reliable information on this disease available through the internet and recommended sites are listed below. Prusiner (1995) has written a review of the prion diseases of which BSE is an example.

- The DEFRA website archive about BSE is at http://archive.defra.gov.uk/foodfarm/farmanimal/diseases/atoz/bse
- The CJD surveillance unit website is at www.cjd.ed.ac.uk/index.htm

• The archive of the official UK enquiry into BSE is at http://collections.europarchive.org/tna/ 20090505194948/http:/bseinquiry.gov.uk

This disease has had massive economic and political effects and has had devastating effects on British farming and consumer confidence. For several years, media articles and broadcasts about the possible human consequences of BSE engendered fear, almost amounting to panic, in large sections of the population and certainly affected the mood of the whole nation. The 'BSE crisis' was a stimulus to the establishment of the Food Standards Agency and to the restructuring and renaming of the ministry of agriculture – the Ministry of Agriculture, Fisheries and Food has been replaced by the Department for Environment, Food and Rural Affairs.

The cattle epidemic of BSE is now over and, with no living cases, the much smaller human epidemic of vCJD may also have run its course with very few further deaths likely. The impact of this disease has been enormous considering the low number of human deaths (about 175 since 1995 compared to around 60 000 deaths in road accidents over the same time period). The total cost to the British nation of the BSE epidemic has been many billions of pounds. Some of these costs are ongoing (research costs, testing of slaughtered animals, removal of *specified bovine offal* from cattle destined for consumption, tagging and tracking of cattle, costs to the blood transfusion service, and so on).

Overview of the disease

Bovine spongiform encephalopathy is an apparently new disease of cattle that first appeared in British cattle in 1985. The affected animals are excitable, aggressive, easily panicked, have an abnormal gait and a tendency to fall down. These symptoms gave rise to the popular name 'mad cow disease'. Around 180 000 British cattle have developed this disease and millions more have been slaughtered and burnt in order to try to eradicate it. Over 80 per cent of cases of BSE have been in dairy cows and most of these in older animals. Only a handful of symptomatic cases have been recorded in cattle under 3 years old. The cattle epidemic peaked in 1992 when around 37 000 confirmed cases were recorded. Figure 19.4 charts the rise and fall of the BSE epidemic in cattle. It now appears to be over, with no

recorded cases in the last 2 years and only three cases since the start of 2008. In addition to those who have developed the disease, millions of cattle have been culled and their carcasses incinerated.

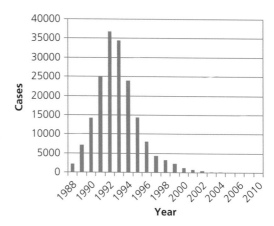

Figure 19.4 Annual number of confirmed cases of bovine spongiform encephalopathy (BSE) in British cattle.

The symptoms of BSE and the spongiform lesions seen in the brains of affected animals are similar to those seen in other *transmissible spongiform encephalopathies* (TSEs) such as those listed below. These diseases are all inevitably fatal.

• *Scrapie* of sheep and goats has been endemic in British sheep since the eighteenth century without any apparent effect on human health.
• *Creutzfeldt–Jakob disease* (CJD) is a rare disease that kills around 30–70 elderly people in the UK each year.
• *Kuru* is a disease that was prevalent among the Fore tribe in Papua New Guinea.

All these diseases are potentially transmissible by injecting extracts of diseased brain into healthy animals. The 'infective agent' is resistant to heat and radiation and, unlike any other infective agents or any living organism, appears to contain no nucleic acid. Stanley Prusiner proposed that transmission was caused by an infective protein or prion and he was awarded a Nobel Prize for this work.

Transmissible spongiform encephalopathies can be acquired in the three ways listed below.

• *Spontaneous sporadic cases.* Most cases of conventional CJD fall into this category. CJD affects around one in a million people in most populations. It almost always occurs in elderly people. It is unrelated to the presence of scrapie in the sheep flock.

- *Genetic cases.* A few cases of CJD are familial.
- *By transmission:*
  - experimentally induced by injecting infected brain into healthy animals
  - iatrogenically induced (caused by medical treatment), for example by injections of contaminated growth hormone or gonadotropins extracted from the pituitary glands of human cadavers, by the use of contaminated surgical instruments, or by transplants of infected corneal tissue, and more recently perhaps by transfusions of infected blood
  - through eating infected tissue (kuru is thought to have been caused by eating infected human brains in cannibalistic rituals).

The incubation period of these transmissible encephalopathies is long. In kuru and iatrogenic CJD, the average time from exposure to onset of clinical symptoms is thought to be around 20 years.

In 1996 it was formally announced that a new variant of CJD (vCJD) had been identified in Britain. It now seems certain that it was caused by eating contaminated beef products. The symptoms of vCJD are different from those of sporadic CJD. It also has different histological characteristics, a different time course, a different EEG pattern and, most significantly, it affects much younger people. Sporadic CJD rarely affects people aged under 60 years but almost all cases of vCJD have been in younger age groups, including teenagers.

What caused the epidemic of BSE in British dairy cattle?

Since the 1920s, cattle – and especially dairy cows – have been fed a protein supplement made by rendering animal remains, including cattle remains. It now seems certain that this feed was the cause of the epidemic, but it is unclear how this feed initially became contaminated with the BSE agent. A once popular theory was that a change in the rendering process of this feed in the late 1970s and early 1980s allowed large amounts of sheep scrapie prion to remain in the feed. This scrapie prion then triggered some cows to develop BSE. The disease was then spread by recycling of BSE-infected cattle material in the feed. This theory offered much reassurance because scrapie had been around for hundreds of years and not been transmitted to people by eating sheep products. Although the scrapie prion had apparently crossed the species barrier it was to another ruminant.

The official inquiry into BSE concluded that this theory was incorrect. Rather, BSE was probably present in cattle several years before 1985 but went undetected, and recycling of infective cattle material in feed spread the disease. It was suggested in this report that the original source of the epidemic may have been a single animal with a mutation in the prion protein gene.

In 1988, the inclusion of ruminant protein in feeds for ruminants was banned and this should have eliminated the source of infection in cattle. However, some animals born long after this feed ban came into force still developed BSE and there are several reasons for this, listed below.

- Existing stocks of banned feed were used up on some farms.
- Use of ruminant protein remained legal for pig and poultry feed and this allowed cross-contamination of ruminant feeds to occur during production. The feed ban was extended in 1996. It became illegal to feed mammalian meat and bone meal (MBM) to any farm animal or to fish. The primary purpose of this reinforced ban was to prevent cross-contamination of cattle feed.
- There is some vertical transmission (from cow to calf) of the disease. It is estimated that a calf born within 1 year of the mother developing clinical symptoms of BSE has a 10 per cent chance of being infected by the mother. Infection occurs either in the womb or during delivery. There is no transmission from paternal semen. There is no evidence of horizontal transmission (from cow to cow).
- A very small number of cattle born after the reinforced MBM feed ban came fully into force have developed BSE and this is probably due largely to cross-contamination of feed occurring outside the UK. In 2001, an EU-wide ban on feeds containing MBM was introduced.

The infective agent in TSEs

The predominant theory is that the infective agent is a protein or prion (Prusiner, 1995). This prion protein (PrP) is a normal protein found in the brain and other tissues of animals. It is suggested that in normal healthy animals the normal PrP protein is present largely in α-helical form and this is easily broken down by proteases. In TSEs, large amounts of this PrP protein are present in a different configuration (β-pleated sheet form) and this is extremely resistant to proteases. It is also very resistant to heat and radiation. When the abnormal PrP comes into contact with the normal form it causes the normal form to change shape. A chain reaction is established and a large amount of abnormal protein accumulates and destroys brain cells, leading to the clinical symptoms and spongiform lesions in the brain. According to Prusiner there are three likely ways in which TSEs can develop.

- *Spontaneous.* Some spontaneous production of abnormal PrP can occur and this will occasionally trigger the chain reaction, as in spontaneous CJD in elderly people.
- *Genetic.* A mutation in the PrP gene may occur which makes the protein more likely to flip to its abnormal structure. There are rare examples of a familial form of CJD in people. It may be that brain tissue from a cow with such a PrP mutation, when fed back to other cows, triggered off the BSE epidemic.
- *Transmission.* If abnormal PrP protein is introduced into the brain via the diet or via direct injection of infected brain material, this can trigger the chain reaction.

Transmission of BSE to humans

Scrapie has long been prevalent in British sheep but is not transmitted to humans via the diet and it is hard to transmit sheep scrapie to rodents. There was a general belief in the 1980s and early 1990s that BSE would probably not jump the species barrier and affect humans. This view was encouraged by the widespread belief that BSE was scrapie that had been transmitted to cows. In 1990, cases of BSE-like diseases were reported in several exotic species in zoos and these had been given feed containing ruminant protein. More disturbingly, the first of several cases of a TSE in domestic cats was identified. These observations suggested that BSE had jumped the species barrier and affected species other than ruminants and even carnivores. It is this 'species barrier' that has limited the spread of BSE to humans. Even though millions of people (and cats) may have been exposed to some bovine prion, the numbers of cases of vCJD and feline spongiform encephalopathy have been low.

In general, the more differences there are in the amino acid sequences of the prion proteins of two species, the more difficult it is to transmit the disease experimentally. Cow prion protein has about 30 amino acid differences from the human protein, and it is already clear that normal genetic variation in the human prion protein affects susceptibility to vCJD. It is also clear that transmission of TSEs is most efficient when infective material is injected directly into the brain and less efficient when it is given orally.

In experimental transmission studies, only some tissues in kuru and BSE contain infective quantities of abnormal PrP – brain, spinal cord and lymphatic tissues. Milk and muscle meat do not contain infective quantities of prion protein in such studies. Steaks and joints of beef from young beef cattle should have been unlikely sources of human infection even at the peak of the BSE epidemic. Concern has focused on meat products, including baby foods, which often included the potentially infected tissues and were often made from meat obtained from elderly dairy cows. A number of measures were introduced by the British government in order to protect the human population from BSE. The most important of these measures are listed below.

- In 1988, it was ordered that all clearly infected animals should be destroyed and their carcasses incinerated. Milk from infected animals was also removed from the food chain.
- In 1989, a ban on specified bovine offal (SBO) entering the human food chain was introduced. It was required that all of the likely infective tissues should be removed from all cattle at slaughter – brain, spinal cord, spleen, thymus, tonsils and intestines. This measure, if properly

enforced, should have afforded almost complete protection to people eating beef. It has been claimed that up until 1996 the enforcement of this measure was not rigorous enough and that significant amounts of these tissues entered the human food chain between 1989 and 1996 (largely by contamination of edible meat with SBO during the removal process). In 1997 these controls were extended to cosmetics, pharmaceuticals and medical products.

- In 1996, it was made illegal to sell cattle aged over 30 months (OTM) for human consumption. Very few young animals have developed BSE and so this measure ensured that little infective material actually reached the slaughterhouse. Animals up to 42 months old could be sold if they came from specialist beef producers whose animals had been fed only on grass and who met very strict criteria under the Beef Assurance Scheme. In November 2005, this 'OTM rule' was replaced by compulsory testing of the carcasses of slaughtered animals over 30 months of age, and the meat from these older tested animals can now be legally sold.
- For a time it was forbidden to sell beef with bone in it, largely because of concerns that it might have nervous tissue adhering to it.

In 1996, the European Union instituted a worldwide ban on British beef exports. This ban was lifted in 1999 but the recovery in British beef exports was initially very slow. There have been no recorded cases of BSE since 2009.

The human 'epidemic' of vCJD

It was in the spring of 1996 that the British government formally announced that a new variant of CJD (vCJD) had been discovered and that this was probably linked to eating contaminated beef before the bovine offal ban was introduced in 1989.

Figure 19.5 shows the annual numbers of deaths from vCJD since 1995. Experience with kuru and iatrogenic CJD suggests that the incubation period of vCJD may be much more than 20 years in some individuals and so occasional cases may continue to occur. Some possibilities that may extend the epidemic of vCJD are mentioned below.

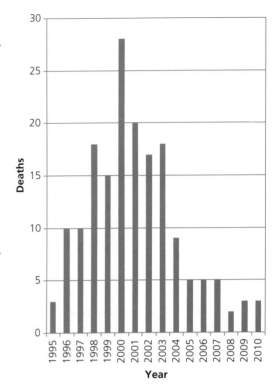

Figure 19.5 Annual deaths from variant Creutzfeldt–Jakob disease (vCJD) in the UK.

- There might be transmission by non-food means, such as by transfusion of contaminated blood, transplantation of infected tissue or use of contaminated surgical instruments. Note that since 1999 all blood for transfusion has had the white cells removed (leucodepletion) which should greatly lessen the risk of transmission of vCJD. More recently, anyone who has themselves received a blood transfusion after January 1980 is prevented from donating blood for transfusion. These measures have considerably increased the costs of supplying blood for transfusions.
- All the early cases of vCJD have occurred in people with a particular variant of the human prion protein which about 40 per cent of people have (they are homozygous for a methionine code at codon 129 of the prion protein gene). It is just conceivable that a second epidemic will occur in those with other genotypes because they have a longer incubation period (there may have been one or two such examples). It seems

reasonable to expect that if these genotypes substantially delay the onset of the disease then they are also likely to reduce the chances of acquiring the disease at all, and thus that any second wave of cases, if it occurs, will probably be markedly smaller than the first wave illustrated in Figure 19.5.

Key points

- Bovine spongiform encephalopathy (BSE) or 'mad cow disease' is a new and fatal neurological disease of cattle.
- BSE produces spongiform lesions in the brain similar to those seen in sheep scrapie and human Creutzfeldt–Jakob disease (CJD) and kuru.
- The British cattle epidemic appears now to be over but it has affected 180 000 cattle, mostly in dairy herds and especially older cows.
- Around 176 people have died from a new form of CJD (vCJD) which is the human form of BSE mainly contracted through eating contaminated beef products.
- BSE and vCJD belong to a group of so-called prion diseases that can be transmitted by injecting or eating infected tissue.
- The infective agent (prion) in these prion diseases is thought to be a normal protein that has undergone a conformational change from α-helix to β-pleated sheet.
- When abnormal prion protein is introduced into the brain it causes other normal prion protein molecules to change shape, and this begins a chain reaction which ultimately destroys large areas of brain tissue.
- The abnormal prion protein is very resistant to protease enzymes and to heat and radiation, so it is not destroyed by cooking or by the body's natural defences.
- Contaminated animal feed made from rendered ruminant remains was almost certainly the source of the cattle epidemic.
- It was at first thought that the initial trigger for BSE was sheep scrapie protein that had survived the rendering process. The belief that BSE was essentially 'scrapie in cows' was reassuring because scrapie has been endemic

→

Key points *continued*

in British sheep for centuries without affecting human health.

- A more recent theory is that BSE is a completely new disease that may have been propagated by the recycling of the infected remains of a single animal with a mutant prion protein. The initial source of the infection is not and may never be definitely established.
- The British government banned the use of ruminant protein in ruminant feed in 1988, but some incidentally contaminated feed continued to be fed to cattle until 1996 and this prolonged the cattle epidemic.
- The use of feeds containing meat and bone meal for farm animals and fish was banned in the UK in 1996 and later banned in the rest of the EU.
- There is occasional transmission of BSE from cow to calf but not apparently from cow to cow or bull to calf.
- Milk and meat from symptomatic animals have been destroyed since 1988.
- All beef sold after 1989 in the UK should have had all of the infective tissues (the specified bovine offal, SBO) removed, but there are claims that this measure was not enforced rigorously enough prior to 1996.
- Between 1996 and 2005, only cattle under 30 months old and free from SBO have been permitted to be sold in the UK (with a few specified exceptions). This over-30-months rule has now been relaxed and meat from older animals can be sold if the carcass is tested for BSE. As there have been no recorded cases of BSE in cattle since 2009, this should guarantee the safety of current beef sales.
- A great deal of infected cattle material probably entered the human food chain prior to 1996 and millions of people may have been exposed to it.
- The human epidemic of vCJD has been at the very low end of earlier predictions. It peaked in 2000 and fell to a small trickle of new cases each year (less than five) by 2005. There are currently (early 2012) no living cases of this disease and so no new diagnoses have been made for a year.

→

Key points *continued*

- The 'species barrier' has limited the spread of the cattle disease to humans who have eaten contaminated beef products.
- It is possible that a second wave of cases of vCJD will occur in people whose prion protein structure has delayed the onset of the disease. It seems reasonable to expect that if this second wave does materialize it will be even smaller than the first wave.

FOOD PROCESSING

Some general pros and cons of food processing

The term 'food processing' covers a multitude of actions to which food may be subjected. They might be traditional or modern and they might occur in the home, catering unit or factory. Unless one eats only raw, home-grown foods then it is impossible to avoid 'processed foods'. It would be impossible to feed a large urban industrial society without some commercial processing of foods. For example, around 50 per cent by value of all food purchases in the UK are frozen or chilled. Processing includes cooking, smoking, drying, freezing, pasteurizing, canning, irradiation, and so on.

Processing of foods, particularly preparation of ready-to-eat foods, 'adds value' to the ingredients and increases their commercial potential for retailers and processors. Food processors and retailers represent some of the most commercially successful businesses in developed countries. This high profitability has tended to politicize food processing issues, sometimes to the detriment of constructive critical debate. The term 'processed food' is often used to convey very negative connotations about modern food and food suppliers. However, it is such an all-embracing term, covering foods across the whole spectrum of composition, that its use in this way is unhelpful and probably warns of the prejudice or political motivation of the critic. Each processed food should be judged on its own merits and should be considered within the context of the whole diet rather than purely in isolation. The recent large and fatal outbreak of *E. coli* VTEC food poisoning in Germany referred to earlier in the chapter was caused by consuming a raw unprocessed food (sprouted seeds) and would

have been prevented by heat treatment of the sprouts.

Commercial processing of food has a number of objectives, in addition to the obvious commercial ones. Some are noted here.

- Processing reduces or prevents the chemical deterioration and microbial spoilage of foods. It thus increases the shelf life of foods and increases food availability, reduces waste and may reduce the cost of food.
- By destroying pathogens or preventing their growth, processing lowers the risk of food-borne diseases.
- It can increase the palatability of foods.
- Processing enables new varieties of foods to be created.
- Commercially prepared food products reduce the time that individuals need to spend on food preparation. Even those unable or unwilling to spend much time on preparation can eat an interesting and varied diet if they can afford to buy high-quality prepared foods.

Commercial processing usually, but not always, has some negative effects on the nutrient content of the unprepared food. These losses may be very similar to, or even less than, those involved in home preparation of food. The losses may not be very significant in the diets of many North Americans and western Europeans who have ample intakes of the essential nutrients. Imbalance of selection from the major food groups is a more significant threat to dietary adequacy in western industrialized countries. In many cases the nutrient content of processed foods (e.g. vitamins in frozen vegetables) may actually be higher than in stale versions of the same food bought 'fresh'. It is often argued that food processors encourage people to consume foods high in fat, sugar and salt but low in complex carbohydrate and thus are partly responsible for the increased prevalence of the diseases of industrialization. It seems probable, however, that even without the encouragement of food processors, our natural inclination to consume such a diet would have prevailed. Nevertheless, it is true that, for example, most of the salt in the UK diet is added by food manufacturers and reductions in the salt of commercially processed foods would have a major impact on total salt intakes. Although sales of sugar have dropped considerably in recent years in the UK, there has been a smaller fall in total sugar intake because more sugar is consumed within commercially prepared foods. Commercial processing tends to reduce the consumer's ability to monitor and regulate their intakes of sugar, salt and fat, despite attempts at making the composition of processed foods more transparent by labelling.

Commercial processors and food retailers provide what they think they can profitably sell. They have, for example, been quick to recognize the commercial opportunities offered by the demand for 'healthy foods'. Many highly processed foods have a very healthy image – for example, some margarine and low-fat spreads, some breakfast cereals, low-fat salad dressings, low-fat yoghurts, low-calorie drinks and certain meat substitutes of vegetable or microbial origin. Some of the modern functional foods that are marketed on their proposed health benefits are the products of modern food processing, such as margarines with high levels of plant sterols that lower blood cholesterol.

Key points

- The term 'processed food' covers a huge and diverse range of food products and so general discussion of their merits and flaws is of limited usefulness.
- Commercial processing often extends the shelf life of foods and may increase their microbiological and chemical safety.
- Commercial processing can improve the palatability of individual foods and increase variety by making foods more accessible and even allowing the creation of new foods.
- The availability of commercially prepared foods decreases the time individuals need to spend on food preparation, although this may increase food costs.
- Nutrient losses during commercial processing of foods may be comparable to losses during home preparation.
- Many commercially prepared foods are high in fat, salt and/or sugar but low in complex carbohydrate.
- Food manufacturers will, at least superficially, respond to consumer demands for healthier processed foods if it is profitable for them. Many highly processed foods are marketed on their image as healthier options.

Specific processing methods

Canning

This is a very good method for the long-term preservation of food. The food is maintained in sealed containers and thus protected from oxidative deterioration or growth of aerobic micro-organisms. The food is subjected to a vigorous heat treatment after canning that is designed to ensure that there is no practical possibility that even heat-resistant bacterial spores will survive. The so-called 'botulinum cook' ensures the destruction of all spores of the potentially lethal toxin-producing, anaerobic organism C. *botulinum* in at-risk foods. If commercially canned food is consumed soon after opening, there is negligible risk of it being associated with food poisoning.

Pasteurization

Mild heat is applied to a food that is sufficient to destroy likely pathogenic bacteria and to reduce the number of spoilage organisms without impairing the food itself. It is usually associated with milk, but other food such as liquid egg, liquid ice cream mix and honey may be pasteurized. Pasteurization of milk traditionally involved holding it at 63°C for 30 minutes. This was designed to ensure the destruction of the organism responsible for tuberculosis, but it also kills *Salmonella* and the other heat-sensitive pathogens usually found in milk. The same result can be achieved by the modern high-temperature short-time method in which the milk is raised to 72°C for 15 seconds (see below).

Ultra-high-temperature treatment

Once again this is most often associated with milk, but it is applied also to other foods like fruit juice. Traditionally, milk was sterilized by heating it to temperatures of 105–110°C for 20–40 minutes. Such severe heat treatment causes chemical changes in the milk that impair its flavour, appearance, smell and nutrient content. The ultra-high-temperature (UHT) method relies on the principle that the rate of chemical reactions only doubles with a 10°C rise in temperature whereas the rate of bacterial killing increases about 10-fold. Thus full sterilization can be achieved by holding the milk at 135°C for just 2 seconds with relatively little chemical change in the milk. Two seconds at 135°C has approximately the same bacterial killing effect as 33 minutes at 105°C but results in chemical changes equivalent to only 16 seconds at this lower temperature. After UHT treatment the milk is placed aseptically into sterile containers and will keep for up to 6 months. Chemical deterioration rather than microbial spoilage limits the duration of storage of UHT products.

Cook–chill processing

In this process, foods are cooked separately as they would be in the home kitchen. Bacterial cells will be killed by this process but spores will survive. The food is then chilled rapidly to temperatures below 5°C to minimize growth of the surviving spore-forming bacteria. The food is then divided into portions and packaged. Rigorous standards of hygiene are required during this portioning stage to prevent re-contamination with spoilage and food poisoning organisms. Most cook–chill foods have a maximum permitted shelf life of 6–8 days partly because of the difficulty of preventing contamination by the ubiquitous *Pseudomonas* group of spoilage organisms.

The introduction of cook–chill foods into hospitals is an area of particular concern. Many groups who are very vulnerable to organisms like *Listeria* are concentrated in hospitals – pregnant women and infants in maternity units, people whose immune systems have been suppressed by disease (e.g. AIDS) or by treatment (e.g. immunosuppressant drugs), and those weakened by injury, disease or old age.

Food irradiation

Irradiation involves exposing food to ionizing radiation which can either be X-rays or more usually γ-rays emitted from a radioactive source such as cobalt-60. This has been reviewed by Hawthorn (1989) and key issues are summarized on the Food Standards Agency website at www.food.gov.uk/safereating. There is no contact between the radioactive source and the food, so the latter does not itself become radioactive.

Irradiation of food is not a new idea – its potential was recognized and demonstrated over 100 years ago. It is only more recently, however, that the widespread application of irradiation in food processing has become economically viable because of the ready availability of γ-ray emitters like cobalt-60. Many countries have now approved the use of irradiation for some categories of foods.

In the USA, irradiation is classified with the food additives because it causes chemical changes in food. Its use is permitted on a wide range of foods including onions, potatoes, herbs and spices, nuts and seeds, wheat, fish, poultry and meat. Irradiated food must be clearly labelled as such.

In the UK prior to 1990, irradiation was forbidden for all foods with the exception of herbs and spices. At the beginning of 1991 this ban was withdrawn. Irradiation of a wide range of foods is now theoretically permitted in properly licensed centres. For example, fruits, vegetables, cereals, fish, shellfish and poultry may all now be legally irradiated in the UK. There is, however, currently only one site in the UK licensed to irradiate human food and it is only licensed to irradiate spices and condiments. The only source of radiation currently used for food irradiation in the UK is γ-rays from cobalt-60. Irradiated foods must be labelled as such.

European Union regulations mean that even where a prepared food contains only a small amount of irradiated ingredient, this must be declared on the label. The only foods that can be freely traded across EU boundaries are those within the categories currently licensed for irradiation in the UK.

The effects of irradiation on the food vary according to the dose used (Figure 19.6). Some of these changes are used to extend the shelf life of foods such as the inhibition of sprouting, delay in ripening and reducing the numbers of spoilage organisms.

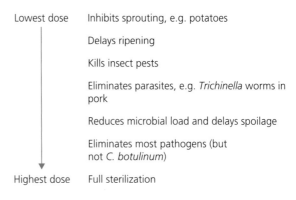

Figure 19.6 Effects of varying doses of ionizing radiation on food.

The killing of insect pests reduces losses and damage to food from this cause and reduces the need to fumigate with chemical insecticides. The elimination of food poisoning organisms should reduce the risks of food poisoning, and sterilization of food by irradiation may be particularly useful in ensuring the safety of food intended for immunosuppressed patients.

Despite these apparent advantages of food irradiation, its introduction has been vigorously opposed by certain pressure groups within the UK. It has been suggested that the full effects of irradiation are not yet well enough understood to be totally confident of its safety. However, the Food Standards Agency (FSA, 2012) states unequivocally that properly irradiated foods are safe and that irradiation is a consumer choice and food labelling issue rather than a safety issue.

Some potential problems of irradiated foods are listed below. Note that these are potential hazards suggested by those who oppose irradiation rather than the views of the author.

- The ionizing radiation induces certain chemical changes within the food, it increases free radical production and chemical species known as radiolytes (see Chapter 13 for a discussion of free radicals and anti-oxidants). The free radicals and radiolytes produced by irradiation are short-lived species and they are responsible for the killing of micro-organisms produced by irradiation. While there may be natural concern that these chemical changes might have detrimental effects on health, it must be added that all processing methods produce some chemical changes in food. For example, smoking and barbecuing lead to production of small amounts of potentially carcinogenic chemicals in food. The chemical changes induced in food by irradiation are less than those produced by heat processing. The low level of chemical change induced by irradiation is illustrated by the extreme difficulty in chemically identifying whether or not a food sample has been irradiated. The FSA (2012) states that methods have been validated for the detection of different irradiated foods, including herbs and spices, meat and poultry containing bone, and foods containing fats, and methods for detecting other irradiated foods are under development.

- Some bacterial and fungal toxins will not be destroyed by irradiation, so if irradiation is used to compensate for earlier poor hygiene then food poisoning from these toxins may result.

- At the doses usually used on foods, spores will survive and may later grow in the food. Irradiation is known to increase mutation rates and so conceivably new and dangerous mutants of micro-organisms might be produced in food.

- At high doses (e.g. those required to achieve sterilization) there may be adverse effects on the palatability of the food and major losses of some nutrients such as thiamin and vitamin E. At dose levels likely to be used for 'pasteurization' of food, irradiation produces almost no change in flavour or nutrient content, unlike other methods of food processing and preservation.

- There is concern about the safety of workers at establishments where food irradiation takes place. There is thus a clear need to regulate and license facilities for food irradiation. Only one site in the UK is currently (early 2012) licensed for food irradiation and this is subject to stringent regulation and inspection by the Food Standards Agency.

Key points

- Rigorous heat treatment and sealed containers ensure that properly canned food will often remain in good condition and microbiologically safe for many years.
- The mild heat treatment of pasteurization should eliminate likely pathogens and reduce levels of spoilage organisms without significant adverse effects on the flavour or nutrient value of the food.
- Sterilization using ultra-high-temperature (UHT) for very short periods results in far less chemical change than traditional sterilization techniques and so has much less effect on flavour and nutrient loss.
- Cook–chill processing does not kill all spore-forming bacteria, and food may also be contaminated with other spoilage and pathogenic organisms during packaging.

Key points *continued*

- *Listeria monocytogenes* can still grow in chilled foods and this can have serious consequences for pregnant women and other vulnerable groups.

- Irradiating foods with varying doses of X-rays or γ-rays has a variety of potential uses that are summarized in Figure 19.6.

- Consumer resistance has limited the marketing of irradiated foods, although many countries permit it. In the UK, only one site is currently licensed for food irradiation and only to irradiate herbs, spices and condiments.

- Irradiation can extend the shelf-life of many foods and/or improve their microbiological safety.

- High doses of radiation do induce potentially adverse chemical changes in food and can reduce palatability and lead to significant losses of nutrients.

- Mild irradiation produces imperceptible changes in flavour or loss of nutrients and it is difficult to chemically detect whether or not a food has been irradiated.

- Some microbial toxins will survive irradiation.

- Some micro-organisms will survive mild irradiation. It has been argued that theoretically this might increase mutation rates in organisms that survive the irradiation process.

- Expert committees have concluded that irradiation is a safe food processing method. The UK Food Standards Agency regards irradiation as a consumer choice and labelling issue rather than a safety issue.

THE CHEMICAL SAFETY OF FOOD

Overview of chemical hazards

There are three potential sources of chemical hazard in food.

- *Food additives*. Chemicals are deliberately added to food during processing.
- *Natural toxicants*. These are compounds naturally present in the food that may have toxic effects.
- *Contaminants*. These are substances that are incidentally or inadvertently added to foods

during agricultural production, storage or processing. Examples are residues of drugs given to food animals, pesticide or fertilizer residues, contaminants leaching into food from packaging or containers, and fungal toxins.

One dilemma facing those trying to ensure the chemical safety of food is to decide what level of any particular chemical substance represents a real hazard to consumers. Total absence of all traces of potentially hazardous chemicals from all foods is, and always has been, an impossible ideal. Almost every chemical, including most nutrients, is toxic if the dose is high enough:

> All substances are poisonous; there is none which is not a poison. The right dose differentiates a poison and a remedy.

Paracelsus, 1493–1541

More substances are being subjected to rigorous toxicological testing, which usually involves exposing animals to high doses of the chemical for prolonged periods. Many chemicals that are ubiquitous in our diet and environment can be shown to have toxic potential by such tests. Analytical procedures are also becoming increasingly sophisticated and sensitive, making it possible to detect infinitesimal amounts of potentially hazardous chemicals in foods. This combination of factors, especially when distorted by popular journalists, can lead to the impression that the chemical hazards in our food are increasing at an alarming rate. At least some of this apparent increase in chemical danger from food is artefact caused by increased awareness of the potential hazards of chemicals and increased ability to detect small amounts.

The Institute of Food Technologists (IFT, 1975) made a distinction between *toxic*, which it defined as 'being inherently capable of producing injury when tested by itself', and *hazard*, defined as 'being likely to produce injury under the circumstances of exposure' as in food.

Food naturally contains thousands of toxic substances, including many nutrients, but very few of these represent a real hazard. For example, the average US consumer ingests around 10 grams of solanine from potatoes each year, which is enough of this atropine-like alkaloid to kill the person if consumed in a single dose. The same average US consumer ingests about 40 mg of lethal hydrogen cyanide in his or her annual kilogram of lima beans and 14 mg of arsenic from seafood.

Most natural toxins are present in low concentrations in natural foods and they do not usually accumulate. They are usually metabolized and/or excreted by a variety of mechanisms that are also involved in the disposal of ingested manufactured chemicals like food additives, drugs and residues of agricultural chemicals. There are a variety of mechanisms and sites through which the different toxicants induce their effect, and so generally the effects of small amounts of many individual toxicants are unlikely to be additive. One per cent of a toxic dose of 100 different toxins will almost certainly not produce ill-effects.

Key points

- Natural toxicants, contaminants and food additives must all be considered potential sources of chemical hazard in food.
- Sensitive analytical techniques can detect numerous substances in food that have toxic potential, but few of them represent a real hazard to consumers who eat a varied diet.

Natural toxicants and contaminants

Circumstances that may increase chemical hazard

The chance of toxic potential becoming a real hazard is likely to be increased if there is exaggerated consumption of one food for a prolonged period. This is true whether the toxin is naturally present, a contaminant or a deliberate additive. This is yet one more reason for encouraging diversity in the diet. Examples of natural toxicants in food producing serious illness may occur when abnormally high amounts of a particular food are consumed. The plant *Lathyrus sativus* has been widely grown in Asia and North Africa and the seeds (chickling peas or khesari dhal) regularly consumed. However, during very dry seasons it was consumed in very large quantities because the plant is very drought resistant. When consumed in very large quantities it can produce a severe disease of the spinal cord

(lathyrism) which can lead to permanent paralysis. When only small quantities are consumed as part of a mixed diet they do not constitute a hazard and are nutritious.

Chemical hazard from food may arise if individual susceptibility causes increased sensitivity to a particular toxin. The common broad bean *Vicia faba* contains a substance that causes haemolysis (red cell breakdown). This can lead to a severe anaemia (favism) in those who are genetically susceptible because they are deficient in a particular enzyme (glucose 6 phosphate dehydrogenase). As many as 35 per cent of some Mediterranean peoples and 10 per cent of black Americans have this particular genetic deficiency. Vomiting, abdominal pain and fever are the acute symptoms. Jaundice and dark urine may occur as a result of the haemolysis, and severe anaemia is a possible consequence of long-term exposure.

Traditional methods of preparing, processing and selecting foods often minimize any potential hazard they may represent. Cassava is one of the most important staple foods for millions of people in the tropics; it may, for example, provide up to 60 per cent of the calorific intake in some Nigerians. Cassava contains certain alkaloids that release cyanide when acted on by an enzyme in the cassava. The traditional method of preparing cassava involves peeling and soaking for several days, and most of the cyanide is lost during fermentation. Cases of sometimes fatal cyanide poisoning are associated with inadequate processing of the cassava (particularly shortening of the fermentation time) and increased use of lower quality 'bitter' cassava which has a higher cyanide content (Akintowa and Tunawashe, 1992). As another example, polar bear liver contains toxic concentrations of retinol, so Inuits avoided eating the liver but unwary polar explorers have been poisoned by eating it.

Some natural toxicants in Western diets

Few natural toxicants are thought to represent significant hazards to Western consumers. Some potential natural chemical hazards in UK food are listed below.

- Scombrotoxic poisoning is caused by heat-stable toxins liberated by the action of bacteria on fish protein during spoilage. The toxin is thus produced by bacterial action but is not in itself a bacterial toxin. Symptoms occur shortly after eating the contaminated fish and include a peppery taste in the mouth, flushing of the face and neck, sweating and sometimes nausea and diarrhoea.

- Eating raw red kidney beans leads to short-lasting symptoms of nausea, vomiting and diarrhoea. These symptoms are thought to be due to a toxin that causes red cells to agglutinate (stick together) – a haemagglutinin. The symptoms are probably due to damage to intestinal cells caused by this toxin. The haemagglutinin is destroyed by vigorous boiling but it may persist if the beans are cooked by prolonged gentle heating in a slow cooker. These beans should always be subjected to 10 minutes of vigorous boiling before being eaten. Cases are always caused by eating raw or inadequately heat-treated beans. As a general rule, raw or undercooked beans should not be eaten as they contain several mildly toxic factors as well as factors that interfere with the proper digestion of protein.

- Some cheeses contain the substance tyramine, which can cause a rise in blood pressure. This may be dangerous for those taking certain antidepressant drugs because they sensitize the individual to the effects of tyramine. (These drugs, called monoamine oxidase inhibitors, are the oldest type of antidepressant and have largely been replaced by more modern drugs which do not sensitize people to tyramine.)

- Solanine is an atropine-like substance found in potatoes. In high enough doses it will cause headache, vomiting and diarrhoea and may perhaps even result in circulatory collapse and neurological disturbances. Levels of solanine in potatoes are rarely enough to produce illness and established outbreaks of potato poisoning are rare.

- Many species of Brassicae (the cabbage family) contain goitrogens, chemicals that induce goitre. These do not represent a real hazard at levels of consumption normally found in industrialized countries. Cassava also contains goitrogens which, if eaten in large amounts, may significantly increase the risk of goitre.

- Mussels that have ingested the plankton species *Gonyaulux tamarensis* may contain hazardous amounts of a heat-stable neurotoxin – *saxitoxin*. At certain times the sea may turn red ('red tides') owing to large numbers of *Gonyaulux* in the water. These red tides may occasionally occur even off the coasts of the UK and the USA, and at such times it is dangerous to eat mussels.

- Some fungi produce toxic chemicals – *mycotoxins*. Some mycotoxins represent a hazard to the inexperienced gatherer of wild fungi and some fungal toxins are deliberately consumed because they contain hallucinogenic agents. The death-cap mushroom *Amanita phalloides* is responsible for the majority of fatal cases of mushroom poisoning. This mushroom is similar in appearance to some edible species and it is reported to have a pleasant taste. Symptoms do not occur until 8–24 hours after ingestion, by which time irreparable liver damage may have occurred and death typically occurs after 7–10 days. Around half a cap (30 g) is enough of this mushroom to kill a human being, and even with modern medical care (including liver transplant in some cases) the death rate from accidental poisoning is still around 10–15 per cent and many of the survivors have permanent liver damage. Moulds also grow on many foods that will not support the growth of bacteria, because fungi are more tolerant of low water activity and low pH than bacteria. Dry foods like nuts and bread, sugary foods like jam (jelly), and salty foods like cheese may all go mouldy. Several of the toxins produced by moulds are potent carcinogens. *Aflatoxins* produced by *Aspergillus flavus* have been responsible for outbreaks of fatal poisoning in Taiwan, India and Uganda. It causes gastrointestinal bleeding, liver damage and pulmonary oedema. It has been shown to cause liver cancer in animal studies. Mouldy nuts would be a likely source of aflatoxin in the USA and UK. Mouldy grain may contain the toxin *ergot* which is produced by the ergot fungus (*Claviceps purpurea*), and this has caused serious outbreaks of poisoning in the past and still does in some countries – a condition referred to as St Vitus' Dance or St Anthony's Fire because the symptoms of poisoning include hallucinations, nervous spasms, convulsions, psychotic delusions and spontaneous abortion. The well-known psychedelic drug lysergic acid diethylamide

(LSD) is made from ergot, and ergot has been used in the past to induce abortions. The last recorded outbreak of ergot poisoning in Europe was in a village called Pont St Esprit in France in 1951 when contaminated bread from the village bakery caused 135 people to be hospitalized and resulted in six deaths. Mouldy food should therefore be regarded as potentially hazardous and should be discarded. In the early 1990s, the detection of very small amounts of the mycotoxin *patulin* in some brands of apple juice received great publicity in the UK.

Mould growth is deliberately encouraged in the production of some foods, including blue cheese and mould-ripened cheese. These are not thought to represent a hazard at usual levels of consumption.

Residues of agricultural chemicals

Expert opinion is that the residues of agricultural chemicals in foods represent no significant hazard to consumers when current regulations are adhered to. Most cases of acute poisoning resulting from ingestion of agricultural chemicals have arisen because of their misuse, including the examples listed below (after Taylor, 2006).

- *Mistaken identification.* There can be confusion of an agricultural chemical with a common, harmless food ingredient like sugar or salt.
- *Eating of seeds intended for planting and treated with a fungicide.* Most fungicides are of low toxicity to people, but those containing mercury and a substance called hexachlorobenzene are exceptions to this general rule. In the late 1950s more than 3000 people in Turkey were affected by hexachlorobenzene poisoning after eating seed grain intended for planting. The symptoms included hair loss, ulcerated skin lesions, and liver and thyroid enlargement. There was 10 per cent mortality.
- *Agricultural misuse of a chemical.* In 1985 in the USA, almost 1400 people became ill after eating watermelons that had been treated with an insecticide called aldicarb. Symptoms included nausea, diarrhoea, headache, blurred vision and disturbances of balance. It is actually illegal to use this insecticide on watermelons because it is known to become concentrated in the edible part of the fruit.

While most toxicologists assert that these chemicals pose no threat to long-term health, these assurances have been insufficient to convince a significant minority of the population who are willing to pay considerably higher prices for *organic produce* that has been grown without the aid of modern agricultural chemicals which include insecticides, herbicides, fungicides, fertilizers and antibiotics, as well as other drugs given to farm animals. These consumers are also willing to accept the less than perfect appearance of their fruits and vegetables that organic farming practices sometimes produce. Many producers and suppliers have been quick to recognize the commercial opportunities afforded by this new market. People who can afford it clearly have the right to choose food grown in this way, but the practicability of supplying the whole population with organic food is doubtful and there are no scientifically quantifiable health benefits. There may be more convincing environmental arguments for farming in this way. Organic growers may well use different varieties of fruits and vegetables, and factors like slower growth with longer maturation/ripening may have effects on texture and flavour. Strain or variety differences, variation in access to sunlight and exercise space may also have some effects on the taste, appearance or texture of milk, meat, eggs and even farmed fish.

Key points

- Food naturally contains small amounts of many toxic substances that, because they are eaten in such small doses, do not cause illness.
- The risk of a natural toxicant causing illness is increased by:
  - abnormally high consumption of the toxin-containing food
  - increased susceptibility to the toxin (e.g. genetic)
  - inadequate removal of the toxin during processing.
- Some toxins present in many Western diets are:
  - scombrotoxin produced by bacterial action on fish protein
  - haemagglutinins and other toxins in raw or undercooked beans

→

Key points *continued*

- – tyramine in cheese which interacts with older antidepressant drugs
- – an atropine-like alkaloid, solanine, normally present in minute amounts in potatoes
- – goitrogens present in minute amounts in plants of the cabbage family
- – mussels contaminated with a neurotoxin produced by the red plankton *Gonyaulux tamarensis*
- – mycotoxins produced by fungi and by mould growth on food.
- Most but not all scientists believe that, when used in permitted amounts, residues of agricultural chemicals do not represent a significant hazard to consumers. Acute cases of poisoning caused by agricultural chemicals (insecticides, herbicides, fungicides, fertilizers and veterinary drugs) have arisen because of accidents or misuse of the chemical.
- Most scientists therefore do not believe that more expensive organic food produced without agricultural chemicals is healthier. Indeed, trading standards officials may find it difficult to distinguish between organic and conventionally grown products by laboratory analysis.
- Many consumers do not accept the scientific consensus about organic food and there may well be stronger ecological arguments for less chemical-dependent food production methods.
- Variety differences and other incidental differences between 'mass produced' food and that produced by smaller organic producers may have effects on the taste, texture or appearance of organic food.

Food additives

Around 300 food additives are used in the UK together with a further 3000 flavourings. The average British person probably consumes several kilograms of these in a year.

Uses of additives

Chemicals are deliberately added to food for a variety of purposes, such as:

- as processing aids (e.g. emulsifiers, flour improvers and anti-caking agents)
- to improve the sensory appeal of foods (e.g. colours, flavours and sweeteners)
- to improve the nutritional value of foods (e.g. vitamins and/or minerals added to bread, breakfast cereals and drinks)
- to prevent the growth of food poisoning and spoilage organisms (e.g. nitrites and nitrates in meat products)
- to inhibit the growth of moulds (e.g. propionic acid or vinegar in bread)
- to inhibit the chemical deterioration of foods (e.g. anti-oxidants like vitamins C and E).

Some arguments against the use of food additives

Those who are opposed to the use of food additives or the scale of their current usage have used all of the arguments below to criticize them.

- They are dangerous chemicals *per se*. In particular, chronic exposure to them could lead to an increase in cancer risk.
- They could be used to disguise faulty or inferior products and thus deceive the consumer. Colourings, flavouring and emulsifiers can disguise the highly fatty and low-grade meat used in some meat products. Colourings and flavourings can disguise the lack of fruit in 'fruit' drinks and yoghurts. Polyphosphates can be used to artificially increase the weight of meat and poultry by increasing its water content.
- Even generally safe additives may trigger adverse reactions in some individuals, examples being allergy to the yellow food colourant tartrazine and to sulphites (sulphur dioxide) used to preserve many foods.
- Preservatives can be used by manufacturers to compensate for poor hygiene standards.
- Many of the cosmetic additives are unnecessary or perhaps even imposed on the consumer by food producers and retailers.

Some counterarguments

Additives with food preserving functions are a necessity if large urban populations are to be supplied with a variety of safe, nutritious and affordable foods. Traditional preservatives have long been used for these purposes – salt, sugar, woodsmoke, vinegar, alcohol, nitrites and nitrates.

When evaluating the safety of modern preservatives or when judging the merits of foods claiming to be 'free from all artificial preservatives', it should be borne in mind that most of these traditional preservatives have been implicated in disease. For example, salt has been linked to hypertension, nitrites lead to the generation of potentially carcinogenic nitrosamines, and small amounts of potential carcinogens are found in smoked foods.

Some additives are essential as processing aids or otherwise necessary for the manufacture of a considerable number of supermarket foods. Some of these foods are considered to be 'healthy foods' and seen as important in helping consumers to comply with current nutrition education guidelines. Emulsifiers and stabilizers are essential for the production of many 'reduced-fat' products like low-fat spread and polyunsaturated margarine. Anti-caking agents are needed for the manufacture of many powders that are to be instantly rehydrated, such as coffee whitener. Artificial sweeteners or sugar replacers are necessary for the production of many 'low-calorie' and 'reduced-sugar' foods.

The additives that are most vulnerable to criticism are those that serve cosmetic purposes – to enhance the appearance or palatability of the food. These may even be claimed to be doing a positive disservice to Western consumers by encouraging over-consumption and obesity. If a purely scientific model of food function is used, then appearance and palatability of food could almost be regarded as a decadent irrelevance. Few people would, however, really want to regard positive sensory appeal of food as an optional extra – although, as already noted, these do have the potential to allow manufacturers to dupe the public into buying prepared foods made from lower quality ingredients.

Food additive regulation

Different countries have differing regulations governing the use of food additives. The common purpose of such regulations is to ensure that they are used safely, effectively, honestly and in the minimum amounts necessary to achieve their objectives.

The Food and Drug Administration (FDA) regulates the use of food additives in the USA. In order to get approval to use a new additive, a manufacturer is required to provide evidence that the additive is effective, is safe, and can be detected and measured in the final product. The approval of the additive is then considered after a public hearing at which experts testify for and against its use. Very few new additives have been submitted for approval in recent years because of the considerable costs involved in acquiring the extensive safety data required by the FDA; only for substances like new artificial sweeteners (e.g. sucralose) or calorie-free fat substitutes (e.g. olestra) does the potential scale of use justify the costs involved. Additives that were in use before this procedure was adopted in the 1950s were put on a list of substances *generally recognized as safe* (GRAS). The GRAS list is subject to a continuing process of review and revision. Almost five decades ago, Congress approved the so-called Delaney clause: 'no additive shall be deemed to be safe if it is found to induce cancer when ingested by man or animal'. This requirement is now regarded as unreasonably absolute in its prohibition and the FDA deems additives to be safe if the risk of human cancer is less than one in a million. Saccharin is a permitted sweetener in the USA despite being reported to cause bladder cancer when administered in very large doses to animals; so, although shown to have toxic potential, it is not thought to represent a hazard to the US consumer.

In the UK, responsibility for regulating the use of food additives lies with the Food Standards Agency, although the European Food Safety Authority is responsible for evaluating food additive safety across the whole of the EU. The European committee comprises independent experts and they would have to consider and advise on any proposed new additive or new usage of an additive. They would consider whether this new additive or additive use was necessary and safe. Grounds for necessity would be factors like:

- increased shelf life of a product
- reduced cost
- an improved product for the consumer
- necessity for the manufacture of a new product or for the introduction of a new manufacturing process.

European Union law states that food additives can only be used if:

- they present no hazard to health at the levels used in foods
- a reasonable need for the additive can be demonstrated (as examples above)
- they do not mislead the consumer.

E numbers have been used for many years to designate food additives in the UK and the rest of the EU. They were introduced as part of efforts to harmonize legislation within the EU and to overcome language barriers. They were originally envisaged as something that would help to engender consumer confidence. If an additive had an E number then the consumer could be totally assured of its safety. In reality, however, the effect was quite the opposite. E numbers on food labels evoke suspicion and have been used to epitomise everything that is unwholesome about 'modern, adulterated and artificial food'.

A full listing of E numbers can be found in the web pages of Dr David Jukes at www.reading.ac.uk/foodlaw. A quick perusal of this extensive list shows that several nutrients and compounds that would be familiar (and perhaps less threatening by name) are included:

- E101 is riboflavin
- E300 is vitamin C
- E302 is calcium carbonate
- E307 is vitamin E
- E120 is cochineal
- E140 is chlorophyll
- E150 is caramel
- E160a is carotene
- E260 is acetic acid (vinegar)
- E553b is talc
- E901 is beeswax.

In the UK there are three sets of regulations – incorporated into UK law in 1995 – dealing with the regulation of sweeteners, colours and miscellaneous food additives (those not covered by the first two categories). These regulations are designed to incorporate EU legislation into national legislation, and they stipulate:

- which additives are permitted for use in food (and for direct sale to the consumer)
- the purity specifications for permitted additives
- conditions of additive use, including in many cases setting the maximum level of use.

Flavourings are not included in these particular regulations. The regulation for all types of additives other than flavourings could be described as a 'positive list system' – only things listed as being approved can be used under the conditions specified in the regulations and other additives within these categories are by default not therefore permitted. In the case of flavourings, the regulation could be said to be a 'negative list' approach, whereby certain things are not permitted or restricted but there is no list of specified, approved flavourings. The long-term objective within the European Union is to produce a positive list for flavourings. Many flavours are natural extracts or synthetic versions of substances within natural extracts that are 'nature identical'.

There are few examples of food additives causing acute adverse symptoms, but some are identified here.

- *Sorbitol* is an alcohol of glucose and, together with some other hexose alcohols, is used as a sweetener for drinks, sweets and chewing gum that is non-cariogenic (does not cause dental decay). These substances are absorbed relatively slowly from the gut, so if large amounts are consumed they can remain within the gut and cause diarrhoea owing to their osmotic effects. Foods containing these sugar alcohols usually carry a warning that high consumption can cause diarrhoea.
- *Sulphites* are added to foods for a variety of reasons, such as bleaching, prevention of browning and as antimicrobials. Under acidic conditions these produce sulphur dioxide in the food. A small number of people are sensitive to this sulphur dioxide and it produces asthma-type symptoms in them. Many foods carry warnings that they contain a source of sulphur dioxide, to alert those susceptible to sulphite-induced asthma.
- *Tartrazine* is a yellow dye and it has been claimed to cause asthma and hives in some sensitive people, although this has not been established with absolute certainty.

- *Olestra* is a synthetic substance used as a calorie-free fat substitute for frying certain savoury snacks in the USA (although not, as at January 2012, permitted in the EU). It can cause gastrointestinal symptoms in some people, such as anal leakage, oily stools and urgency of defecation.

Testing the safety of food additives

Listed below are the four potential sources of information which might be used to evaluate the safety of food additives:

- human experiments
- human epidemiology
- in-vitro tests
- animal experiments.

One of the major concerns relating to the safety of food additives is that lifetime exposure to an additive may increase the risk of chronic disease and especially of human cancer. Human experiments are inevitably either short term or small scale and subject to ethical restrictions that would preclude heavy and prolonged exposure to an additive. Such human experiments can be of no real use in identifying even relatively large increases in cancer risk due to particular additives. Neither can epidemiology be expected to pinpoint harmful effects of individual additives. Epidemiology involves relating exposure to changes in disease rates, yet we are all exposed to hundreds of additives in amounts that would be difficult to quantify on an individual basis, and even in a worst-case scenario the increased cancer rate due to the additive is likely to be small. It proved difficult to show convincingly with epidemiological methods that smoking causes lung cancer even though the association is strong, the level of exposure is relatively easy to establish and there is an identifiable matched but unexposed population.

In-vitro tests involve the use of isolated mammalian cells or micro-organisms. The best established of these test are those, like the Ames test, that use the ability of compounds to cause mutation in bacteria as an indicator of their likely carcinogenicity in mammals. Mutagenesis, carcinogenesis and teratogenesis (causing fetal abnormalities) may all be caused by damage to the genetic material DNA. Such tests are a useful way of screening out some potential carcinogens or teratogens and thus of reducing the number of compound that need to undergo full animal testing. In-vitro tests are, however, not able to provide positive assurance that a compound or one of its metabolites is going to be safe in higher animals. Such tests are, in any case, validated by comparison of the mutagenic effects of chemicals with their carcinogenic effect when used in animal tests.

Animal tests on food additives can be categorized under four main headings: acute and subacute toxicity tests; absorption, distribution, metabolism and excretion tests; teratogenicity tests; and long-term carcinogenicity tests.

Acute and subacute toxicity tests

These seek to establish just how much of the additive is required to produce acutely toxic and fatal effects. In the subacute tests, animals are exposed to very high doses for 3 months and tissues are examined microscopically at autopsy for signs of damage.

Absorption, distribution, metabolism and excretion tests

These seek to establish how much of the additive is absorbed, where it goes after absorption, how it is chemically processed after absorption, and how quickly it is excreted. Such studies can give important pointers to the dangers likely to be associated with consumption of the additive (see examples below).

- If the compound is not absorbed from the gut then any adverse effects are likely to be confined to the gut.
- If a water-soluble substance is absorbed and then excreted unchanged in the urine, the bladder is the likely danger organ if the substance is carcinogenic.
- If the substance is absorbed but only slowly excreted or metabolized, it will tend to accumulate. Chronic low intakes may lead to build-up of high levels.
- If the substance is metabolized, metabolites need to be identified and their potential toxicity also needs to be assessed.

- If substances are absorbed and detoxified in the liver, and then excreted in the bile or urine, the liver may be likely to be affected if the compound is carcinogenic.

Teratogenicity testing

This involves feeding large amounts of the compound to pregnant animals to see whether the compound causes birth defects or in any way harms the developing fetuses.

Long-term carcinogenicity testing

This usually involves exposing test animals to relatively high doses of the additive over their whole lifespan. The tumour rates in exposed animals are then compared to those of control animals who have been maintained under identical conditions but have not been exposed to the additive. Such controlled experiments mean that experimenters are able to confidently attribute any increased tumour rate in the test group to the carcinogenic effect of the additive. There are a number of potential criticisms of these tests, such as those noted here.

- Substances that are not carcinogenic in laboratory animals may be carcinogenic in people.
- The controlled conditions of testing are very different from those of use. In the tests, genetically homogeneous animals are used; animals are usually fed single additives and are not usually exposed to other chemicals (e.g. drugs, cigarette smoke or alcohol). Animals are also maintained on defined laboratory diets. In use, the additive will be fed to genetically diverse people – perhaps only certain genotypes will be sensitive to its toxic effects. In use, there is the possibility that the additive may only become toxic if it interacts with other chemicals, or perhaps it becomes harmful under particular dietary or environmental conditions (e.g. deficiency of anti-oxidant vitamins or minerals).
- Laboratory animals have relatively high background tumour rates. This means that the additive needs to produce relatively large increases in tumour rate to be detected with the comparatively small numbers of animals used in the tests. The signal (increase due to additive) must be large to detect it against the background noise (spontaneous tumours not due to additive and occurring randomly in both groups). Thus these tests may be insensitive indicators of carcinogenicity and even small increases in risk can be significant if hundreds of millions of people are to be exposed.

Safety testing of additives depends very much on animal experiments because they are the only practical methods available. In order to try to ensure safety in use, despite the potential flaws discussed, wide safety margins are used. A '*no observable effect*' level is identified in animal experiments; that is, a dose of lifetime exposure that produces no detectable effects in any species used. This no-effect level is then divided by a safety factor (usually 100) to determine an acceptable daily intake (ADI) for people. It is, of course, difficult to control the additive intakes of individuals by regulating the maximum amounts permitted in particular foods. The difficulty of converting dosages between species of different sizes is discussed in Chapter 4.

Most food additives have been subjected to extensive safety testing. Many substances naturally present in foods would probably fail such tests and, of course, a number of additives are naturally present in some foods. Nevertheless the inevitable flaws in the testing procedures do suggest the need to use the minimum effective amounts and for there to be a continuing critical review of which additives are to continue to be recognized as safe. Millstone (1985) critically reviewed the testing and regulation of food additives from a British perspective, and although that paper is now over 25 years old the arguments and principles are essentially unchanged.

> ### Key points
>
> - Hundreds of food additives and thousands of flavourings are in general use.
> - Additives are used:
>   - as processing aids
>   - to preserve food and increase its microbiological safety
>   - to improve its taste, texture or appearance
>   - to increase its nutrient content.
>
>

Key points *continued*

- Some criticisms applied to food additives are:
  - they may be toxic or have carcinogenic potential
  - they can be used to disguise low-quality ingredients or poor standards of hygiene
  - idiosyncratic reactions may occur even with additives that are generally safe
  - flavourings and colourings are unnecessary.
- However:
  - preservatives are necessary for safe mass production of food and even traditional preservatives have their problems
  - food additives are necessary to produce some modern foods that are marketed as healthy options.
- In the USA, use of food additives is regulated by the FDA and in the UK by the Food Standards Agency, although the European Food Safety Authority has an EU-wide role in this respect.
- Regulatory authorities try to ensure that additives are necessary, are used in minimum amounts to achieve their purposes, and are safe when used in permitted amounts.
- In the EU, all additives have a designated E number to be used on food labels.
- Even if huge doses of a chemical produce adverse effects in laboratory animals, that does not necessarily mean that small amounts represent a hazard to people.
- Safety testing of additives is inevitably very dependent on animal tests. Differences between species, the defined conditions of lab tests and the high spontaneous tumour rates in lab animals all tend to reduce confidence in the validity of these as tests of human safety.
- A large safety margin is used when the dose that is demonstrably safe in animals is translated into an acceptable intake for people.

FUNCTIONAL FOODS

Functional foods can be defined as those that have components or ingredients incorporated into them in order to give a specific medical or physiological benefit in addition to their purely nutritional value.

These foods often carry some form of health claim on the packaging or in their advertising. They are also sometimes referred to as *nutraceuticals*, a term that implies that they have both nutritional and pharmaceutical functions. The term functional food could encompass some ordinary foods that have been fortified with a nutrient, such as bread or breakfast cereals fortified with high levels of folic acid to reduce incidence of neural tube defects (see Chapter 13 for a brief discussion of food fortification and Chapter 14 for details of this particular example). Many of the 'active' ingredients of functional foods are found in ordinary foods such as the secondary plant metabolites found in fruits and vegetables (see Chapter 13). This section is based on a chapter in Webb (2011a) and an extended discussion of these topics and further references can be found in that source.

Functional foods are legally classified as foods rather than medicines. In the UK and the EU, they are not permitted to carry claims that they are able to prevent or cure specific diseases; only substances legally classified as medicines are permitted to carry such claims. Certain general health claims have traditionally been permitted but these are currently being evaluated by the European Food Safety Authority with the aim that only scientifically substantiated claims will in future be allowed (health claims are discussed earlier in this chapter and the evaluation process and examples of rulings are further discussed in Chapter 13). The rules are essentially the same for foods, dietary supplements and functional foods. Permitted health claims on food labels in the USA were discussed earlier in the chapter.

Although estimates of the size of the functional food market will vary according to precise inclusion criteria, there can be no doubt that the market for these foods has increased rapidly in the last few years. In the UK it was estimated that the market for functional foods increased more than 10-fold in real terms between 1998 and 2007, from £137 million to £1.72 billion (IGD, 2007). In the USA, annual sales of functional foods were estimated to represent around 5 per cent of the total food market and were growing at an annual rate of 10–20 per cent, compared with a growth rate of just 1–4 per cent for the food industry as a whole (PWC, 2009).

This short section of the chapter will be restricted to discussion of just three categories of functional foods as listed below, followed by a brief note on so-called 'superfoods'.

- *Probiotics, prebiotics and synbiotics.* Probiotics are fermented dairy products that contain living cultures of *Lactobacillus* or *Bifidobacterium* which alter the microbial balance of the gut. Prebiotics are food ingredients (like the plant polysaccharide inulin) that selectively promote the growth of some bacteria within the gut and thus have similar effects to probiotics. Synbiotics are a combination of the previous two.
- *Phyto-oestrogens.* Foods made from soybeans or a few other foods contain substantial amounts of substances called phyto-oestrogens which, although not steroids (they are categorized as isoflavones), do have significant oestrogenic activity and are marketed on that basis.
- *Plant sterols or phytosterols.* Products can contain plant sterols (phytosterols) that are said to lower blood LDL concentrations when used in place of butter, margarine and other 'dairy' products.

Note that in each of these examples it is also possible to buy similar products in the form of dietary supplements to be taken in pill or potion form. I will not attempt to differentiate between these modes of consumption.

Probiotics, prebiotics and synbiotics

Probiotics are live cultures of micro-organisms that are intended to survive passage through the gut and then to adhere to and colonize the large intestine. By colonizing the large bowel they favourably alter the microbial balance, for example by displacing potential pathogens and creating an acidic environment that is unfavourable to pathogen growth. They are mainly so-called *lactic acid bacteria* like the lactobacilli, bifidobacteria and some streptococci which produce lactic acid as an end-product of their metabolism. Over 20 bacteria and a few fungi have been used as probiotics and they are consumed in the form of fermented milk drinks, yoghurts and some other foods or in capsules.

According to RTS (2005), the western European market for probiotics grew by an annual rate of 12 per cent between 2000 and 2005 and amounted to €1.45 billion in 2005. They predicted a continuing annual growth rate of 8 per cent so that the market should have been worth €2 billion in 2010. This compares with a growth rate of just 1–2 per cent in the total food market.

Prebiotics are indigestible oligosaccharides that enter the large bowel where they are fermented and enhance the growth of the types of bacteria used as probiotics. Several of these prebiotics are oligomers of fructose (fructo-oligosaccharides, FOS, and the slightly larger fructose polymer inulin). Gibson *et al.* (1995) were able to show that FOS, when taken by volunteers for 15 days as a replacement for sucrose in a controlled diet, increased the proportion of bifidobacteria in the faeces from 17 to 82 per cent and halved the proportion of *Clostridia*. Inulin has a similar effect. Synbiotics contain probiotic bacteria and prebiotics, and this is aimed at improving the survival and colonization of the lactic acid bacteria. The rest of the discussion refers largely to probiotics, but if prebiotics produce similar changes in gut flora to probiotics then they might be expected to have similar general effects. RTS (2005) also reported rapid growth (around 10 per cent a year) in the market for prebiotics and estimated that by 2010 the western European market would be €1.4 billion.

Goldin (1998) has suggested that a good probiotic has the following characteristics:

- compatibility with the host
- ability to survive gut transit and reach the colon in a viable state
- good ability to adhere to the intestinal epithelium
- rapid rate of multiplication
- not pathogenic
- good survival in foods or supplements
- production of antimicrobial agents that will inhibit or kill potential pathogens
- antimutagenic, anticarcinogenic effects (e.g. by reducing production of mutagens by other organisms in the intestine).

Many suggestions and claims have been made about the potential benefits of regular long-term consumption of probiotics. Several of these are listed below.

- They may increase nutrient availability by fermentation within the gut or even produce available vitamins within the gut. According to Gibson (1998), probiotics increase weight gain in young animals and bottle-fed babies and increased nutrient availability may be a contributing factor to this extra weight gain.

- They may reduce the symptoms of lactose intolerance. Bacterial lactase may contribute to lactose breakdown in the intestine even if viable bacterial cells do not survive passage though the stomach. Montalto *et al.* (2006) found that the lactose content of ordinary live yoghurt was reduced by up to 50 per cent during the fermentation process and this continues after ingestion. Adding probiotic bacteria to unfermented milk probably does not reduce objective measures of lactose intolerance, although there is some suggestion that specific strains might have an effect (Levry *et al.*, 2005).
- They may reduce the number and severity of intestinal infections and so reduce diarrhoea.
- They may reduce plasma LDL cholesterol, although in a review of this topic Taylor and Williams (1998) concluded that any effect, if it exists, is very weak and difficult to detect. A more recent 2-month trial found that consuming a mixture of *Lactobacillus acidophilus*, *Bifidobacterium longum* and a prebiotic had no effect on blood lipid levels in healthy young adults (Greany *et al.*, 2008).
- They may reduce the prevalence of vaginal infections caused by the yeast *Candida albicans* (thrush). Lactic acid bacteria in the normal microflora of the vagina create an acid pH which protects against colonization by *C. albicans*. There is little evidence to support their effectiveness, but oral consumption of probiotics does influence the vaginal microflora (Reid *et al.*, 2004).
- It has been claimed that long-term consumption might reduce the risk of bowel cancer.
- When taken by pregnant women and infants, it is claimed that probiotics can reduce the prevalence of atopic (allergic) disease, especially childhood eczema.

Three of the above suggestions, the effects on intestinal infections and diarrhoea, bowel cancer risk and childhood eczema, are briefly discussed below. The EFSA has so far not approved any health claims relating to probiotic consumption.

The normal gut microflora protects against colonization by pathogenic organisms that cause diarrhoea. In breast-fed babies, up to 99 per cent of the bacterial population in the gut may be bifidobacteria. Bottle-fed babies have a much more diverse gut microflora, including some organisms that are potential pathogens or some that may produce potential mutagens or increase intestinal putrefaction. The stools of breastfed babies are paler, looser, have a less offensive odour and have a much lower pH than those of bottle-fed babies. Rates of intestinal infections and mortality from diarrhoeal diseases are lower in breastfed than in bottle-fed babies (see Chapter 16). These observations are suggestive of a protective effect of lactic acid bacteria against colonization of the gut by potential pathogens.

Several potential mechanisms by which lactic acid bacteria might protect against gut infection have been suggested:

- production of an acidic environment
- competition with other bacteria for key nutrients
- secretion of substances that kill or inhibit growth of other bacteria
- competition with pathogens for intestinal adhesion sites
- provocation of an immune response
- breakdown of toxins produced by pathogens.

A major problem with trying to assess the efficacy is that there are many types and causes of diarrhoea and there are also many different probiotic bacteria. While the evidence is by no means conclusive, there are grounds for believing that some probiotics may be beneficial in treating and/or preventing at least some types of diarrhoea. Szajewska and Mrukowicz (2001) did a systematic review of controlled trials of probiotic use in the treatment of infectious diarrhoea in infants and young children. The 10 trials they reviewed did suggest that probiotics significantly reduced the duration of diarrhoea, especially that caused by *rotavirus* (a very common cause of infant diarrhoea). Their analysis of studies testing for a preventive benefit of probiotics found that the evidence was inconclusive and conflicting. More recently, Saavedra *et al.* (2004) gave formula containing live probiotic bacteria to babies for up to a year and they found reduced reports of colic, irritability and less antibiotic use in the group receiving the probiotic compared to those receiving the placebo. Binns *et al.* (2007) reported that milk containing both probiotics and prebiotics reduced the days on which loose stools were reported by 20 per cent in Australian toddlers attending childcare centres.

The organism *Clostridium difficile* has attracted much media attention in the last few years and is responsible for more deaths among hospital patients than the much better known MRSA (methicillin-resistant *Staphylococcus aureus*). In 2005 it caused around 3800 deaths in the UK, more than double the number attributed to MRSA. It is often present in the gut without producing symptoms, but after antibiotic treatment it may proliferate and cause severe diarrhoea and inflammation of the bowel. In a meta-analysis of nine randomized controlled trials, D'Souza *et al.* (2002) concluded that probiotics did help to prevent this type of antibiotic-associated diarrhoea. The *Lactobacilli* and the yeast *Saccharomyces boulardii* were seen as particularly promising probiotics for this purpose. A more recent meta-analysis seemed to confirm the effectiveness of *S. boulardii* and suggested that other probiotics may be effective (McFarland, 2010).

Earlier in the chapter it was noted that diarrhoea is frequently experienced by those who travel abroad on holiday or business. Studies of the preventive effects of probiotics have yielded very mixed results, with some studies reporting no benefits and others suggesting marked benefits. Mixed results are probably to be expected given the range of organisms that can cause 'travellers' diarrhoea' and the wide range of potential probiotics. See Webb (2011a) for further details.

Allen *et al.* (2003) reviewed 23 trials that had used probiotics in normal adults and children in cases of acute diarrhoea caused by an infective agent. They found that probiotics reduced the chance of diarrhoea still being present after 3 days and reduced the average duration of diarrhoea by 30 hours.

The evidence that probiotics may have some short-term benefits on diarrhoea and gut health has helped to encourage speculation that they might afford some longer term protection against bowel cancer. There are some animal studies that suggest that probiotics can reduce the incidence of chemically induced cancers in animal models (e.g.

Reddy, 1998), but there is little direct evidence as yet for a protective effect in humans. Fotiadis *et al.* (2008) confirmed that there is still no direct evidence for a protective effect in humans, and epidemiological studies linking high fermented milk consumption to bowel cancer produced inconsistent results. There are several theoretical mechanisms by which probiotics might help to reduce bowel cancer risk (see the two examples below), but at present they are merely speculative suggestions. See Fotiadis *et al.* (2008) for further discussion of this issue.

- The acidic conditions produced in the bowel by probiotics might reduce the production of mutagens from food breakdown and/or bile acid degradation.
- Fermentation products like butyrate may have an anti-proliferative effect which might inhibit tumour development.

The incidence of childhood eczema has doubled in Britain in the last few decades and there have also been large increases in the incidence of other atopic (allergic) diseases such as hay fever and asthma. It has been hypothesized that optimizing the gut microflora might help prevent such diseases by preventing the increases in gut permeability and thus antigen penetration that occurs during infection or by stimulating anti-allergenic responses. In a double-blind placebo-controlled trial involving over 150 women, Kalliomaki *et al.* (2001) gave a probiotic bacterium (*L. rhamnosus*)in capsule form to women with a history of atopic disease from 2–4 weeks before their due date until 6 months after delivery. In those babies who were bottle fed the probiotic was added to the formula. Frequency of atopic eczema was halved in those receiving the probiotic compared to those receiving the placebo, and this was a highly statistically significant effect. Follow-up studies have indicated that the benefits on eczema were still apparent at 4 years, although there was no evidence of benefit for other atopic conditions, asthma and hay fever (Kalliomaki *et al.*, 2003). Recent studies are not unequivocal in their support of the protective effect of *L. rhamnosus* and a general reduction rate of 50 per cent now seems unlikely. For further discussion see Webb (2011a) and the meta-analysis by Osborn and Sinn (2007).

The phyto-oestrogens

There are some substances in plants, called phyto-oestrogens, that have a low level of oestrogenic activity. These bind with the human oestrogen receptor and exert a weak oestrogen-like effect, and they are thus termed *partial agonists*; they have less than one ten-thousandth of the activity of the body's main endogenously produced oestrogen. Agonists are compounds that bind to a receptor and mimic the effect of the normal ligand, whereas those that bind to the receptor and exert no effect are termed *antagonists* and these therefore block the effects of the normal ligand by competing with it for the receptor binding sites. The phyto-oestrogens, as partial agonists, may increase total oestrogen activity when endogenous levels are very low (e.g. after the menopause). Even though their activity is very low they can be eaten in substantial quantities and so the oestrogenic effect is significant. Paradoxically they may decrease total oestrogen activity when it is high by competing with endogenous oestrogen for the receptor sites but exerting a much lower oestrogenic effect.

The isoflavones in soy products with the most oestrogenic activity are called *diadzein* and *genistein*. These are found at levels of 2–4 mg of isoflavone per gram of soy protein, and they are found in other legumes but at levels that are orders of magnitude less. Clover and alfalfa sprouts contain *coumesterol* which is another phyto-oestrogen. The chemical structures of diadzein, genistein and coumesterol and the main mammalian oestrogen (oestradiol) are shown in Figure 19.7. Other classes of phyto-oestrogens are *lignans* found in whole grains, vegetables, fruits and flaxseeds; these are structurally similar to the isoflavones and, although usually present only in small amounts in individual foods (except flaxseeds), they may be consumed in substantial amounts because of their wide distribution in plant foods.

The approximate amounts of phyto-oestrogens in some soy foods are:

- soy flour – 5 mg/g of soy protein
- tofu – 2 mg/g
- soy milk – 2 mg/g
- textured soy protein used as a meat substitute – 5 m/g
- soy sauce – none.

Figure 19.7 The structures of oestradiol, the major mammalian oestrogen, and three phyto-oestrogens.

Phyto-oestrogens may be consumed in several ways:

- as soy foods
- as dietary supplements containing extracts of soy protein
- as natural extracts, particularly of red clover and black cohosh

• as other phyto-oestrogens in foods (e.g. lignans in whole grains, fruits, vegetables and flaxseeds and as isoflavones found in alfalfa sprouts).

Phyto-oestrogens have been claimed to offer the following potential benefits:

• relief of acute menopausal symptoms in older women
• reduction in the bone loss (and consequently reduced risk of osteoporosis) in elderly women that is associated with the menopausal decline in oestrogen production
• reduced rates of breast cancer and possibly other cancers when consumed by younger women
• reduced levels of LDL cholesterol in the blood – clinical trials suggest that large supplements of some soy protein extracts do reduce LDL cholesterol but that this is not due to the phyto-oestrogen content as purified phyto-oestrogens are ineffective (Webb, 2011a).

Hormone (oestrogen) replacement therapy (HRT) is an accepted and effective way of reducing the unpleasant acute symptoms caused by declining oestrogen production at the menopause. These symptoms include hot flushes, night sweats, insomnia, depression and vaginal dryness. Several reports have highlighted concerns about the safety of HRT (e.g. Nelson *et al.*, 2002; Beral, 2003), so many women have sought to use supplements containing phyto-oestrogen of soy, black cohosh or red clover as 'natural' alternatives to HRT. Vincent and Fitzpatrick (2000) found evidence that these supplements do produce reductions in symptoms like hot flushes although they are less effective than conventional HRT. The reported reductions in some trials are quite high but they are often not substantially higher than that caused by a placebo even though in some cases they are statistically significant. The 'placebo effect' is often very high in any trials where the outcome is a patient's subjective perception of changes in symptom severity. A more recent systematic review found no convincing evidence that phyto-oestrogens were any more effective than a placebo in alleviating menopausal symptoms (Lethaby *et al.*, 2007).

Hormone replacement therapy has also been widely used to reduce post-menopausal bone loss in older women and thus to reduce the prevalence of fractures due to osteoporosis (discussed more fully in Chapter 14 in the section on calcium). Once again it has been suggested that phyto-oestrogens might offer a 'natural and safer' alternative to HRT. Most of the evidence supporting a positive effect of phyto-oestrogens on bone health has come from in-vitro studies, animal experiments and epidemiological associations. Branca (2003) and COT (2002) summed up the various lines of evidence as noted below.

• Genistein seems to reduce bone resorption by osteoclasts and stimulate bone formation by osteoblasts in in-vitro studies. Silwinski *et al.* (2005) have shown that genistein from soy reduces the formation of osteoclasts when added to in-vitro cultures of bone marrow cells, as does a drug with known oestrogenic activity.
• Soybean feeding increases bone density in female rats that have had their ovaries surgically removed (Mathey *et al.*, 2007).
• In high soy-consuming areas, cross-sectional studies suggest that women with the highest soy intakes have higher bone densities. This effect is not seen in areas where soy consumption is generally lower, suggesting that perhaps a relatively high threshold dose is needed before any effect is detectable.
• Earlier short-term trials (about 6 months) lend some support for a positive influence of phyto-oestrogens on bone mineral density in the lumbar spine. However, a recent meta-analysis of 10 eligible studies found that a mean dose of 87 mg/day of soy isoflavones taken for a year did not have significant effects on bone density; there was some suggestion of a positive effect at the lumbar spine with higher doses (Liu *et al.*, 2009).

The suggestion that high intakes of phyto-oestrogens might reduce the risk of breast cancer when consumed by younger women is probably the most speculative of their suggested benefits, and evidence currently available is far from conclusive or even persuasive.

Rates of breast cancer are low in Far Eastern countries like Japan and China where average intakes of soy foods are around 15–20 times higher than in Western countries with high rates of breast cancer. In women who migrate from high soy-consuming areas to low soy-consuming areas, the rates of breast cancer tend to remain low in the migrants but rise in subsequent generations. This has been interpreted as indicating that exposure to soy products (i.e. phyto-oestrogens) early in life or even *in utero* affords later protection against breast cancer. Note also that migrants may take time to acculturate and to adopt the dietary and lifestyle patterns of their new homeland. Recent epidemiological studies that have attempted to relate phyto-oestrogen intakes to breast cancer risk have been inconclusive and contradictory. There is some evidence that phyto-oestrogens may afford some protection against chemically induced breast tumours in animals. The present state of evidence does not support the use of phyto-oestrogen supplements or even support the use of foods rich in phyto-oestrogens for this purpose. Further discussion may be found in COT (2002) and Limer and Spiers (2004).

Concerns about the safety of foods and supplements high in phyto-oestrogens were first raised in the 1940s when it was observed that some Australian sheep grazing on red clover became infertile. Babies fed on soy-based infant formula have the highest exposure to dietary phyto-oestrogens; their daily consumption is around 4 mg/kg of body weight, which is at least four times higher than that consumed by adults in the high soy-consuming countries of the Far East. Soy-based formulas have been in use for around 80 years without any obvious harmful effects, although there are few published studies that have specifically addressed this issue. As a precautionary measure, COT (2002) recommended that soy-based infant formulas should be fed to UK babies only when it is clinically indicated (for example, allergy to cow milk would be a clinical indication if the baby could tolerate soy milk). Merrit and Jenks (2004) and the Canadian Paediatric Society (2009) have since both concluded that soy-based formulas do not adversely affect human growth, development or reproduction for most babies. However, the Canadian Paediatric Society did not recommend their use in premature infants.

Another theoretical concern about high intakes of phyto-oestrogens is that they might exert a proliferative effect on existing oestrogen-sensitive breast tumours. There is limited evidence from animal studies that phyto-oestrogens can exert such an effect. It is paradoxical that this concern co-exists with the suggestion that phyto-oestrogens may help prevent breast cancer. The safety of phyto-oestrogens has been reviewed by COT (2002) and Barnes (2003).

Plant sterols or phytosterols

Plants do not produce cholesterol but they do produce a range of steroids that are very similar in chemical structure and are collectively termed *phytosterols*. The most prevalent of these plant sterols are called β-*sitosterol* and *campesterol* which make up over 80 per cent of total dietary phytosterols. Other phytosterols include *stigmasterol* and the fungal steroid *ergosterol* which, when irradiated with ultraviolet light, yields vitamin D_2. The average daily intake of these plant sterols is normally around 100–300 mg in the UK, with the highest intakes naturally recorded in vegetarians.

These plant sterols are structurally very similar to cholesterol. For example, the only difference between cholesterol and β-sitosterol is that the latter has an extra ethyl (CH_3CH_2) group attached to carbon 24 of cholesterol. Cholesterol and most plant sterols have a double bond in one of the rings of the steroid nucleus (between carbons 5 and 6). A tiny proportion of the plant sterols in the diet do not have this double bond and are sometimes termed the *saturated phytosterols* or the (phyto)stanols; these structures are exemplified in Figure 19.8.

All phytosterols, whether saturated or not, are poorly absorbed from the gut – up to 5 per cent of the majority of unsaturated plant sterols, and less than 1 per cent of the saturated phytostanols. (The terms phytosterol or plant sterol are used from this point to refer to both the saturated and unsaturated forms.) While poorly absorbed themselves, plant sterols do inhibit the absorption of cholesterol – both the cholesterol present in food and that secreted into the gut in bile, much of which is normally reabsorbed. These plant sterols increase faecal losses of both ingested cholesterol and biliary cholesterol and thus have the potential to lower blood cholesterol levels, specifically plasma LDL cholesterol (see Chapter 12). Other suggested mechanisms by which they might reduce LDL

Figure 19.8 The chemical structures of cholesterol, β-sitosterol and β-sitostanol.

cholesterol include an effect on cholesterol metabolism within gut and liver cells that might lead to increased expression of the LDL receptor and thus more rapid clearance of cholesterol from blood (Plat and Mensink, 2005; Calpe-Berdiel *et al.*, 2009).

The basic science of this has been established for decades and β-sitosterol was used as a cholesterol-lowering drug as far back as the 1970s. In 1995, a new brand of margarine was launched in Finland that contained large amounts (*c*12 g/100 g) of β-sitostanol esters which can be produced from by-products of the wood-pulping and paper-making industries; see Webb (2011a) for further details. This margarine has since been marketed in many other countries and a number of rival margarines and other foods containing plant sterols have been launched.

There have been a series of controlled trials of these plant sterols (Law listed 14 in 2000), and these studies confirm their potential to lower blood cholesterol levels by clinically significant amounts. According to Law (2000), intakes of 2–3 g/day of these phytosterols in margarine or other functional foods leads to a significant reduction in plasma LDL cholesterol within weeks in both men and women. Law suggested that universal consumption of this amount of plant sterol might reduce heart disease risk by up to 25 per cent. More recent meta-analyses tend to confirm their cholesterol-lowering effect (Katan *et al.*, 2003; Demonty *et al.*, 2009). Inclusion of around 2 g/day of phytosterols in the diet reduces LDL cholesterol by around 10 per cent, and by double this amount if combined with a diet that is low in saturated fat and cholesterol. They enhance the effect of statin-type drugs, and combining statins and phytosterols seems to be more effective than just increasing the statin dose. Demonty *et al.* (2009) were able to establish a dose-dependent cholesterol-lowering effect of statins.

Webb (2011a) discusses issues (see below) which may indicate a need for caution and further research before phytosterols are given unqualified endorsement for universal usage. Many discussed in Law (2000) and in the correspondence arising from that paper can be viewed via the BMJ website at www.bmj.com/content/320/7238/861?view=long&pmid=10731187.

- There is a limited supply of phytosterols and so the products fortified with them are relatively expensive. Law (2000) estimated that, at that time, available sources of phytosterols could supply only around 10 per cent of people in Western countries.
- While the evidence of the cholesterol-lowering effects of phytosterols in controlled trials is very persuasive, the impact of casual product replacement is not clear.
- There is as yet no substantial evidence that any fall in cholesterol levels due to casual consumption of phytosterol-containing products will ultimately translate into significant

reductions in cardiovascular or total mortality rates. Nonetheless, by analogy, substantial falls in cholesterol levels brought about by statin-type drugs do lead to falls in these mortalities.

- Phytosterols may interfere with the absorption of some other lipid-soluble substances such as β-carotene and vitamin E.
- Some people with rare genetic defects may be adversely affected by large phytosterol intakes. The amounts being advocated are at least an order of magnitude greater than intakes from normal diets, so the effects of lifetime consumption of these amounts need to be monitored and assessed.

Superfoods

The term 'superfood' seems to have originated in the USA around 2003 and was first used in a UK national newspaper in 2005 to describe a range of 'ordinary' foods (e.g. green tea, tomato products and many, sometimes exotic, fruits and vegetables) that were marketed on the basis that their consumption confers some particular health benefits (Bender, 2007).

The name evolved initially as a marketing term to enhance the consumer appeal of particular foods and so there is no official definition or definitive list of superfoods. Bender (2007) defined them as:

> a range of ordinary foods that are marketed as being particularly rich in conventional nutrients, antioxidants, polyunsaturated fatty acids, dietary fibre or specific phytochemicals or secondary plant metabolites.

He also generated a list of 40 foods that would be covered by this term by synthesizing other lists derived from an internet search. The number of foods to which the term is applied is growing and would now include several exotic fruits and vegetables that would not previously have been seen on the shelves of ordinary British supermarkets – such as goji berries, acai berries, pomegranate juice as well as the more familiar foods like broccoli and tomatoes.

Webb (2011a) contains an illustrative list of some of the best known of these superfoods with an indication of the rationale for their claimed beneficial effects. This is summarized below.

- *Broccoli and several other Cruciferous vegetables like cabbage and sprouts.* These vegetables are a source of the sulphur-containing secondary metabolites known as *glucosinolates*. It is suggested that substances generated from these glucosinolates may reduce cancer risk by reducing the activation of certain potential carcinogens in food.
- *Garlic and other members of the Allium or onion family.* These all contain S-alkyl cysteine sulphoxides which are also sulphur-containing secondary plant metabolites. In particular, the allicin in garlic has been claimed to have antibacterial activity, anti-cancer effects, and anti-thrombotic and blood cholesterol-lowering effects.
- *Several berry fruits* – including blueberries, cranberries, strawberries and several other more recently introduced types like goji berries and acai berries. These are marketed on their high content of anthrocyanins which have anti-oxidant activity.
- *Foods that are rich in pigments from the carotenoid group of tetraterpenoids.* These include carrots (β-carotene), tomatoes (lycopene), and red peppers (lutein). A few carotenoids like β-carotene have vitamin A activity but all of them have anti-oxidant activity; lycopene is seen as the most powerful anti-oxidant and has no vitamin A activity.
- *Salmon and some other oily fish* – because of their high content of long-chain n-3 (ω-3) polyunsaturated fatty acids (see Chapter 12).
- *A variety of other fruits* – such as apples, kiwi, mango and red grapes, usually as a combination of anti-oxidant effects due to the presence of anti-oxidant nutrients and flavonoids of various types.
- *Olive oil* – because of its high level of monounsaturated fatty acids and also because of the presence of lipid-soluble anti-oxidants.
- *Soy* – largely because of the presence of isoflavones which have low oestrogenic activity (as discussed under phyto-oestrogens earlier in the chapter). Flaxseeds and other cereal seeds also contain lignans which have oestrogenic activity.
- *Green tea* – because of the presence of polyphenols which may have anti-oxidant and

anti-mutagenic effects. Cocoa is also rich in phenolic compounds.

- *Red wine* – is said to have cardioprotective effects because of its content of polyphenols (including resveratrol) which act as anti-oxidants. As discussed in Chapter 5, there is evidence that moderate alcohol consumption may protect against cardiovascular disease and moderate consumption of red wine in particular may be associated with reduced all-cause mortality. There are, however, severe deleterious health and social effects of excess alcohol consumption.
- *Walnuts and several other types of tree nuts* – there is epidemiological evidence to link high nut consumption with reduced risk of cardiovascular disease and most are rich in polyunsaturated fatty acids. Brazil nuts are considered to be a rich source of selenium.

It must be emphasized that these are *claims*, and in some cases the claim is based on little more than a chemical analysis that shows high levels of a particular nutrient or phytochemical.

Extra intake of a nutrient or phytochemical is beneficial only if it is consumed by someone who would benefit from consuming more of the substance. It seems probable that the people most likely to consume superfoods (and any supplement), particularly new exotic or expensive ones, are those whose diet is already high in micronutrients and phytochemicals. For many of these ingredients of superfoods there is no real evidence that increased consumption will benefit anyone. Despite decades of research and extravagant claims about increasing life expectancy, there is no convincing evidence that high anti-oxidant intake confers any long-term benefits. The European Food Safety Authority has not approved any health claims for anti-oxidants (see Chapter 13).

Key points

- Functional foods or neutraceuticals have components that are intended to confer specific health benefits. The worldwide market for functional foods is growing much more rapidly than the food market generally.
- Functional foods usually carry some health claim on their packaging, although in the UK they cannot claim to cure or prevent a specific disease.
- Probiotics are fermented dairy products containing live bacteria. They are intended to alter the microbial balance in the intestine and hinder the growth of pathogens. Prebiotics are indigestible food components that are intended to enhance the growth of certain bacteria within the gut.
- It has been proposed that probiotics may alleviate or help prevent gut infections and diarrhoea.
- There is a body of evidence to support probiotics reducing the duration of infantile diarrhoea due to human rotavirus and to reduce antibiotic-associated diarrhoea due to *Clostridium difficile*.
- Conclusive evidence of beneficial effects of probiotics on diarrhoea is hindered by the large number of organisms that can cause diarrhoea and the wide range of organisms that have been used as probiotics.
- There are speculative grounds for suggesting that probiotics may reduce bowel cancer risk but little direct evidence to support this proposition.
- Probiotics create an acidic environment in the intestine which may hinder pathogen colonization and prevent production of mutagens from food and bile acids.
- Probiotic bacteria may also compete with potential pathogens for adhesion sites in the intestine and again reduce the risk of colonization.
- Probiotics taken in late pregnancy and during breastfeeding (or added to bottle feeds) have been reported (2001 and 2003) to significantly reduce the later risk of the baby developing eczema, although more recent studies are less than conclusive.
- Phyto-oestrogens are plant substances like diadzein and genistein from soy products that have very weak oestrogenic activity – they are partial oestrogen agonists.

→

Key points *continued*

- In post-menopausal women, large intakes of phyto-oestrogens may enhance total oestrogen response and thus may possibly reduce menopausal symptoms and reduce post-menopausal bone loss.

- In younger women, it is claimed that large intakes of phyto-oestrogens might reduce breast cancer risk by moderating the response to endogenous oestrogen.

- There is a theoretical possibility that phyto-oestrogens might have a proliferative effect on existing breast tumours.

- Infants fed on soy-based formula receive the highest exposure to phyto-oestrogens. Several expert groups have recommended that, as a precaution, soy-based formula should not be given to infants unless this is clinically necessary (e.g. cow milk allergy) although there is no evidence of harm to babies after 80 years of use.

- Phytosterols are cholesterol-like sterols produced in plants and fungi that are very poorly absorbed from the gut. They inhibit the absorption of dietary cholesterol and the reabsorption of biliary cholesterol.

- In controlled trials, phytosterols have been convincingly shown to have an LDL cholesterol lowering effect.

- Long-term benefits of prolonged casual use of phytosterol-containing margarine and other foods have yet to be formally demonstrated but by analogy, substantial falls in blood cholesterol levels caused by statins do yield long-term holistic benefits.

- Phytosterol-containing foods are relatively expensive. At present, production capabilities are limited so they could only be used by a relatively small proportion of people in affluent countries.

- Superfoods are ordinary foods that are promoted on the basis that their consumption confers some health benefit because they are rich in conventional nutrients, anti-oxidants, unsaturated fatty acids, dietary fibre or some secondary plant metabolites.

INDEX

abdominal obesity (excess fat) 215, 216, 312, 516
absorption 162–4
  ageing effects 472
  calcium 413, 456
    in pregnancy 411, 445
    vitamin D and 359, 368, 419
  fat 163–4, 301–2
  food additives 571–2
  iron (inorganic) 406, 408
    inhibitors and promoters of 407
  see also malabsorption
acceptable macronutrient distribution range 77
acesulfame K 250
acetyl coenzyme A 159, 160
acid–base balance and ageing 472
acrodermatitis enteropathica 401
adaptive thermogenesis 187–8, 187–8, 190–1
additives see food additives
adenosine phosphates see ADP; AMP; ATP
s-adenosylmethionine (SAMe) 352
adequacy (of diet or food supplies) 5–7
  micronutrients
    assessment 330–4
    improvement strategies 333–4
  protein 273
  vegetarianism 508–12
  yardstick of 65
adequate intake (AI) 77
adipose tissue (body fat)
  anatomical location and relative harmfulness 215–16
  abdominal 215, 216, 312, 516
  brown, and adaptive thermogenesis 190–1
  dietary fat excess converted to 226
  fat-cell theory and children 231–2
  health promotion focusing on 218
  satiety signals (liposstat) 194, 196–7
  surgical removal 240
adolescence 462–9
  activity levels 523–4
ADP (adenosine diphosphate) 157
  creatine phosphate and 528
β_3-adrenergic agents 239
aerobic capacity assessment 520

aerobic metabolism of pyruvic acid 159–60
aesthetic taboos 58
affective disorder, anorexia nervosa as 184
affluence see wealth and affluence
aflatoxins (of A. flavus) 566
Africa
  cereal production, stagnation 47
  meat craving in 37
Africans and Afro-Caribbeans see black people
age 449–83
  bone density and fracture risk related to 414–15
  cholesterol plasma levels related to (UK) 305, 306
  height related to, children 92–3
  maternal, and infant weaning 460
  physical activity levels and 522
  reference nutrient intakes by see reference nutrient intake
  standardization in epidemiological studies 106
age-related macular degeneration (ARMD) 335, 356
ageing
  coenzyme Q10 and 350–1
  effects 472
    on health 470–1
  see also elderly
Agency for Healthcare Research and Quality (AHRQ) report anti-oxidant supplements 343
Agouti-related peptide 194
agriculture
  chemicals 567
  farm workers and heart disease 311
air displacement plethysmography 91
alanine 269
alanine aminotransferase test, erythrocyte 380
alcohol consumption 143–5
  blood pressure and 430, 431
  energy from 173
  guidelines and recommendations 143–5
  heart disease and 104, 145, 312
  milk thistle and 11
  osteoporosis risk and 418
  vitamin deficiency 360–1
    thiamin 162, 361, 375, 376

algal extracts 298, 323, 381, 510
alimentary tract see gastrointestinal tract
alkaloids 354
allergy (food) 4, 485–6
Allied Dunbar National Fitness Survey 521, 523
  elderly 480
Allium see onion family
Alzheimer's disease and Ginkgo biloba 346
Amanita phalloides 566
Ames test 571
amino acids 268–84
  essential/non-dispensable 274–6
    conditionally 4, 348
  functions/uses 272–3
  infant feeding, breast milk and formulas 455
  limiting 275–6
  metabolism 161
  nitrogen-containing compounds synthesized from 272
  non-essential/dispensable 275
  quantifying requirements 275–6
  selenium-containing 400
  sulphur-containing see sulphur-containing compounds
aminopeptidase 270
AMP (adenosine monophosphate) 157
amphetamine 237
α-amylase 162, 255
  pancreatic 152, 246
  weaning and 459
  starches resistant to 257, 260–1
amylopectin 255
  structure 256
amylose 255
  structure 256
anaemia
  aplastic 407
  folic acid-deficiency 359, 385
  iron-deficiency 393, 405, 406, 407–10
  pernicious 4, 360, 383, 484
  vitamin B_{12}-deficiency 359, 381, 382, 510
anaerobic bacterial growth 545
anaerobic metabolism 159
  glycogen 528

analytical epidemiology of disease–diet links 103
anandamide 194
animal(s), experimental
  disease–diet linkage 103, 118–21
    species differences to be considered 119, 120–1
  energy balance and its regulation 120, 189, 190, 191, 192–3
  hypertension and salt intake 428–9
  inappropriate extrapolation of results to humans 118–19, 278, 281–2
  nutrient requirements 84
    protein/amino acids 275, 281–2
  obesity models 190–1, 195, 196–7, 198, 199, 200, 221
    behavioural characteristics 222
  see also species differences
animal fats 289–90
anorexia, hospital patients 500
anorexia nervosa (AN) 182
  causes 183–5
  characteristics and consequences 182, 183
  incidence 183
anthropological classification of foods 35–8
anthropometry 65, 86–94
  children 92–4
  elderly 477
  obesity and overweight definitions 202
antibiotic-associated diarrhoea, probiotics 575
antidepressant drugs
  anorexia treatment 184
  tyramine and monoamine oxidase inhibitors 120, 566
antihypertensive drugs 423
anti-inflammatory effects of fish oils 318
anti-oxidants 138, 324, 335–46
  alcoholic drinks 145
  plant secondary metabolites 337, 355, 581
  protective effects 341–6
  supplements 11, 326
  vitamin C as 390, 391, 391–2
  vitamin E as 372
aplastic anaemia 407
apoproteins 300
appetite
  regulation 194, 195, 196, 200
    appestat 193, 194, 195, 196, 197, 198
  suppressants 237–8, 241
  see also anorexia; anorexia nervosa

arcuate nucleus (of hypothalamus) 194, 195
arginine 269
arm circumference (mid-arm) 87, 92
arrhythmias and fish oils 318
arthritis
  chondroitin sulphate 346, 349–50
  fish oils 320
  glucosamine in see glucosamine
artificial sweeteners 250–2
ascorbic acid see vitamin C
Asian people in UK see South Asian/Indian subcontinent people
asparagine 269
aspartame 250
aspartate aminotransferase test, erythrocyte 380
aspartic acid 269
assessment, nutritional 64–101
  biochemical methods see biochemical assessment
  at hospital admission 503–4
  micronutrient adequacy 330–4
  strategies 64–5, 85–98
atherogenesis and atherosclerosis 304, 310
  cholesterol levels and 312
  epidemiological studies 311, 312
  fats and 307, 309
  fish oils and 319
  free radicals and 339
athletic performance 526–30
  body weight and energy intake and 526–30
  coenzyme Q10 and 350
  creatine and 351, 528
  see also training
Atkin's diet 225
atorvastatin 315
ATP (adenosine triphosphate) 156, 157
  in glycolysis 159
  in oxidative phosphorylation 158
  in substrate-level phosphorylation 157
atropine 354
attention-deficit hyperactivity disorder and fish oils 320–1
attitudes in BASNEF model of behavioural change 27, 28
availabilities (of food)
  healthy foods as alternatives to less-healthy foods 149–50
  hierarchy of 41–63
  hospital patients, lack 500
aversion therapy 223

babies see infants; neonates
Bacillus cereus 541, 542, 543, 553
bacteria
  dental caries and 253
  food-poisoning 541–2
    avoidance of food contamination with 547–8
    growth requirements 545
    maximizing killing 547, 548
    mechanisms of ill effects 542–4
    minimizing storage time in conditions allowing growth 547, 548
bacteriostatic effects of breast milk components 457
balance studies of dietary requirements 81–2
bariatric (weight-losing) surgery 239–40, 241
basal metabolic rate 100
  athletes 526
  elderly 473
BASNEF model 27–9
behavioural change (in diet and other lifestyles) 16–23
  barriers to 25–7, 149–50
    cultural resistance 59–60
    socioeconomic factors 55
  promotion (interventions to induce)
    effecting 23–9
    ineffective 11
    justification 16–23
    secondary consequences 22–3
    unhelpful/harmful effects 10–11, 22, 278
  realistically achievable, and magnitude of benefit 19–20
  willingness to change 147–8
behavioural problems (children) and fish oil supplementation 319, 320–1
behavioural therapy, overweight/obesity 222–3
beliefs influencing dietary change 24
  in BASNEF model 27–9
  older people's traditional beliefs 150
  taboos 56–9
benefit payments/welfare and food selection 51
beriberi (of thiamin deficiency) 3, 359, 360, 375–6
  concurrent with riboflavin deficiency 377
berry fruits 337–8, 581
'best before' date 535

beta-3 (β_3)-adrenergic agents 239
beta-carotene *see* carotene
beta-oxidation 160–1
bicycle ergometer 520
Bifidobacterium as probiotics 574, 575
bile acids and infant feeding 455, 456
bile salts 164, 301, 302
binge-eating *see* bulimia nervosa
biochemical assessment (incl. markers) of nutrient status 65, 83, 94–5
  minerals
    iodine 402
    iron 83, 95–6, 406
    magnesium 397
    manganese 397
    potassium 399
    selenium 400
    zinc 401
  toxicity 366
  vitamins
    biotin 389
    pantothenic acid 389
    vitamin A 361, 363
    vitamin B_1 (thiamin) 374
    vitamin B_2 (riboflavin) 376
    vitamin B_3 (niacin) 378
    vitamin B_6 (pyridoxine) 380
    vitamin B_9 (folate) 384, 385
    vitamin B_{12} (cobalamin) 381
    vitamin D 365
    vitamin E 372
bioelectrical impedance 87, 91
biological markers of nutrient status 83–4
biological model (function) of food 31–2
biological variations and food tables 73
biotin 389
birth defects (congenital)
  neural tube defects in folate deficiency 22, 125, 385–6, 386–7, 446–7
  other than neural tube in folate deficiency 386
birth weights
  dieting in pregnancy and effects on 442
  energy aspects of pregnancy and 442–3
  infant mortality rate and, associations 439
bisphosphonates, osteoporosis 420
Bitot spots 364
black people (incl. Afro-Caribbeans), health and nutrition
  Americans 514
  UK 514, 516, 517, 518
blackcurrant seed oil 298

bleeding (blood loss) leading to iron deficiency 409
blind challenge in food allergy 485
blood
  calcium levels 411, 412
  clotting *see* clotting
  lipoproteins *see* lipoproteins
  loss leading to iron deficiency 409
  nutrient measurements 82, 95–6, 97–8
    micronutrients in elderly 478
  substrate levels influencing satiety 194, 195–6
blood pressure, high (hypertension) 8
  causes/associations 109, 427–31
    obesity 214, 430
    salt intake 9, 19–20, 107, 108–9, 111, 124–5, 422–3, 427–30, 431
    vitamin D insufficiency 370
  elderly 482
  heart disease risk in 312
    potassium protecting against 399, 430
  interventions
    drugs 423
    magnesium supplements 397
    salt intake 124–5, 429
body
  composition and ageing 472
  density assessment 87, 91
body builders, BMI 88–9
body image foods 37
body mass index (BMI) 86–7, 88–9
  alternative (to height measurement) in assessment of 89
  children 93–4
  elderly *see* elderly
  health risks of high BMI 216, 217–18
  life expectancy and 211–13
  obesity and overweight defined by 202
bomb calorimeter 171
bonding and breastfeeding 457
bone 414–15
  calcium and 411, 412
  calcium content in food tables affected by pieces of 74
  density 414–15
    age and sex impact on 414–15
    measurement 415
    physical activity impact on *see* physical activity
  fractures *see* fractures
  phyto-oestrogen effects on 417, 578
  thinning *see* osteoporosis
  vitamin D and calcitriol and 368
    deficiency effects on bone 368–9
  see also mammalian meat and bone meal

borage (starflower) oil 298, 299, 322
bottle (formula)-feeding
  breastfeeding vs 449
  composition 455
    based on cow milk 455
  cost 458
  factors influencing choice 451–5
  follow-on formulas 456
  gut microflora and 456, 575
  hygiene problems 457–8
  soy-based formulas 579
botulinum cook 553, 561
bovine spongiform encephalopathy (BSE) 554–60
bowel (intestine)
  bypass surgery in obesity 240
  cancer (colorectal cancer) 114
    folate and 387, 388–9
    probiotics and 575, 576
    protective diets 107, 262–6
    vegetarian diets and 512
    vitamin D and 370
  digestion and absorption *see* absorption; digestion
boys
  obesity 209, 210
  reference nutrient intakes 436, 464
  sex hormones and puberty 463
brain
  damage *see* neurological damage
  in energy intake regulation 194
  fish oils and 319, 320–1
  in starvation 179
bran and bowel cancer risk 263
brand variations and food tables 73
Brassica (cabbage family)
  goitrogenic substances 405, 566
  secondary metabolites
    in carcinogen detoxification 355
    sulphur-containing 354
bread
  as European superfood 36
  obesity and 11
  wholemeal 148
bread and cereals group 151
breast cancer
  breastfeeding and 458
  soy products and 112
breast milk 456
  composition 281, 435, 449, 455, 456
breast pain (mastalgia), evening primrose oil 322, 323, 346
breastfeeding 449–59
  benefits 455–9
  bottle-feeding vs 449
  factors influencing choice 451–4
  social class *see* social status
  taboos 57, 453

gut microflora and 456, 575
prevalence 450–1
UK immigrants 60
weaning from *see* weaning
see also lactation
Britain *see* United Kingdom
broad bean and favism 565
broccoli 581
brown fat and adaptive thermogenesis
190–1
BSE (bovine spongiform
encephalopathy) 554–60
bulimia nervosa (BN) and binge-
eating 182
causes 183, 184
characteristics and consequences
182, 183
incidence 183
butyrate from fibre fermentation
258, 263

cabbage family *see Brassica*
cachexia, cancer 185–6
calcitonin in osteoporosis 420
calcitriol (1,25-dihydroxyvitamin D;
1,25-dihydroxycholecalciferol)
365, 367–8, 369, 370, 412
calcium 410–21
adequate intake
assessment in UK 333
vegetarian diet 510–11
availability 412–13
children
intakes 465
recommendations/requirements
463, 464
content in food tables affected by
pieces of bone 74
deficiency/low intake
effects 411
hypertension risk 430
prevalence 411
risk factors 411
distribution 411–12
functions/roles 411, 411–12
guidelines and recommendations 147
children 463, 464
elderly 474
on high intakes 411
hormonal regulation of homeostasis
412
infant feeding 456
pregnancy 445
requirements 412–13
sources 410–11
standards 410
supplements 411
in osteoporosis (and its
consequences) prevention and
treatment 369, 419–20, 420

toxicity 411
typically highest intakes 411
vitamin D and 368
calories
balancing, recommendations and
guidelines 136
consumer use of foods high in 34–5
obesity/overweight and intake of
111, 136
see also kilocalories
calorimeter, bomb 171
campesterol 579
Campylobacter (incl. *C. jejuni*) 540,
541, 542, 543, 546, 551
cancer
antioxidants and 341–6
carotenoids 19, 341, 342
vitamin A and 116–17, 364–5
vitamin D and *see* vitamin D
cachexia 185–6
diet and 19, 113, 341–6
antioxidants *see subheading above*
bowel cancer *see* bowel
breast cancer and *see* breast
cancer
fruit and vegetable consumption
and 9, 19, 138, 263, 265, 342–5
garlic 20
obesity and 213
ovarian cancer and galactose 116
plant secondary metabolites 355–6
salt intake and gastric cancer
423, 428
thyroid 403
see also carcinogen; carcinogenesis
candidiasis, vaginal, and probiotics 575
cannabinoids, endogenous *see*
endocannabinoids
canned foods 561
food poisoning risk 546
production 561
carbohydrate (including sugars)
245–67
absorption 162–3
diets low in *see* low-carbohydrate
diets
digestion 162–3, 246, 255
as energy source 172, 173
glycaemic index of foods containing
see glycaemic index
guidelines and recommendations
on dietary intake 136, 140–2
metabolism 158–60
nature and classification 246–7
obesity and dietary levels of 11,
224–6
protein combined with (food-
combining diets) 234
sources of 247–8
structures 256

carbohydrate–fat (sugar–fat) seesaw
149, 173
carbon dioxide evolution,
measurement 99
carboxylated glutamic acid residues 373
carboxypeptidase 270
carboxypeptidases 163
carcass analysis of fatness 94–5
carcinogen detoxification and plant
secondary metabolites 355
carcinogenesis
food additive testing 571
long-term carcinogenicity 572
free radicals and 335
vitamin A deficiency and 364
cardiomyopathy in Keshan disease
339, 400
cardiopulmonary exercise testing 520
cardiovascular disease *see* heart
disease
CARET trial 344
carnitine 4, 348, 349, 484
deficiency 349
therapeutic use 484
β-carotene (and other carotenoids)
341–2, 344–5, 581
supplements or high intake 15–16,
344
cancer and 19, 341, 342
cardiovascular disease and 130, 344
smoking and 11, 328, 344
casein, infant feeding 455–6
case–control studies of disease–diet
linkage 103, 115–17
bowel cancer 264–6
cassava
cyanide release 565
goitrogenic substances 405, 566
catabolic response 501
catalase 337
catering managers as gatekeepers 63
cattle and BSE 554–60
cause–effect relationship with diet
and disease 18–19, 104
cells
disease due to free radical damage
in 338
energetics 156–64
in starvation 179
organic substances with vitamin-
like roles in 324, 326, 337
centiles in anthropometry 93
cereals
energy density 174
as energy source 178, 273, 274
food group of bread and 151
production, and Green Revolution
47
protein content 273
Chandra, Dr Ranjit 480

change in behaviour *see* behavioural
    change
cheese tyramine *see* tyramine
chemical changes in irradiated
    food 563
chemical environment for bacterial
    growth 545
chemical safety of food 564–73
chemiosmotic theory of oxidative
    phosphorylation 158
children 462–9
    anthropometry 92–4
    behavioural problems and fish oil
        supplementation 319, 320–1
    diarrhoea (young children) and
        pre- or probiotics 575–6
    eczema, probiotics 575, 576
    energy density of foods 176, 463,
        465
    food allergy 485, 486
    Indian childhood cirrhosis 396
    iron deficiency 408
    obesity 209–10
        anti-obesity measures 231–2
        nature vs nurture in cause of
            220–1
        socioeconomic disadvantages
            214–15
        TV viewing/physical inactivity
            and 228, 231
    osteoporosis (in later life) and
        preventive measures in 419
    phenylketonuria treatment 488
    physical activity levels 231, 523–4
        obesity and 228, 231
    requirements 435–6
        protein/amino acid 275, 278,
            280, 281, 282
        reference nutrient intakes 436,
            462–3, 464
    zinc deficiency 401
    see also infants
chilled (cook–chilled) foods 562
    listeriosis risk 554, 562
    production 562
chimpanzee, hypertension and salt
    intake 428–9
Chinese system of food classification
    34
chips (French fries) in UK 37
Chlorella 381, 383
chloride, requirements and function
    421, 424
    see also salt
cholecalciferol *see* vitamin D
cholecystokinin (CCK) 195, 239
    antiobesity potential 239
    leptin and 199–200
cholesterol 302, 310–11

dietary content
    influence on plasma levels 118–
        19
    various foods 12
functional foods effects on plasma
    levels of
    plant sterols 579–81
    probiotics 575
    soy products 578
guidelines and interventions aimed
    at reducing plasma levels 11,
        142
    drugs 14, 314–16, 482, 580
    in prevention of coronary disease
        20–2
guidelines and recommendations
    on dietary intake 136, 140–1
health images (regarding heart
    disease) 309
high blood/plasma levels
    (hypercholesteraemia) 8, 304,
        310–11
    elderly 482
    familial 118, 304–5
    fat types consumed and 9, 122
    heart disease and *see* heart
        disease
    influence of dietary cholesterol
        intake 118–19
    obesity and 214
    in lipoproteins 300
    non-starch polysaccharides
        reducing level of 259
    UK population plasma levels
        305, 306
cholesterol-lowering drugs 14,
    314–16, 482, 580
choline 351–2
chondroitin sulphate, arthritis 346,
    349–50
chromium 394–5
    deficiency 394, 395
    supplements 394
chromomodulin 394–5
chronic disease *see* disease
chylomicrons 164, 300, 301–2
chymotrypsin 163, 270
circulatory disease *see* heart disease
cirrhosis, Indian childhood 396
cis-fatty acids 287–8
citric acid cycle 160
clinical signs of nutritional problems
    65, 85–6
clinical trials, disease–diet linkage
    103–4, 124–6
Clostridium botulinum 542, 543, 545,
    553, 561
Clostridium difficile and probiotics
    575

Clostridium perfringens 541, 542,
    543, 552
clotting (coagulation)
    alcohol and 145
    fish oils and 318, 321
    plant secondary metabolites and
        356
    vitamin K and 373
coagulation *see* clotting
cobalamin *see* vitamin B$_{12}$
cocaine 354
Cochrane Library and Cochrane
    Collaboration 132
coconut oil 290
codeine 354
Codex Alimentarius Commission 535
coding errors in food intake
    assessment 71
coeliac disease (gluten-sensitive
    enteropathy) 4, 484, 486–7
    dietary management 486–7
    weaning and 462
coenzyme(s) (cofactors) 156–7
coenzyme A 160
    pantothenic acid as precursor of
        390
coenzyme Q10 (ubiquinone) 350–1
    supplements 350–1
    and cardiovascular disease 343
cohort studies of disease–diet linkage
    103, 112–15
    bowel/colon cancer 114, 264–6
    heart disease 313–14
cold (common)
    vitamin C supplements 392
    zinc supplement 401–2
cold and hot classification system 34
cold stress, old people 472
collagen 414
collagenase 270
colorectal cancer *see* bowel
colostrum 347
colourings 568
COMA *see* Committee on Medical
    Aspects of Food and Nutrition
    Policy
Committee on Medical Aspects of
    Food and Nutrition Policy
    (COMA) 75, 76, 77, 79, 81,
        82, 83
    energy requirements 168–9
compliance with in human
    experimental studies of
    disease–diet links 122
conception *see* contraceptive effect;
    preconceptual period;
    pregnancy
conditionally essential nutrients
    4–5, 324, 348–63

conflict and war 7
congenital defects *see* birth defects
conjugated linoleic acid (CLA) 288–9
consumers
   food classification by 33–5
   on food safety and quality 533–40
      food labelling *see* labelling
      low-fat claims 295
consumption *see* intake
contamination of food
   chemical 564, 565–8
   food poisoning-bacteria 547–8
contraceptive effect of breastfeeding
   458
control group in trials, ethics of
   withholding treatment 126
cook–chill *see* chilled (cook–chilled)
   foods
cooking temperature for killing
   bacteria 543, 548
   see also heat treatment
cooking utensils and water affecting
   food tables 74
copper 394–5
   adequate intake in UK 333
   deficiency 394, 394–5
copper–zinc superoxide dismutase
   337
core foods 35
Cori cycle 159
corn milling and niacin deficiency
   379
coronary disease *see* heart disease
cosmetic additives 568, 569
cost
   formula feeds 458
   healthy foods/diet 52–6, 150
   see also economic and financial
      dimensions
cot death (sudden infant death
   syndrome)
   breastfeeding and 457
   sleeping position and 11–13, 111
coumesterol 577
cow milk 456
   composition 455, 456
creatine 351
   athletic performance and 351, 528
cretinism 403
Creutzfeldt–Jakob disease (CJD)
   555, 555–6
   spontaneous/sporadic 555–6, 557
   variant (vCJD) 554, 557
      epidemic 558–9
cross-cultural studies of disease–diet
   links 103, 107–10
cross-sectional studies of disease–diet
   linkage 117–18
cruciferous vegetables 354, 581

culinary style and dietary changes 24
culture 23, 56–62
   acceptability affecting availability
      of food 42, 56–62
   dietary changes and cultural
      values 24
   dietary prejudice and 32–3
   gatekeepers and 63
   resistance to change 59–60
   superfoods 36, 37
   see also cross-cultural studies
curare 354
cyanide release, cassava 565
cyanocobalamin *see* vitamin B_{12}
cycle ergometer 520
cysteine 4, 269, 348
   infant feeding 455
   selenium replacing sulphur in 400
cystic fibrosis 493–4
cytokines
   cancer cachexia and 186
   injury/illness and 501

daidzein 354, 577
dairy food 510–11
   energy density 175
   vegetarians eating
      (ovolactovegetarians) 507,
      509, 510
data sources and quality in disease–
   diet linkage studies 104–5
deaths *see* mortalities
deficiency diseases (in general) 6, 393
   developed/industrialized countries
      7, 435
   dietary change advice and curing
      of 24
   early 20th century curing of 3
   vitamin 358–9, 388
deforestation 47
DEFRA data on food selection 48,
   50, 51, 66, 67, 68
dehydration
   athletes, prevention 529
   hypernatraemic, and infant feeding
      with cow milk 456
dehydration and BMI 88
delayed hypersensitivity 4, 486–7
Δ (Delta) notation system for fatty
   acids 287
dementia and *Ginkgo biloba* 346
Demiquet index 87, 89
demi-span measurement 89
density
   body assessment 87, 91
   energy *see* energy
   nutrient 176–7
dental caries
   diet (sugars) and 107, 252–5

fluoride and *see* fluoride
deoxyribose 246
deprivation studies of requirements
   80–1
dermatitis (eczema) in childhood and
   probiotics 575, 576
desaturase and desaturation 297, 299,
   322
descriptive epidemiology of disease–
   diet links 103
   bowel cancer 263–4
   heart disease 312–13
developed (industrialized/Western/
   affluent) countries
   consumer classification of foods in
      34
   disease–diet linkage in 107–8
   Eastern diet in 40
   food selection 48–56
      poverty/low-income and 48–56,
      150
   health promotion in, at expense of
      poorer countries 154–5
   migration from developing
      countries to 60–1
   obesity 204–9
   suboptimal nutrition and deficiency
      disorders 7, 435
      iron deficiency 408–9, 410
   see also Western diet and lifestyle
developing (less-developed/less-
   industrialized) countries
   deficiency disorders 6
      iron 410
   health promotion in wealthier
      countries at expense of 154–5
   infant feeding 456–7
      bottle-feeding 453, 456–7
      breastfeeding prevalence 451
   migration to developing countries
      60–1
dexfenfluramine 237
diabetes 488–93
   British Asians 516–17
   diagnosis 489
   historical treatments 490
   in pregnancy 440
   principles of management 490–1
   symptoms and long-term
      complications 489–90
      cardiovascular disease 312, 490,
      492
   type 1 488–9, 491
      vitamin D insufficiency and 370
   type 2 312, 489, 491
      chromium and 395
      obesity/overweight and 8, 214,
      216, 219, 491
      South Asian migrants in UK 59

Diabetes Control and Complications
    Trial 489
diabetes model (*db/db*) of obesity
    196, 197, 198, 199, 200
diarrhoea (from food-borne bacteria)
    antibiotic-associated, and
        probiotics 575
    haemorrhagic 542
    infant/child, and pre- or probiotics
        575–6
    travellers' 543, 549, 576
    treatment 549
diet
    change in *see* behavioural change
    disease and *see* disease
    prejudice in 32–3
    recommendations and guidelines
        see recommendations and
        guidelines
    requirements *see* requirements
    standards *see* standards
    taboos *see* taboos
    treatment via *see* treatment
    weight-reducing *see* dieting
    Western *see* Western diet and
        lifestyle
Dietary Goals for the United States
    135
Dietary Guidelines for Americans
    135
dietary reference intakes (DRIs) 77
    energy in older adults 473
dietary reference values (DRVs) 65
    children 462, 463–4
    fat types 293
    minerals 393
dietetic care of general hospital
    patients 502
dieting (meal replacement) 232–4
    consumer books on 224–5, 233–4
    eating disorders and 183
    in pregnancy 442
    yo-yo 183, 217
digestion 162–4
    carbohydrate 162–3, 246, 255
    drugs blocking 238–9
    enyzmatic *see* enzymes
    fat 163–4, 301–2
    proteins 163, 268–70
    see also gastrointestinal tract
1,25-dihydroxyvitamin D (1,25-
    dihydroxycholecalciferol) 365,
    367–8, 369, 370, 412
dipeptidases 270
disability, expectation of life without
    471
    see also physical difficulties
disaccharides 246
discrimination, obesity 215

disease and illness (long-term/
    chronic/in general)
    ageing and 470–1
    evidence linking diet and 16,
        18–19, 102–33
    elderly 479–83
    methods of obtaining 102–33
    minerals and 393, 402–32
    obesity and 213, 214, 216, 217
    oxidant theory of *see* anti-oxidants;
        oxidant theory
    prevention of/protection from
        disease
        anti-oxidants 341–6
        changes in diet 7–16, 25
        plant secondary metabolites
            355–6
    sodium and 421–6
    starvation and malnutrition in 178
        hospital patients 500
    see also specific diseases
distribution (in body), food additives
    571
diterpenes 353
docosahexaenoic acid (DHA) 290,
    297, 298, 317
    algal extracts 298, 323
    brain and 297, 319
    cardiovascular deaths and 320
    fish oil 317
docosapentaenoic acid (DPA) in fish
    oil 317
doctors, nutritional education 503
double-blinding in trials 124, 125
Douglas bag 99
drugs
    blood pressure-lowering 423
    cholesterol-lowering 14, 314–16,
        482, 580
    obesity treatment 200, 237–9
        side-effects 241
    osteoporosis treatment 420
    thermogenesis induced by 188, 239
dual-centre hypothesis of energy
    intake 193–4
Dutch Hunger Winter (1944-5) 437,
    441, 443

E numbers 570
Eastern countries
    import to Western countries of diet
        from 40
    import of Western diet to 40
eating disorders 182–5
    causes 183–4
    characteristics and consequences
        182–3
    females *see* women
    incidence 183

treatment 184–5
    see also feeding; intake; overeating
ecological basis of taboos 58
economic and financial dimensions
    behavioural change 28
    food availability 41, 43–56
    obesity 214–15
    see also cost; income; poverty;
        social status
eczema (childhood), probiotics
    575, 576
education (nutritional) 3–29
    cultural significance of food 36
    current priorities 7–16
    of doctors and nurses 503
    on food selection 33, 150–4
    traditionally priorities 5–7
    weight control 230
    willingness to change and 147–9
educational attainment and obesity
    levels 209
eggs
    protein quality 282
    Salmonella and 551–2
eicosanoids 285, 297
    essential fatty acids and 298–9
    fish oil effects on production 318
eicosapentaenoic acid (EPA) 287, 297
    in cancer cachexia 186
    chemical structure 286, 287
    eicosanoid production and 318
    from fish oil 186, 290, 317
elastase 163, 270
elderly (older adults) 469–83
    BMI 477
        assessment 88
        prognostic significance 481
    demographic and social trends
        469–71
    diets and nutritional status 475–9
    disease and diet in 479–83
    osteoporosis and its prevention 416,
        417, 418–19, 419–20, 474
    physical activity levels 480, 522,
        523, 524, 525
    requirements and guidelines 473–5
    reference nutrient intakes for
        males 436
    supplementation (in general),
        dishonest/fraudulent results
        133
    traditional beliefs 150
    see also ageing
electron transport chain 158
elongase (elongation enzymes) 297,
    299
employment *see* work
enabling factors in BASNEF model of
    behavioural change 27, 28–9

endergonic reactions 157
endocannabinoids 194
    receptors 238
        antiobesity drug targeting 238
endocrine system (and hormones)
    in calcium homeostasis 412
    in energy balance regulation 198
    gut hormones and satiety
        signalling 194
    starvation affecting 181
endopeptidases 163, 269–70
endurance training 527, 528
energy 167–201
    balance *see* energy balance
    cellular energetics *see* cells
    content of food/macronutrients
        171, 292
    density 174–6
        children 176, 463, 465
        fat *see* fat
    expenditure
        drugs increasing 239
        matching intake to 139–40
        measurement 98–100
        regulation 189–90
    intake 187, 188
        athletic performance and 526–30
        decline in recent decades 7, 227
        elderly 476–9
        guidelines and recommendations
            139–40
        hospital patients, depressed 500
        matching expenditure to
            139–40
        National Dietary and Nutritional
            Surveys of *see* National Dietary
            and Nutritional Surveys
        in lactation 82
    low-energy diets *see* low-energy
        diets
    marasmus attributed to deficit of
        282–3
    negative 188
    percent energy as fat 146
        in various foods 12, 292, 293
    percent energy in macronutrients
        (other than fat) 172
        British diet 146
        protein 273, 274
    positive 188
    pregnancy and 436, 441–3
    requirements 168–72
        children 462–7
        elderly 473, 474–5
        estimation 168–70
        lactation 82, 448–9
        UK *see* United Kingdom
        US 160, 168, 169
        variations/general trends 170–2

    see also dietary reference values;
        estimated average requirement
    sources of 167
        elderly 476
        fat as 294–5
        by food groups *see* food groups
        by (macro)nutrient type 172–4
        in starvation 179
        units 167
        weaning foods 461
    see also protein–energy
        malnutrition
energy balance 187–201
    animal studies 120–1
    concepts 187–8
        set-point theory 189
    non-starch polysaccharides and 259
    physical activity levels and 168,
        169, 235
    regulation 120, 188–201
        external factors 192
        physiological 188–9
England *see* United Kingdom
enrichment of foods *see* fortification
enteral (tube) feeding 502, 503
    outcomes 504–5
environment
    for bacterial growth 545
    disease associations with 113
    free radical generation by factors
        from 335
    obesity associations with 220–1
    taboos relating to 58
    see also nature
Environmental health Officers
    (EHOs) 534
enzymes 156–7, 246
    digestive (GI tract)
        carbohydrate digestion 162–3,
            246
        fat digestion 163, 301–2
        pancreatic *see* pancreatic
            enzymes
        protein digestion 163, 269–70
    mineral-containing
        chromium 395
        copper 337, 396
        magnesium 396, 397
        manganese 397, 398
        molybdenum 398
        selenium 337, 400
        zinc 400, 401
    in pentose phosphate pathway 162
    see also specific enzymes
EPIC (European Prospective
    Investigation into Cancer and
    Nutrition) 113, 265, 516
epidemiological studies of disease–
    diet links 103, 104–15

bowel cancer 107, 114, 263–6
    features and problems 104–7
    heart disease 312–13
    hypertension and salt 427–8
ergosterol 309, 579
ergot poisoning 566–7
erythrocytes (red cells)
    aspartate or alanine
        aminotransferase test 380
    folate concentrations, assessment
        384, 385
    glutathione reductase activation
        test 83, 96–7, 377
Escherichia coli 543, 552
    O157 541, 542, 543, 545, 549,
        552
    verocytotoxin-producing (VTEC)
        541, 542, 546, 552, 560
essential nutrients
    conditionally 4–5, 324, 348–63
    identification 3–5
    see also specific nutrients
estimated average requirement (EAR)
    76–7, 77
    energy (EER) 168, 170
        by age and other lifecycle groups
            436, 473
        in lactation 82, 448
        in pregnancy 441–2
    protein 271, 273, 281
        in pregnancy 444
ethics 38
    withholding treatment in control
        groups 126
ethnic minorities 513–19
    specific, health and nutrition
        514–17
    UK 513, 514–18
        Asians *see* South Asian/Indian
            subcontinent people
        dietary comparisons of different
            groups 514–18
        four generation concept of food
            choices 61–2
        obesity 207–8
ethnicity (race)
    breastfeeding and 452
    weaning from 460
    obesity and 207
    osteoporotic fractures and 417
ethnocentrism 32–3
Europe
    bread as superfood 36
    obesity prevalence 206
    see also European Union
European Food Safety Authority on
    additives 569–70
European Food Standards Agency
    539, 569

European Prospective Investigation into Cancer and Nutrition (EPIC) 113, 265, 512
European Union
  health claims of foods 539
  micronutrient supplements 325, 327, 328
    Food Supplements Directive 328, 393
  RDAs on food labels 78, 79
evening primrose oil 298, 299, 321, 322, 323, 346
evolutionary selection pressure and obesity 219–20
excretion, food additives 571
exercise see physical activity
exergonic reactions 157
exopeptidases 163, 270
Expenditure and Food Survey 66, 67, 68
experimental studies
  animals see animals
  disease–diet links 103, 103–4, 118–32
    heart disease 122, 313–14
    humans 103, 121–32
    hypertension–salt 428–9
    in-vitro 132–3
  natural see natural experiments
extrinsic non-milk sugar 249
eye
  age-related macular degeneration 355, 356
  retinopathy see retinopathy
  vitamin A and vision in the 362–3
    effects of deficiency on night vision 357, 359, 361, 363–4

factorial calculation of nutrient requirements 82
FAD (flavin adenine dinucleotide) 377
faeces, calcium fluxes 412
  see also diarrhoea
falls in elderly, prevention of/ protection from 419
family (families), obesity running in 220–1
Family Expenditure Survey 66–7, 68
family therapy, eating disorders 184
farmers, heart disease 311
  see also agriculture
fasting see dieting; hunger; starvation
fat (dietary lipid) 285–323
  absorption 163–4, 301–2
  chemical structure 286, 287
  childhood diets 465
  content of various foods 12, 292

effect of adding small amounts of fat 294–5
weaning 296, 459, 460–1
definition 285
digestion 163–4, 301–2
disease risk related to types of 9
  colon cancer 114, 115
energy density 174, 176, 226
  altering fat content of food affecting 294–5
as energy source 172, 173, 294–5
fattening potential compared to carbohydrate 224–6
guidelines and recommendations 140–2
  expert reports 135, 136
health images 306–9
  heart disease and see heart disease
intake, UK 292–4
intake reduction
  aim 11
  barriers 230–1
  see also low-fat diet
metabolism 161–2
  oxidation see oxidation
natural, supplements 326
palatability 226, 230, 295–6
peroxidation 335, 372
purchase for home consumption, 1975/1996 comparisons 148
role in diet 294–300
satiety and see satiety
saturated see saturated fat
sources 291–4
substitute (olestra) 238–9, 571
transport 301–2, 303–4
types 287–91
  disease risk related to see subheading above
  see also hyperlipidaemia
fat (tissue/body) see adipose tissue
fat-soluble vitamins 296, 358
fat–sugar seesaw 149, 173
fatness, assessment
  in animals 94–5
  methods 87, 89–90, 91–2
fatty acids (dietary)
  chemical structure 286, 287
  cholesterol levels and 11
  essential 297–9
    deficiency 297
    eicosanoids and 298–9
  health images (regarding heart disease) 307–9
  metabolism 160–1
    oxidation see oxidation
  saturation degree and chain length effects on melting points 288

short-chain, from fibre and starch 258, 263
sources 291–4
  proportion of fatty acid types in various sources 289–90
types 287–91
  distribution in dietary fat 289–90
  saturated see saturated fat and fatty acids
  unsaturated see monounsaturated fatty acids; polyunsaturated fatty acids; unsaturated fatty acids
fatty streaks 304
favism 565
feeding/eating
  glycaemic response 262
  habit 192
  of hospital patients 502–3
  hospital patients, physical difficulties 500
  hunger and, weakening link between 221–5
  infants see infants
  thermogenesis 188
  see also dieting; intake; overeating
females see girls; women
fenfluramine 237
fermentation of non-starch polysaccharides 258–9
ferritin 406
  plasma/serum, measurement 406, 407–8
fertility, breastfeeding reducing 458
fetus
  alcohol syndrome 376, 447–8
  famine exposure in Dutch Hunger Winter (1944-5) 437
  glucose availability 442–3
  growth see growth
  vitamin A and development in 363
  see also teratogenicity
fibre (incl. non-starch polysaccharides; NSPs) 246, 257–61
  bowel cancer and 107, 262–6
  current intakes 257–8
  diabetics 491
  elderly 482
  as energy source 171
  guidelines and recommendations on intake 136, 141, 142
  heart disease and 266
  infant weaning and 461
  short-term physiological effects of increasing intake 258–9
  see also high-fibre diets; lignin; low-fibre diets; starches, resistant

fibrinogen (plasma) and obesity 214
fifths (quintiles) in cohort studies 114
filling foods, inexpensive, consumer
    attitudes to 35
finance *see* economic and financial
    dimensions
fish
    consumption
        guidelines and recommendations
            139
        income in industrialized
            countries and 49
        World's fish stocks and 154–5
    energy density 174, 175, 226
    oily 139, 581
    vegetarians avoiding 507
fish oil (incl. fish liver) and other
        marine oils 290, 292, 298,
        317–22
    in cancer cachexia 186
    consumption
        guidelines and recommendations
            139, 321–2
        myocardial infarction (previous)
            and effect on deaths of 127–8
    disease and 319–21
        health images of fish oil 308
        heart 308, 319–20, 346
        protective effect mechanisms
            318–19
    eicosapentaenoic acid from 186,
        290, 317
    sources 292
flavin adenine dinucleotide (FAD)
    377
flavin mononucleotide (FMN) 377
flavonols 354
flavourings 568, 570
flaxseed oil 298, 299, 323
flour enrichment/fortification
    folic acid 386, 388, 446
    niacin 379
fluoridation, water 127
fluoride 393, 396–7
    dental caries and 127, 254
    infants and 461–2
    guidelines and recommendations
        147
    supplements 396
FMN (flavin mononucleotide) 377
foam cells 304
folate/folic acid (vitamin B$_9$) 383–9
    adequate intake in UK, assessment
        331, 332
    assessment of status 384
    childhood RNI 464
    deficiency/biochemical
        insufficiency 359, 382
        anaemia 359

British Asians 515
elderly 478
preconceptual/early pregnancy,
    and neural tube defects 22,
    125, 385–6, 386–7, 446–7
functions 383
hazards/toxicity 384, 387, 387–8
nature 384–5
prevalence 384
recommendations on high intakes
    384
risk factors 383
sources 383, 384–5
standards 383
supplements 22, 125, 384, 385–7
    preconceptual 22, 125, 385–6,
        386–7, 440, 446–7
typical highest UK intakes 384
folk medicine 39
follow-on formulas 456
food(s)
    allergy 4, 485–6
    availabilities *see* availabilities
    biological model (function) of 31–2
    classification systems 33–8
    composition tables *see* food tables
    fortification *see* fortification
    functional 39, 309, 328, 539, 561,
        573–83
    glycaemic index *see* glycaemic
        index
    hospital, unacceptability 500
    intake *see* intake
    labelling *see* labelling of foods
    non-nutritional (non-biological) uses
        23–4, 30, 31, 38–9, 39–40
    palatability *see* palatability
    preparation, safe 544–7
    processed *see* processed food
    production
        domestic, estimation (for food
            balance sheets) 65
        worldwide 46, 47
    recommendations 137–9
    safety and quality *see* safety and
        quality
    selection 30–63
        aids 33, 150–4
        poverty/low-income and
            (industrialized countries)
            48–56, 150
    storage *see* storage
    variety, obesity and 223–4
food additives 564, 568–73
    animal toxicology studies 119–20
    uses 568
        arguments for and against 568–9
Food and Drug Administration
    (FDA) on additives 569

food balance sheets 65–6
food diaries
    in household budget surveys 66, 67
    individuals 69
        allergy 485
        energy sources 177
food groups 33, 151
    source of energy by 177–8, 292
        childhood–adult comparisons
            467
    source of fat by 292
    source of starch by 247
food intolerance 484
    lactose intolerance 575
    therapy 484
food plates (tilted plate model) 33,
        153–4
    sources of energy 178
food poisoning (food-borne diseases)
        540–54
    organisms causing 541–4, 551–4
    outbreaks, causes 545–6
        pinpointing 549–51
    prevention/avoidance of 544–9
    treatment 549
    see also diarrhoea
food pyramids 33, 151–3
    sources of energy 178
Food Safety Act (1990) 534
Food Standards Agency (FDA) 534
    labelling 536
    salt reduction targets 425–6
    supplements 327, 345
    see also European Food Standards
        Agency
Food Supplements Directive 328, 393
food tables (of composition) in
        nutritional assessment 72–4
    problems and errors 71, 73–4
foreign travel, diarrhoea 543, 549,
        576
forest destruction 37
formula feeding *see* bottle-feeding
fortification (enrichment) of foods
        329–30, 334
    folic acid 386, 387, 388, 446
    iron 409–10, 410
    niacin 379
    vitamin D 371
four food group plan 151
fractures
    hip (non-osteoporotic or in
        general), nutritional treatment
        504
    osteoporotic 369, 414–20
        factors impacting on risk of 414–
            19
        hip 415, 416, 418
        prevention 419–20

Framingham study 113–14
free radicals 335–41
    disease due to *see* oxidant theory
    physiological mechanisms limiting
        damage by 336–8
    reactions 335
        peroxidation of fat 335, 372
    situations increasing damage by
        338–9
    see also respiratory burst
Freudian theory, eating disorders 184
fructose 246
    oligomers, as prebiotics 574
fruit
    costs 150
    disease and levels of consumption
        of 138–9, 342–5
        cancer 9, 19, 138, 263, 265,
            342–5
    energy density 174, 175
    as energy source 178
    guidelines and recommendations
        on intake 138–9
        elderly 483
    as superfoods 337–8, 581–2
    Western (industrialized)
        countries consumption of
        effects on poorer countries 155
        income and 49
fruit and vegetable group 151
functional foods 39, 309, 328, 539,
    561, 573–83
fungi
    protein products 279–80
    toxins 563, 566
fungicide-treated seeds, eating of 567
funnel plot 129

galactosaemia 4, 248
galactose 246
    ovarian cancer and 116
gamma (γ)-ray treatment of food
    562
garlic 354–5, 581
    heart disease and cancer and 20
gastric... *see* stomach
gastroenteritis 541, 542
    foreign travel and 543
    infants 457–8, 459
gastrointestinal tract (alimentary
        tract/gut)
    calcium fluxes 412
    digestion and absorption in *see*
        absorption; digestion
    food-borne infections *see* food
        poisoning
    macronutrient handling 162–4
    microflora, and infant feeding
        method 456, 575

non-starch polysaccharide effects
    258–9
    satiety signals and 194, 194–5
    see also specific parts/regions
gatekeepers controlling food supply
    34, 42, 62–3
gender *see* sex
'generally recognized as safe' (GRAS)
    list 569
genetic cases of CJD 556, 557
genetic factors, obesity 220–1
genistein 354, 577, 578
ghrelin 195, 200, 239
gingivitis 254
Ginkgo biloba 346, 347, 353, 354
girls
    obesity 209, 210
    reference nutrient intakes 436, 464
    sex hormones and puberty 463
    WHO standards for height 93
Gla proteins 373
global/worldwide/international
        dimensions
    economic availability of food 44–8
    obesity 204–7
    protein deficiency/crisis (false
        indication) 14, 18, 119, 278–83
glucagon-like peptide 1 (GLP-1) 195
gluconeogenesis 1161
glucosamine and arthritis 346, 349–
    50
    in-vitro studies 132
glucose 246
    absorption (and transporters) 163
    blood concentrations *see* glycaemia;
        glycaemic index
    metabolism 158–60
        carbohydrate consumption and
            its effects on 226
    structure 256
    tolerance
        fibre improving 258, 266
        testing 489
glucosinolates 354, 581
    chronic disease prevention 355
GLUT-5 163
glutamic acid 269
    carboxylated residues 373
    in folic acid structure 384
glutamine 4, 269, 348
glutathione peroxidase and selenium
    337
glutathione reductase 337
    activation test, erythrocyte 83,
        96–7, 377
gluten-sensitive enteropathy *see*
    coeliac disease
glycaemia (blood glucose
        concentrations) 489

in diabetes
    control 491–2
    in diagnosis 489
    obesity and 214
    satiety and (the glucostat) 194,
        195–6
    see also hyperglycaemia;
        hypoglycaemia
glycaemic index (GI) 261–2, 492
    diabetes and 492
    high 261
    low 233, 261
    medium 261
glycerol 285
    metabolism 160–1
glycine 269
glycocholic acid 455
glycogen 255
    anaerobic metabolism 528
    stores and endurance sports
        528–9
glycolysis 158–9
glycosylation in diabetes 490
goitre 402, 403–4
    foods inducing 405, 566
gold thioglucose, satiety studies 195
GRAS (generally recognized as safe)
    list 569
Green Revolution 47
green tea 354, 581–2
groups (food) *see* food groups
groups (people)
    nutritional assessment 65–8
    special/specific 435–83, 507–30
        in disease–diet linkage studies
            110
        targeting of recommendations at
            137
growth
    bacterial
        minimizing storage time in
            conditions allowing 547, 548
        requirements 545
    children 463
        zinc deficiency and 401
    fetal 440
        and glucose availability 442–3
    guideline(s) *see* recommendations and
        guidelines
    guideline daily amounts (GDAs)
        536–7
    gum disease 254
    gut *see* gastrointestinal tract

habitual eating 192
haem iron 407
    vegetarian diet 511
haemagglutinin, red kidney bean 566
haemochromatosis 407

haemodilution, iron deficiency with 409
haemoglobin
   concentration, measurement 83, 95–6, 406
   glycosylation in diabetes 490
haemorrhage (blood loss) leading to iron deficiency 409
haemorrhagic diarrhoea 542
haemorrhagic disease of newborn and vitamin K deficiency 359, 373
Hartnup disease 269, 484
Hawaii, Japanese immigrants 61
HDL see high-density lipoprotein
healing of wounds and zinc deficiency 401–2
health
   ageing and 470–1
   beliefs and taboos about 58
   food law in consumer health protection 533
   physical activity long-term benefits 524–6
   specific ethnic minority groups, and nutrition 514–17
   see also disease
health claims on food labels
   low-fat foods 295
   UK 536, 539
   US 538, 539
Health of the Nation 106, 139, 153, 521
health promotion and campaigns
   barriers to success 25–7
   body fat-focused 218
   bone health (in osteoporosis prevention and treatment) 419, 420
   diet as means to 7–16, 230
   iron sufficiency 409
   P:S ratio, overemphasis 312
   in wealthier countries at expense of poorer ones 154–5
   weight control in populations 230
   willingness to change and 147–9
   see also behavioural change; education
Health survey for England 203, 208, 210, 227
Healthy Eating Pyramid (UK) 153
healthy foods and diet 52–6
   availability (as alternatives to less-healthy foods) 149–50
   minimum cost 52–6, 150
   refreshing, consumer attitudes to 35
Healthy People 2000, breastfeeding 450
Healthy People 2010, exercise 521, 522

children/adolescents 523–4
heart
   cardiomyopathy in Keshan disease 339, 400
   rhythm, fish oil effects 318
heart disease, coronary (and circulatory/cardiovascular disease) 266, 304–16
   alcohol consumption and 104, 145, 312
   antioxidants and 341–6
      carotenoids/β-carotene 130, 341–2
      vitamin E 130, 342, 343, 344
   Asians in UK 311–12, 516–17
   cholesterol levels and 304–16
      evidence for cholesterol involvement 312–16
      interventions to reduce cholesterol in prevention of disease 20–2
   diabetics 312, 490, 492
   evidence linking diet with 311–16
   fat and 304–16
      saturated 107, 108, 122, 306–7, 307, 311, 312, 313, 314
      fibre and 266
      fish oil and 308, 319–20, 346
      folate and 387
      free radicals and 339
      fruit/vegetable consumption and 138
      garlic and 20
      key tenets of hypothesis linking diet with 310–11
   Multiple Risk-Factor Intervention Trial 127, 314
   obesity and 213, 216, 312
   physical activity levels and 312, 525
   plant secondary metabolites and 356
   smoking as confounding variable in epidemiological studies of diet and 19
heat
   conservation, animals 121
   generation see thermogenesis
heat treatment of foods
   insufficient 548
   ultra-high 561–2
height/stature 87–8
   in BMI assessment 88
   children (related to age) 92–3
   measurement 87–8
   alternative to 89
Helicobacter pylori 423
herbal medicines 5, 325, 326, 346, 347, 355
hexose 246

hierarchies (in food choice models)
   of availabilities 41–63
   of human needs 39–41
high-density lipoprotein (HDL) and HDL cholesterol 300
   alcohol consumption and 145
   heart disease and 307
high-fat diet in diabetes 490
high-fat milk (whole fat), switch to low-fat from 148, 150, 293
high-fibre diets 142, 259
   bowel cancer and 263, 264, 265
   coronary disease and 266
   palatability 149
high-protein foods, problems in development 279
Hindus 515
   taboos 56, 58
hip fractures
   nutritional treatment 504
   osteoporotic 415, 416, 418
      fall prevention/protection 419
histidine 269
Holland, 1944–5 Hunger Winter 437, 441, 443
homeostasis and ageing 472
homocysteine levels and folate deficiency 387
honesty
   in individual food intake measurement 70
   scientific 133
hormone(s) see endocrine system
hormone replacement therapy (HRT) 417
   phyto-oestrogens as alternative 417, 578
hospital patients
   listeriosis risk with cook–chill foods 562
   malnutrition 496–505
hot and cold classification system 34
household (in food selection)
   gatekeepers 62–3
   income and budget 48–56
      surveys 66–8
housewife as gatekeeper 62–3
humans
   experiments on disease–diet linkage 103, 121–32
   hierarchies of needs 39–41
hunger
   eating and, weakening link between 221–5
   poverty and 47
   see also starvation
hyaluronic acid and free radicals 335
hydroxyapatite 411, 414
hydroxyl radical 335

5-hydroxytryptamine (serotonin)-reuptake inhibitors as appetite suppressants 237
25-hydroxyvitamin D (25-hydroxycholecalciferol) 367
hygiene
  bottle-feeding and 457–8
  food 548
    legislation 549
hypercalcaemia (high blood calcium) 411
hypercholesteraemia see cholesterol
hyperglycaemia in diabetes
  persistent, consequences 490
  repeated measurements in diagnosis 489
hyperlipidaemia
  diabetes 491
  familial 301
hypermetabolism in injury see injury
hypernatraemic dehydration and infant feeding with cow milk 456
hypersensitivity
  acute/immediate 4, 485–6
  delayed 4, 486–7
hypertension see blood pressure
hyperthyroidism 403
hypocalcaemia (low blood calcium) 411
hypoglycaemia in diabetics 491, 492
hypothalamus and energy intake 192–3, 193, 194, 195, 196, 197, 198, 199
hypothermia, old people 472

IDL (intermediate-density lipoprotein) 300, 303, 304
illness see disease and illness
immediate (acute) hypersensitivity 4, 485–6
immune system
  ageing effects 472
  breast milk immune-functioning components 457
  fish oil immunosuppressive effects 321
  malnutrition effects 498–9
  supplement effects in elderly on, dishonest/fraudulent results 133
  vitamin A and 363
    deficiency 46–7, 363, 498
  vitamin D and 368, 369, 370
  in zinc deficiency 401, 498
immunoglobulin A in malnutrition 498
immunoglobulin E and food allergy 485

in-vitro studies
  disease–diet links 132–3
  food additive toxicology 571
incidence of disease 105
income (and its effects on food selection) 48–56
  UK immigrants 60
  see also poverty
Indian childhood cirrhosis 396
Indian subcontinent migrants in UK see South Asian/Indian subcontinent migrants
individual (person)
  availability of food to 42
  dietary change at level of 20–2
  as enabling factor in behavioural change 28
  in food intake assessments 68–70
    in household surveys 67
  relationships between 38–9
  skills and knowledge about diet 150
  see also groups
industrialized countries see developed countries
infants (babies)
  deaths see mortalities
  diarrhoea, and pre- or probiotics 575–6
  feeding 449–62
    factors influencing choice of method 451–5
    see also bottle-feeding; breastfeeding
  lactase deficiency 248
  newborn see neonates
  retinopathy of prematurity 338
  weaning from milk see weaning
infection
  breastfeeding protective effects 457
  gastrointestinal, food-borne see food poisoning
  in malnutrition 181
    hospital patients 497, 498
  vitamin D status and susceptibility to 370
  see also transmissible spongiform encephalopathies
infective dose of food-borne bacteria 543
  high 543
  low 542, 543
inflammatory response
  ageing and 472
  fish oil effects 318
  vitamin D and 368, 369–70
information (nutritional) on labels
  UK 535–6
  US 537

ingredients on packaged food labels
  UK 535–6
  US 537
injury/trauma
  immune system in 498–9
  metabolic response (hypermetabolism) 501, 502
  protein breakdown 271, 501
  nutrient requirements in 500–1
insulin 195, 196, 199
  resistance 219, 489
    heart disease and 311, 312
    metabolic consequences 219, 489
    minority groups in UK 489, 516
  therapy 489, 490, 491
intake (consumption) of nutrients
  energy see energy
  external influences 192
  hospital patients
    depressed 499–500
    monitoring 504
  ideal, current UK diets compared with 146
  measurement 65–72
  recommendations and guidelines on see recommendations and guidelines
  see also adequate intake; dietary reference intakes; feeding; reference nutrient intakes and specific (types of) nutrients and food groups e.g. fruit; meat; vegetables
Integrated Household Survey, Living Costs and Food module 66–7
intermediate-density lipoprotein (IDL) 300, 303, 304
international dimensions see global/worldwide/international dimensions
interpersonal relationships 38–9
intervention trials/studies at population level 104, 126–8
  cancer and anti-oxidants 343–4
  energy supplements in pregnancy 443
  heart disease 127, 314, 344
  hypertension and salt intake 428
  vitamin C status 371
interviewer bias in individual food intake estimation 69
intestine see bowel
intolerance to food and its therapy 484
iodine 402–5
  adequate intake in UK 333
  deficiency 6, 393, 403–4
    effects of 402, 403–4

prevalence 402
  risk factors 402
  fortification 329
  functions 402, 402–3
  requirements and intake 404–5
  supplements 402, 404
ionizing radiation treatment of food
    562–3
Irish people in UK 514
iron 405–10
  adequate intake
    assessment 332
    vegetarian diet 511
  athletes, status and requirements
    527
  balance, regulation 407
  biochemical measure of status (Hb
    concentration) 83, 95–6, 406
  catalase and 337
  children
    intakes 465, 466
    requirements/recommendations
      464
  deficiency/poor status 405, 407–10
    anaemia 393, 405, 406, 407–10
    elderly 478
    prevalence 406, 408
    prevention 409
    risk factors 405
    vegetarians 511
  fortification of foods 409–10, 410
  functions 405
  guidelines and recommendations 147
    children 464
    on high intakes 406
  menstrual loss 406, 474
  overload 407
  in pregnancy see pregnancy
  requirements 406–7
  sources 405, 410
  supplementation 406, 409, 410
    pregnancy 14–15, 445–6
  toxicity 406
  typical highest intakes in UK 406
irradiation of food 562–3
irrigation overuse 47
isoflavones 354, 577, 581
isoleucine 269
isomaltase 163, 246, 255
Israel, immigrants to 60

J-curve (of mortality)
  alcohol consumption 143
  body mass index 212
Jadad score 125
Japan
  disease–diet linkage 111
  Hawaiian migrants from 61
  superfoods 36

jaw-wiring 240
Jewish food restrictions 39, 43, 58
  see also Israel
joint inflammation see arthritis
joule 167

kelp, iodine in 404
Keshan disease 339, 400
ketones/ketone bodies 160, 179–80
kidney (renal...)
  calcium and 412
  chronic failure 495–6
  diabetic disease 490
  salt/sodium handling and essential
    hypertension 422
kidney bean poisoning 566
kilocalories 167
  see also calories
kinky hair (Menke's) disease 395–6
Kjeldahl method 271
knee height measurement 89
knowledge (individual) and skills
    about diet 150
Krebs cycle 160
kuru 555, 556, 557, 558
kwashiorkor 280, 282–3

labelling of foods 535–40
  RDAs in EU on 78, 79
lactase 163, 246
  deficiency (congenital and
    secondary) 248
  primary lactase non-persistence
    248
lactation 448–9
  energy requirements (incl. EAR)
    82, 448–9
  nutritional preparedness for 439–
    40
  reference nutrient intakes 436, 448,
    449
  species variations in relative
    burdens 438
  see also breastfeeding
lactic acid production 158, 159
  lactic acid-producing bacteria (incl.
    lactobacilli)
    infant feeding methods and 456
    in probiotics 574, 575, 576
lactoferrin 457
lactose 248
  intolerance 248, 575
lathyrism 565
law/legislation (and regulations) on
    food 533–5
  food additives 569–71
  hygiene legislation 549
  labelling in US 537
LDL see low-density lipoprotein

lecithin 351–2
legislation see law
leptin 196–7, 198–200
  congenital deficiency 200
  therapeutic use (incl. analogues)
    200, 239
less-developed countries see
    developing countries
leucine 269
life expectancy 471
  body mass index and 211–13
  England and Wales 469
lifecycle 435–83
  see also age
lifestyle
  infant feeding choices and 452–3
  in old age, active 471
  osteoporotic (and fracture) risk and
    416–18
  promoting lifestyle change 419
  Western see Western diet and
    lifestyle
lignans 577, 580
lignin 257
lingual lipase 301
  breast milk 456
linoleic acid 287
  chemical structure 286, 287
  conjugated (CLA) 288–9
linolenic acid 297, 298, 299, 322, 323
linseed (flaxseed) oil 298, 299, 323
lipases 163, 164, 301–2
  lingual see lingual lipase
  lipoprotein 301, 303
  pancreatic, drug blocking 238
lipid see fat; hyperlipidaemia
α-lipoic acid 351
lipoprotein(s) (blood/plasma) 300–1
  fish oil effects 318
  in lipid transport 303–4
  see also specific types
lipoprotein lipases 301, 303
lipostat 194, 196–7
liposuction 240
Listeria monocytogenes 541, 554
  cook–chill foods and 554, 562
liver
  glycogen stores and endurance
    sports 528–9
  Indian childhood cirrhosis of 396
Living Costs and Food module of
    Integrated Household Survey
    66–7
low birth weight 439
  maternal energy and 442, 443, 444
low-carbohydrate diets 225, 233–4
  diabetics 491
low-density lipoprotein/LDL (and
    LDL-cholesterol) 300

free radicals and 335
functional foods effects on levels of
    plant sterols 579–81
    probiotics 575
    soy products 578
    heart disease and 304–5, 307, 312
    plant secondary metabolites and
        356
    receptor 303
        gene defect 304
        reduced synthesis 304
    recommendations on reducing
        plasma levels 142
low-energy diets
    children 176
    unlimited access to low energy
        foods 234
    very 240–1
low-fat (fat-reduced) diets 225, 230,
    233, 295
    orlistat and 238
    very 225, 295
low-fat foods (in general), health
    claims 296
low-fat milk, switch from high-fat to
    148, 150, 293
low-fibre diets
    bowel cancer and 262, 263–4, 265
    type 2 diabetes and 489
low-protein diet in chronic renal
    failure 495
low-salt diet
    in BP reduction 429
    traditional 427, 428
lower reference nutrient intake
    (LRNI) 76, 79
    children 464, 468
    micronutrients 78, 332, 468
    minerals 394, 468
lycopene 337, 341, 342, 581
lysine 269
    synthetic, for food supplementation
        280
lysozyme in breast milk 457

macrocytic (incl. megaloblastic)
    anaemia
    folic acid deficiency 359, 385
    iron deficiency 407
    vitamin B_{12} deficiency 359, 381,
        382, 510
macronutrients (essential) 3, 243–323
    childhood–adults comparisons in
        diets 467
    current UK diets compared with
        ideal intakes of 146
    energy content see energy
    guidelines and recommendations
        134–42

gut handling 162–4
    see also acceptable macronutrient
        distribution range and specific
        types of macronutrient
macular degeneration, age-related
    335, 356
magic foods, sympathetic 37
magnesium 396–7
    adequate intake in UK 333
    deficiency 396, 397
    supplements 396, 397
maize (corn) milling and niacin
    deficiency 379
malabsorption
    injured/sick patients 500–1
    vitamin B_{12} 4
males see boys; men
malnutrition (and suboptimal
    nutrition)
    ageing and 472
    in disease see disease
    hospital patients 496–505
    industrialized countries 435
    infection see infection
    pregnancy 437
    protein–energy see protein–energy
        malnutrition
    screening tool (MUST) 505
    wasting in starvation or 179, 497,
        498
    see also starvation
maltase 162, 246, 255
Malthus, Thomas 45
maltose, structure 256
mammalian meat and bone meal and
    BSE 556
manganese (and deficiency and
    supplements) 397–8
manganese superoxide dismutase 337
    deficiency 337
mannose and retinol 363
marasmus 282–3
margarines (and their health images)
    hard/trans-fatty acid containing
        288, 292, 293, 294, 308
    soft 288, 292, 293, 307
marine oils see fish oil and other
    marine oils
Masai diet 311
Maslow's hierarchy of needs 40
mastalgia, evening primrose oil 322,
    323, 346
maternity hospital (UK) changes in
    practice on breastfeeding
    (1990 to 2000) 454
meal see dieting; feeding
meat
    craving in Africa for 37
    energy density 174, 175

fat 291
    food poisoning outbreaks in UK
        546
    fungal protein as substitute for 280
    income in industrialized countries
        and consumption of 49
    red, and bowel cancer 265
    vegetarians avoiding 507
    see also mammalian meat and bone
        meal
meat group 151
megaloblastic anaemia see macrocytic
    (incl. megaloblastic) anaemia
α-melanocyte-stimulating hormone
    194
melting points of fatty acids,
    saturation degree and chain
    length effects on 288
memory errors in individual food
    intake estimation 69
men (males)
    cholesterol plasma levels in (UK)
        305, 306
    obesity 208
        defined by high waist-to-hip
            ratio 202
    reference nutrient intakes in the
        elderly 436
    skinfold thickness charts 90
    starvation experiment (Minnesota)
        184
    see also boys; sex (gender)
Menke's disease 395–6
menopausal oestrogens and
    osteoporotic fracture risk 417
menstrual period
    absence in female athletes 527
    iron loss 406, 474
mental development and
    phenylketonuria 250, 487
meta-analyses of disease–diet linkage
    103, 128–32
metabolic syndrome 219, 489
metabolism 156–64
    in cancer, disturbances 185–6
    carbohydrate 158–60
    fat see fat
    food additives 571
    injury response see injury
    protein/amino acid 161
    rate measurement 98–100
    see also basal metabolic rate
metabolizable energy 171
methionine 269, 352
    infant feeding 455
    selenium replacing sulphur in 400
methotrexate and folate 388
N'-methylnicotinamide, urinary
    excretion assessment 378

Mexican Americans, obesity 207
mice *see* mouse
micelles 164, 301
microbial flora in gut and infant
    feeding method 456, 575
microbiological safety of food *see* food
    poisoning
microcytic anaemia in iron deficiency
    407
micronutrients 324–432
    adequate intake
        assessment 330–4
        athletes 527
    childhood intakes and
        recommendations 462, 464,
        466, 467, 468
    dietary standards (RNI/LNRI/
        RDA) 78, 330–4
    elderly intakes and
        recommendations 477–8
    essential 3
    fortification *see* fortification
    pregnancy 438, 445–7
    supplements *see* supplementation
    see also minerals; vitamins
microvascular disease, diabetics 490
mid-arm circumference 87, 92
migration
    disease–diet linkage studies 103,
        112
        heart disease 312
        hypertension and salt 427–8
    eating habits and 58–62
    see also ethnic minorities
milk 248
    cow *see* cow milk
    fat 291
        switch to low-fat from high-fat
            148, 150, 293
    human *see* breast milk
    interspecies comparisons of
        composition 281
milk group 151
milk sugar 248
milk thistle and alcohol consumption
    11
mindex 89
minerals 393–432
    adequate intake
        assessment in UK 332, 333
        athletes 527
    biochemical tests of status 96
    chelation by non-starch
        polysaccharide 259
    childhood intakes and
        recommendations 464, 466,
        467, 468
    dietary standards 78, 79
    disease and 393, 402–32

in food tables
    adhered soil and 74
    bioavailability 74
    cooking water and 74
income in industrialized countries
    and intake of 49
infant feeding 456
pregnancy 438, 445–6
supplementation 326
mitochondria, oxidative
    phosphorylation 157–8
moisture and bacterial growth 545
molybdenum (and deficiency and
    supplements) 398
monoacylglycerol 163, 164
monoamine oxidase inhibitors and
    tyramine 120, 566
monosaccharides 246
    metabolism 158–60
monoterpenes 353
monotony in dieting 234
monounsaturated fatty acids
    cholesterol levels and 11
    health images (regarding heart
        disease) 307–8
    structure 286, 287
mood (affective) disorder, anorexia
    nervosa as 184
morality 38
morphine 354
mortalities/deaths
    alcohol consumption and 143–4
    data (on disease in general) 105,
        106
        Japanese people 111–12
        migrants (incl. ethnic groups in
            UK) 112, 516
    elderly BMI and 481
    exercise levels impacting on 526
        see also physical fitness
    fish oil supplements effects in
        cardiovascular disease 319–20
    infant
        birth weight correlations with
            rate of 439
        cot death *see* cot death
        feeding choices and 457
    myocardial infarction (previous),
        effect of dietary interventions
        127–8
    obesity/high BMI and 212, 213,
        217
    preoperative nutritional
        interventions and 501
    salt reduction and its effects on
        429–30
mothers as gatekeepers 62–3
mouse, obesity model (*ob/ob*) 190,
    191, 196, 197, 198, 199, 200

MRFIT (Multiple Risk-Factor
    Intervention Trial) 127, 314
multiple publishing of trials 130
multiple risk-factor interventions in
    trials 126–7
    MRFIT 127, 314
multiple sclerosis and vitamin D
    deficiency 370
muscle
    glycogen stores, and endurance
        sports 528–9
    in malnutrition 497, 498
    mid-arm, circumference 87, 92
mushroom poisoning 566
Muslims in UK 515
mussels, saxitoxin (from plankton) in
    566
MUST (Malnutrition Universal
    Screening Tool) 505
mutagenicity testing of food additives
    571
mutual supplementation of protein
    276
mycotoxins 279–80
myocardial infarction (previous),
    dietary intervention effects on
    deaths 127–8
myoglobin 406

n system for fatty acids 287
n-3 (ω-3) polyunsaturated fatty acids
    11, 297–8, 299, 308, 317, 318,
    319
    in cancer cachexia, benefits 186
    in fish oil 317–18
    health images (regarding heart
        disease) 308, 312, 319–40
    in rheumatoid arthritis 320
n-6 (ω-6) polyunsaturated fatty acids
    11, 297, 298, 299, 308
    health images (regarding heart
        disease) 308
    UK recommendations 140
NAD and NADP *see* nicotinamide
    adenine dinucleotide;
    nicotinamide adenine
    dinucleotide phosphate
National Advisory Committee on
    Nutrition Education (NACNE,
    1983) 135, 144, 147
National Dietary and Nutritional
    Surveys (NDNSs) 51, 71, 88,
    106, 146
    childhood and adolescence 465,
        466–8, 523
    cholesterol concentrations 306
    cross-sectional studies 117
    energy intake 227
        by food groups 177, 467

fat intake 293
    micronutrients 330, 331
    older adults 476, 477
National Food Survey 51, 66, 67, 68
    calculation of minimum
        subsistence level 52
    carbohydrate 247
    energy intakes 227
    fat intake 292
National Institute for Health and
        Clinical Excellence, waist
        circumference 216
natural experiments (experiments of
        nature) 103, 118
    heart disease 313
natural fat supplements 326
natural medicines 346–56
natural toxicants 564, 565–7
nature
    disease–diet linkage studies and
        experiments of 103, 118
    obesity and nurture versus 220–1
    see also environment
needs (human), hierarchies of 39–41
neonates (newborn babies)
    birth weights see birth weights
    fetal alcohol syndrome 376, 447–8
    haemorrhagic disease and vitamin
        K deficiency 359, 373
nephropathy, diabetic 490
net iron cost of pregnancy 446
net protein utilization 277
Netherlands, 1944-5 Hunger Winter
        437, 441, 443
neural tube defects (NTDs) and folic
        acid 22, 125, 385–6, 386–7,
        446–7
neurological (brain) damage
    phenylketonuria 250, 488
    vitamin B_{12} deficiency 383, 388
    see also brain; mental development
neuropeptide Y 194, 195
neutrophils, respiratory burst see
        respiratory burst
newborns see neonates
niacin (vitamin B_3; nicotinic acid)
        158, 357, 377–9
    adequate intake in UK 332
    childhood RNI 464
    deficiency (and pellagra) 3, 59,
        360, 379
    endogenous synthesis 360
    in food tables 74
    sources 360, 377
    supplements
        in multivitamins 378
        warnings 328
NICE, waist circumference 216

nicotinamide adenine dinucleotide
        (NAD)
    in glycolysis 159
    in Krebs cycle 160
    in oxidative phosphorylation 157–8
nicotinamide adenine dinucleotide
        phosphate (NADP) 158
    in pentose phosphate pathway
        161–2
nicotine 354
nicotinic acid see niacin
night blindness 357, 359, 361, 363–4
Nightingale, Florence, on
        malnutrition 496
nitrogen
    balance 271–4
        concept 272–3
        negative 272
        positive 273
        requirements 272–3
    in cow vs breast milk 455
nitrosamines and gastric cancer 423
non-starch polysaccharides see fibre
norovirus 542, 543
nurses, nutritional education 503
Nurses' Health Study 114
nut(s) 582
    energy density 175
    fats/oils 291–2
    as superfoods 582
nutraceuticals (functional foods) 39,
        309, 328, 539, 561, 573–83
nutrients
    bacterial growth 545
    humans 243–432
        density 176–7
        deprivation studies 80–1
        intake, determining 65
        requirements see requirements
        supplementation see
            supplementation
    see also specific (types of) nutrient
Nutrition Labelling and Education
        Act of 1990 (NLEA) 537
Nutrition Task Force 153

obesity/overweight 202–42
    animal studies see animals
    caloric intake and 111, 136
    causes (possible) 219–29
        carbohydrate content of foods 11,
            224–6
    children see children
    consequences 211–19
        blood pressure increases 214, 430
        heart disease 213, 216, 312
        type 2 diabetes 8, 214, 216, 219,
            491

definition 202–3
    elderly 477, 480, 481
    individual treatment 229–41,
        232–42
        aggressive measures 237–42
        behavioural 222–3
        drug see drugs
        surgical 239–40
    physical activity levels and see
        physical activity
    population interventions 229–32
    prevalence 203–11
        Pima Indians 200, 207, 221
    prevention 229–30
    vigilance in 235–6
obligatory nitrogen loss 272
observational studies and methods
    disease linked to diet 102–3
        hypertension and salt intake
            427–8
    nutritional assessment 65
occupation see work
odds ratio 117
oedema and BMI 88
oestrogens
    menopausal, and osteoporotic
        fracture risk 417
    plant (phyto-estrogens) 574, 577–9
        breast cancer and 112, 578–9
        as HRT alternative 417, 578
oils 322–3
    energy density 175
    see also fish oil; nuts; seeds;
        vegetable oils
oily fish 139, 581
older adults see ageing; elderly
oleic acid 287
    chemical structure 286, 287
olestra 238–9, 571
olive oil 11, 290, 308, 581
omega-3 and -6 fatty acids see n-3
        polyunsaturated fatty acids;
        n-6 polyunsaturated fatty acids
onion family (Allium) 354–5, 581
    chronic disease prevention 355
operator bias in human experimental
        studies of disease–diet links
        122
    clinical trials 124
opsin 362
organic produce free from
        agricultural chemicals 567
organic substances with vitamin-like
        roles 324, 326, 337
orlistat 238
Orwell, George, and Road to Wigan
        Pier 54
osteoarthritis

fish oils 320
  glucosamine and chondroitin
      sulphate 349–50
osteomalacia and vitamin D
      deficiency 368–9
  British Asians 515
osteoporosis 414–20, 423, 474
  female athletes 527
  fractures in *see* fractures
  incidence 415–16
  prevention of (and its
      consequences) 369, 419–20
  physical activity in 418, 525
  phyto-oestrogens as alternative
      to HRT 417, 578
  risk factors for 414–19
  salt intake and 423
  treatment 420
  vitamin D status and 369, 419
outcome measures in human
      experimental studies of
      disease–diet links 122, 126–7
ovarian cancer and galactose 116
over-30-month (OTM) rule 558
overeating/overfeeding 188, 190
  experimental animals 192–3,
      195–6
overweight *see* obesity
ovolactovegetarians. 507, 509, 510
oxidant (free radical) theory of
      disease 122, 335–46
  fraudulent results 133
  see also respiratory burst
oxidation of foodstuffs 98–9
  cholesterol, adverse effects of
      oxidized cholesterol 309
  fat/fatty acids 321
    β-oxidation 160–1
    carbohydrate consumption
        lowering 226
    fish oil effects 321
oxidative phosphorylation 157–8
  uncoupling proteins (UCPs)
      158, 191
oxygen
  bacterial growth without 545
  consumption/uptake (VO$_2$)
      measurement 98–9
    maximum (VO$_{2max}$), in exercise
        520
oxygen free radicals *see* free radicals;
      oxidant theory of disease
oxyntomodulin (oxm) 195
  antiobesity potential 239

packaged food, ingredients on *see*
      ingredients on packaged food
      labels
paediatric population *see* children

palatability 149, 192
  fat increasing 226, 230, 295–6
palm oil 290
palmitic acid 287
  chemical structure 286, 297
pancreatic enzymes
  carbohydrate digestion *see* amylase
  fat digestion *see* lipase
  protein digestion 163, 269, 270
  supplements in cystic fibrosis 494
pancreatic peptide (PP) 195
pantothenic acid 389–90
para-amino benzoic acid (PABA) in
      folic acid 384
parathyroid hormone, recombinant
      (teriparatide) 420
parenteral feeding 503
parents, fatness levels correlating
      with children 220
pasteurized foods 561
  food poisoning risk 546
  production 561
    irradiation 563
pellagra 3, 359, 360, 379
pentose 246
pentose phosphate pathway 161–2
pepsin 163, 269
peptidases 163, 269–70
periodontal disease 254
peripheral foods 36
pernicious anaemia 4, 360, 383, 484
peroxidation, lipid/lipoprotein 335,
      372
person *see* individual
personality changes in starvation 181
pesco-vegetarian 507
phagocytic cells, free radical
      generation *see* respiratory burst
phase I and II enzymes and
      carcinogen detoxification 355
phenols 353–4, 581–2
phenylalanine 269
  intolerance *see* phenylketonuria
phenylketonuria 4, 275, 484, 487–8
  aspartame avoidance 250
  pregnancy and 440
phosphatidic acid 285
phosphatidylcholine (lecithin) 351–2
phospholipids 285
  in lipoproteins 300
phosphorus (and deficiency and
      supplements) 398
phosphorylation
  oxidative *see* oxidative
      phosphorylation
  substrate-level 157
    creatine phosphate and 528
phylloquinone *see* vitamin K
physical activity/exercise 519–30

ageing and decline in levels (PAL)
      of 473
blood pressure and 430, 431
bone density and levels of 418, 525
  females 527
children *see* children
  elderly 480, 522, 523, 524, 525
  energy requirements and levels
      (PAL) of 168, 169, 235
  guidelines and recommendations
      140
  heart disease and levels of 312, 525
  interventions increasing level (PAL)
      of 234–5
    schoolchildren 231
  long-term health benefits 524–6
  obesity/overweight and levels of
      111, 136, 140, 227–9, 230
    barriers to being more active 230
    interventions, *see subheading
        above*
  in osteoporosis prevention in older
      people 418
  setting targets for 521
  thermogenic effects 187
  UK
    British Asians' levels of 517
    current levels 521–5
    setting targets 521
  see also athletic performance
physical availability of food 41, 42–3
physical difficulties in eating by
      hospital patients 500
physical fitness 519–24
  mortality risk and 526
  obesity-related 218
  survey in UK 521, 523
    elderly 480
physical resources and behavioural
      change 28
physiologic group foods 37
phytochemicals *see* oestrogens; plants
Pima Indians, obesity 200, 207, 221
placebo effect in human experimental
      studies of disease–diet links
      122
  clinical trials 124
plants
  as functional foods 574, 577–81
    superfoods 337–8, 581–2
  secondary metabolites
      (phytochemicals) 5, 325,
      353–6
    anti-oxidant 337, 355, 581
    chronic disease prevention 355–6
    oestrogens *see* oestrogens
    sterols 309, 353, 574, 579–81
    sulphur-containing 254–5, 581
    supplements 326

toxicants 565, 566
  see also herbal medicines
platelet aggregation
  fish oils and 318
  plant secondary metabolites and
    356
plates *see* food plates
plethysmography, air displacement 91
political control of food supply 39
polypeptide YY (PPY) 195
polyphenols 337, 353–4, 581–2
  red wine 145, 583
polysaccharides 246
  non-starch *see* fibre
polyunsaturated fatty acid(s)
  cholesterol levels and 11, 122–3
  health images (regarding heart
    disease) 308
  n-3 and n-6 *see* n-3 (ω-3)
    polyunsaturated fatty acids;
    n-6 (ω-6) polyunsaturated
    fatty acids
  WHO recommendations on intake
    136
polyunsaturated fatty acid to
    saturated fatty acid (P:S) ratio
    11, 122–3, 290
  overemphasis in health promotion
    312
  various foods 12
populations
  anomalous, in cross-cultural
    studies 109–10
  cross-sectional studies (of disease–
    diet linkage) 117–18
  dietary change at level of 20–2
  growth 45–6
  interventions trials on level *see*
    intervention trials
  nutritional assessment 65–8
    sampling bias 70–1
  obesity prevention at level of
    229–32
  quintiles of, in cohort studies 115
  special groups *see* groups
portion/serving size
  UK 69
  US 537
postmenopausal HRT *see* hormone
    replacement therapy
postprandial thermogenesis 188
potassium 398–9
  adequate intake in UK 333
  blood pressure and 399, 430
  deficiency 399
  guidelines and recommendations
    147
    children 464
  supplements 399

potatoes
  obesity and 11
  solanine poisoning 566
  see also chips
poultry, food poisoning outbreaks in
    UK 546
poverty (poor/low-income people)
  birth weight and 443
  elderly 470
  in Expenditure and Food
    Survey 68
  food selection and, industrialized
    countries 48–56, 150
  hunger and 47
pravastatin 315
prebiotics 574, 575, 576
preconceptual period 440
  folate supplements 22, 125, 385–6,
    386–7, 440
pregnancy 437–48
  alcohol and 376, 447–8
  dietary allowance 438–9
  energy aspects 436, 441–3
  estimated requirements for 82,
    436, 440
  folic acid (planned pregnancy or in
    pregnancy) 440–1
    and neural tube defects 22, 125,
      385–6, 386–7, 440, 446–7
  iron in 445, 445–6
    deficiency, and associated
      anaemia 408, 409
    supplementation 14–15, 445–6
  malnutrition in 437
  micronutrients (in general) 438,
    445–7
  outcomes 439–40
  protein in 444–5
  reference nutrient intakes *see*
    reference nutrient intake
  scale of increased nutritional needs
    437–8
  species variations in relative
    burdens 438
  vitamin A and D contents of fish
    oil preparations, cautions 322
  see also preconceptual period
prematurity, retinopathy of 338
premenstrual syndrome, vitamin B$_6$
    administration 381
prestige foods 37
prevalence of disease 105
primary intervention trials 127
prion diseases 554
prion protein (PrP) 556, 557, 558
probiotics 574, 574–6
processed food 560–4
  energy density 174
  production 560–4

methods 561–2
  pros and cons 560–1
  salt reduction in 23, 426
proline 269
promoters (cancer) and phyto-
    oestrogens 355–6
prospective methods
  case–control studies using 116
  individual food intake estimation
    69–70
  compared with retrospective
    methods 70–1
prostaglandins 285, 297
  fish oil effects on production 318
protein 268–84
  absorption 163
  adequacy 273
  athletes, intake and requirements
    527–8
  carbohydrate combined with (food-
    combining diets) 234
  chemistry 268–9
  in chronic renal failure, diets low in
    495
  content in foods 273, 274
    estimation 271–2
  copper-containing 396
  deficiency 280, 282–3
  digestion 163, 268–70
  as energy source 172
  first-/second-class 276
  free radicals effects 335
  guidelines and recommendations
    140–2, 270–1, 273
  infant feeding 455–6
  intakes 270–1
  metabolism 161
  mutual supplementation of 276
  post-translational modification 273
  pregnancy and 444–5
  quality 274–8
    egg and wheat 282
    measurement 276–7
  ruminant, BSE transmission 556,
    557
  significance in human nutrition
    278–83
    historical overview 278–80
  sources 270–1
  standards 270–1
  turnover 272
    in injury 271, 501
  world crisis of deficiency (false
    indication) 14, 18, 119, 278–83
  see also enzymes
protein–energy malnutrition 283
  immune system in 498
prothrombin levels and vitamin K
    status 83–4

psychological causes
    eating disorders 184
    starvation 178
psychological effects
    of exercise 521
    of starvation 181
psychological function of food 23
psychological response to illness/
        hospitalization/diagnosis,
        anorexia resulting from 500
psychological treatments
    eating disorders 184
    obesity 222–3
pteridine in folic acid structure 384
puberty 463
public places, breastfeeding 57, 453,
        454
publishing of trials
    bias 129
    multiple 130
pyramids see food pyramids
pyridoxine see vitamin B$_6$
pyruvic acid, aerobic metabolism
        159–60

quality of food, safety and 533–83
quality of life
    elderly 471
    obesity and 213–15
quantification errors in individual
        food intake estimation 69
quinine 354
quintiles in cohort studies 114
Quorn 279–80

race see ethnic minorities; ethnicity
radioactive tracer studies of nutrient
        pools 81
radio-allergosorbent test 485
rapeseed oil (oilseed rape) 155, 290,
        298
rats
    behavioural characteristics in obese
        rats 222
    energy balance and its regulation
        189, 190, 191, 192–3,
        194–5
    fatness estimates 95
    protein/amino acid requirements
        275, 281–2
raw food, risk of food poisoning
        543
    reducing 546, 547, 548
reactive species of oxygen see free
        radicals; oxidant theory of
        disease
recipe variations and food tables 73
recommendations and guidelines
        (dietary) 134–55

questions for advisors to consider
        31
    range of expert reports and their
        consistency 134–6
    variations in presentation 136–7
    vegetarian diet 512–13
    see also specific nutrients and dietary
        standards
recommended dietary/daily
        allowance (RDA - mainly
        USA) 65
    calcium in children 463
    energy 168, 169, 177
        children 462–3
    food labels in EU 78, 79
    iodine 404
    micronutrients in general (in USA)
        78, 446
    older and younger adults 474
    origin 75
    pregnancy 438
        vitamin A 447
        vitamin D 447
    protein 270, 280
    vitamin D 367
        pregnancy 447
RECORD trial 369
red blood cells see erythrocytes
red kidney bean poisoning 566
red wine 145, 583
reference nutrient intakes (RNIs) 76,
        79
    age and other lifecycle groups 436
        children 436, 462–3, 464
        older and younger adults 474
    lactation 436, 448, 449
    lower see lower reference nutrient
        intake
    micronutrients (in general) 78
    minerals 332, 333, 393, 398, 404,
        406
        children 462, 463, 464
        lactating women 448, 449
        in pregnancy 445, 447
    pregnancy 436, 438–9
        minerals 445, 447
        protein 444
        vitamins 331, 367, 447
    protein 270–1, 273, 280
        lactating women 449
        in pregnancy 444
    vitamins 78, 331, 332, 367
        children 462, 464
        lactating women 448, 449
        in pregnancy 331, 367, 447
    see also dietary reference intakes
refreshing healthy foods, consumer
        attitudes to 35
regulations see law

relationships, interpersonal 38–9
religion 38, 39
    ethnic minorities in UK 515
    taboos 56, 57, 58, 58–9
    vegetarianism 264, 509, 510, 512
renal... see kidney
requirements (dietary/nutrient)
    animal experiments see animals
    balance studies 81–2
    defining 80
    energy see energy
    estimated average see estimated
        average requirement
    factorial calculation 82
    variations in 435–530
    see also specific nutrients/food groups
research 18
residential homes, elderly living in 470
resources as enabling factors in
        behavioural change 28
respiration chambers 99, 100
respiratory burst/oxidative pulse
        (phagocytic cells/neutrophils)
        336
    malnutrition and 498
respiratory quotient 99
respirometers, portable 99
resveratrol 145, 582
retina, vitamin A and 362–3
retinal 362
retinoic acid 362
retinoids, therapeutic uses 365
retinol see vitamin A
retinopathy
    diabetic 490
    of prematurity 338
retrospective methods
    case-control studies using 115
    individual food intake estimation
        68–9
        compared with prospective
        methods 70–1
rheumatoid arthritis, fish oils 320
rhodopsin 362–3
riboflavin (vitamin B$_2$) 376–7
    adequate intake assessment in UK
        331
    biochemical markers of status 83,
        96–7
    childhood intakes and
        recommendations 464, 466
    deficiency/biochemical
        insufficiency 83, 331, 376, 377
    elderly 478
    supplements 376, 377
ribose 246
rice
    beriberi and 375–6
    as Japanese superfood 36

rickets 3, 357, 359, 368–9
  South Asian migrants in UK 59,
    515–16
rimonabant 238
rodents
  behavioural characteristics in obese
    rats 222
  energy balance and its regulation 120,
    189, 190, 191, 192–3, 194–5
  protein/amino acid requirements
    275, 281–2
  ruminant protein, BSE transmission
    556, 557
Russian Federation, obesity
  prevalence 206

saccharin 250
safety and quality of food 533–83
  phyto-oestrogens 579
  see also toxicology testing
St Johns wort 355
saliva, carbohydrate digestion 162,
  246
salmon 581
Salmonella 541, 542, 543, 546,
  551–2
  S. enteriditis 541, 547, 551
salt (sodium chloride) 422–32
  assessing requirement 424–6
  balance, and ageing 472
  declining intake over time 110–11
  in food tables, and its addition in
    cooking 74
  guidelines and recommendations
    on intake 140–2, 146
  habitual intake 425
  historical importance 422
  problems with/diseases associated
    with high intake of 9, 19–20
    hypertension/high BP 9, 19–20,
      107, 108–9, 111, 124–5, 422–
      3, 427–30, 431
  in processed food, reducing levels
    23, 426
  reduction/restriction of intake 399,
    422, 425–6, 428
    effects on morbidity and
      mortality 429–30
    extreme 429
  sources and amounts in diet 424–5
  weaning foods 461
  see also sodium
salt-reduced versions of foods 425
Samoans, obesity prevalence 206–7
sampling bias (population) in
  nutritional assessment 70–1
sanitation and taboos 58
satiety
  fat 296

compared to carbohydrate
  (calorie-for-calorie) 226
  mechanisms 193–6, 198, 199–200
  sensory-specific 223–4
saturated fat and fatty acids 287
  chemical structure 286, 287
  childhood diets 465
  heart disease and 107, 108, 122,
    306–7, 307, 311, 312, 313, 314
  percent energy as, in various foods
    12
  recommendations on intake
    UK 140
    WHO 136
  see also polyunsaturated fatty acid
    to saturated fatty acid (P:S)
    ratio
saturated phytosterols 579
saturation of fatty acids and melting
  points 288
saw palmetto 346, 347
saxitoxin 566
school, interventions 231
  physical education 231, 524
scombrotoxic poisoning 565–6
scrapie 555, 556, 557
scurvy see vitamin C
Second World War, Dutch Hunger
  Winter 437, 441, 443
secondary foods 35–6
secondary intervention trials 127
secondary metabolites of plants see
  plants
sedentary lifestyle (physical
  inactivity)
  British Asians 517
  obesity and 111, 136, 140, 227–9,
    230
  osteoporotic fracture risk and 417–
    18
seeds
  energy density 175
  fats/oils 291–2
  fungicide-treated, eating of 567
selection of subjects (human
  experimental studies of
  disease–diet links) 121, 126
  bias 130–2
selenium 399–400
  children, RNI 464
  deficiency 338, 400
    Keshan disease and 339, 400
    glutathione peroxidase and 337
    supplements 338–9, 400
sensory nerves and satiety 194
sensory-specific satiety 223–4
serine 269
serotonin-reuptake inhibitors as
  appetite suppressants 237

service provision adversely impacting
  on intake in hospital patients
  500
  minimizing 504
serving size see portion/serving size
sesquiterpenes 353
set-point theory (energy balance) 189
Seventh Day Adventists 110
  bowel cancer rates 264
  heart disease rates 312
  vegetarianism 264, 509, 510, 512
sex (gender)
  bone density and fracture risk
    related to 414–15
  elderly male:female ratio in
    population by age 469
  physical activity levels and 522
sex hormones and puberty 463
SGLT1 163
short-chain fatty acids from fibre and
  starch 258, 263
sibutramine 237–8
Sikhs in UK 515
simvastatin 315
β-sitosterol 309, 579, 580
skills (individual) and knowledge
  about diet 150
skin
  calcium and 412
  prick tests 485
  vitamin D synthesis see sunlight
    exposure and vitamin D
    synthesis
skinfold calipers 87, 89
  calibration 89, 90, 91
smoking
  β-carotene supplements and 11,
    328, 344
  as confounding variable in
    epidemiological studies of diet
    and heart disease 19
  education effecting reductions in
    147–8
  hip fracture risk in elderly
    and 418
social factors in elderly affecting
  nutritional status 475–6
social function of food 23
social morbidity, obesity 214–15
social status/class (socioeconomic
  group) 38
  breastfeeding and 40, 452
  weaning from 460
social trends, elderly 469–71
sodium 421–6
  deficiency
    effects 421
    risk factors 421
  disease 421–6

functions 421
infant feeding 456
recommendations 421
sources 421
standards 421
see also salt
sodium (ion)/glucose transporter 1
    (SGLT1) 163
solanine poisoning 566
sorbitol 570
sorghum and pellagra 379
South Asian/Indian subcontinent
    people in UK 514–18
    eating habits 59–62
    heart disease 311–12, 516–17
    obesity 207–8
    vegetarianism 515, 516, 518
    vitamin D insufficiency 371, 515–16
soy products 578–9, 581
    alternative to HRT 417, 578
    amounts of phyto-oestrogen in 577
    breast cancer and 112, 578–9
specialist nutritionist in hospitals 504
speciality meal items, consumer
    attitudes to 35
species differences/comparisons
    animal studies of disease–diet
        linkage 119, 120–1
    milk composition 281
    pregnancy and lactation, variations
        in relative burdens 438
specified bovine offal (SBO) and BSE
    557–8
spina bifida
    famine and 437
    preconceptual or maternal folate
        status 22, 385, 386
spinal cord damage in vitamin B$_{12}$
    deficiency 383
spirometer, static 99
Spirulina 381, 383, 510
sportspersons *see* athletic
    performance; training
sprouts 581
standardized mortality ratios 106
standards, dietary 75–85
    definitions and explanations 75–8
    inaccurate/overestimated 79–80,
        278
    minerals
        calcium 410
        chromium 394
        copper 395
        iron 405
        magnesium 396
        manganese 397
        molybdenum 398
        potassium 398
        selenium 399

sodium 421
zinc 400
origin 75
protein 270–1
uses 78–9
    micronutrients 78, 330–4
vitamins
    biotin 389
    pantothenic acid 389
    vitamin A 361
    vitamin B$_1$ (thiamin) 374
    vitamin B$_2$ (riboflavin) 376
    vitamin B$_3$ (niacin) 378
    vitamin B$_6$ (pyridoxine) 380
    vitamin B$_9$ (folate) 383
    vitamin B$_{12}$ (cobalamin) 381
    vitamin C 390
    vitamin D 365
    vitamin E 371
    vitamin K 372
Staphylococcus aureus 541, 542, 543,
    546, 548, 550, 552–3
starches 246, 255–7
    resistant 257, 260–1
    sources 247
starchy staples and products, energy
    density 174, 175
starflower/borage oil 298, 299, 322
starvation/fasting 178–81
    adverse effects 180–1
    in disease *see* disease
    immediate causes 178–9
    marasmus due to 282
    Minnesota experiment on men 184
    physiological responses and
        adaptations 179
    in pregnancy in Dutch Hunger
        Winter (1944-5) 437, 441, 443
    wasting in malnutrition or 179,
        497, 498
    see also dieting; hunger;
        malnutrition
state benefit payments and food
    selection 51
static bicycle ergometer 520
static spirometer 99
statins 14, 315–16, 482, 580
stature *see* height
status (social) *see* social status
sterilization
    by irradiation 563
    by ultra-high heat treatment 561–2
sterols, plant (phytosterols) 309, 353,
    574, 579–81
stigmasterol 309, 579
stomach (gastric...)
    acid depletion leading to iron
        deficiency 409
    cancer, and salt intake 423, 428

surgery for obesity 239–40
    see also gastroenteritis
stools *see* diarrhoea; faeces
storage
    in conditions allowing bacterial
        growth, minimizing time 547,
        548
    nutrient content changing with 73–4
Streptococcys mutans 253
stroke and salt intake 428
subject in human experimental
    studies of disease–diet links
    allocation bias, avoidance 125
    selection *see* selection
subjective norm in BASNEF model of
    behavioural change 27, 28, 29
substrates
    blood, influencing satiety 194,
        195–6
    phosphorylation *see*
        phosphorylation
    utilization in exercise 528–9
sucralose 250–1
sucrase 163, 246, 248
sucrose 248–9
sugar(s) 246, 248–50, 249
    added/extrinsic (and its
        consumption)
        childhood 465
        dental caries and 107, 252–5
        elderly 482–3
        guidelines and recommendations
            135, 136, 141, 148
        income in industrialized
            countries and 49
        weaning foods 461
    sources 247
    substitutes 250–2
    see also carbohydrate
sugar alcohols as sweeteners 251
sugar–fat seesaw 149, 173
sugar units 246
sulphites 570
sulphur-containing compounds
    amino acids 269, 352
        infant feeding 455
        selenium replacing sulphur in
            400
    secondary plant metabolites 254–5,
        581
sunlight (UV) exposure and vitamin
    D synthesis 360, 366, 370
    British Asians 515
    elderly 474, 477
    improving exposure 371, 420
superfoods 581–2
    cultural 36, 37
    fruits and vegetables (and extracts)
        as 337–8, 581–2

image of vegetable oils and soft
    margarines as 307
superoxide dismutase 337
    deficiency 337
superoxide radical 335
supplementation, dietary
        (predominantly micronutrient)
    adequate intake improved by 334
    definition of supplements 326
    elderly, dishonest/fraudulent results
        133
    food tables and 73
    hazards see toxicity
    hospital patients 502
        outcomes 504–5
    non-essential substances 346–56
    overview 325–9
    see also specific nutrients
surgery
    immune system following 499
    nutritional considerations 501, 502
    obesity 239–40, 241
sweeteners, artificial 250–2
sympathetic magic foods 37
symptomatic relief, therapeutic diet
        giving 25
synbiotics 574
syndrome X 219, 489
systematic reviews of disease–diet
        links 103, 128–32

taboos, dietary 56–9
    breastfeeding 57, 453
Takahara's disease 337
tartrazine 570
taste, agreeable see palatability
taurine, infant feeding 455
taurocholic acid 455
tea, green 354, 581–2
teeth decay see dental caries
television viewing 228, 231
temperature
    with food poisoning bacteria
        for growth 545
        for killing 543, 548
    regulation in old people 472
    see also chilled foods; heat
        treatment; thermogenesis
teratogenicity
    food additive testing 572
    retinol/vitamin A 317, 364, 365,
        439, 447
teriparatide 420
terpenoids 353
thalassaemia 407
thermogenesis (heat generation)
        187–8
    adaptive 187–8, 190–1
    animals 121

defects causing obesity 190–1
    drugs inducing 188, 239
thermoregulation, old people 472
thiamin (vitamin B₁) 37405
    adequate intake in UK 332
    deficiency/biochemical
        insufficiency 3, 162, 360, 374,
        375–6
        alcoholics 162, 361, 375, 376
        beriberi see beriberi
        elderly 478
    functions 374, 375
    nature and sources 374
    requirements 375
    status assessment 83
    supplements 374, 375
thiamin pyrophosphate 357
threonine 269
thrombosis risk and fish oils 318
thrush, probiotics 575
thyroid carcinoma 403
thyroxine 402
tilted plate model see food plates
time aspects
    bacterial growth 545
    trends in disease–diet linkage
        studies 103, 110–12
    weaning 459–60
tissues, measurement of nutrient
        levels 82
tocopherol see vitamin E
tolerable upper intake levels (ULs) 77
tooth decay see dental caries
toxicity (and its risk)
    food additives see toxicology testing
    supplements or high intakes 326–7
        chromium 394
        copper 306, 395
        iodine 402
        iron 406
        magnesium 397
        molybdenum 398
        selenium 400
        zinc 401
    vitamins
        biotin 389
        vitamin A 362
        vitamin B₂ (riboflavin) 376
        vitamin B₃ (niacin) 378
        vitamin B₆ (pyridoxine) 381
        vitamin B₉ (folate) 384, 387,
            387–8
        vitamin C 390, 392
        vitamin D 366, 371
        vitamin E 372
        vitamin K 373
toxicology testing 564
    food additives 571
        animal studies 119–20, 572

toxins (in food poisoning)
    bacterial 541–2, 542, 543, 545,
        546, 549, 550, 552, 553, 561,
        563, 565–6
    fungal 563, 566
    natural 564, 565–7
Trading Standards Officers (TSOs)
        534
Traditional Herbal Medicines
        Directive 325
traffic light system 536
training
    benefits 520–2
    energy and nutrient intake and 526,
        527, 528, 529
trans-fatty acids (trans configuration)
        286, 287–8
    health images (regarding heart
        disease) 308–9
    intake and sources 294
transaldolase 162
transamination 161, 275
transferrin, plasma 406
    assessment 408
transketolase 162
transmissible spongiform
        encephalopathies (TSEs) 554–
        60
trauma see injury
travellers' diarrhoea 543, 549, 576
treatment (by diet or nutrition) 484–
        506
    deficiency diseases 4
    diet as complete therapy 484–8
    diet as specific component of
        therapy 488–96
    in human experimental studies of
        disease–diet links
        compliance with 122
        withheld in control group, ethics
            126
triacylglycerol (triglyceride) 160, 285
    digestion 163, 164
    in lipoproteins 300
    melting points 288
    structure 286
trials
    clinical, disease–diet linkage 103–
        4, 124–6
    interventions at population level see
        intervention trials
tricarboxylic acid (Krebs) cycle 160
triglyceride see triacylglycerol
triiodothyronine 402
tripeptidases 270
trypsin 163, 270
tryptophan 269
TV viewing 228, 321
twin studies of obesity 220

tyramine 566
  monoamine oxidase inhibitors and 120, 566
tyrosine 4, 269, 348
  deficiency in phenylketonuria 487

ubiquinone see coenzyme Q10
UCPs (uncoupling proteins) 158
UHT (ultra-high heat treatment) 561–2
UK see United Kingdom
ultra-high heat treatment 561–2
ultraviolet light exposure see sunlight
UN
  Codex Alimentarius Commission 535
  protein gap and 279
uncoupling proteins (UCPs) 158, 191
underweight, elderly 477, 480
UNICEF and breastfeeding 451, 457
United Kingdom (Britain; UK - and incl. England)
  breastfeeding in
    maternity hospital changes in practice (1990 to 2000) 454
    policy (vs bottle-feeding) 449
    prevalence 450
  changes in diet from 1930s 7
  childhood dietary surveys 464–6
  chip consumption 37
  cholesterol plasma levels in 305, 306
  consumer classification of food 34
  current diets compared with ideal intakes 146
  dietary standards 75, 75–7, 76, 77, 78
  energy requirement/guidelines/recommendations 168
    lactation 448–9
    older adults 473
  ethnic minorities see ethnic minorities
  fat sources and intakes 292–4
  fibre (non-starch polysaccharide) intakes 257–8
  food law and regulations 533–4
    additives 569–70
    labelling (incl. health claims) 535–7, 539
  food poisoning outbreaks 545–6
  food selection 48–62
    aids to 33, 153–4
  guidelines and recommendations 137, 138, 139, 140–1
    children and adolescents 462, 464
    DRVs see dietary reference values
    elderly 474

energy see subheading above
  expert reports in 134, 135
  on physical activity and weight management 140
  protein 270–1
  RNI see reference nutrient intakes
life expectancy 469
micronutrients, adequate intake assessment 330–4
mineral intakes (typical highest)
  calcium 411
  chromium 394
  copper 395
  iodine 402
  iron 406
  manganese 397
  molybdenum 398
  selenium 400
  zinc 401
obesity prevalence 203, 204, 207, 208
  children 209–10
physical activity see physical activity
pregnancy and iron supplementation 446
South Asian populations in see South Asian/Indian subcontinent people
supplements and their regulation in 325, 326, 327
vegetarianism 512–13
vitamin intakes (typical highest)
  biotin 389
  pantothenic acid 390
  vitamin A 362
  vitamin B_1 (thiamin) 374
  vitamin B_2 (riboflavin) 376
  vitamin B_3 (niacin) 378
  vitamin B_6 (pyridoxine) 380
  vitamin B_{12} (cobalamin) 382
  vitamin D 366
  vitamin E 372
  vitamin K 373
United Kingdom Prospective Diabetic Study (UKPDS) 491
United Nations see UN; UNICEF
United States (USA)
  breastfeeding
    infant mortality rates and 457
    prevalence 450–1
  dietary standards 75, 77, 79
    micronutrients 78
    origin 75
    see also recommended dietary/daily allowance
  food additives 569

food labelling (incl. health claims) 537–9, 539
  guidelines/recommendations/requirements 137, 138, 139
    elderly 474
    energy 160, 168, 169
    expert reports in 134, 135
    food guide pyramid 33, 151–3
    on physical activity and weight management 140
    RDA see recommended dietary/daily allowance
  healthy life in old age, increasing span of 471
  obesity, prevalence 203, 204, 207
  physical activity levels 521, 522
unsaturated fatty acids
  chemical structure 286, 287
  health images (regarding heart disease) 307–8
  see also monounsaturated fatty acids; polyunsaturated fatty acids
uraemia in chronic renal failure 495
urine, nutrient measurements 97
USA see United States
'use by' date 535
UV light exposure see sunlight

vaginal candidiasis and probiotics 575
vascular disease see heart disease; microvascular disease
vegans 507, 508, 509, 510
  vitamin B_{12} supplements in pregnancy 447
vegetable(s)
  cruciferous 354, 581
  disease risk and levels of consumption 138, 342–5
    cancer 9, 19, 138, 263, 265, 342–5
  energy density 174, 175
  as energy source 178
  expense 150
  guidelines and recommendations 138–9
    elderly 482
  Seventh Day Adventists 264, 509, 510, 512
  as superfoods 337–8, 581–2
  Western (industrialized) countries consumption of
    effects on poorer countries 155
    income and 49
vegetable and fruit group 151
vegetable oils 290, 298
  flaxseed oil 298, 299, 323
  health images 307
  olive oil 11, 290, 308, 581
  rapeseed oil 155, 290, 298

vegetarianism 507–13
    adequacy of diet 508–12
    guidelines 512–13
    heart disease rates 312
    hostility to or from vegetarians 32,
        57
    meat substitutes 280
    reasons for adopting 507–8
    see also vegans
verocytotoxin-producing *E. coli*
        (VTEC) 541, 542, 546, 552,
        560
very low-density lipoprotein (VLDL)
        300–1, 303
very low-energy diets 240–1
very low-fat diets 225, 295
Vibrio parahaemolyticus 541, 542, 543
Vicia faba and favism 565
vigilance, obese people 235–6
vincristine 354
viruses causing food poisoning 542,
        543
vitamin(s) (general aspects) 357–92
    adequate intake
        assessment in UK 330–2, 333
    athletes 527
    biochemical tests of status 96
    chelation by non-starch
        polysaccharide 259
    childhood intakes and
        recommendations 462, 464,
        466, 467, 468
    classification 358
    deficiency
        circumstances precipitating 360–1
        diseases due to 358–9, 388
    definition 357
    dietary standards 78, 79
    elderly intakes and
        recommendations 462, 464,
        466, 467, 468, 474, 477–8
    fat-soluble 296, 358
    food tables and 74
    general concepts and principles
        357–61
    income in industrialized countries
        and intake of 49
    infant feeding 456
    precursors and endogenous
        synthesis 359–60
    pregnancy 438, 439, 446–7
    supplementation 326
        in pregnancy 439, 446–7, 447
    water-soluble 358
vitamin A (retinol) 296, 361–5
    adequate intake
        assessment in UK 331, 332
        vegetarian diet 510

assessment of status 361, 363
    biosynthesis 360
    blood and tissue levels,
        measurement 82
    cancer and 116–17, 364–5
    childhood intakes and
        recommendations 464, 466
    deficiency/low intake 6, 46–7, 296,
        331, 357, 359, 363 4
        effects 46–7, 361, 363–4, 498
        prevalence 361–2
        risk factors 361, 364
    food tables 74
    functions 361, 362–3
    pregnancy 447
        cautions (incl. possible
            teratogenicity) 317, 364, 365,
            439, 447
    recommendations on high intakes
        362
    requirements 363
    sources 361, 362
        beta-carotene 15
        fish oil 317
    supplements and their benefits
        362, 364–5
    toxicity/adverse effects 362, 364
    typical highest intakes 362
vitamin B₁ *see* thiamin
vitamin B₂ *see* riboflavin
vitamin B₃ *see* niacin
vitamin B₆ (pyridoxine) 380–1
    adequate intake assessment in UK
        331
    deficiency/low intake 331, 332,
        380–1
    elderly 474
    supplements 380, 381
        warnings 328
vitamin B₉ *see* folate
vitamin B₁₂ (cobalamin incl.
        cyanocobalamin) 381–3
    adequate intake assessment in UK
        331
        functions 381, 382
        sources 381, 382
    deficiency/low intake 331, 332,
        359, 360
        British Asians 515
        effects 381
        prevalence 381–2
        risk factors 381
        vegetarians 510
    malabsorption 4
    pregnancy 447
    requirements and assessment of
        status 381, 382
    supplements 382, 383

vitamin C (ascorbic acid) 343, 390–2
    animal studies of synthesis 84
    blood and tissue levels,
        measurement 82
    childhood RNI 464
    deficiency/biochemical insufficiency
        (and scurvy) 359, 360, 391
        elderly 478
        prevalence 390
        prevention 81
        risk factors 390
    endogenous synthesis 360
    free radicals and 339
    functions 390, 391
    iron absorption and 407
    radiotracer studies of pool size 81
    sources 177, 390, 390–1
    supplements 391–2
        cardiovascular disease prevention
            343
        warnings 328
    toxicity 390, 392
vitamin D (cholecalciferol) 365–71
    adequate intake
        assessment in UK 331, 332
        vegetarian diet 509–10
    biochemical assessment of status
        365
    biochemical functions 365
    cancer and 370
        bowel/colorectal cancer 266, 360
    deficiency/low intake 3, 35, 331,
        359, 360, 365, 368–70
        acute states 368–9
        British Asians 371, 515–16
        effects 365
        elderly 420, 474, 477, 478
        prevalence 365
        risk factors 365
        see also rickets
    dietary sources 365, 366–7
    dietary standards 365
    elderly intake and
        recommendations 474, 477
    endogenous synthesis 360, 366–7
        sunlight in *see* sunlight
    in fish oil 317
        pregnancy and cautions with fish
            oil preparations 322
    nature 366
    osteoporosis and 369, 419
    population status and its
        improvement 371
    pregnancy 447
    recommendations on high intakes
        366
    requirements 366–7
    supplementation 366, 369

osteoporosis management 419–
    20, 420
    targeted 371
    toxicity 366, 371
    typical highest intakes in UK 366
vitamin E (tocopherol) 339, 345,
    371–2
    deficiency 372
        experimental 338
    free radicals and 339
    supplements 371
        and cardiovascular disease 130,
            342, 343, 344
vitamin K (phylloquinone) 372–4
    deficiency 83–4, 360, 373–4
        haemorrhagic disease of newborn
            359, 373
    supplements 373
vitamin-like organic substances 324,
    326, 337
VLDL (very low-density lipoprotein)
    300–1
volume (body), measuring 91

waist circumference 202
    raised/high 202, 204, 205, 208
        health risks 216
waist-to-hip ratio 202
    raised/high 202, 204, 205, 207,
        208, 215
        health risks 215, 216
walnuts 582
war 7
wasting in starvation/malnutrition
    179, 497, 498
    see also cachexia
water
    body
        balance disturbances in old age
            472
        predicting body fat content 91–2
    cooking, affecting food tables 74
    doubly-labelled, in energy
        expenditure estimation
        99–100
    fluoridation 127, 254
water-soluble vitamins 358
watercress 347
waxes 285
wealth and affluence 38
    education reversing dietary changes
        accompanying 42
    see also developed (industrialized/
        Western/affluent) countries
weaning (foods) 459–62
    choice of foods 460
    fat in foods 296, 459, 460–1

priorities 460–1
    timing 459–60
weighed inventory method if
        individual food intake
        estimation 69
weight 87, 87–8
    athletic performance and 526–30
    at birth see birth weights
    in BMI assessment 88
    cycling (yo-yo dieting) 183, 217
    elderly 477, 480–1
    gain 86
    loss/reduction (unintentional - over
        3 months) 86, 88
        elderly 481–2
    loss/reduction in obesity
        realistic rates 232–6
        surgical methods 239–40, 241
    management, recommendations
        and guidelines 136, 139–40,
        142
    pre-pregnant, breastfeeding and
        restoration of 458
    see also dieting; obesity;
        underweight
weight-bearing exercise in older
        adults 418
welfare and benefit payments 51, 52
Wernicke–Korsakoff syndrome 162,
        361, 375, 376
Western diet and lifestyle (causing
        disease) 7–16
    disease (in general) and 107–8
        risk factors for 8–9
    export of diet to Eastern countries
        40
    low-fibre content see low-fibre diets
    natural toxicants 565–6
    obesity management and changes in
        229–31
    osteoporosis and associated
        fractures 417
        promoting lifestyle change 419
    recommendations offered to alter
        9–10
    salt reduction advice 422
    simple changes and their possible
        harm 10–11
    see also developed countries
Western Samoa, obesity prevalence
        206–7
wheat protein quality 282
whey, infant feeding 455–6
WHO see World Health Organization
wholemeal bread 148
Wilson's disease 396
wine, red 145, 583

women (females)
    athletes, with low body
        weight 527
    cholesterol plasma levels in (UK)
        305, 306
    eating disorders
        athletes 527
        causes 183, 184
    energy balance and physical activity
        levels 235
    as household gatekeepers 62–3
    obesity 208
        defined by high waist-to-hip
            ratio 202
        socioeconomic impact 215
    skinfold thickness charts 90
    see also girls; sex (gender)
work (occupation/employment)
    physical activity levels in 525–6
    weaning and return to 460
World Health Organization (WHO)
    height standards for girls 93
    infant mortality rates and feeding
        methods 457
    marasmus and its neglect 283
    nutritional guidelines and
        recommendations 136
    obesity prevalence 204–6
        children 209
World War II, Dutch Hunger Winter
        437, 441, 443
worldwide issues see global/
        worldwide/international
        dimensions
wound healing and zinc deficiency
        401–2

X-ray treatment of food 562
xerophthalmia and vitamin A
        deficiency 364

yoghurt and ovarian cancer 116
yo-yo dieting 183, 217
Yudkin, John 224–5

zinc 400–3
    adequate intake
        in UK 333
        vegetarians 511
    children, RNI 464
    deficiency 338, 401
        elderly 478
        immune system 401, 498
        inherited 401
    supplements 338–9, 400, 401–2
zinc–copper superoxide dismutase
        337